Magnetic Nanomaterials for Hyperthermia-Based Therapy, Imaging, and Drug Delivery

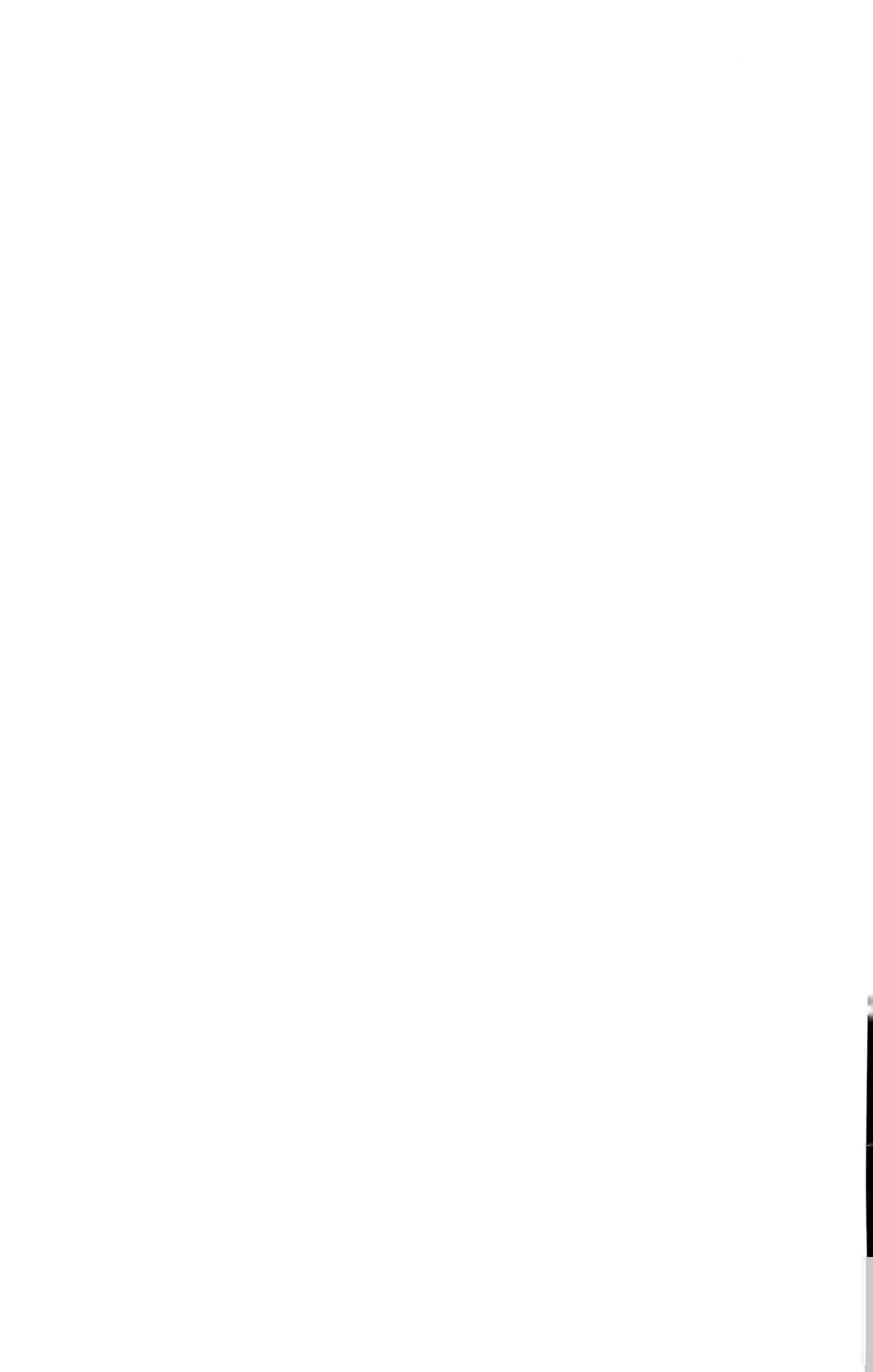

Magnetic Nanomaterials for Hyperthermia-Based Therapy, Imaging, and Drug Delivery

Editor

Constantin Mihai Lucaciu

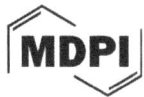

Basel • Beijing • Wuhan • Barcelona • Belgrade • Novi Sad • Cluj • Manchester

Editor
Constantin Mihai Lucaciu
"Iuliu Hatieganu" University
of Medicine and Pharmacy
Cluj-Napoca
Romania

Editorial Office
MDPI
St. Alban-Anlage 66
4052 Basel, Switzerland

This is a reprint of articles from the Special Issue published online in the open access journal *Pharmaceutics* (ISSN 1999-4923) (available at: https://www.mdpi.com/journal/pharmaceutics/special_issues/2123RIR422).

For citation purposes, cite each article independently as indicated on the article page online and as indicated below:

Lastname, A.A.; Lastname, B.B. Article Title. *Journal Name* **Year**, *Volume Number*, Page Range.

ISBN 978-3-7258-0633-1 (Hbk)
ISBN 978-3-7258-0634-8 (PDF)
doi.org/10.3390/books978-3-7258-0634-8

© 2024 by the authors. Articles in this book are Open Access and distributed under the Creative Commons Attribution (CC BY) license. The book as a whole is distributed by MDPI under the terms and conditions of the Creative Commons Attribution-NonCommercial-NoDerivs (CC BY-NC-ND) license.

Contents

About the Editor vii

Constantin Mihai Lucaciu
Magnetic Nanomaterials for Hyperthermia-Based Therapy, Imaging, and Drug Delivery
Reprinted from: *Pharmaceutics* **2024**, *16*, 263, doi:10.3390/pharmaceutics16020263 1

Sandor I. Bernad, Vlad Socoliuc, Izabell Craciunescu, Rodica Turcu and Elena S. Bernad
Field-Induced Agglomerations of Polyethylene-Glycol-Functionalized Nanoclusters: Rheological Behaviour and Optical Microscopy
Reprinted from: *Pharmaceutics* **2023**, *15*, 2612, doi:10.3390/pharmaceutics15112612. 6

Cristina Chircov, Iulia Alexandra Dumitru, Bogdan Stefan Vasile, Ovidiu-Cristian Oprea, Alina Maria Holban and Roxana Cristina Popescu
Microfluidic Synthesis of Magnetite Nanoparticles for the Controlled Release of Antibiotics
Reprinted from: *Pharmaceutics* **2023**, *15*, 2215, doi:10.3390/pharmaceutics15092215 28

Costica Caizer, Isabela Simona Caizer-Gaitan, Claudia Geanina Watz, Cristina Adriana Dehelean, Tiberiu Bratu and Codruța Soica
High Efficacy on the Death of Breast Cancer Cells Using SPMHT with Magnetite Cyclodextrins Nanobioconjugates
Reprinted from: *Pharmaceutics* **2023**, *15*, 1145, doi:10.3390/pharmaceutics15041145 43

Perihan Ünak, Volkan Yasakçı, Elif Tutun, K. Buşra Karatay, Rafał Walczak, Kamil Wawrowicz, Kinga Żelechowska-Matysiak, et al.
Multimodal Radiobioconjugates of Magnetic Nanoparticles Labeled with ^{44}Sc and ^{47}Sc for Theranostic Application
Reprinted from: *Pharmaceutics* **2023**, *15*, 850, doi:10.3390/pharmaceutics15030850 63

Relton R. Oliveira, Emílio R. Cintra, Ailton A. Sousa-Junior, Larissa C. Moreira, Artur C. G. da Silva, Ana Luiza R. de Souza, Marize C. Valadares, et al.
Paclitaxel-Loaded Lipid-Coated Magnetic Nanoparticles for Dual Chemo-Magnetic Hyperthermia Therapy of Melanoma
Reprinted from: *Pharmaceutics* **2023**, *15*, 818, doi:10.3390/pharmaceutics15030818 82

Stefan Nitica, Ionel Fizesan, Roxana Dudric, Felicia Loghin, Constantin Mihai Lucaciu and Cristian Iacovita
Doxorubicin Loaded Thermosensitive Magneto-Liposomes Obtained by a Gel Hydration Technique: Characterization and In Vitro Magneto-Chemotherapeutic Effect Assessment
Reprinted from: *Pharmaceutics* **2022**, *14*, 2501, doi:10.3390/pharmaceutics14112501 101

Aisha H. A. Alsenousy, Rasha A. El-Tahan, Nesma A. Ghazal, Rafael Piñol, Angel Millán, Lamiaa M. A. Ali and Maher A. Kamel
The Anti-Obesity Potential of Superparamagnetic Iron Oxide Nanoparticles against High-Fat Diet-Induced Obesity in Rats: Possible Involvement of Mitochondrial Biogenesis in the Adipose Tissues
Reprinted from: *Pharmaceutics* **2022**, *14*, 2134, doi:10.3390/pharmaceutics14102134 119

Alexandra Pusta, Mihaela Tertis, Izabell Crăciunescu, Rodica Turcu, Simona Mirel and Cecilia Cristea
Recent Advances in the Development of Drug Delivery Applications of Magnetic Nanomaterials
Reprinted from: *Pharmaceutics* **2023**, *15*, 1872, doi:10.3390/pharmaceutics15071872 140

Sayan Ganguly and Shlomo Margel
Bioimaging Probes Based on Magneto-Fluorescent Nanoparticles
Reprinted from: *Pharmaceutics* **2023**, *15*, 686, doi:10.3390/pharmaceutics15020686 . . . . **177**

Ming-Hsien Chan, Chien-Hsiu Li, Yu-Chan Chang and Michael Hsiao
Iron-Based Ceramic Composite Nanomaterials for Magnetic Fluid Hyperthermia and Drug Delivery
Reprinted from: *Pharmaceutics* **2022**, *14*, 2584, doi:10.3390/pharmaceutics14122584 . . . . **211**

Lidia Gago, Francisco Quiñonero, Gloria Perazzoli, Consolación Melguizo, Jose Prados, Raul Ortiz and Laura Cabeza
Nanomedicine and Hyperthermia for the Treatment of Gastrointestinal Cancer: A Systematic Review
Reprinted from: *Pharmaceutics* **2023**, *15*, 1958, doi:10.3390/pharmaceutics15071958 . . . . **235**

About the Editor

Constantin Mihai Lucaciu

Constantin Mihai Lucaciu earned his Physics degree from Babes-Bolyai University in Cluj-Napoca and completed his Ph.D. in Biophysics at the same institution. He gained professional experience at the Institute of Isotopic and Molecular Technologies. In 1991, he became a member of the "Iuliu Hatieganu" University of Medicine and Pharmacy in Cluj-Napoca, where, since 2005, he has held the position of Professor of Biophysics and served as the Head of the Biophysics Department. He was awarded the Romanian Academy award for physics in 1989. His research focuses on the transport of ions through biological membranes, the study of free radicals in biological systems, and the application of IR, Raman, and SERS techniques. Additionally, he explores the biomedical applications of magnetic, plasmonic, and hybrid nanoparticles.

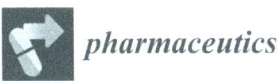

Editorial

Magnetic Nanomaterials for Hyperthermia-Based Therapy, Imaging, and Drug Delivery

Constantin Mihai Lucaciu

Department of Pharmaceutical Physics-Biophysics, Faculty of Pharmacy, "Iuliu Hatieganu" University of Medicine and Pharmacy, 6 Pasteur St., 400349 Cluj-Napoca, Romania; clucaciu@umfcluj.ro; Tel.: +40-744647854

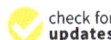

Citation: Lucaciu, C.M. Magnetic Nanomaterials for Hyperthermia-Based Therapy, Imaging, and Drug Delivery. *Pharmaceutics* 2024, 16, 263. https://doi.org/10.3390/pharmaceutics16020263

Received: 16 January 2024
Accepted: 7 February 2024
Published: 11 February 2024

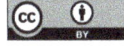

Copyright: © 2024 by the author. Licensee MDPI, Basel, Switzerland. This article is an open access article distributed under the terms and conditions of the Creative Commons Attribution (CC BY) license (https://creativecommons.org/licenses/by/4.0/).

In recent years, nanomedicine has experienced remarkable advancements, due to the development of new nanomaterials with outstanding properties that have demonstrated significant advantages over traditional medicines.

Among various nanoparticles, magnetic nanoparticles (MNPs) have emerged as promising candidates for a wide range of biomedical applications, particularly due to their responsiveness to external magnetic fields, enabling remote control and manipulation [1]. Their first medical applications were related to their role in changing water proton magnetic relaxation times, being used as contrast agents in magnetic resonance imaging (MRI) [2]; iron oxide MNPs are FDA-approved for imaging purposes and anemia treatments. While numerous studies are dedicated to improving the contrast in both T_1 and T_2 weighted MRI images using MNPs, magnetic particle imaging (MPI) has emerged in the last decade as an alternate technique, with tremendous potential in medical imaging [3], featuring multiple advantages such as linear quantitation, no tissue background, deep penetration, and no use of ionizing radiation.

Another important medical application of MNPs in the treatment of solid cancer tumors is magnetic hyperthermia (MH), a technique based on the heating of MNPs when submitted to radiofrequency alternating magnetic fields upon their loading in the tumor area. MH has achieved significant recognition, representing the first ever medical device to receive European approval for the treatment of glioblastoma multiforme (GBM), a form of brain tumor. Furthermore, ongoing clinical trials for U.S. Food and Drug Administration (FDA) approval are under way, specifically focusing on the treatment of prostate and pancreatic cancers. Despite the promise demonstrated in clinical trials where MH therapy was combined with standard chemotherapy and/or radiotherapy, achieving complete tumor regression remains elusive. Various factors contribute to this outcome, with the heat performance of injected MNPs playing a pivotal role. Therefore, a large number of studies have been conducted in the past few decades aiming to understand the role of composition, shape, size, structure, and surface functionalization in the heating performance of MNPs in MH [4]. Direct heat effects contribute to cell death; however, the elevated temperatures of MNPs open avenues for further exploration. In many preclinical and clinical studies, authors have initially hypothesized that the therapeutic impact observed was primarily attributed to the induction of tumor necrosis during hyperthermia applications. However, the potential effects on the tumor microenvironment, specifically the induction of antitumor immune responses, have not been thoroughly examined. Contemporary perspectives now suggest that a crucial element contributing to the therapeutic efficacy of hyperthermia is the initiation of a heat-mediated immune response against the tumor. This immune response enhances the tumor's visibility to the immune system, suggesting that MH treatment can facilitate spatially and temporally controlled temperature increases, acting as an immune trigger. This recognition of hyperthermia as an immune modulator underscores its potential in not only targeting tumors directly, but also in harnessing the body's immune system for a more comprehensive and effective therapeutic approach [5]. This highlights the evolving landscape of MNPs as a promising tool in the realm of cancer therapeutics.

By surface functionalization or through the creation of hybrid formulations with polymers, fluorophores, liposomes, and plasmonic or silica shells, MNPs acquire multifunctional capabilities. These multifaceted nanomaterials hold the potential to both diagnose and treat medical conditions, offering the ability to remotely control their positioning and activation, thus positioning them as a highly investigated class of theranostic materials. Among the numerous applications of such hybrid nanostructures, here we focus on controlled drug delivery. Drug delivery systems utilizing MNPs present a range of advantages, enhancing the precision and efficiency of therapeutic interventions. Some key benefits include the ability to target specific anatomical locations within the body, a reduction in the required drug dosage to achieve a specific concentration at the target site, and the mitigation of potential side effects. By leveraging the magnetic properties of MNPs, these delivery systems enable a more focused and controlled release of therapeutic agents, optimizing the therapeutic outcome while minimizing the impact on non-target sites. This targeted drug delivery approach holds promise for enhancing treatment efficacy and minimizing undesirable effects associated with systemic drug administration.

This Special Issue, entitled "Magnetic Nanomaterials for Hyperthermia-Based Therapy, Imaging, and Drug Delivery", provides a platform for researchers to share their latest experimental and theoretical findings related to the development and application of magnetic nanomaterials in the medical field, assembling both reviews (four) and research papers (seven) focused on the distinct aspects of MNP medical applications and written by recognized experts in the field.

In the first review paper, Gago et al. (contribution 11) conducted a systematic search of in vitro and in vivo studies published in the last decade that employ hyperthermia therapy mediated by magnetic nanoparticles for treating gastrointestinal cancers. The results revealed that iron oxide is the preferred material for magnetism generation in nanoparticles, and colorectal cancer is the most widely studied gastrointestinal cancer. Interestingly, novel therapies employing nanoparticles loaded with chemotherapeutic drugs, in combination with magnetic hyperthermia, demonstrated an excellent antitumor effect.

Ganguly and Margel (contribution 9) explored the most recent developments in synthetic methodologies and methods for the fabrication of magneto-fluorescent nanocomposites. The primary applications of multimodal magneto-fluorescent nanoparticles in biomedicine, including biological imaging, cancer treatment, and drug administration, are covered in this article, together with an overview of the future possibilities for these technologies.

Pusta et al. (contribution 8) performed a critical overview of the recent literature concerning advancements in the field of magnetic nanoparticles used in drug delivery, with a focus on their classification, characteristics, synthesis and functionalization methods, limitations, and examples of magnetic drug delivery systems incorporating chemotherapeutics or RNA.

Chan et al. (contribution 10) reviewed potential improvements in the magnetic properties of iron-based nanoparticles in the preparation of multifunctional composite materials through their combination with ceramic materials. They demonstrate the potential of ferromagnetic enhancement and multifunctional composite materials for MRI diagnosis, drug delivery, MH therapy, and cellular imaging applications.

An interesting study was reported by Alsenousy et al. (contribution 7) on the potential of superparamagnetic iron oxide nanoparticles (SPIONs) as anti-obesity agents. For the first time, the authors reported promising ameliorating effects of SPION treatments against weight gain, hyperglycemia, adiponectin, leptin, and dyslipidemia in obese rats. At the molecular level, surprisingly, SPION treatments markedly corrected the disturbed expression and protein content of inflammatory markers and parameters controlling mitochondrial biogenesis and functions in both brown and white adipose tissue.

The combination of magnetic hyperthermia with chemotherapy is considered a promising strategy in cancer therapy due to the synergy between high temperatures and chemotherapeutic effects, which can be further developed for targeted and remote-controlled drug release. Nitica et al. (contribution 6) reported a simple, rapid, and reproducible method for the preparation of thermosensitive magnetoliposomes (TsMLs) loaded with doxorubicin (DOX), consisting of a lipidic gel formation from a previously obtained water-in-oil microemulsion with fine aqueous droplets containing magnetic nanoparticles (MNPs) dispersed in an organic solution of thermosensitive lipids (transition temperature of ~43 °C), followed by gel hydration with an aqueous solution of DOX. The obtained thermosensitive magnetoliposomes (TsMLs) were around 300 nm in diameter and exhibited 40% DOX incorporation efficiency. The most suitable MNPs to incorporate into the liposomal aqueous lumen were Zn ferrites, with a very low coercive field at 300 K (7 kA/m), close to the superparamagnetic regime, exhibiting a maximum specific absorption rate (SAR) of 1130 W/gFe when dispersed in water and 635 W/gFe when confined inside TsMLs. No toxicity of Zn ferrite MNPs or TsMLs was noticed against the A459 cancer cell line after 48 h incubation over the tested concentration range. The passive release of DOX from the TsMLs after 48 h incubation induced toxicity, starting with a dosage level of 62.5 mg/cm^2. Below this threshold, the subsequent exposure to an alternating magnetic field (20–30 kA/m, 355 kHz) for 30 min drastically reduced the viability of the A459 cells due to the release of incorporated DOX. These results strongly suggest that TsMLs represent a viable strategy for anticancer therapies using the magnetic-field-controlled release of DOX.

Oliveira et al. (contribution 5) reported the development of paclitaxel-loaded lipid-coated manganese ferrite magnetic nanoparticles (PTX-LMNPs) as synthetic magnetosome analogs, envisaging the combined chemo-magnetic hyperthermia treatment of melanoma. Their results showed that PTX-LMNP-mediated MHT triggers PTX release, facilitating its thermal-modulated local delivery to diseased sites within short timeframes. Moreover, half-maximal PTX inhibitory concentration (IC$_{50}$) could be significantly reduced relatively to free PTX (142,500×) and Taxol® (340×). Therefore, the dual chemo-MHT therapy mediated by intratumorally injected PTX-LMNP stands out as a promising alternative to efficiently deliver PTX to melanoma cells, consequently reducing systemic side effects commonly associated with conventional chemotherapies.

Unak et al. (contribution 4) obtained MNPs surrounded by silica and an organic layer, labeled with ^{44}Sc for SPECT and ^{47}Sc for radiotherapy. The radiobioconjugate exhibited high affinity and cytotoxicity toward the human prostate cancer LNCaP (PSMA+) cell line, much higher than for PC-3 (PSMA-) cells. High cytotoxicity of the radiobioconjugate was confirmed by radiotoxicity studies on LNCaP 3D spheroids. In addition, the magnetic properties of the radiobioconjugate should allow for its use in guiding drug delivery driven by a magnetic field gradient.

Caizer et al. (contribution 3) reported an in vitro study on the human breast adenocarcinoma cell line (MCF-7) by applying superparamagnetic hyperthermia (SPMHT), using novel Fe$_3$O$_4$–PAA–(HP-γ-CDs) (PAA is polyacrylic acid and HP-γ-CDs is hydroxypropyl gamma-cyclodextrins) nanobioconjugates, obtaining >95% cell deaths in specific alternating magnetic field conditions.

Chircov et al. (contribution 2) presented a microfluidic device to obtain a series of antibiotic-loaded MNPs. The results proved a considerable uniformity of antibiotic-containing nanoparticles, good biocompatibility, and promising antimicrobial properties against *S. aureus*, *P. aeruginosa*, and *C. albicans* strains.

Bernad et al. (contribution 1 investigated the agglomeration processes of magnetoresponsive functionalized nanocluster suspensions in a magnetic field, as well as how these structures impact the behavior of these suspensions in biomedical applications. Their results show that the applied magnetic field aligns the magnetic moments of the nanoclusters, resulting in the formation of chains, linear aggregates, or agglomerates of clusters aligned along the applied field direction. The design of chain-like structures can cause considerable changes in the characteristics of ferrofluids, ranging from rheological differences to colloidal stability changes.

The diverse topics covered in this Special Issue span the spectrum from drug delivery to hyperthermia-based therapy and cancer and other disease treatments, showcasing the versatility of magnetic nanoparticles in addressing multifaceted challenges in medicine.

A notable aspect highlighted in the contributions is the potential for synergistic effects, particularly in conjunction with other therapeutic modalities such as chemotherapy. This emphasizes the pivotal role that magnetic nanomaterials can play in shaping the landscape of medical treatments.

Acknowledgments: As Guest Editor of this Special Issue, "Magnetic Nanomaterials for Hyperthermia-Based Therapy, Imaging, and Drug Delivery", I would like to express my deep appreciation to all the authors whose valuable work has been published herein. Their significant contributions, showcased in this Special Issue, have played a pivotal role in its success. I also want to acknowledge the dedicated efforts of the editorial staff for their support and guidance throughout the publication process and their role in bringing this issue to completion.

Conflicts of Interest: The author declares no conflicts of interest.

List of Contributions

1. Bernad, S.I.; Socoliuc, V.; Craciunescu, I.; Turcu, R.; Bernad, E.S. Field-Induced Agglomerations of Polyethylene-Glycol-Functionalized Nanoclusters: Rheological Behaviour and Optical Microscopy. *Pharmaceutics* **2023**, *15*, 2612. https://doi.org/10.3390/pharmaceutics15112612.
2. Chircov, C.; Dumitru, I.A.; Vasile, B.S.; Oprea, O.-C.; Holban, A.M.; Popescu, R.C. Microfluidic Synthesis of Magnetite Nanoparticles for the Controlled Release of Antibiotics. *Pharmaceutics* **2023**, *15*, 2215. https://doi.org/10.3390/pharmaceutics15092215.
3. Caizer, C.; Caizer-Gaitan, I.S.; Watz, C.G.; Dehelean, C.A.; Bratu, T.; Soica, C. High Efficacy on the Death of Breast Cancer Cells Using SPMHT with Magnetite Cyclodextrins Nanobioconjugates. *Pharmaceutics* **2023**, *15*, 1145. https://doi.org/10.3390/pharmaceutics15041145.
4. Ünak, P.; Yasakçı, V.; Tutun, E.; Karatay, K.B.; Walczak, R.; Wawrowicz, K.; Żelechowska-Matysiak, K.; Majkowska-Pilip, A.; Bilewicz, A. Multimodal Radiobioconjugates of Magnetic Nanoparticles Labeled with 44Sc and 47Sc for Theranostic Application. *Pharmaceutics* **2023**, *15*, 850. https://doi.org/10.3390/pharmaceutics15030850.
5. Oliveira, R.R.; Cintra, E.R.; Sousa-Junior, A.A.; Moreira, L.C.; da Silva, A.C.G.; de Souza, A.L.R.; Valadares, M.C.; Carrião, M.S.; Bakuzis, A.F.; Lima, E.M. Paclitaxel-Loaded Lipid-Coated Magnetic Nanoparticles for Dual Chemo-Magnetic Hyperthermia Therapy of Melanoma. *Pharmaceutics* **2023**, *15*, 818. https://doi.org/10.3390/pharmaceutics15030818.
6. Nitica, S.; Fizesan, I.; Dudric, R.; Loghin, F.; Lucaciu, C.M.; Iacovita, C. Doxorubicin Loaded Thermosensitive Magneto-Liposomes Obtained by a Gel Hydration Technique: Characterization and In Vitro Magneto-Chemotherapeutic Effect Assessment. *Pharmaceutics* **2022**, *14*, 2501. https://doi.org/10.3390/pharmaceutics14112501.
7. Alsenousy, A.H.A.; El-Tahan, R.A.; Ghazal, N.A.; Piñol, R.; Millán, A.; Ali, L.M.A.; Kamel, M.A. The Anti-Obesity Potential of Superparamagnetic Iron Oxide Nanoparticles against High-Fat Diet-Induced Obesity in Rats: Possible Involvement of Mitochondrial Biogenesis in the Adipose Tissues. *Pharmaceutics* **2022**, *14*, 2134. https://doi.org/10.3390/pharmaceutics14102134.
8. Pusta, A.; Tertis, M.; Crăciunescu, I.; Turcu, R.; Mirel, S.; Cristea, C. Recent Advances in the Development of Drug Delivery Applications of Magnetic Nanomaterials. *Pharmaceutics* **2023**, *15*, 1872. https://doi.org/10.3390/pharmaceutics15071872.
9. Ganguly, S.; Margel, S. Bioimaging Probes Based on Magneto-Fluorescent Nanoparticles. *Pharmaceutics* **2023**, *15*, 686. https://doi.org/10.3390/pharmaceutics15020686.
10. Chan, M.-H.; Li, C.-H.; Chang, Y.-C.; Hsiao, M. Iron-Based Ceramic Composite Nanomaterials for Magnetic Fluid Hyperthermia and Drug Delivery. *Pharmaceutics* **2022**, *14*, 2584. https://doi.org/10.3390/pharmaceutics14122584.
11. Gago, L.; Quiñonero, F.; Perazzoli, G.; Melguizo, C.; Prados, J.; Ortiz, R.; Cabeza, L. Nanomedicine and Hyperthermia for the Treatment of Gastrointestinal Cancer: A Systematic Review. *Pharmaceutics* **2023**, *15*, 1958. https://doi.org/10.3390/pharmaceutics15071958.

References

1. Khizar, S.; Elkalla, E.; Zine, N.; Jaffrezic-Renault, N.; Errachid, A.; Elaissari, A. Magnetic nanoparticles: Multifunctional tool for cancer therapy. *Expert Opin. Drug Deliv.* **2023**, *20*, 189–204. [CrossRef] [PubMed]
2. Blanco-Andujar, C.; Walter, A.; Cotin, G.; Bordeianu, C.; Mertz, D.; Felder-Flesch, D.; Begin-Colin, S. Design of iron oxide-based nanoparticles for MRI and magnetic hyperthermia. *Nanomedicine* **2016**, *11*, 1889–1910. [CrossRef] [PubMed]
3. Xie, X.; Zhai, J.; Zhou, X.; Guo, Z.; Lo, P.-C.; Zhu, G.; Chan, K.W.Y.; Yang, M. Magnetic Particle Imaging: From Tracer Design to Biomedical Applications in Vasculature Abnormality. *Adv. Mater.* **2023**, 2306450. [CrossRef] [PubMed]

4. Gavilan, H.; Avugadda, S.K.; Fernandez-Cabada, T.; Soni, N.; Cssani, M.; Mai, B.T.; Chantrell, R.; Pellegrino, T. Magnetic nanoparticles and clusters for magnetic hyperthermia: Optimizing their heat performance and developing combinatorial therapies to tackle cancer. *Chem. Soc. Rev.* **2021**, *50*, 11614–11667. [CrossRef] [PubMed]
5. Carter, T.J.; Agliardi, G.; Lin, F.-Y.; Ellis, M.; Jones, C.; Robson, M.; Richard-Londt, A.; Southern, P.; Lythgoe, M.; Thin, M.Z.; et al. Potential of Magnetic Hyperthermia to Stimulate Localized Immune Activation. *Small* **2021**, *17*, 2005241. [CrossRef] [PubMed]

Disclaimer/Publisher's Note: The statements, opinions and data contained in all publications are solely those of the individual author(s) and contributor(s) and not of MDPI and/or the editor(s). MDPI and/or the editor(s) disclaim responsibility for any injury to people or property resulting from any ideas, methods, instructions or products referred to in the content.

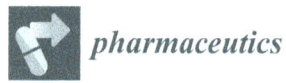

Article

Field-Induced Agglomerations of Polyethylene-Glycol-Functionalized Nanoclusters: Rheological Behaviour and Optical Microscopy

Sandor I. Bernad [1,*], Vlad Socoliuc [1], Izabell Craciunescu [2], Rodica Turcu [2] and Elena S. Bernad [3]

[1] Centre for Fundamental and Advanced Technical Research, Romanian Academy—Timisoara Branch, Mihai Viteazul Str. 24, RO-300223 Timisoara, Romania; vsocoliuc@gmail.com

[2] National Institute for Research and Development of Isotopic and Molecular Technologies (INCDTIM), Donat Str. 67-103, RO-400293 Cluj-Napoca, Romania; izabell.craciunescu@itim-cj.ro (I.C.); rodica.turcu14@gmail.com (R.T.)

[3] Department of Obstetrics and Gynecology, Faculty of General Medicine, University of Medicine and Pharmacy "Victor Babes" Timisoara, P-ta Eftimie Murgu 2, RO-300041 Timisoara, Romania; ebernad@yahoo.com

* Correspondence: sandor.bernad@upt.ro

Abstract: This research aims to investigate the agglomeration processes of magnetoresponsive functionalized nanocluster suspensions in a magnetic field, as well as how these structures impact the behaviour of these suspensions in biomedical applications. The synthesis, shape, colloidal stability, and magnetic characteristics of PEG-functionalized nanoclusters are described in this paper. Experiments using TEM, XPS, dynamic light scattering (DLS), VSM, and optical microscopy were performed to study chain-like agglomeration production and its influence on colloidal behaviour in physiologically relevant suspensions. The applied magnetic field aligns the magnetic moments of the nanoclusters. It provides an attraction between neighbouring particles, resulting in the formation of chains, linear aggregates, or agglomerates of clusters aligned along the applied field direction. Optical microscopy has been used to observe the creation of these aligned linear formations. The design of chain-like structures can cause considerable changes in the characteristics of ferrofluids, ranging from rheological differences to colloidal stability changes.

Keywords: magnetoresponsive nanocomposite; particle aggregation/agglomeration; magnetic particle targeting; chain formation; magnetorheological properties; optical microscopy

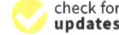

Citation: Bernad, S.I.; Socoliuc, V.; Craciunescu, I.; Turcu, R.; Bernad, E.S. Field-Induced Agglomerations of Polyethylene-Glycol-Functionalized Nanoclusters: Rheological Behaviour and Optical Microscopy. *Pharmaceutics* 2023, 15, 2612. https://doi.org/10.3390/pharmaceutics15112612

Academic Editors: Donato Cosco, Natalia L. Klyachko, Xiaowei Zeng and Sofia Lima

Received: 12 September 2023
Revised: 1 November 2023
Accepted: 9 November 2023
Published: 10 November 2023

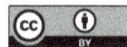

Copyright: © 2023 by the authors. Licensee MDPI, Basel, Switzerland. This article is an open access article distributed under the terms and conditions of the Creative Commons Attribution (CC BY) license (https://creativecommons.org/licenses/by/4.0/).

1. Introduction

The potential for preventing thrombotic events and limiting post-angioplasty restenosis with rapid endothelium recovery and restoring its normal activities [1–3] justifies the development of techniques for quickening arterial re-endothelialization.

For the treatment of chronic diseases, localized therapies that use pharmaceuticals targeted by magnetic carriers are particularly appealing since they can get around the dose limit toxicity constraint while increasing drug efficacy [4]. Using a static magnetic field (SMF), magnetic guiding improves the deposition of drug carriers that are magnetically responsive when injected [5,6].

Magnetically guided medication delivery is impacted by three vital biophysical processes: (i) drug-loaded particle transport through the arteries, (ii) extravasation via blood vessel walls, and (iii) interstitial transport inside tissue.

It is crucial to note that when using magnetic drug targeting (MDT), medications are administered only by touching the artery wall. Magnetic nanoparticles (MNPs) are only captured from the blood flow when the following applies:

(a) They are in contact with the artery wall.

(b) They hold in place. In this situation, the magnetic force component must be vital enough to counteract the drag force and keep a particle in place.

Iron oxide particles (IONPs), particularly magnetite (Fe_3O_4) and maghemite (γ-Fe_2O_3), are the most widely employed magnetic materials among the many classes of MNPs, particularly in biomedical applications [7]. Their surface alterations, in addition to their inherent physicochemical characteristics, control this potential.

Numerous recent studies on the advantages of using magnetic iron oxide nanocomposites made with various functional coatings as potential magnetic carriers for biomedical applications concluded that clusters of magnetic nanoparticles could be superior to single nanoparticles in some applications [8–10].

Applications of magnetic nanoparticles in biomedicine are affected in different ways by the creation of linear aggregates. The magnetophoretic mobility of the system will be considerably altered as aggregates form. When paired with the size and acicular shape of the aggregates, larger particles' increased magnetophoretic mobility may drastically modify their behaviour for use in magnetically targeted medication delivery. The toxicity of magnetic particles considerably rises after applying a magnetic field, according to recent studies by Bae et al. [11]. Their research revealed that the more significant cytotoxicity was probably caused by the increased cellular absorption caused by the creation of field-induced aggregates. Therefore, for applications with static magnetic fields, attention should be paid to building systems that limit field-induced aggregations.

Agglomerates are created when a single physical entanglement occurs between the aggregated particles and van der Waals forces, resulting in loose bonding. Because the fundamental particles that make up an aggregate are firmly bound or fused, it is stated in the ISO standards that the aggregate's external specific surface area is less than the aggregate's total surface area. It is also stated that because agglomerate constituents are weakly or loosely linked, the shallow specific surface area of agglomerates is equivalent to the entire surface area of those constituents.

It is important to note that IONPs in aqueous suspensions can undergo a phase transition caused by the magnetic field even at low magnetic flux density values. To do this, they can either assemble into elongated aggregates (with micrometric dimensions along the direction of the applied magnetic field) [12] or form fractal groups under the combined action of magnetic dipolar and colloidal interactions [13].

Individual nanoparticles or clusters of nanoparticles can combine to create irreversibly bound aggregates through close contact or reversibly bound agglomerates [14,15] that can be dispersed with sonication or other mixing techniques [16]. The relative strengths of the attractive and repulsive nanoparticle interactions determine whether particles agglomerate permanently or reversibly [14].

The delicate subject of flow recirculation from stents on drug release has been the subject of numerous investigations. According to Zunino et al.'s research [17], persistent recirculation emerges downstream of struts oriented transversally to the flow under steady flow circumstances. This concludes that these areas only contribute to drug accumulation in the artery despite the lengthened drug residence period. The endothelium of the blood vessel, which is made up of a thin, continuous layer of cell lining, is where nanoparticles will first come into contact after intravascular delivery, which is vital to note. As the primary focus in treating disease, including inflammatory cardiovascular disorders [18,19], the interaction of multifunctional nanoparticles with the endothelium is crucial. By allowing specific solutes and molecules to pass through, the vascular endothelium plays a selective role in the transfer of drug carriers. According to Qiu et al. [20], the vascular endothelium was more permeable when using an external magnetic field.

Problem Description

In our previous work [21], the magnetic nanoclusters produced chain-like structures in a stented vascular model during the stent targeting process (Figure 1). These magnetically built structures around the stent geometry have a significant length at the end of the targeting, with an average chain size of 0.56 mm. Removing the magnetic field at the end of the targeting procedure did not affect the spontaneous disintegration of the produced filaments into a small structure or cluster the same size as those in the injected suspension.

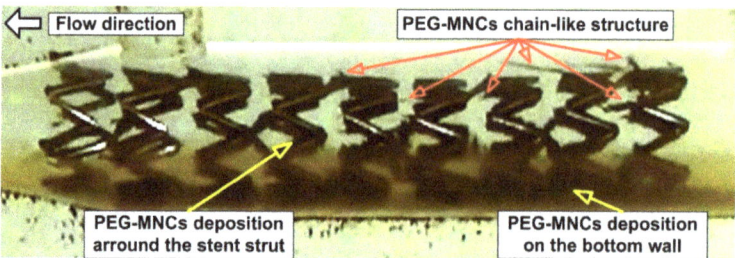

Figure 1. Chain-like structure development during the stent targeting processes. Magnetically induced aggregation of the PEG_MNCs in the targeted region (red arrows) at the end of the injection period of 30 s. Magnetic cluster depositions on the bottom wall of the artery model and stent struts' coverage with magnetic clusters (yellow arrows) at the end of the injection period of 30 s. The chain-like magnetic particle structure was generated in a different part of the stent geometry in the presence of the external magnetic field. Permanent magnet positions correspond to the distance of 15 mm from the artery model bottom wall. The used magnet: rectangular NdFeB50 permanent magnet, with dimensions of 30 mm × 20 mm × 20 mm (length × width × thickness). White arrow—flow direction.

Without a magnetic field, the fluid flow creates a hydrodynamic force that causes these structures to disintegrate into many smaller fragments. The fluid stream picks up the resultant pieces; some are deposited distally in the stent or transmitted distally in the test circuit. From a medical standpoint, these washed particles can clog the distal capillary network and serve as a potential site for thrombus formation, which would be lethal to the patient.

The observation of agglomeration formation throughout the targeting process prompted the need to understand the cause of the formation of these structures. Thus, in study [22], based on the results of multiple experiments in the same conditions as in work [21], we determined that the agglomeration phenomenon observed during targeting is not random but rather the result of an external magnetic field. We also discovered that the stent design, particularly the presence of an external magnetic field, influences agglomeration formation.

Optical microscopy was used to comprehend the chain-like structure generations. Also, we investigated colloidal interaction among the MNC clusters.

Our prior work established that long-range magnetic dipolar interactions emerge in an external field and prevail over colloidal ones (van der Waals, steric, and electrostatic forces). However, several questions remain unanswered, including how different magnets or field intensity influence chain generation, how the magnetorheological properties of the suspension influence structure generation, how the polydispersity index can be correlated with the behaviour and rheology of the suspension in the presence of a magnetic field, and how sonication of the samples and the density of the working fluid influence the behaviour of the suspension.

To answer the questions mentioned above, we conducted a series of new studies in addition to those undertaken in prior publications [21,22], as follows:

1. We used a new type of permanent magnet. This magnet has a length to cover the size of the stent strictly.
2. Detailed DLS investigations were performed to study the cluster distribution and polydispersity index to highlight connections with suspension magnetorheological behaviour and agglomerate generation.

3. We performed detailed optical microscopy investigations for two magnetic field intensities. It is essential that we perform the optical microscopy investigation for the same period used in the targeting processes to understand the chain development observed in the in vitro study.

2. Materials and Methods

2.1. Magnetoresponsive Nanocluster Synthesis

Our earlier works [21,22] present the PEG-coated magnetic nanoclusters. Briefly, for the preparation of PEG-MNCs, the oil-in-water mini-emulsion method was used, which involves, in the first step, the mechanical mixing of two different, non-miscible phases, an aqueous phase containing the stabilizing surfactant, PEG (PEG-2000) (1.795 g, 2% wt%), and an organic, oily phase containing the hydrophobic magnetic nanoparticles (0.5 wt% Fe_3O_4) (ferrofluid—magnetic nanoparticles dispersed in toluene). By using an ultrasonic finger (U.P. 400S), the two phases of emulsification take place (50% amplitude, 2 min), and very fine droplets of organic solvent (toluene) containing the magnetic nanoparticles are formed in the aqueous medium. The stabilizing surfactant (PEG) in the aqueous medium allows the formation of micelles of specific sizes in which the surfactant molecules arrange themselves with the polar end to the aqueous medium and the non-polar end to the organic phase. The formed stable mini emulsion is transferred to a larger beaker and heated (100 °C) in an oil bath under magnetic solid stirring (500 rpm) for 30 min to release the organic solvent, toluene, inside the micelles using evaporation. The as-formed magnetic clusters are magnetically separated from the reaction medium using a strong magnet, washed successively three times with a water–methanol mixture (100 mL/wash) to remove traces of reactants, and then redispersed in distilled water at known concentrations. Following that, the PEG-coated MNCs were dispersed in an aqueous carrier at preset weights to produce the investigated suspensions.

2.2. Characterization

2.2.1. TEM Investigation

The morphology of the magnetic clusters was examined using scanning electron microscopy (STEM). For this, a microscope equipped with a cold-field emission gun, the Hitachi HD2700 (Hitachi High-Tech Corporation, Tokyo, Japan), was used. ImageJ (https://imagej.nih.gov/ij/) (accessed on 20 July 2023) was used to obtain the PEG_MNC diameter distribution. A total of 200 PEG_MNCs from three TEM images were evaluated to establish the average size distribution.

2.2.2. X-ray Photoelectron Spectroscopy (XPS)

By using an XPS spectrometer with the dual-anode X-ray source Al/Mg, a PHOIBOS 150 2D CCD hemispherical energy analyser, and a multi-channel Tron detector with a vacuum maintained at 1×10^{-9} torr, researchers were able to determine the chemical composition (atomic concentrations) of the surface as well as the chemical state of the atoms of the coated nanoclusters PEG-MNC. XPS research used the AlKa X-ray source (1486.6 eV) running at 200 W. To enable the XPS measurements, the dispersion of particles was dried on an indium foil. The XPS survey spectra were captured at 0.5 eV/step and 30 eV pass energy. Ten scans were accumulated at a pass energy of 30 eV and a step energy of 0.1 eV to create the high-resolution spectra for the individual elements (Fe, C, and O). The Gaussian–Lorentzian product function and a non-linear Shirley background subtraction were used in CasaXPS v10 software for data processing and curve fitting.

2.2.3. Dynamic Light Scattering (DLS) Measurements

A Malvern Zetasizer Nano-ZS device (Malvern Panalytical Ltd., Malvern, UK) outfitted with a He-Ne laser (λ = 633 nm, max 5 mW) and operating at a scattering angle of 173° was used to quantify the particles' hydrodynamic size and zeta potential. Before the measurements, the samples were diluted to a 0.1 mg/mL concentration. One millilitre of particle suspension was used in each measure.

2.2.4. Magnetic Characterization

The magnetization curves of the PEG-coated clusters were measured using a vibrating sample magnetometer (VSM 880-ADE Technologies, Westwood, MA, USA) at room temperature in the field range of 0–1000 kA/m.

2.2.5. Rheology

The magneto-viscous characteristics of the pegylated nanoparticles were tested at 25 °C in both the presence and absence of a magnetic field using a rotating rheometer (Anton Paar MCR 300 Physica, Anton Paar GmbH, Graz, Austria) with a 20 mm diameter plate–plate magnetorheological cell (MRD 170/1T-SN80730989). In this cell, a perpendicular magnetic field is applied to the sample layer situated between the plates. A Hall probe installed under the bottom plate of the MR cell measures the magnetic flux density of the applied magnetic field.

2.3. Magnetic Field Generation

MNC retention can be measured in vitro to estimate what would happen in vivo. Thus, it is possible to investigate the effects of several factors on the efficiency of magnetic targeting [23], including magnet configuration, flow velocity, particle surface features, separation from the magnetic pole, and particle size.

The concept of the present study, which is based on our prior findings [24,25], is to use a single external permanent magnet system to create a strong magnetic field that will be used to magnetize, direct, and deliver the MNCs in the stented vascular segment.

The rectangular NdFeB52 permanent magnet (commercial notation N52: Neodymium 52), which has dimensions of 20 × 10 × 5 mm (length × width × thickness) and a maximum energy product (BxH) of 52 MGOe, was utilized to create the magnetic field in our experiment (Figure 2).

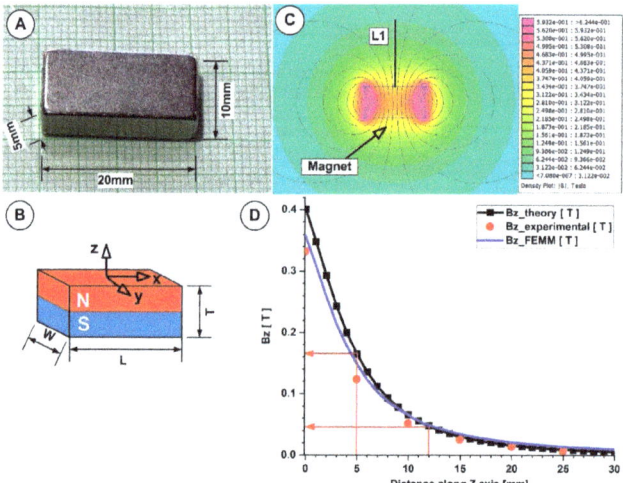

Figure 2. A magnetic field generated with the NbFeB52 permanent magnet was used in the experimental investigation. (**A**) The dimension of the used magnet and axis association. (**B**) A used permanent magnet has polarization along the Z-axis. (**C**) Numerical investigations of the magnetic field generated with the NdFeB52 magnet. (**D**) B_z evolution function of the magnet surface distance. Comparison between theoretical, experimental, and numerical results.

B-Field Measurement

Using a Tesla meter (Model 5080, F.W. Bell Gaussmeter, Milwaukie, OR, USA) placed using a micrometre, the actual B-field strength was measured along the magnet's central axis at various points. The measurement error of the micrometre was calculated to be 0.15 mm, while the measurement error of the B-field was taken from the Tesla meter manual. With a peak magnitude of 405 mT and a drop-off to 0.08 mT at 3 cm from the magnet's base, the B-field magnitudes along the central axis of the interest fell exponentially with distance (Figure 2D). The magnetic field's most significant spatial gradient was close to the magnet's edges (Figure 2D). In the present experiment, to investigate the influence of the magnetic field on MNC targeting and the agglomeration phenomena, the magnet position ranged between 5 and 12 mm from the vessel wall (corresponding to magnetic field intensity of 0.42 and 0.183 T, respectively; Figure 2D, red arrows).

We compare the B-field distribution obtained from analytical solutions, numerical simulations, and experimental investigations to obtain a clearer picture of the generated magnetic field.

With [26], Equation (1) was used to obtain the analytical solution for the B-field distribution along the magnet's central axis at different distances (Line L1 in Figure 2C).

$$B(z) = \frac{B_r}{\pi} \left(\tan^{-1} \frac{WL}{2z\sqrt{4z^2 + W^2 + L^2}} - \tan^{-1} \frac{WL}{2(z+T)\sqrt{4(z+T)^2 + W^2 + L^2}} \right), \quad (1)$$

where W is the magnet width, L is the magnet length, T is the magnet thickness, B_r is the magnet residual flux density, and z is the distance from the magnet surface (where $z \geq 0$) on the magnet's centreline.

The examined permanent magnet was numerically simulated using the freeware Finite Element Method Magnetism (FEMM) version 4.2 (accessed on 10 June 2023, at http://www.femm.info/wiki/HomePage).

The experimentally obtained B-field values and the corresponding analytically and numerically calculated values were in good agreement, as shown in Figure 2D.

3. Results

3.1. PEG-MNC Size and Morphology

The nanoclusters possess a well-defined spherical shape with a core–shell structure consisting of a cluster core with closely packed magnetite nanoparticles (Figure 3A,B). The PEG_MNCs' size was measured with direct counting from TEM micrographs and showed diameters ranging from 40 to 120 nm. In turn, the morphologies of the small nano-chain aggregates (Figure 3A, bottom chain) magnetically assembled from MNCs and chemically fixated show predominantly single-particle chains of a few nanoclusters. Counting particle lengths from TEM micrographs yields a distribution of nano-chains in the range of 4–8 nanoclusters with a mean of 6 ± 3 nanoclusters.

Also, the micrographs indicate that the visualized structures had arbitrary morphologies ranging from chain-like to closely packed, creating both small and large aggregates (Figure 3A). Furthermore, TEM micrographs showed that the dimensionality and size of these structures varied greatly and could contain many MNCs.

ImageJ was used to obtain the PEG_MNC and the core (magnetite nanoparticles) diameter distribution (imagej.nih.gov/ij/; accessed on 15 June 2023). Each sample's histogram, created by measuring 200 clusters over three TEM images, was fitted to a lognormal distribution function.

Figure 3C displays the diameter distribution of the core magnetic nanoparticles. With an average core size of 7 ± 1.5 nm and an average cluster size of 62 ± 17 nm (presented in our previous work [22]), TEM observations support the multicore flower-like shape of synthesized particles.

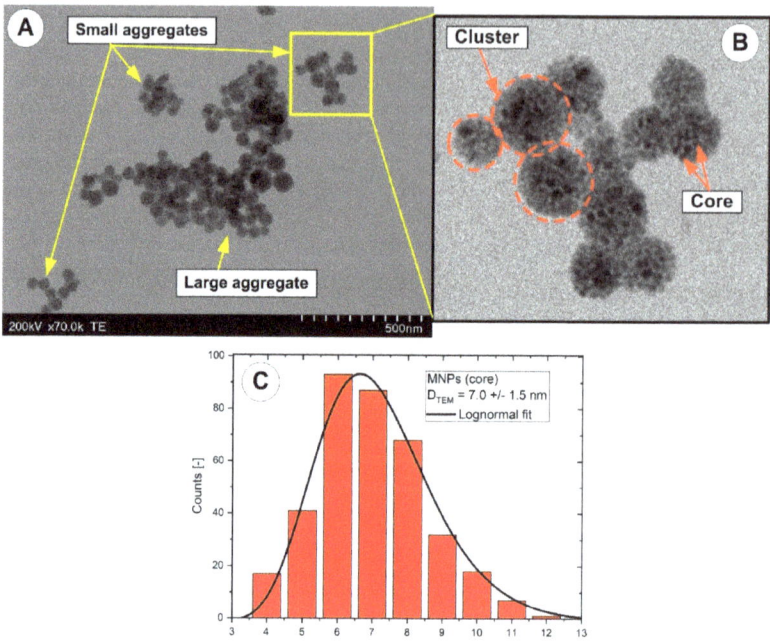

Figure 3. (**A**) Representative TEM image of the PEG-MNC clusters and aggregates. The aggregates show chain-like and close-packed morphologies (yellow arrows). (**B**) Detail regarding the spherical clusters (red circle) and core inside the cluster. TEM size histograms for core nanoparticles (**C**).

It is vital to note that the sample drying process greatly influences TEM micrographs. Dewetting reduces the contact area between clusters, and attractive interparticle forces cause aggregation, aided by drying [27].

During the TEM sample preparation, the polymer chains' conformation may alter because of the increasing pressure, which could cause the coating layer to contract.

In the present work, we use the term "aggregate" for this structure because the investigated structure results from the formation of compact masses of irreversibly linked clusters, per the definition presented in [13].

It is critical to distinguish between 'real' aggregates in the sample and 'developed' aggregates developed during sample processing. For this, DLS was used to evaluate the materials in their suspended natural condition, and the results were compared to those of TEM. The results are presented in the following sections.

3.2. The Surface Chemical Analysis of the Magnetic Cluster

The successful coating of the magnetic clusters with PEG was shown with the XPS analysis (detailed investigations were presented in [22]). The C 1s, O 1s, and Fe 2p core-level XPS high-resolution spectra for PEG_CMC were investigated. The contributions from the peaks corresponding to specific groups of the surfactant, oleic acid, and the PEG coating of the clusters are seen in the deconvolution of the C 1s and O 1s spectra. Three components, corresponding to C-C, C-H (284.7 eV), C-O (286.6 eV), and O-C=O (288.9 eV), were found to suit the C 1s spectrum best. Three elements that are attributed to Fe-O (530.2 eV), C-O (531.8 eV), and O-C=O (533 eV) may be seen in the O 1s spectrum. The doublets Fe 2p3/2 and Fe 2p1/2 can be found in the Fe 2p spectrum.

3.3. DLS Characterization of the PEG-MNCs' Suspension

The PEG-MNC's stability was assessed using DLS measurements. The Malvern Zeta Sizer evaluated the studied samples for zeta size and potential. Three crucial properties of the final PEGylated MNC are revealed with dynamic light scattering (DLS): size distribution, zeta potential (ZP), and hydrodynamic diameter (zeta-average of the MNC).

ZP levels typically fall within the −100 to +100 mV range [28]. Colloidal stability can be predicted based on ZP magnitude. A high level of stability is naturally present in the ZP of NPs with values of −25 or + 25 mV. High ZP denotes powerfully charged particles, which inhibit particle aggregation by preventing electric repulsion. Attraction triumphs over repulsion when the ZP is low, and the mixture is likely to agglomerate, coagulate, or flocculate because of van der Waals interparticle attraction [28].

The MNCs used in our studies were coated with a PEG2000 layer, giving them unique surface charges and chemical characteristics. In deionized water, the PEG-MNC assumed a dispersed colloidal state with an average hydrodynamic diameter of 4527 nm (Figure 4A time T = 0 min) and a negative surface charge of −7.22 mV (Table 1, Figure 4B). The sample's aggregation was measured using the polydispersity index (PDI), which was discovered to be 0.229.

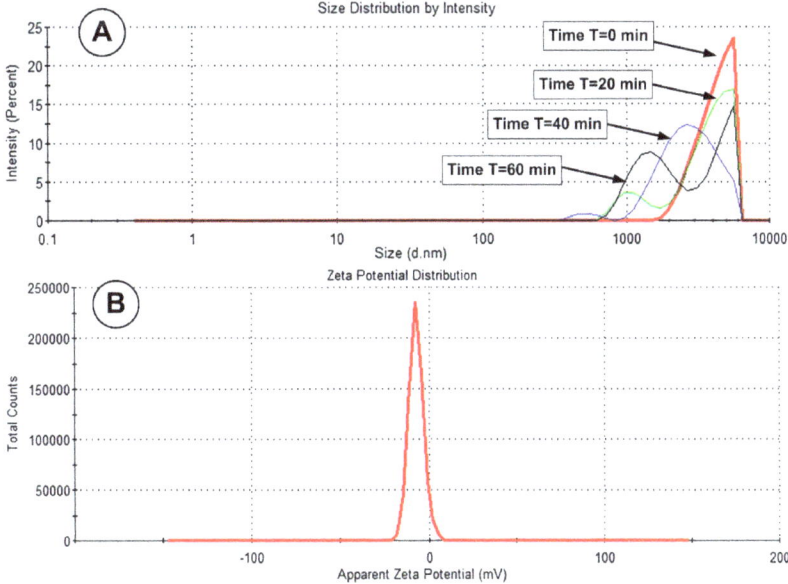

Figure 4. (**A**) Size distribution by intensity for the PEG-MNC aqueous dispersion corresponding to different time steps after the vigorous stirring of the suspension. (**B**) Zeta potential corresponding to the investigated PEG-MNCs' suspension.

Table 1. Zeta potential and size distribution by Intensity of the PEG-MNCs in water.

Hydrodynamic Diameter, D_H (nm)	Zeta Potential (mV)	Polydispersity Index, PDI
4572	−7.22	0.229

The hydrodynamic size is substantially more significant when compared to the matching TEM observations, indicating the existence of aggregates in this solution. Furthermore, the polydispersity index (PDI), calculated as the ratio of the standard deviation square to the mean size, was discovered to be 0.229. Due to the existence of bigger aggregates, the PDI of the PEG_MNC solution is relatively high.

In Figure 4A, it is evident that there are large agglomerates (micro-size structures) in the PEG-MNC aqueous dispersion, which exhibits a monomodal distribution and polydispersity. According to descriptions in the literature, a polydispersity index (PDI) value of less than 0.1 may indicate a high degree of homogeneity in the particle population, whereas high PDI values indicate a wide size range or possibly multiple populations [29].

It is crucial to give precise feedback regarding the time frame involved in this process to employ the DLS to monitor the aggregation kinetics of MNCs [30]. In our investigations, the DLS measurements track the PEG-coated MNCs' colloidal stability in an aqueous dispersion over 60 min (Figure 4A).

As seen in Figure 4A, during the first DLS measurement, which was performed precisely after vigorous stirring, vast clusters of agglomeration occurred with an average hydrodynamic diameter of about 4572 nm. Stronger magnetic attraction exists within the groups because the magnetic attraction between particles grows with a particle radius to the sixth power, further causing flocculation. The intensity-weighted size distribution shifts to bimodal after 20 min, as seen in Figure 4A. The size of the individual agglomerates (first peak) that remain suspended decreases over time (4572 nm at the time T = 0 min, ≈3400 nm at the time T = 20 min compared to ≈2600 nm at the time T = 60 min), indicating that the initial clusters take some time to form large agglomerates with a bimodal distribution (such as that at time T = 60 min).

3.3.1. PEG-MNCs' Sedimentation Kinetics

As shown in the next paragraph, sedimentation kinetics were studied using DLS measurements of the hydrodynamic diameter in two stages.

Stage one: The settling behaviour of the suspensions of PEG-MNCs in the distilled water was checked using DLS measurements at 60 min after manual stirring (Figure 5), with measurements of the hydrodynamic diameter distributions of the suspended PEG_MNC population in the different segments of the investigated tube (the test tubes contain 20 mL of a 5% mass concentration PEG-MNC aqueous suspension).

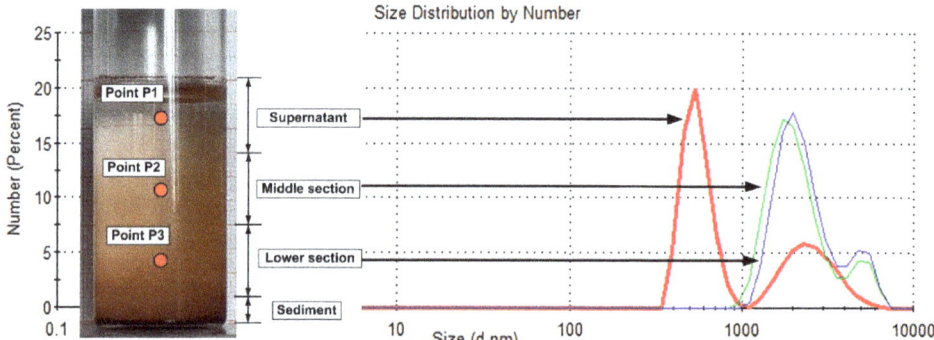

Figure 5. Particle size distribution by number obtained using DLS measurements at 60 min after manual stirring. Measurements were performed at three points corresponding to different stages of cluster sedimentation. Points P1, P2, and P3 represent the position where the samples were taken and used colloid: PEG_MNCs dispersed in distilled water.

Figure 5 shows that the peak position moved to be smaller for the supernatant region, demonstrating that the sedimentation processes are progressing. Small and large aggregates and agglomerates are present in the supernatant, but the number of the small structures is much larger than the large ones. The particle size distribution in the middle section and the lower area is very similar but indicates the presence of the gravitational sedimentation processes with the bimodal size distribution. More important is that, at the end of 60 min, a consistent layer of PEG-MNCs was deposited on the bottom of the tube.

Phase two: DLS measurements checked the settling behaviour of PEG-MNC suspensions every 10 min for 60 min after vigorous manual stirring. The measurement was performed for samples from the position corresponding to Point 2 in Figure 5.

The PEG-MNC suspensions' sedimentation kinetic curve is shown in Figure 6. In Figure 6, the sedimentation profile is divided into three areas: agglomeration, sedimentation-1, and sedimentation-2, according to the findings presented in [31]. When the aggregates or agglomerates reach a threshold size, they rapidly deposit ("sedimentation-1" segment in Figure 6). After a while, the sedimentation rate can decline, consistent with the sedimentation of various structures that fail to reach the required critical size [31].

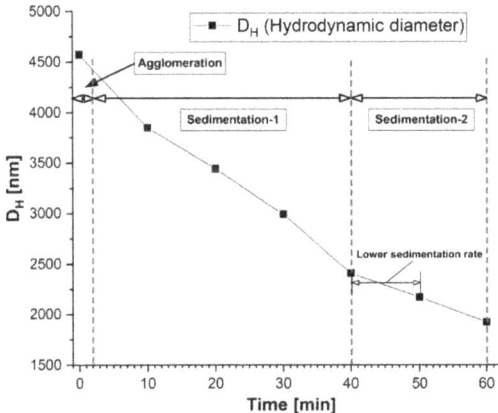

Figure 6. Sedimentation curve for the 5% mass concentration PEG-MNCs dispersed in distilled water.

After the investigation period, the DLS measurement verified the presence of a structure with an approximate hydrodynamic diameter of 1800 nm (Figure 6), showing that a significant portion of the PEG-MNC agglomeration or aggregate population had settled on the cuvette's bottom.

3.3.2. Effects of Sonication on Aggregate Size

As was previously mentioned, a stable colloid may be mostly made up of individual clusters, aggregates, and agglomerates; all these structures tend to clump together and settle over time. The sonication process was used in this work as a method to enhance the dispersion of nanoparticles in liquids. It is well recognized that a properly timed treatment can aid in dispersion and uniformity of the suspension, but extended sonication times can also cause ultrasound-driven aggregation [32].

A bath-type sonicator (Bandelin RK 100 H ultrasonic bath, Bandelin electronic GmbH & KG, Berlin, Germany, 320 W) operating at room temperature distributed the PEG-MNCs in the base fluid. The sample received 2880 J of energy during the 15 min sonication process. DLS measurement is used to track the colloidal stability of the PEG-coated MNCs in the aqueous dispersion after 15 min of bath sonication for over 60 min (Figure 7).

As shown in Figure 7, the initial suspension (time T = 0 min, performed exactly after sonication) exhibited a broad polydisperse and multimodal size distribution primarily in the 530 nm–3 µm range, with two minor fractions of particles, the first of which had a peak centre near 230 nm (range of 190 to 530 nm) and the second of which had a peak centre near 5.5 µm (range of 3.5 to 6.4 µm). As can be seen in Figure 7, the initial PEG-MNCs' profile changed throughout the investigation from a multimodal distribution (times T = 0 min and T = 60 min) to a bimodal distribution (T = 20 min) and a monomodal distribution (T = 40 min), displaying both a microscale agglomerate and a nanoscale fraction.

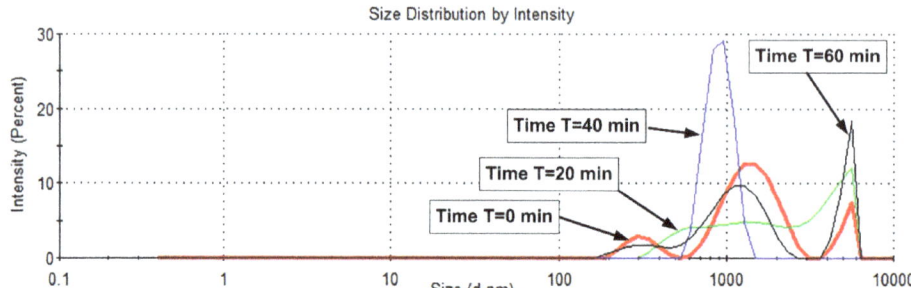

Figure 7. Particle size distribution by intensity of the 5% mass concentration PEG-MNCs dispersed in the distilled water at different time intervals after 15 min of bath sonication.

Contrary to the literature [29,32], bath sonication in our situation does not result in uniformly sized particle dispersions or a considerable reduction in the PEG-MNC aggregate size.

3.4. Magnetic Properties of the Magnetoresponsive Nanocluster

One of the most crucial conditions for successful applications in biomedicine, including magnetic targeting, is the strong magnetic moment of the functionalized multicore carriers [33].

Magnetic experiments with a vibrating sample magnetometer (VSM) reveal that the synthesized nanostructures' colloidal and powder forms behave superparamagnetically, as demonstrated in our prior work [22]. Also, measurements show no hysteresis, and it suggests that the magnetic moments of the nanoparticles packed into the centres of nanoclusters and nano-chains are unblocked using heat.

The saturation magnetization for the PEG-coated MNCs is 55 emu/g, and for the water-based suspension, it is 142 memu/g. These are both less than the values for bulk magnetite, 92 emu/g. These are the consequences of the PEG layer, water, and the induced non-magnetic layer (due to the surface effects of the nanoparticles embedded in the cluster) [34].

3.5. PEG-MNC Aqueous Dispersion Rheological Properties

The start and course of many cardiovascular diseases are influenced by the mechanical blood vessel wall behaviour and blood flow properties [35]. While operating more like a Newtonian fluid in the large arteries, blood behaves differently in the small/capillary arteries [36]. The wall shear stress (WSS) results from friction between the flowing blood and the endothelial surface of the artery wall.

In the current study, the possibility of particle targeting for a stented artery was explored for the WSS value in a range of $0.1~\text{s}^{-1}$ to $1000~\text{s}^{-1}$, corresponding to the blood flow in the stented artery [37].

3.5.1. Rheological Properties of the PEG_MNCs' Aqueous Dispersions

Parallel plate geometry was used to apply steady shear strain to the suspensions. A shear rate ramp up in the 0.1–$1000~\text{s}^{-1}$ range was used to obtain the viscosity curves of apparent viscosity (η) vs. shear rate ($\dot{\gamma}$). The magnetorheological accessory produced a perpendicular external magnetic field to the shear flow. The temperature for all rheological testing was 25 °C. The variations in the shear viscosity of PEG_MNCs' aqueous suspension as a function of the shear rate without the magnetic field and for two distinct magnetic field intensities, 42 and 183 mT, were presented in our previous work [22].

Viscosity Changes in the Absence of the Magnetic Field

The PEG_MNC aqueous suspension shows the shear thinning typical of multicore particle suspensions [38,39], brought on with the clusters' aggregation or agglomeration. The van der Waals attraction force between the clusters is what propels the agglomeration in the absence of a magnetic field. As can be seen, as the field intensity increases, the magnetic force takes precedence over the hydrodynamic force, increasing viscosity as the field-induced aggregates get more robust and resist shear. The characteristics of the viscosity curves indicate areas of varying slopes that represent the distinct structural evolution in the sample. Also, these characteristics exhibit a non-Newtonian nature with a progressively emerging typical shear thinning behaviour. Because the investigated suspensions were non-Newtonian [39,40], we used the Carreau model [41] (Equation (2)) to fit the measured viscosity curves.

$$\eta(\dot{\gamma}) = \eta_\infty + (\eta_0 - \eta_\infty)\left[1 + \left(C\dot{\gamma}\right)^2\right]^{-p} \qquad (2)$$

where C (s) is the Carreau constant (the slope of the viscosity curve on the log–log scale at high values of the shear rate), p (−) is the Carreau exponent, and η_0 and η_∞ (Pas) are the viscosities at infinitely low and infinitely high shear rates, respectively.

As presented in our previous work [22], the increased viscosity of the PEG_MNC suspensions at low shear (0.1–10 s^{-1}) is caused by this network of agglomerated particles. Shear forces break up the particle network once the suspension starts to flow and the shear rate rises. As a result, as the shear rate increases, the agglomerates' size continuously decreases, which causes the viscosity to decrease. When the viscosity reaches a constant value, only shear forces can shrink the size of the clusters.

Magnetorheological Investigations

Both the magnetorheological effect (MRE), which increases shear stress when an external magnetic field is applied, and the magneto-viscous effect (MVE), which increases viscosity when an external magnetic field is used, were studied in the presence of the magnetic field. These effects are critical to developing a strategy for utilizing these intelligent fluids.

This network of agglomerated clusters contributes to the greater viscosity ($\eta \approx$ 1–10 Pas) of the MNC suspensions at low shear. On the other hand, viscosity in the low shear rate area rapidly dropped, which indicates that the structures of the dispersed PEG_MNCs formed under the external magnetic field persisted until the shear rate reached the value of 1000/s.

The MVE on the range of low shear rates (0.01 s^{-1} to 10 s^{-1}) is found to be almost independent of the shear rate, but it significantly decreases at high speeds as cluster agglomerations are destroyed. Figure 8A shows the MVE's dependence on the strength of the magnetic field for various shear rate values. The MNC agglomerates are destroyed for higher shear rates, and the MVE decreases. The observed MVE behaviour is a consequence of the multicore nature of the magnetic component, resulting in a high induced magnetic moment of particles, favouring their structuring in a magnetic field corresponding to the findings presented in [42].

Figure 8B illustrates the test results aiming at the viscosity behaviour as a function of time or the quickness of the development or destruction of cluster agglomerations while applying or halting the external magnetic field. The test contains three intervals at which a low shear rate is kept constant—so as not to disturb the formation of particle agglomerations too much. The torque has values high enough (>5 µNm) for the reproducibility of experimental data. On the first and the last interval, the magnetic field intensity was fixed at the value of 0 (with six experimental points each); on the second interval, the values of field intensity B were 20, 42, and 183 mT and were fixed in turn. The temperature was set as T = 25 °C. The magnetic field intensity was chosen following the results presented in Figure 2.

To better understand how quickly cluster agglomeration occurs when an external magnetic field is applied, the measurement time in this test was set at 6 s/point for intervals with no magnetic field and 8 s/point for intervals with one. Due to low sample viscosity values, shorter measurement periods or points could not be specified. The structures are seen to form within 6 s. In the absence of a magnetic field, slow agglomeration persists throughout the application of a magnetic field, and for a field intensity of 183 mT, the agglomeration phenomenon reaches saturation 150 s after the magnetic field application.

The formation or destruction of particle agglomerations happens very quickly. For all investigated magnetic field intensities, the suspension viscosity practically returns to its value before applying it after the magnetic field is turned off.

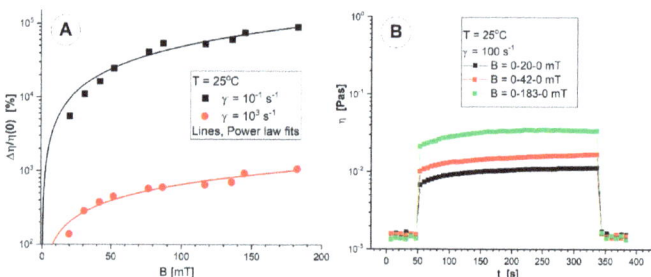

Figure 8. Rheological properties of the PEG_MNCs' aqueous suspension at the temperature of 25 °C. (**A**) Magneto-viscous effects' function of different magnetic flux densities for two different shear rates (0.1 and 1000 s^{-1}); (**B**) viscosity curve function of time for different magnetic flux densities.

3.5.2. Effects of the Carrier Fluid Density

From a macro-rheological perspective, it is known that the haematocrit (concentration of red blood cells) and blood viscosity are directly correlated [43], which means that an increase or decrease in the RBC concentration affects blood viscosity values as well as its non-Newtonian behaviour [44]. At a shear rate of 0.1 s^{-1}, the viscosity of the same blood can be 60 cP (0.06 Pas), whereas, at a shear rate of 200 s^{-1}, it would be 5 or 6 cP (0.005 or 0.006 Pas) [45]. This indicates that blood viscosity varies in the microcirculation, major arteries, and veins, where shear rates can range from a few to more than 1000 s^{-1} [46]. At low shear rates (such as veins) as opposed to high shear rates (such as arteries), the effect of haematocrit on blood viscosity is significantly more significant [47].

Considering the previous, we sought to determine how the variation in the carrier fluid (CF) density affected the rheological characteristics of the model suspension. We produced CF with 1055 and 1068 kg/m^3 densities to conduct this, respectively. The density was changed by adjusting the glycerine–water ratio in the CF composition. Our study's carrier fluid (CF) consisted of glycerol–water solutions with a density (1055 kg/m^3) equivalent to blood. The rheological characterization of CF was detailed in our previous work [20,21].

Figure 9A depicts the rheological properties of CF, PEG_MNC aqueous suspension (distilled water + 5% PEG_MNC), and model suspensions (CF + 5% PEG_MNC). The presence of PEG_MNC has a considerable influence on the suspension viscosity curve for the aqueous suspension in the low and high shear regions. Still, the viscosity curve for model suspensions exhibits a progressive increase over the whole inquiry range. Also, Figure 9A shows that all the examined suspensions exhibit shear thinning behaviour at relatively low shear rates (<10 s^{-1}). Figure 9B demonstrates that the model suspension's (CF + 5% PEG_MNCs) rheological behaviour is essentially unaffected by changes in the CF density. At low levels of the shear stress, a variation in behaviour between the suspension model and the CF is seen. It is significant to note that increasing the carrier fluid's density does not impact the model suspension's magnetic viscous behaviour (Figure 9C,D).

The glycerol–water PEG_MNC dispersions were selected because they allowed us to assess a slight change in viscosity when a magnetic field was applied and examine the magnetorheological properties. This is the most intriguing aspect of how we conducted this experiment.

We employed this blood analogue fluid (water–glycerol solutions) during the experimental examination to guarantee that the rheological features of the carrier fluid accurately recreated blood rheology. The flow field across the test portion must exhibit the same characteristics as normal blood flow (a viscous flow). Fluid flow is an essential predictor of PEG_MNC aggregation surrounding the implanted stent, as demonstrated in our early works [21,22]. Our investigations showed that these dispersions are stable for 1 h, which is long enough for targeted experiments and viscosity measurements.

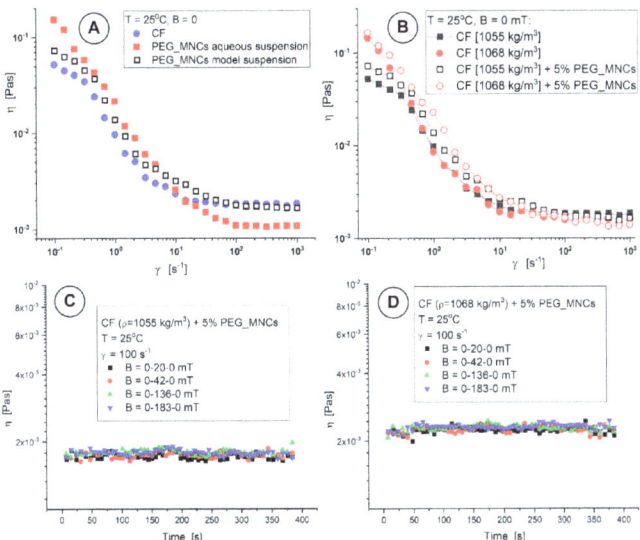

Figure 9. (**A**) Comparison between CF, aqueous, and model suspension viscosity curves at T = 25 °C. (**B**) CF and model suspension viscosity curves at T = 25 °C for different density values. (**C,D**) Viscosity curve function of time for different densities of the carrier fluid (CF) for the model suspension (CF + 5% PEG_MNC) corresponding to different magnetic flux densities.

Because the viscosity of a glycerol aqueous solution is highly sensitive to temperature changes, neither the temperature nor the applied magnetic field must vary during the targeting and measuring time. As a result, all experimental measurements are carried out in an air-conditioned room. Furthermore, to prevent working fluid temperature change, measurements are taken in an open circuit where the fluid is not recirculated. Also, we used DC (direct current) magnetic fields, which do not transmit heat to the test section.

3.6. Kinetics of the PEG_MNC Chain Formation in the Magnetic Field

Any ferrofluid will inevitably have particle-size polydispersity, which is crucial for creating structures generated with the field [48]. In a polydisperse fluid, the particle size, shape, or strength of the interaction between the components might differ [49].

The field-induced microstructures created with the magnetic field were examined using an optical microscope.

We investigated two approaches for optical microscopy research. In the first case, we used a low-intensity magnetic field (42 mT); in the second, we used a magnetic field with a strength of 124 mT. Each field intensity corresponds to the different positions of the permanent magnet, as shown in Figure 2. This technique was designed to investigate the effect of external magnetic field intensity on aggregate and agglomerate formation. Both scenarios used an aqueous suspension containing 5% mass concentration PEG_MNC. All solutions were vigorously stirred before testing, and the investigated samples were collected from the same region of the tube (middle section, as shown in Figure 5). More importantly, these analyses were conducted in both situations for the same injection period (30 s) employed in the targeting methods to understand agglomeration development better.

As shown in Figure 10A, without a magnetic field, the dispersion's superparamagnetic nanoparticles move randomly according to Brownian motion. When exposed to an external magnetic field, the nanoparticles' induced magnetic moments align with the magnetic field's direction.

Figure 10B shows the formation of magnetically induced large MNC filaments (agglomerates) that are field-oriented. The initial suspension is subjected to the magnetic field for 30 s, the same amount of time employed for stent particle targeting. During this time, the PEG-coated MNCs self-assembled into linear agglomerates in the magnetic field's direction (see Supplemental Video). Also, the filaments do not spontaneously disintegrate once the magnetic field is removed; instead, they become randomly orientated, as presented in Figure 10C. Figure 10C shows that these large structures did not shrink or fragment once the magnetic field was removed. The Supplemental Movie provides a detailed presentation of the creation and development of these structures.

Given the size of these large structures in the range of several micrometres generated under the influence of magnetic fields, it is reasonable to assume that the observed behaviour is closely related to the magneto-viscous properties outlined in earlier sections. As a result, quantifying structure formation is critical to analyse the influence of external magnetic field intensity and duration on the size of chain-like shapes.

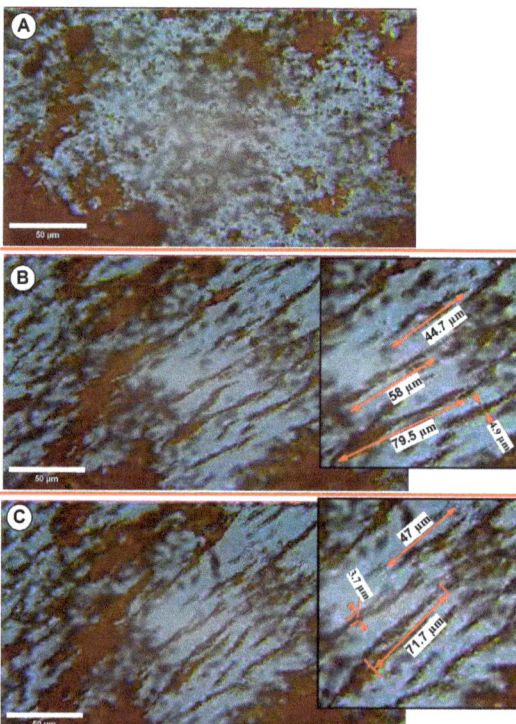

Figure 10. Optical microscopy investigations of the PEG-MNC aqueous suspension phase condensation phenomena induced in the presence of the external magnetic field. (**A**) Suspension without a magnetic field. (**B**) The figure shows the large PEG_MNC agglomerates generated under the action of the externally applied magnetic field of intensity H = 47 mT—detail regarding the length and thickness of these large, generated structures (chains). (**C**) The PEG_MNC agglomerates after turning off the magnetic field. Detail shows that the suspension contained large, micro-sized cluster agglomerates after turning off the magnetic field. All measurements of the agglomerate's length were processed using ImageJ software—scale bar: 50 μm.

Effect of the Magnetic Field Intensity

We used optical microscopy to learn more about the interaction of PEG_MNCs in the presence of a magnetic field. This experiment aims to demonstrate the effect of the increasing magnetic field strength on agglomeration processes.

The optical microscopy experiments were carried out under the following conditions: a magnetic field intensity of 124 mT (corresponding to a magnet position of 7 mm from the artery bottom wall), a magnetic field application period of 30 s (same as in the previous experiment), and a vigorously stirred sample of the PEG_MNC aqueous suspension.

Figure 11 shows images of PEG_MNC clusters in aqueous suspension after field application. The PEG_MNC appears diffused in the carrier fluid without a magnetic field (Figure 11A). When the magnetic field is activated, the MNCs migrate and form agglomerates directed in the field direction, as seen in Figure 11B–F.

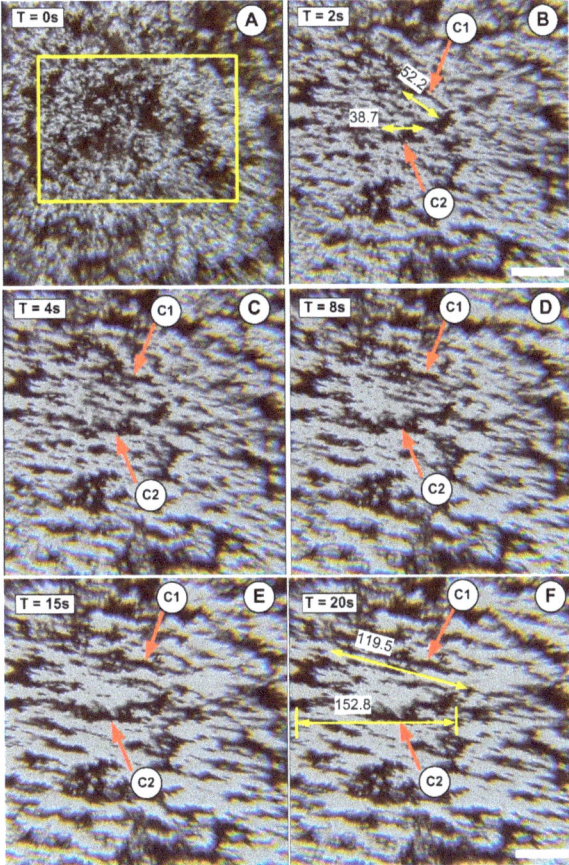

Figure 11. Optical microscopy images of the PEG_MNC transition from a dispersed stage to chain-like structures in the presence of the external magnetic field. (**A**) Suspension in the absence of the magnetic field. (**B–F**) Stages of the chain structure's development after the magnetic field was switched on. The investigated period is 30 s, under the action of the externally applied magnetic field of intensity H = 124 mT. (**B,F**) detail the length and thickness evolution during the investigated period for two agglomerates (chains), C1 and C2. (**F**) shows the sizeable micron-size chain structure oriented in the field direction at the end of the investigation period—scale bar: 50 μm.

Figure 11A demonstrates that the sample initially showed no agglomerates but showed pre-existing cluster aggregates. The size distribution and volume fraction of particles and the applied field's strength determine the kinetics of field-induced aggregation in ferrofluids. A ferrofluid system will be thermodynamically stable without a magnetic field [38]. When subjected to a magnetic field, however, the stability is lost, and to re-establish equilibrium, both clusters and aggregates begin to aggregate/agglomerate to produce two distinct phases, namely carrier fluid and the formed structures.

This separation begins with a brief nucleation step in which a few particles or pre-existing aggregates initiate particle agglomeration in the presence of an external magnetic field.

As shown in Figure 11B and more clearly in the Supplemental Video, a short but thick structure emerges a few seconds after the rapid initiation of the magnetic field. These formations (agglomerates) are oriented in the field direction and move in the carrier fluid. During the following several seconds, these primary agglomerates adhere together head to tail to create large (>150 μm) and practically stationary needle-like secondary agglomerates (Figure 11F). The agglomerate's size grows with time (Figure 11B–F). Individual agglomerates develop relatively quickly (between 2 and 8 s), owing to the adsorption of magnetic clusters or tiny aggregates from the surrounding fluid. Because of their dipolar contacts, the surrounding aggregates consolidate and form a long-size structure (agglomerates) in the following period (between 10 and 20 s, Figure 11D,F).

The shape and size of the created agglomerates remain nearly constant between 20 and 30 s. These findings underline that the generated structures have achieved their maximum length and are in equilibrium.

4. Discussion

The investigated PEG_MNC suspensions possess significantly larger particles, as evidenced with DLS results. The larger particles have stronger dipolar strength [38]. This system's initial susceptibility and magnetization curve strongly depend on the number of bigger particles. When the number of bigger particles rises, the magnetization of the system grows quicker, even in weak fields, resulting in a higher initial susceptibility [38,48]. Larger particles have been shown to play a significant function as condensation centres in the production of nuclei [12,50]. When the chain length exceeds a certain threshold, it attracts the next tiny cluster (including both big and small particles). It creates a thicker column, which might be considered the nucleation location (according to [12]). As a result, even at modest field strengths, aggregates act as nucleation sites, initiating chain development. As field strength increases, the chains lengthen, increasing the aspect ratio. Chain zippering produces long and dense columnar formations.

However, in a system with high polydispersity, the larger particles can operate as nucleation centres even at very low field strengths, implying that aggregation kinetics are much faster with significantly lower activation energy, resulting in a higher nucleation rate.

In conclusion, the created agglomerates were developed around the existing large structure. These initial large structures functioned as condensation sites for heterogeneous nucleation of free clusters and existing aggregates.

Given that our ferrofluids contain oleic-acid-capped magnetic nanoparticles (as described in [21]), we hypothesized that the occurrence of cluster aggregations (as shown with the TEM observations, Figure 3A) is most likely owing to a non-uniform surfactant coating on their surface. Our idea is consistent with the findings provided in [51]. Furthermore, because the particles are functionalized, they cannot come into direct contact with one another, even in an external magnetic field. As a result, solvent molecules will become trapped between the nanoparticles, forming an aggregation. More solvent molecules are trapped between aggregates when the chain density is large [51]. This idea is consistent with that, as stated before in [22], MNCs are soldered in aggregates due to strong contacts between polyethylene glycol (PEG) shells or the collective encapsulation of many MNCs within PEG.

Rheological studies of the PEG_MNC suspension at low field strength (42 mT, Figure 8A) revealed a considerable increase in viscosity across the whole examined shear domain. Furthermore, even at a fixed shear rate, when the field intensity increases, the magnetic force prevails over the hydrodynamic force, increasing viscosity as the field-induced aggregates grow stronger and resist shear. These findings emphasize the unfavourable influence of polydispersity and higher aggregate size on rheological behaviour and agglomerate formation.

Larger magnetic carriers, as is known, enhance magnetic force on the carriers, boosting targeting efficiency. On the other hand, this increased structure and targeting efficiency may be helpful for various medicinal applications [52].

In our previous investigations [22], to find an explanation for the observed aggregation process, the colloidal interaction among the MNC clusters was investigated. Also, the electrostatic repulsion energy, van der Waals, and magnetic dipole–dipole attraction were calculated in the absence and presence of the external magnetic field to examine the colloidal interaction between the PEG_MNC clusters. Moreover, the field-induced microstructures created with the magnetic field were analysed using an optical microscopic technique.

Based on our findings, we conclude that an external magnetic field induces aggregation, and MNCs are soldered in aggregates, most likely due to bridge contacts among PEG shells or collective engulfment in the PEG of many MNCs.

To demonstrate that the agglomerate generation during targeting is not a particular phenomenon caused by the stent geometry (precisely the local strut arrangement), in this study, during optical microscopy investigations, we evaluated the effect of the two different magnetic field intensities on the structure generation. The morphology and dimensions of the generated agglomerates were compared with the size of the structures found in our earlier investigation (Table 2).

Table 2. Comparison between the dimensions of the generated agglomerate during optical microscopy in the presence of the different magnetic field intensities.

References	Magnet Type	Dimension (l × w × t) (mm)	Magnet Position Relative to the Microscope Plate (mm)	Field Intensity (mT)	Investigation Period (s)	Maximum Average Length of the Agglomerates (μm)
Early results [22]	NdFeB50	30 × 20 × 20	16	110	5	41
Present investigations	NdFeB52	20 × 10 × 5	7	124	30	146
			12	47	30	69

Where l × w × t = length × width × thickness.

The results in Table 2 demonstrate that even when exposing the suspension to the magnetic field for the same duration, different field intensities generated agglomerates with different shapes and lengths.

For a better understanding of aggregate growth, we display the length history of chain C2 (from Figure 11) over the research period of 30 s.

Figure 12 depicts the experimental dependence of the maximum aggregate length L on elapsed time t for a sample containing 5% PEG_MNC mass concentration in a magnetic field strength of 124 mT. As presented in the section Effect of the Magnetic Field Intensity, the aggregate length increased with time, a fact confirmed with Figure 12. As the figure shows, the experimental L(t) curves shift in the slope at t = 8 s. Furthermore, the agglomeration process approaches saturation 20 s after applying the magnetic field. After this period, the aggregates' form and length remain constant. This observed behaviour is strongly connected to the magneto-viscous features described in previous sections.

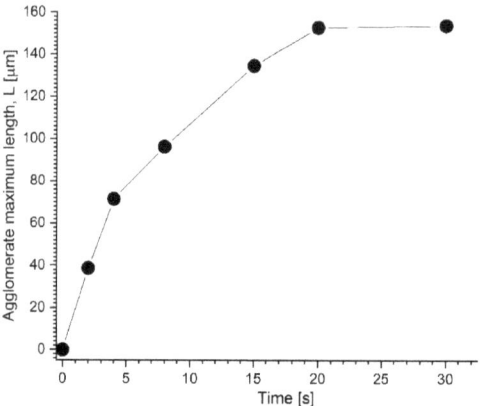

Figure 12. Magnetic-field-induced aggregate maximum length evolution occurred during the investigated period of 30 s. The field intensity is 124 mT, corresponding to the magnet distance from the microscope plate of 7 mm. The experimental L(t) curve corresponds to chain C2 plotted in Figure 11.

5. Conclusions

According to [38], most ferrofluid systems are stable without a magnetic field. Stability is compromised when exposed to a magnetic field, and the nanoparticles or nanoclusters assemble or agglomerate to regain equilibrium. The consequence was the formation of two separate phases: the carrier fluid and the aggregates.

The processes above were thoroughly examined in the current paper. In this work, we investigated the possible influence of cluster size distribution and polydispersity on agglomerate generations, the correlation between suspension magnetorheological behaviour and agglomerate formations, and the effect of sonication, carrier fluid density, and sedimentation profile on agglomeration processes, in addition to the parameters measured in our previous paper.

Optical microscopy was used to analyse aggregation and agglomeration processes for various magnetic field intensities, and the results related to both the suspension polydispersity index and rheological behaviour.

The size and polydispersity characterization of PEG-coated MNC suspensions using DLS reveals that this suspension contains single clusters and pre-existing aggregates. We hypothesized that MNCs are soldered in aggregates, most likely due to bridge connections between PEG shells or collective engulfment in PEG of numerous MNCs, based on the acquired results and analysis of the PEG_MNC synthesis technique. Furthermore, dispersed particles aggregate or agglomerate, even after ultrasonic treatment, forming sizable structures. This outcome is closely related to the hypothesis previously mentioned.

Rheological studies show that changes in suspension density do not affect the suspension's rheological and magneto-viscous (MVE) behaviour. According to optical microscopy imaging, only large clusters or pre-existing aggregates produce agglomerates. This assumption is linked to the original polydispersity of the colloid.

The observed MVE behaviour is due to the magnetic component's multicore nature, resulting in a high induced magnetic moment of particles, favouring their structuring in a magnetic field. The magneto-viscous measurement results are aimed at the viscosity behaviour as a function of time and the rapid formation or destruction of cluster agglomerations when applying or stopping the external magnetic field.

Finally, the generation and development of the chain-like structure are related to the synthesis of PEG-MNC, the colloidal stability of MNC, and the rheological and magnetic properties of the model suspensions.

Supplementary Materials: The following supporting information can be downloaded at: https://www.mdpi.com/article/10.3390/pharmaceutics15112612/s1, Video S1: Agglomeration in the presence of the external magnetic field.

Author Contributions: Conceptualization, Writing—original draft, Writing—review and editing, Visualization, Investigation, S.I.B.; Conceptualization, Investigation, V.S.; Methodology, Validation, S.I.B., V.S. and E.S.B.; Investigation, Validation, R.T. and I.C. All authors have read and agreed to the published version of the manuscript.

Funding: This research received no external funding.

Institutional Review Board Statement: Not applicable.

Informed Consent Statement: Not applicable.

Data Availability Statement: Data are contained within the article and Supplementary Materials.

Acknowledgments: For S.I. Bernad, this work was supported by the RA-TB/CFATR/LHC multiannual research program 2023–2024. For V. Socoliuc, this work was supported partially by the RA-TB/CFATR/LMF multiannual research program 2023–2024 and with a grant from the Ministry of Research, Innovation and Digitization, CNCS/CCCDI—UEFISCDI, project number PN-III-P2-2.1-PED-2021-2049, within PNCDI III. For I. Craciunescu, R. Turcu, and E. Bernad, this work was supported partially with a grant from the Ministry of Research, Innovation and Digitization, CNCS/CCCDI—UEFISCDI, project number PN-III-P2-2.1-PED-2021-2049, within PNCDI III.

Conflicts of Interest: The authors declare no conflict of interest.

References

1. Douglas, G.; Van Kampen, E.; Hale, A.B.; McNeill, E.; Patel, J.; Crabtree, M.J.; Ali, Z.; Hoerr, R.A.; Alp, N.J.; Channon, K.M. Endothelial cell repopulation after stenting determines in-stent neointima formation: Effects of bare-metal vs. drug-eluting stents and genetic endothelial cell modification. *Eur. Heart J.* **2012**, *34*, 3378–3388. [CrossRef]
2. Fuchs, A.T.; Kuehnl, A.; Pelisek, J.; Rolland, P.H.; Mekkaoui, C.; Netz, H.; Nikol, S. Inhibition of restenosis formation without compromising reendothelialization as a potential solution to thrombosis following angioplasty? *Endothelium* **2008**, *15*, 85–92. [CrossRef]
3. Van Belle, E.; Bauters, C.; Asahara, T.; Isner, J.M. Endothelial regrowth after arterial injury: From vascular repair to therapeutics. *Cardiovasc. Res.* **1998**, *38*, 54–68. [CrossRef]
4. Tibbitt, M.W.; Dahlman, J.E.; Langer, R. Emerging Frontiers in Drug Delivery. *J. Am. Chem. Soc.* **2016**, *138*, 704–717. [CrossRef]
5. Shapiro, B.; Kulkarni, S.; Nacev, A.; Muro, S.; Stepanov, P.Y.; Weinberg, I.N. Open challenges in magnetic drug targeting. *Wiley Interdiscip. Rev. Nanomed. Nanobiotechnol.* **2015**, *7*, 446–457. [CrossRef]
6. Schleich, N.; Danhier, F.; Préat, V. Iron oxide-loaded nanotheranostics: Major obstacles to in vivo studies and clinical translation. *J. Control. Release* **2015**, *198*, 35–54. [CrossRef]
7. Xie, W.; Guo, Z.; Gao, F.; Gao, Q.; Wang, D.; Liaw, B.; Cai, Q.; Sun, X.; Wang, X.; Zhao, L. Shape-, size- and structure-controlled synthesis and biocompatibility of iron oxide nanoparticles for magnetic theranostics. *Theranostics* **2018**, *8*, 3284–3307. [CrossRef]
8. Lu, Z.D.; Yin, Y.D. Colloidal nanoparticle clusters: Functional materials by design. *Chem. Soc. Rev.* **2012**, *41*, 6874–6887. [CrossRef]
9. Boles, M.A.; Engel, M.; Talapin, D.V. Self-assembly of colloidal nanocrystals: From intricate structures to functional materials. *Chem. Rev.* **2016**, *116*, 11220–11289. [CrossRef]
10. Bunge, A.; Porav, A.S.; Borodi, G.; Radu, T.; Pîrnău, A.; Berghian-Grosan, C.; Turcu, R. Correlation between synthesis parameters and properties of magnetite clusters prepared by solvothermal polyol method. *J. Mater. Sci.* **2019**, *54*, 2853–2875. [CrossRef]
11. Bae, J.E.; Huh, M.I.; Ryu, B.K.; Do, J.Y.; Jin, S.U.; Moon, M.J.; Jung, J.C.; Chang, Y.; Kim, E.; Chi, S.G.; et al. The effect of static magnetic fields on the aggregation and cytotoxicity of magnetic nanoparticles. *Biomaterials* **2011**, *32*, 9401–9414. [CrossRef] [PubMed]
12. Ezzaier, H.; Alves Marins, J.; Razvin, I.; Abbas, M.; Ben Haj Amara, A.; Zubarev, A.; Kuzhir, P. Two-stage kinetics of field-induced aggregation of medium-sized magnetic nanoparticles. *J. Chem. Phys.* **2017**, *146*, 114902. [CrossRef] [PubMed]
13. Vikesland, P.J.; Rebodos, R.L.; Bottero, J.Y.; Rose, J.; Masion, A. Aggregation and sedimentation of magnetite nanoparticle clusters. *Environ. Sci. Nano* **2016**, *3*, 567–577. [CrossRef]
14. Vikesland, P.J.; Heathcock, A.M.; Rebodos, R.L.; Makus, K.E. Particle size and aggregation effects on magnetite reactivity toward carbon tetrachloride. *Environ. Sci. Technol.* **2007**, *41*, 5277–5283. [CrossRef]
15. Rubasinghege, G.; Lentz, R.W.; Park, H.; Scherer, M.M.; Grassian, V.H. Nanorod dissolution quenched in the aggregated state. *Langmuir* **2010**, *26*, 1524–1527. [CrossRef]
16. Lin, M.Y.; Lindsay, H.M.; Weitz, D.A.; Ball, R.C.; Klein, R.; Meakin, P. Universality in colloid aggregation. *Nature* **1989**, *339*, 360–362. [CrossRef]

17. Zunino, P.; D'Angelo, C.; Petrini, L.; Vergara, C.; Capelli, C.; Migliavacca, F. Numerical simulation of drug eluting coronary stents: Mechanics, fluid dynamics and drug release. *Comput. Methods Appl. Mech. Eng.* **2009**, *198*, 3633–3644. [CrossRef]
18. Lu, Y.C.; Luo, P.C.; Huang, C.W.; Leu, Y.L.; Wang, T.H.; Wei, K.C.; Wang, H.E.; Ma, Y.H. Augmented cellular uptake of nanoparticles using tea catechins: Effect of surface modification on nanoparticle-cell interaction. *Nanoscale* **2014**, *6*, 10297–10306. [CrossRef]
19. Onyskiw, P.J.; Eniola-Adefeso, O. Effect of PEGylation on ligand-based targeting of drug carriers to the vascular wall in blood flow. *Langmuir* **2013**, *29*, 11127–11134. [CrossRef]
20. Qiu, Y.; Tong, S.; Zhang, L.; Sakurai, Y.; Myers, D.R.; Hong, L.; Lam, W.A.; Bao, G. Magnetic forces enable controlled drug delivery by disrupting endothelial cell-cell junctions. *Nat. Commun.* **2017**, *8*, 15594. [CrossRef]
21. Bernad, S.I.; Craciunescu, I.; Sandhu, G.S.; Dragomir-Daescu, D.; Tombacz, E.; Vekas, L.; Turcu, R. Fluid Targeted delivery of functionalized magnetoresponsive nanocomposite particles to a ferromagnetic stent. *J. Magn. Magn. Mater.* **2021**, *519*, 167489. [CrossRef]
22. Bernad, S.I.; Socoliuc, V.; Susan-Resiga, D.; Crăciunescu, I.; Turcu, R.; Tombácz, E.; Vékás, L.; Ioncica, M.C.; Bernad, E.S. Magnetoresponsive Functionalized Nanocomposite Aggregation Kinetics and Chain Formation at the Targeted Site during Magnetic Targeting. *Pharmaceutics* **2022**, *14*, 1923. [CrossRef] [PubMed]
23. Liu, J.F.; Lan, Z.; Ferrari, C.; Stein, J.M.; Higbee-Dempsey, E.; Yan, L.; Amirshaghaghi, A.; Cheng, Z.; Issadore, D.; Tsourkas, A. Use of Oppositely Polarized External Magnets to Improve the Accumulation and Penetration of Magnetic Nanocarriers into Solid Tumors. *ACS Nano* **2020**, *14*, 142–152. [CrossRef] [PubMed]
24. Bernad, S.I.; Bernad, E. Magnetic Forces by Permanent Magnets to Manipulate Magnetoresponsive Particles in Drug-Targeting Applications. *Micromachines* **2022**, *13*, 1818. [CrossRef]
25. Bernad, S.I.; Susan-Resiga, D.; Bernad, E. Hemodynamic Effects on Particle Targeting in the Arterial Bifurcation for Different Magnet Positions. *Molecules* **2019**, *24*, 2509. [CrossRef]
26. Camacho, J.M.; Sosa, V. Alternative method to calculate the magnetic field of permanent magnets with azimuthal symmetry. *Rev. Mex. Fis.* **2013**, *59*, 8–17.
27. Michen, B.; Geers, C.; Vanhecke, D.; Endes, C.; Rothen-Rutishauser, B.; Balog, S.; Petri-Fink, A. Avoiding drying-artifacts in transmission electron microscopy: Characterizing the size and colloidal state of nanoparticles. *Sci. Rep.* **2015**, *5*, 9793. [CrossRef]
28. Horie, M.; Fujita, K. Toxicity of Metal Oxides Nanoparticles. *Adv. Mol. Toxicol.* **2011**, *5*, 145–178. [CrossRef]
29. Lim, J.; Yeap, S.; Che, H.; Low, S. Characterization of magnetic nanoparticle by dynamic light scattering. *Nanoscale Res. Lett.* **2013**, *8*, 381. [CrossRef]
30. Yeap, S.P.; Ahmad, A.L.; Ooi, B.S.; Lim, J. Electrosteric Stabilization and Its Role in Cooperative Magnetophoresis of Colloidal Magnetic Nanoparticles. *Langmuir* **2012**, *28*, 14878–14891. [CrossRef]
31. Phenrat, T.; Saleh, N.; Sirk, K.; Tilton, R.D.; Lowry, G.V. Aggregation and Sedimentation of Aqueous Nanoscale Zerovalent Iron Dispersions. *Environ. Sci. Technol.* **2007**, *41*, 284–290. [CrossRef] [PubMed]
32. Zhong, Z.; Chen, F.; Subramanian, A.S.; Lin, J.; Highfield, J.; Gedanken, A. Assembly of Au colloids into linear and spherical aggregates and effect of ultrasound irradiation on structure. *J. Mater. Chem.* **2006**, *16*, 489–495. [CrossRef]
33. Laurent, S.; Saei, A.A.; Behzadi, S.; Panahifar, A.; Mahmoudi, M. Superparamagnetic iron oxide nanoparticles for delivery of therapeutic agents: Opportunities and challenges. *Expert Opin. Drug Deliv.* **2014**, *11*, 1449–1470. [CrossRef] [PubMed]
34. Luigjes, B.; Woudenberg, S.M.C.; de Groot, R.; Meeldijk, J.D.; Torres Galvis, H.M.; de Jong, K.P.; Philipse, A.P.; Erné, B.H. Diverging Geometric and Magnetic Size Distributions of Iron Oxide Nanocrystals. *J. Phys. Chem. C* **2011**, *115*, 14598–14605. [CrossRef]
35. Sankar, D.S.; Hemalatha, K. Pulsatile flow of Herschel–Bulkley fluid through stenosed arteries—A mathematical model. *Int. J. Non-Linear Mech.* **2006**, *41*, 979–990. [CrossRef]
36. Mandal, P.K. An unsteady analysis of non-Newtonian blood flow through tapered arteries with a stenosis. *Int. J. Non-Linear Mech.* **2005**, *40*, 151–164. [CrossRef]
37. Bourantas, C.V.; Papafaklis, M.I.; Kotsia, A.; Farooq, V.; Muramatsu, T.; Gomez-Lara, J.; Zhang, Y.-J.; Igbal, J.; Kalatzis, F.G.; Naka, K.K.; et al. Effect of the Endothelial Shear Stress Patterns on Neointimal Proliferation Following Drug-Eluting Bioresorbable Vascular Scaffold Implantation. *JACC Cardiovasc. Interv.* **2014**, *7*, 315–324. [CrossRef]
38. Ivanov, A.O.; Zubarev, A. Chain Formation and Phase Separation in Ferrofluids: The Influence on Viscous Properties. *Materials* **2020**, *13*, 3956. [CrossRef]
39. Zablotsky, D.; Kralj, S.; Kitenbergs, G.; Maiorov, M. Features of magnetorheology of chain-forming ferrofluids with multicore magnetic nanoparticles: Experiment and simulation. *Colloids Surf. A Physicochem. Eng. Asp.* **2020**, *603*, 125079. [CrossRef]
40. Musikhin, A.Y.; Kuzhir, P.; Zubarev, A.Y. To the theory of magneto-induced flow in thrombosed channels. *J. Magn. Magn. Mater.* **2023**, *587*, 171316. [CrossRef]
41. Carreau, P.J. Rheological Equations from Molecular Network Theories. *Trans. Soc. Rheol.* **1972**, *16*, 99–127. [CrossRef]
42. Linke, J.M.; Odenbach, S. Anisotropy of the magnetoviscous effect in a ferrofluid with weakly interacting 640 magnetite nanoparticles. *J. Phys. Condens. Matter* **2015**, *27*, 176001. [CrossRef] [PubMed]
43. Eckmann, D.M.; Bowers, S.; Stecker, M.; Cheung, A.T. Hematocrit, volume expander, temperature, and shear rate effects on blood viscosity. *Anesth. Analg.* **2000**, *91*, 539–545. [CrossRef] [PubMed]

44. Picart, C.; Piau, J.M.; Galliard, H.; Carpentier, P. Human blood shear yield stress and its hematocrit dependence. *J. Rheol.* **1998**, *42*, 1–12. [CrossRef]
45. Nader, E.; Skinner, S.; Romana, M.; Fort, R.; Lemonne, N.; Guillot, N.; Guthier, A.; Antoine-Jonville, S.; Renoux, C.; Hardy-Dessource, M.D.; et al. Blood Rheology: Key Parameters, Impact on Blood Flow, Role in Sickle Cell Disease and Effects of Exercise. *Front. Physiol.* **2019**, *10*, 1329. [CrossRef]
46. Connes, P.; Alexy, T.; Detterich, J.; Romana, M.; Hardy-Dessources, M.D.; Ballas, S.K. The role of blood rheology in sickle cell disease. *Blood Rev.* **2016**, *30*, 111–118. [CrossRef]
47. Cokelet, G.R.; Meiselman, H.J. Macro- and micro-rheological properties of blood. In *Handbook of Hemorheology and Hemodynamics*; Baskurt, O.K., Hardeman, M.R., Rampling, M.W., Meiselman, H.J., Eds.; IOS Press: Amsterdam, The Netherlands, 2007; pp. 45–71.
48. Camp, P.J.; Elfimova, E.A.; Ivanov, A.O. The effects of polydispersity on the initial susceptibilities of ferrofluids. *J. Phys. Condens. Matter* **2014**, *26*, 456002. [CrossRef]
49. Mohapatra, D.K.; Camp, P.J.; Philip, J. Influence of size polydispersity on magnetic field tunable structures in magnetic nanofluids containing superparamagnetic nanoparticles. *Nanoscale Adv.* **2021**, *3*, 3573–3592. [CrossRef]
50. Ivanov, A.O.; Novak, E.V. Phase separation of ferrocolloids: The role of van der Waals interaction. *Colloid J.* **2007**, *69*, 302–311. [CrossRef]
51. Vinod, S.; Philip, J. Experimental evidence for the significant role of initial cluster size and liquid confinement on thermo-physical properties of magnetic nanofluids under applied magnetic field. *J. Mol. Liq.* **2018**, *257*, 1–11. [CrossRef]
52. Grodzinski, P.; Kircher, M.; Goldberg, M.; Gabizon, A. Integrating nanotechnology into cancer care. *ACS Nano* **2019**, *13*, 7370–7376. [CrossRef] [PubMed]

Disclaimer/Publisher's Note: The statements, opinions and data contained in all publications are solely those of the individual author(s) and contributor(s) and not of MDPI and/or the editor(s). MDPI and/or the editor(s) disclaim responsibility for any injury to people or property resulting from any ideas, methods, instructions or products referred to in the content.

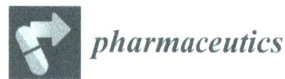

Article

Microfluidic Synthesis of Magnetite Nanoparticles for the Controlled Release of Antibiotics

Cristina Chircov [1,2], Iulia Alexandra Dumitru [3], Bogdan Stefan Vasile [2,4,5], Ovidiu-Cristian Oprea [2,6], Alina Maria Holban [7] and Roxana Cristina Popescu [8,9,*]

[1] Department of Science and Engineering of Oxide Materials and Nanomaterials, National University of Science and Technology Politehnica Bucharest, 011061 Bucharest, Romania; cristina.chircov@yahoo.com
[2] National Research Center for Micro and Nanomaterials, National University of Science and Technology Politehnica Bucharest, 060042 Bucharest, Romania; bogdan.vasile@upb.ro (B.S.V.); ovidiu.oprea@upb.ro (O.-C.O.)
[3] Faculty of Engineering in Foreign Languages, National University of Science and Technology Politehnica Bucharest, 060042 Bucharest, Romania; iulia.dumitru2212@stud.fim.upb.ro
[4] Research Center for Advanced Materials, Products and Processes, National University of Science and Technology Politehnica Bucharest, 060042 Bucharest, Romania
[5] National Research Center for Food Safety, National University of Science and Technology Politehnica Bucharest, 060042 Bucharest, Romania
[6] Department of Inorganic Chemistry, Physical Chemistry and Electrochemistry, National University of Science and Technology Politehnica Bucharest, 1-7 Polizu Street, 011061 Bucharest, Romania
[7] Microbiology and Immunology Department, Faculty of Biology, Research Institute of the University of Bucharest, University of Bucharest, 060101 Bucharest, Romania; alina_m_h@yahoo.com
[8] Faculty of Medical Engineering, National University of Science and Technology Politehnica Bucharest, 1-7 Polizu Street, 011061 Bucharest, Romania
[9] Department of Life and Environmental Science, National Institute for R&D in Physics and Nuclear Engineering Horia Hulubei, 30 Reactorului, 077125 Magurele, Romania
* Correspondence: roxana.popescu@nipne.ro

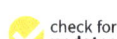

Citation: Chircov, C.; Dumitru, I.A.; Vasile, B.S.; Oprea, O.-C.; Holban, A.M.; Popescu, R.C. Microfluidic Synthesis of Magnetite Nanoparticles for the Controlled Release of Antibiotics. *Pharmaceutics* 2023, *15*, 2215. https://doi.org/10.3390/pharmaceutics15092215

Academic Editors: Constantin Mihai Lucaciu and Natalia L. Klyachko

Received: 20 July 2023
Revised: 5 August 2023
Accepted: 23 August 2023
Published: 27 August 2023

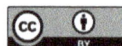

Copyright: © 2023 by the authors. Licensee MDPI, Basel, Switzerland. This article is an open access article distributed under the terms and conditions of the Creative Commons Attribution (CC BY) license (https://creativecommons.org/licenses/by/4.0/).

Abstract: Magnetite nanoparticles (MNPs) have been intensively studied for biomedical applications, especially as drug delivery systems for the treatment of infections. Additionally, they are characterized by intrinsic antimicrobial properties owing to their capacity to disrupt or penetrate the microbial cell wall and induce cell death. However, the current focus has shifted towards increasing the control of the synthesis reaction to ensure more uniform nanoparticle sizes and shapes. In this context, microfluidics has emerged as a potential candidate method for the controlled synthesis of nanoparticles. Thus, the aim of the present study was to obtain a series of antibiotic-loaded MNPs through a microfluidic device. The structural properties of the nanoparticles were investigated through X-ray diffraction (XRD) and, selected area electron diffraction (SAED), the morphology was evaluated through transmission electron microscopy (TEM) and high-resolution TEM (HR-TEM), the antibiotic loading was assessed through Fourier-transform infrared spectroscopy (FT-IR) and, and thermogravimetry and differential scanning calorimetry (TG-DSC) analyses, and. the release profiles of both antibiotics was determined through UV-Vis spectroscopy. The biocompatibility of the nanoparticles was assessed through the MTT assay on a BJ cell line, while the antimicrobial properties were investigated against the *S. aureus*, *P. aeruginosa*, and *C. albicans* strains. Results proved considerable uniformity of the antibiotic-containing nanoparticles, good biocompatibility, and promising antimicrobial activity. Therefore, this study represents a step forward towards the microfluidic development of highly effective nanostructured systems for antimicrobial therapies.

Keywords: magnetite nanoparticles; microfluidics; antibiotics; drug delivery systems

1. Introduction

One of the greatest challenges that concerns society in the 21st century is represented by the increasing occurrence of microbial infections and the development of bacterial mechanisms to resist the activity of conventional antibiotics [1–4]. In this regard, the incidence of nosocomial infections represents a major mortality cause among patients, with severe socio-economic and ecological implications [2,5,6].

Therefore, current research trends focus on the development of alternative antimicrobial systems that could potentiate the effectiveness of antibiotics. Nanoparticles possess promising potential in terms of their use as antimicrobial agents due to intrinsic antimicrobial properties, as well as the possibility of being used as drug delivery carriers for targeted delivery [7–10]. Among them, magnetite nanoparticles (MNPs) are one of the most intensively studied types of nanoparticles owing to their unique functional and biological properties. Specifically, besides their intrinsic antimicrobial properties which makes them more suitable than polymeric nanoparticles, their unique magnetic properties allow for the direct targeting of the disease site using a magnetic field [11]. Therefore, MNPs are used in a wide variety of biomedical applications, ranging from antimicrobial and anticancer treatment alternatives [4,12–16] to diagnosis and imagining applications [17–19]. Nevertheless, the synthesis of MNPs generally involves the co-precipitation of iron ions into an alkaline medium, which poses several disadvantages in terms of control over the outcome properties of the nanoparticles, especially regarding their size and shape uniformity [20–23]. Therefore, different synthesis techniques that could overcome such limitations while maintaining the advantages of low cost, ease of application, and efficiency are required. Examples of non-conventional MNP synthesis techniques include the solvothermal [15,24–27] or microwave-assisted hydrothermal [13,28–31] methods, which allow for the control of the particle size by aging time variations, and the microfluidic approaches [32–35], through which particle size is controlled by varying the microchannel diameters, the flows within the microchannels, and the concentrations of the solutions. In this context, microfluidics has emerged as a promising alternative for obtaining nanomaterials with significantly narrow size distributions and uniform shapes and functional properties [23,36–39].

In this manner, the design of the present study focused on the development of streptomycin- and neomycin-loaded MNPs through the microfluidic synthesis method, which would enhance the uniformity of the nanosystems in terms of size, shape, polydispersity, surface reactivity, and drug loading. The obtained results confirm the potential of microfluidic approaches in the pathway towards their application for obtaining standardized nanoparticle-based drug delivery systems.

2. Materials and Methods

2.1. Materials

Ferric chloride hexahydrate ($FeCl_3 \cdot 6H_2O$), ferrous sulphate heptahydrate ($FeSO_4 \cdot 7H_2O$), sodium hydroxide (NaOH), streptomycin sulfate, and neomycin trisulfate were purchased from Sigma-Aldrich Merck (Darmstadt, Germany) and used as acquired.

The biocompatibility assay involved the use of normal BJ human dermal fibroblast cells (CLS, Heidelberg, Germany).

For the antimicrobial assays, three microbial strains were used (a Gram-negative bacterial species, i.e., *Pseudomonas aeruginosa* ATCC 27853, a Gram-positive bacterial species, i.e., *Staphylococcus aureus* ATCC 25923, and a fungal species, i.e., *Candida albicans* ATCC 10231), which were obtained from the Faculty of Biology, University of Bucharest.

2.2. MNP Synthesis

Both pristine and antibiotic-loaded MNPs were synthesized according to the procedures described in our previous studies [32,33]. Specifically, the nanoparticles were obtained through a microfluidic method involving the co-precipitation of iron ions using a lab-on-chip device [32,33]. The precursor stock solution was prepared by dissolving $FeCl_3 \cdot 6H_2O$ and $FeSO_4 \cdot 7H_2O$ in a 1:2 molar ratio at the final mass concentration of 1%. Subsequently, NaOH was dissolved at a 1 M concentration, followed by the addition of 1, 5, and 10% streptomycin sulfate or neomycin trisulfate. The obtained solutions were simultaneously introduced into the microfluidic device using a peristaltic pump equipped with four channels. The precursor solution was injected through the central inlet at the flow of 30 rpm, while the precipitating solution containing the antibiotics was administered through the side inlets at a flow of 15 rpm each. The obtained nanoparticles were collected, washed with deionized water until a neutral pH, and dried overnight at 40 °C (Table 1).

Table 1. Summary of the obtained pristine and antibiotic-loaded MNPs.

Sample	Type of Antibiotic Used	Antibiotic Concentration (%)
Fe_3O_4	-	-
Fe_3O_4_str_1%		1
Fe_3O_4_str_5%	streptomycin sulfate	5
Fe_3O_4_str_10%		10
Fe_3O_4_neo_1%		1
Fe_3O_4_neo_5%	neomycin trisulfate	5
Fe_3O_4_neo_10%		10

2.3. Morpho-Structural Characterization

2.3.1. X-ray Diffraction (XRD)

The structural features of all samples were investigated using a CuKα radiation-provided PANalytical Empyrean diffractometer (PANalytical, Almelo, The Netherlands). Diffractograms were acquired between the 2θ angle values of 20 and 80°, with a 0.0256° step size and 1 s time per step. Further, the HighScore Plus software (version 3.0, PANalytical, Almelo, The Netherlands) was used for the Rietveld fitting of the acquired diffractograms (goodness of fit < 4 was considered acceptable) in order to determine the unit cell parameters, the average crystallite size, and the crystallinity of each sample.

2.3.2. Transmission Electron Microscopy (TEM), High-Resolution TEM (HR-TEM), and Selected Area Electron Diffraction (SAED)

Sample preparation involved the dispersion of a small amount of nanoparticles into deionized water and placing 10 µL of the suspension into a 400-mesh lacey carbon-coated copper grid. The TEM and HR-TEM images and the SAED patterns were acquired on a high-resolution 80–200 TITAN THEMIS transmission microscope (purchased from FEI, Hillsboro, OR, USA). The microscope was equipped with a column EDXS detector and an image corrector, and it was operated in transmission mode at a voltage of 200 kV. The obtained images were used for the subsequent assessment of particle size distribution by measuring 100 nanoparticles within the ImageJ software (version 1.8.0, University of Wisconsin, Madison, WI, USA).

2.3.3. Dynamic Light Scattering (DLS), Polydispersity Index (PDI), and Zeta Potential

In this study, 5 mg of the pristine and antibiotic-loaded MNPs was added to 15 mL of PBS 1x solution with a pH of 7.4 and dispersed using a Sonorex Digitec DT 514 ultrasonic bath (Bandelin, Berlin, Germany) for 10 min at 25 °C. A small amount of the dispersion was further introduced into the measurement cell and placed inside the DelsaMax Pro equipment (Backman Coulter, Brea, CA, USA). Three measurements were performed for each sample.

2.3.4. Fourier Transform Infrared Spectroscopy (FT-IR)

IR spectra in the 4000–400 cm^{-1} wavenumber range were acquired for all samples in order to assess the functional groups present and, consequently, to demonstrate the presence of the antibiotics within the drug delivery systems. A mercury cadmium telluride detector-provided Thermo Scientific Nicolet iS50 (Thermo Fischer Scientific, Waltham, MA, USA) spectrometer was employed. Measurements were performed in the attenuated total reflectance (ATR) mode. Acquisitions were made at room temperature, with a resolution of 4 cm^{-1} and 64 scans for each sample. The OmnicPicta software (version 8.2, Thermo Nicolet, Thermo Fischer Scientific, Waltham, MA, USA) was used for data processing.

2.3.5. Thermogravimetry and Differential Scanning Calorimetry (TG-DSC)

The amount of loaded antibiotics was assessed through the TG-DSC analysis, using an STA TG/DSC Netzsch Jupiter 449 F3 equipment (Selb, Germany). All samples were heated from 20 to 900 °C at a heating rate of 10 K/min and in a 50 mL/min dynamic air atmosphere.

2.3.6. UV–Vis Spectrophotometry

A Thermo Evolution 600 double-beam UV–Vis spectrophotometer (Thermo Fischer Scientific, Waltham, MA, USA) and a 1 cm optical path glass cuvette were used for the UV–Vis spectroscopy measurements. Measurements were performed using a fixed wavelength of 202 nm for both types of antibiotics in order to assess their release profiles. For this step, 100 mg of each antibiotic-loaded sample was placed inside a dialysis bag, followed by their immersion in 50 mL of PBS 1x solution (pH of 7.4). All samples were maintained at 37 °C. At specific time-points, 1 mL of the supernatant was collected and replaced with fresh PBS. Data were expressed as the amount of antibiotic released (mg).

2.4. Biological Evaluation
2.4.1. Cell Viability and Proliferation

Normal BJ human dermal fibroblast cells were cultured at 37 °C, 5% CO_2, and 90% humidity in 10% fetal bovine serum-supplemented Dulbecco's Modified Eagle Medium (DMEM). The nanoparticles were sterilized using UV radiation overnight and then suspended in deionized water at a concentration of 5 mg/mL via ultrasonic dispersion. Cells were seeded at a concentration of 5000 cells/well in 96-well plates and incubated for 24 h to allow cell attachment. Subsequently, the culture medium was replaced with nanoparticle-containing culture medium at a concentration of 0 and 50 µg/mL and incubated for 24 h. The MTT tetrazolium salts assay was employed for cell viability and proliferation investigations. Specifically, the nanoparticle medium was removed from the cells after the incubation period, and replaced with an MTT solution in complete culture medium and incubated for 2 h. This solution was prepared by dissolving 10% MTT (5 mg/mL in PBS) in complete culture medium. The method involves the ability of cells to metabolize MTT into formazan, which is proportional to cell viability. After the incubation time, the MTT culture medium was removed, and the formazan crystals were solubilized with DMSO. The amount of formazan produced is spectrophotometrically determined by measuring the absorbance at a wavelength of 570 nm. Blank samples, i.e., nanoparticles without cells, at the investigated concentrations, whose absorbance was subtracted from that of the samples with cells were used for all quantitative determinations. For each sample, three experiments were carried out. The obtained values were related to the negative control samples (which was assigned a value of 100%) in order to calculate the cell viability and differentiation ability. Cell viability and differentiation ability values were expressed as ±SEM (standard error of the mean).

Furthermore, the statistical significance was evaluated by the Student *t*-test function, with three levels of significance assigned (i.e., * $p < 0.05$, ** $p < 0.01$, and *** $p < 0.001$)

2.4.2. Antimicrobial Activity

The antimicrobial assays performed are in accordance with previous studies [12,13,40,41]. All samples were sterilized using UV radiation for 20 min, followed by their dispersion in sterile deionized water at a concentration of 2 mg/mL.

An adapted diffusion test from the Clinical & Laboratory Standards Institute (CLSI) guidelines was employed for assessing the inhibition zone diameter. Briefly, Petri dishes containing the Mueller–Hinton agar medium for the *S. aureus* and *P. aeruginosa* bacterial strains and Sabouraud Dextrose broth for *C. albicans* yeast were used for the swab-inoculation of 1–3 × 10^8 CFU/mL microbial suspensions (equivalent to 0.5 McFarland density standard). 10 µL of each nanoparticle suspension was added on the inoculated plates and incubated for 24 h at 37 °C. Subsequently, the diameter of the inhibition zone was measured, and the results were expressed in mm.

To determine the minimum inhibitory concentration (MIC), the microdilution technique in 96-well plates was employed. Each sample was subjected to binary serial dilutions from 2 mg/mL to 0.015 mg/mL in the appropriate nutritive broth, and the plates were inoculated using microbial suspensions of ~10^6 CFU/mL. After the incubation for 24 h at 37 °C, the MIC was assessed through the naked-eye analysis and the lowest nanoparticle concentration that visibly inhibited the growth of the microbial strains was considered [42].

3. Results

The pristine and antibiotic-loaded MNPs obtained through the microfluidic synthesis method were characterized in terms of their morpho-structural and physico-chemical properties through XRD, TEM, HR-TEM, SAED, FT-IR, and TG-DSC. Subsequently, the cytotoxicity of the obtained structures was evaluated through the MTT assay on the BJ cell line, followed by the assessment of their antimicrobial activity through the inhibition zone diameter and MIC assays.

XRD analysis was employed to determine the crystalline phases present within the samples (Figure 1). Within all samples, the XRD patterns reveal the presence of magnetite in the cubic crystallization system and the Fd3m space group as the unique crystalline phase through the characteristic Miller indices (according to JCPDS 01-084-2782 [43]). Therefore, the addition of antibiotics does not lead to the formation of secondary iron oxide phases, such as maghemite or hematite.

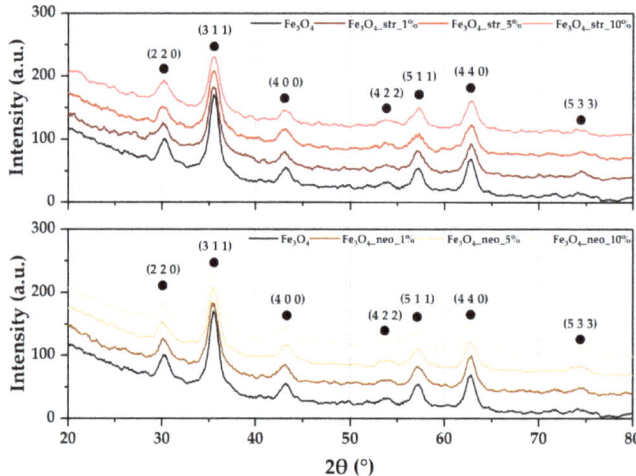

Figure 1. XRD patterns for the pristine and antibiotic-loaded MNPs and the associated Miller indices (●—magnetite).

Furthermore, the acquired diffractograms were subjected to Rietveld refinement in order to determine the unit cell parameters, the average crystallite sizes, and the crystallinity of the samples (Table 2). Results show that the addition of the streptomycin antibiotic gradually decreases the average crystallite size up to the 5% concentration, while the addition of neomycin, up to the 10% concentration. Introducing the antibiotic also influences the crystallinity of the samples, which is inversely proportional to the antibiotic concentration. Nonetheless, the crystallinity of the samples with the highest antibiotic concentration is similar to the pristine nanoparticles. Therefore, it is safe to assume that antibiotic loading does not negatively affect the structural properties but rather acts as an adjuvant in controlling the crystallinity of the nanosystems.

Table 2. Unit cell parameters, average crystallite size, and crystallinity determined through Rietveld refinement.

Sample	Unit Cell Parameters		Average Crystallite Size ± Standard Deviation (SD) [nm]	Crystallinity [%]
	a = b = c [Å]	α = β = γ [°]		
Fe_3O_4	8.35	90	6.71 ± 0.46	12.91
Fe_3O_4_str_1%	8.33	90	5.62 ± 0.57	15.54
Fe_3O_4_str_5%	8.37	90	4.99 ± 0.10	14.62
Fe_3O_4_str_10%	8.34	90	5.78 ± 0.66	12.84
Fe_3O_4_neo_1%	8.34	90	6.23 ± 0.73	13.62
Fe_3O_4_neo_5%	8.35	90	5.80 ± 0.38	13.20
Fe_3O_4_neo_10%	8.37	90	5.46 ± 0.25	12.45

Furthermore, the SAED results confirm the previous observations, as the diffraction rings within the patterns are associated with the Miller indices characteristic for magnetite (Figure 2). The neomycin-containing nanoparticles seem to have a lower degree of crystallinity, as the diffraction rings are more diffused, which is in accordance with the Rietveld refinement results.

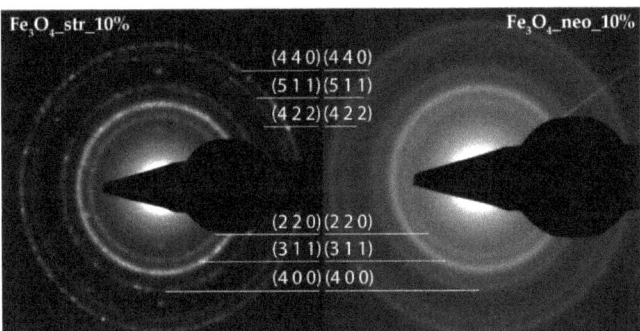

Figure 2. The SAED patterns for the Fe_3O_4_str_10% and Fe_3O_4_neo_10% samples.

The morphology of the nanostructures was assessed through TEM and HR-TEM (Figure 3). As can be observed, the nanoparticles are characterized by a quasispherical shape and an increased agglomeration tendency due to their surface energy. Furthermore, the high degree of crystallinity is demonstrated through the HR-TEM images, where the atomic planes within the nanoparticles are visible. The obtained images were further used to assess the size distribution of the nanosystems (Figure 3). The distributions are significantly narrow, between 2 and 7 nm, which further demonstrates the suitability of the microfluidic method for the synthesis of nanomaterials as it allows for dimensional control. There are no considerable differences between the two types of antibiotics regarding their effect on the morphology and size of the nanoparticles.

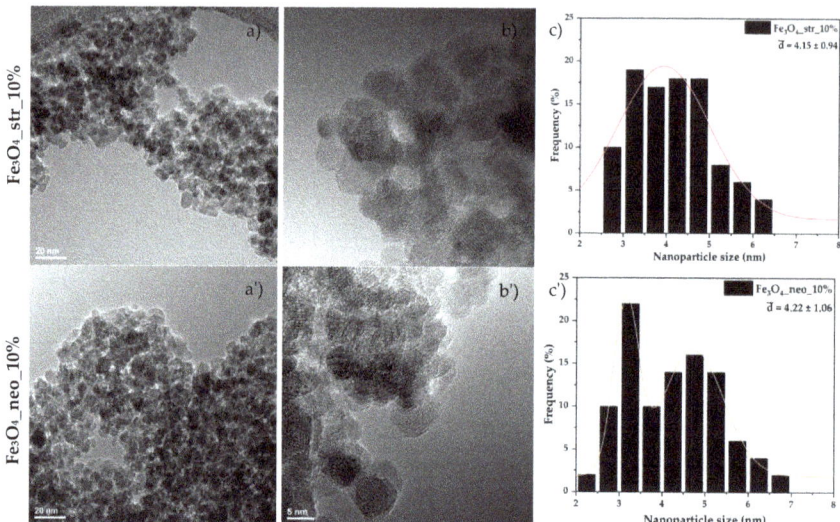

Figure 3. The TEM (**a,a′**), HR-TEM (**b,b′**), and size distributions (**c,c′**) for the Fe$_3$O$_4$_str_10% and Fe$_3$O$_4$_neo_10% samples.

The stability of the developed drug delivery systems was assessed through hydrodynamic diameter, PDI, and zeta potential measurements (Figure 4). As the results show, the hydrodynamic diameter of the nanoparticles decreases after antibiotic loading, which could be caused by the reduction of free hydroxyl groups present on the surface of pristine magnetite. In both cases, increasing the antibiotic amount further leads to proportionally higher hydrodynamic diameter values. Considering that the zeta potential also increases with the antibiotic amount, it could be assumed that the increasingly higher amount of antibiotics on the surface of the MNPs is the cause for higher particle diameters. The hydrodynamic diameter is larger in the case of streptomycin due to a higher degree of interaction with the solvent molecules. All PDI values are lower than 0.7, which generally indicates a narrow particle size distribution [44].

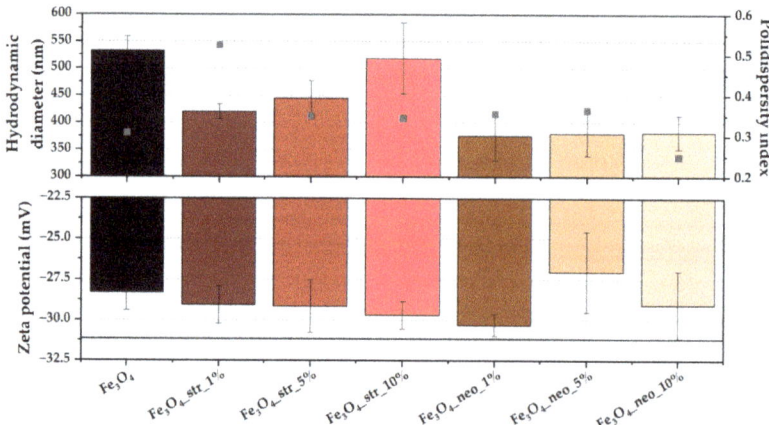

Figure 4. The hydrodynamic diameter (values shown as columns), the PDI (values shown as points), and the zeta potential values for the pristine and antibiotic-loaded MNPs (expressed as mean ± SD, $n = 3$).

The efficiency of the antibiotic loading was further evaluated through the FT-IR analysis (Figure 5). The spectra show the Fe-O bond characteristic for magnetite at the 538 cm^{-1} wavenumber. As it overlaps with C-H bending, the increase in the maximum intensity with the addition of the antibiotics is attributed to the efficient loading of the drug molecules within the nanoparticles. Moreover, as there are no shifts of the maximum for the antibiotic-loaded samples, it is safe to assume that the antibiotics were chemically bound to the nanostructures through hydrogen bonding. The antibiotic loading can also be seen in the wavenumber range of 600–1800 cm^{-1}, where absorption bands specific for the characteristic functional groups are present.

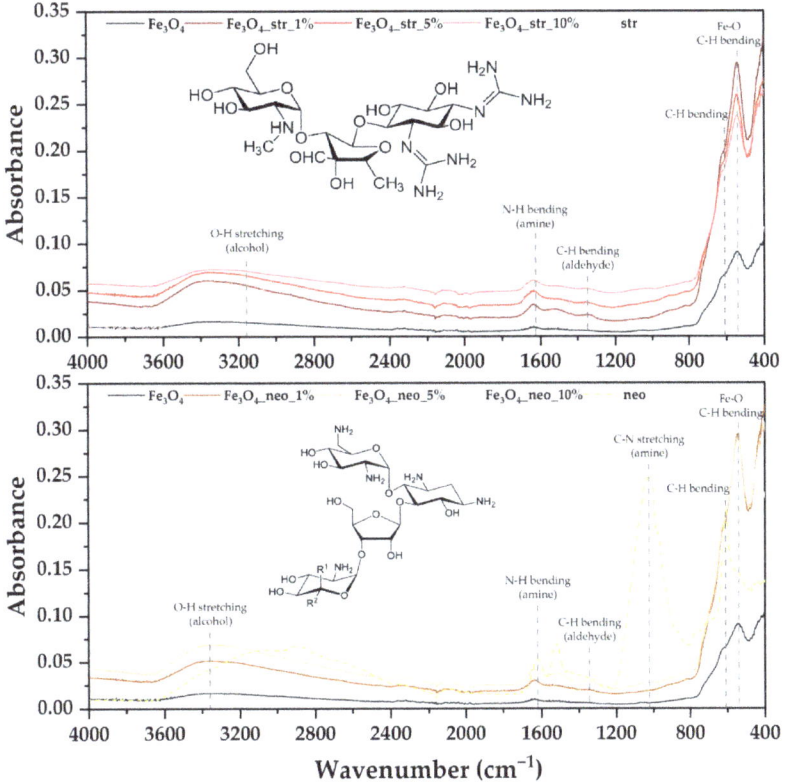

Figure 5. FT-IR spectra for the pristine and the antibiotic-loaded MNPs.

The MNPs were further subjected to TG-DSC analysis in order to determine the mass loss and the associated thermal effects, which allowed for the estimation of the antibiotic loading within the nanoparticles (Figure 6, Table 3). It can be observed that up to 200 °C, all samples are losing residual water molecules, between 2.63 and 4.17%. The minimum solvent quantity can be found in the case of pristine MNPs, with larger quantities retained by the antibiotic-loaded samples. This process is accompanied by an endothermic effect on the DSC curve, with the minimum around 76–89 °C. Between 200 and 400 °C, the samples are losing mass, the processes being associated with some weak exothermic effects, indicating various oxidation reactions. The Fe^{2+} is oxidized to Fe^{3+} as the Fe_3O_4 (magnetite) is transformed to γ-Fe_2O_3 (maghemite) [45]. Concomitantly, the organic substances loaded onto the nanoparticles are being partially oxidized, as indicated by the multiple, different, small exothermic effects. After 400 °C, the small mass loss recorded can be assigned to the condensation of terminal –OH moieties but also to the burning of the residual carbonaceous mass. The strong, typical, exothermic effect around 500 °C is assigned to the transformation of maghemite to hematite [46,47]. The exothermic effect area increases slightly as the percentage of residual carbonaceous mass increases, from 111 to 122 J/g, a similar value being previously reported [46]. Furthermore, the antibiotic loading is proportional to the antibiotic concentration used for the MNP synthesis, with an increased loading efficiency for the streptomycin-loaded samples compared to the neomycin-loaded ones.

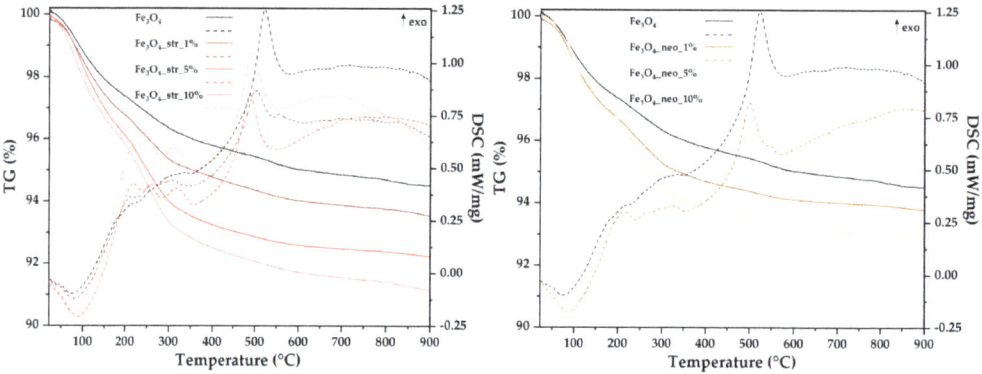

Figure 6. TG-DSC curves the pristine and the antibiotic-loaded MNPs.

Table 3. The thermal effects, mass loss, and estimated antibiotic loading for the pristine and the antibiotic-loaded MNPs.

Sample	Mass Loss (%) 200 °C	Endo (°C)	Mass Loss (%) 200–400 °C	Mass Loss (%) 400–900 °C	Exo (°C)/ Area (J/g)	Estimated Load (%)
Fe_3O_4	2.63	76.8	1.58	1.27	521.9/111.6	-
Fe_3O_4_str_1%	3.14	79.8	1.99	1.22	501.8/111.1	1.03
Fe_3O_4_str_5%	3.87	88.4	2.85	1.00	488.4/112.0	2.40
Fe_3O_4_str_10%	4.17	79.1	3.31	1.35	495.1/122.8	3.55
Fe_3O_4_neo_1%	3.23	86.3	2.02	0.90	500.1/111.3	0.76
Fe_3O_4_neo_5%	3.44	86.9	2.70	1.05	504.4/112.9	1.81
Fe_3O_4_neo_10%	3.29	88.3	3.52	1.25	504.4/122.1	2.73

The drug release profiles were assessed through UV-Vis spectroscopy measurements (Figure 7). In both cases, the amount of released antibiotics is proportional to the concentration of drug loaded, with less significant differences between 5% and 10% than between 1% and 5%. Furthermore, it can be observed that the streptomycin antibiotic is gradually released from the nanoparticles (from ~0.6 to 2.2 mg), reaching a plateau after approximately 3 h that is maintained for the entire 72 h period. However, the drug amount released from the 1% sample decreases after 24 h, which could mean that the entire quantity is released within this timeframe. By contrast, the neomycin-loaded samples are characterized by a burst release that occurs within the first 10 min, reaching a plateau after approximately 6 h. In this case, the plateau is only maintained for 72 h for the 10% sample. In this manner, it could be concluded that the streptomycin-loaded samples provide a more controlled drug release owing to a higher encapsulation efficiency and a stronger interaction between the nanoparticles and the drug molecules.

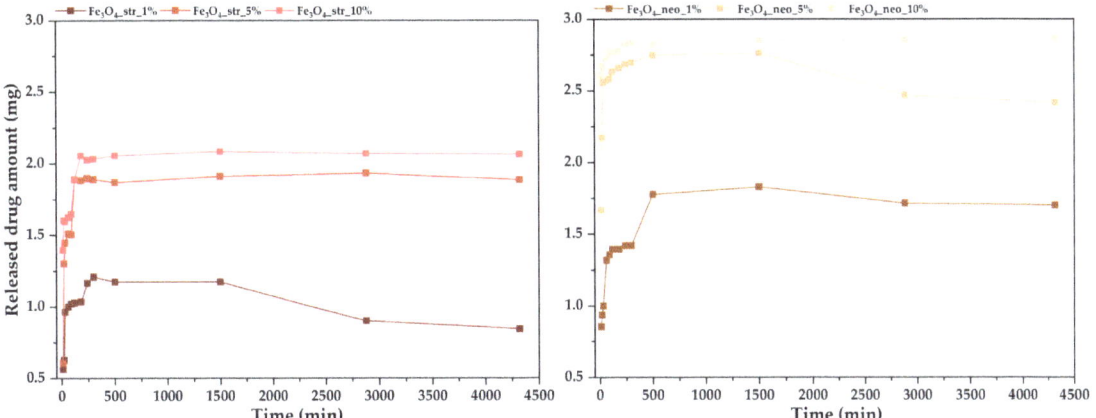

Figure 7. Drug release profiles for the antibiotic-loaded MNPs.

Furthermore, the biocompatibility of the obtained drug delivery systems was determined through the MTT assay on the BJ cell line (Figure 8). On one hand, the cell viability characteristic for the pristine nanoparticles is significantly low, with values of approximately 40%. This effect could be attributed to the highly reduced nanoparticle size that could ensure their internalization within the cells and the production of reactive oxygen species. However, in both cases, the addition of the antibiotics within the nanostructured systems leads to an increase in cell viability, especially in the case of the streptomycin antibiotic. The highest cell viability is registered for the $Fe_3O_4\_str\_5\%$ sample, for which the estimated drug load is around 2.40%. Increasing the streptomycin load to 3.55%, as it is in the case of the $Fe_3O_4\_str\_10\%$ sample, leads to a decrease in cell viability due to possible toxic effects caused by the higher amount of the antibiotic. The presence of the neomycin antibiotic within the nanoparticles does not significantly increase the cell viability compared to the pristine sample, as was observed in the previous case, which could be attributed to the higher amount of drug released, as shown by the UV-Vis measurements.

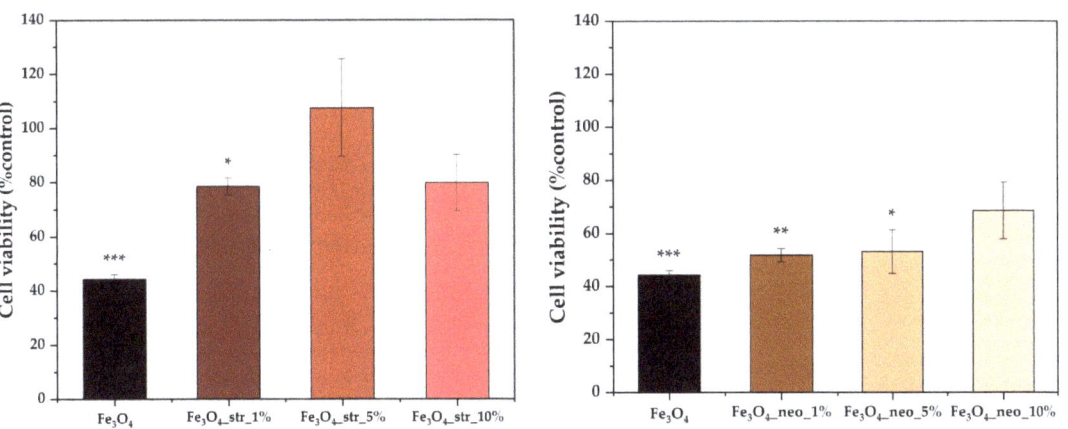

Figure 8. Cell viability values for the pristine and antibiotic-loaded MNPs (BJ cell line; values expressed as mean ± SD, n = 3; different signs indicate significant differences between the control and each sample; *—lower significance; ** and ***—higher significance).

In regard to their antimicrobial properties, the obtained drug delivery systems were subjected to the inhibition zone diameter and MIC assays. With respect to the inhibition zone diameter results (Table 4), it can be seen that the highest antibacterial efficiency was recorded against the *P. aeruginosa* strain, which is a Gram-negative bacterium, with a more pronounced effect registered for the streptomycin antibiotic. While both drugs are known to affect both Gram-positive and Gram-negative bacteria, streptomycin is mostly recommended for Gram-negative strains. Furthermore, the neomycin-loaded samples appear to be more efficient against Gram-positive bacteria, as the highest inhibition zones were measured against the *S. aureus* strain. The results against the *C. albicans* yeast further confirm the antimicrobial potential of the developed drug delivery systems, as the inhibition zone diameters are similar or even higher than the values measured for *S. aureus*. Nevertheless, the pristine MNP sample leads to inhibition zones similar to the antibiotic-loaded samples, thus demonstrating the intrinsic antimicrobial properties of MNPs primarily owing to the significantly small sizes. The MIC assay results (Table 5) confirm previous observations regarding the highest efficiency of the developed systems against the *P. aeruginosa* strain. Additionally, the antifungal effect is comparable to the effect against *S. aureus* bacteria.

Table 4. Inhibition zone diameter measured for the pristine and the antibiotic-loaded MNPs.

Microbial Strain	Inhibition Zone Diameter (mm)						
	Fe_3O_4	$Fe_3O_4\_str\_1\%$	$Fe_3O_4\_str\_5\%$	$Fe_3O_4\_str\_10\%$	$Fe_3O_4\_neo\_1\%$	$Fe_3O_4\_neo\_5\%$	$Fe_3O_4\_neo\_10\%$
S. aureus	2	0	2	2	2	4	4
P. aeruginosa	7	6	6	6	6	5	6
C. albicans	5	2	4	4	5	4	5

Table 5. MIC values determined for the pristine and the antibiotic-loaded MNPs.

Microbial Strain	MIC (mg/mL)						
	Fe_3O_4	$Fe_3O_4\_str\_1\%$	$Fe_3O_4\_str\_5\%$	$Fe_3O_4\_str\_10\%$	$Fe_3O_4\_neo\_1\%$	$Fe_3O_4\_neo\_5\%$	$Fe_3O_4\_neo\_10\%$
S. aureus	2	2	1	2	2	2	1
P. aeruginosa	1	1	1	1	1	2	1
C. albicans	2	2	2	2	2	2	2

4. Discussion

The present study aimed to develop a series of streptomycin/neomycin-loaded MNPs through a microfluidic approach that could further be employed in antimicrobial therapies. The obtained drug delivery systems were characterized by XRD, TEM, HR-TEM, and SAED, FT-IR, and TG-DSC in order to determine their physico-chemical and structural features. The biological evaluation of the obtained structures involved the assessment of their biocompatibility through the MTT assay on the BJ cell line and their antimicrobial effects through the inhibition zone diameter and MIC assays.

In regard to the structural properties of pristine MNPs, it can be seen that the average crystallite size and, consequently, the crystallinity of the nanoparticles is lower than those reported in our previous study, i.e., 6.71 nm and 12.91% and 8.06 nm and 18.53%, respectively [33]. Although the synthesis parameters were maintained constant (flow and concentration of the precursor and precipitating agent solutions), the difference between the two studies resides in the type of precipitator used. Therefore, it could be safe to assume that the use of NaOH as an alkaline agent leads to the formation of nanoparticles with lower crystallite sizes than NH_4OH. One literature study focusing on this subject showed that the use of NaOH leads to an average nanoparticle size of 15.29 nm compared to 33.97 nm for nanoparticles obtained with NH_4OH. This conclusion could be further translated to the crystallite size, as the nanoparticles appeared to be monocrystalline [48]. The mechanism behind this observation resides in the fact that the base amount and final pH are known to directly affect the nucleation and growth of the MNPs and, consequently, particle size. Specifically, it was shown that higher pH values lead to a decrease in nanoparticle size, which is in accordance with the present results [49]. Furthermore, as the antibiotics used for the development of the nanostructured drug delivery systems are alkaline compounds, the decreasing crystallite sizes with increasing concentrations are correlated with the previously described hypothesis. However, the increase in sample crystallinity with the addition of the antibiotic could be attributed to the contribution of the drug molecules to the crystallinity of the samples.

Furthermore, the higher drug loading determined for the streptomycin antibiotic could be attributed to a higher availability of the functional groups within the molecule to interact and form physico-chemical bonds with the hydroxyl groups present onto the surface of MNPs. A similar behavior was also observed in our previous paper, where the yield of sulfanilic acid functionalization was significantly lower than the yield for 4-sulfobenzoic acid [33].

To the best of our knowledge, this study represents the first one to investigate the synthesis and concomitant loading of drug molecules onto the surface of MNPs through a microfluidic approach. Nevertheless, there are other studies focusing on the microfluidic synthesis of MNPs [32,33,35,50,51], which have also obtained significantly narrow size distributions, which are similar to the ones described in the current study. Additionally, there are studies describing the direct synthesis of drug delivery systems through microfluidic devices, which mainly use polymers as the nanocarrier, such as curcumin-loaded shellac nanoparticles [52], liposomes containing plasmid DNA [53], poly(lactic-co-glycolic acid) particles loaded with indomethanic [54], doxorubicin [55], tamoxifen [55], or curcumin [56], 5-fluorouracil-loaded alginate–chitosan nanoparticles [57]. While these studies have reported higher encapsulation efficiencies, i.e., 93% [52], which could prove a higher suitability of using polymeric nanoparticles instead of inorganic nanoparticles, polymeric systems lack the intrinsic antimicrobial/anticancer properties that MNPs possess. This property was highlighted in the present study, as the pristine MNPs exhibited antimicrobial activities similar to the systems containing the antibiotics.

Therefore, the current study demonstrated the potential of microfluidic techniques for the development of drug delivery systems with significantly narrow size distributions. Additionally, the possibility to control and modulate the outcome properties of the systems, especially in regard to their crystallite and particle size and crystallinity, could consequently influence their biological behavior in contact with both cells and microbial species.

5. Conclusions

This study aimed to achieve one-step MNP synthesis and antibiotic loading through a microfluidic approach in order to obtain a series of drug delivery systems that could be applied in antimicrobial therapies. The results obtained demonstrated the presence of magnetite as the unique mineralogical phase and the formation of nanoparticles with significantly narrow size distributions and average nanoparticle sizes of ~4 nm. The results were in accordance with previously available studies, further proving the reproducibility of microfluidic approaches for nanoparticle syntheses. Furthermore, it was shown that the drug loading capacity is dependent upon the type of drug used, as the drug load calculated for streptomycin was higher than neomycin, especially at higher concentrations. The drug loading results were further translated into the biocompatibility assay, which showed cell viability results dependent upon the antibiotic type and concentration but also higher values for the antibiotic-loaded samples compared to the pristine ones. Furthermore, the antimicrobial activity was shown to be dependent upon the microbial strain; additionally, the pristine MNPs showed similar antimicrobial effects as the antibiotic-loaded ones. In this manner, this study successfully demonstrated the potential of the microfluidic method to obtain drug delivery systems that could be applied in antimicrobial therapies for both treatment and prevention of infections.

Author Contributions: Conceptualization, C.C. and R.C.P.; methodology, C.C. and R.C.P.; formal analysis, C.C., A.M.H. and R.C.P.; investigation, C.C., I.A.D., B.S.V., O.-C.O., A.M.H. and R.C.P.; writing, original draft preparation, C.C., I.A.D., A.M.H. and R.C.P.; writing, review and editing, C.C., B.S.V., O.-C.O., A.M.H. and R.C.P. All authors have read and agreed to the published version of the manuscript.

Funding: This research received no external funding.

Institutional Review Board Statement: Not applicable.

Informed Consent Statement: Not applicable.

Data Availability Statement: Not applicable.

Acknowledgments: The authors acknowledge the financial support obtained through PNRR.C9-I8: Aerogel-based magnetic nanocomposites for water decontamination, contract number 760092. Also, the role played by the team and infrastructure of the National Research Center for Micro and Nanomaterials from the University Politehnica of Bucharest and the research grant "UPB—Proof of Concept 2020", Code: PN-III-P1.2-PCCDI-2017-1 are highly acknowledged.

Conflicts of Interest: The authors declare no conflict of interest.

References

1. Prestinaci, F.; Pezzotti, P.; Pantosti, A. Antimicrobial resistance: A global multifaceted phenomenon. *Pathog. Glob. Health* **2015**, *109*, 309–318. [CrossRef]
2. Spirescu, V.A.; Chircov, C.; Grumezescu, A.M.; Vasile, B.Ș.; Andronescu, E. Inorganic nanoparticles and composite films for antimicrobial therapies. *Int. J. Mol. Sci.* **2021**, *22*, 4595. [CrossRef]
3. Spirescu, V.A.; Chircov, C.; Grumezescu, A.M.; Andronescu, E. Polymeric nanoparticles for antimicrobial therapies: An up-to-date overview. *Polymers* **2021**, *13*, 724. [CrossRef] [PubMed]
4. Mihai, A.D.; Chircov, C.; Grumezescu, A.M.; Holban, A.M. Magnetite nanoparticles and essential oils systems for advanced antibacterial therapies. *Int. J. Mol. Sci.* **2020**, *21*, 7355. [CrossRef] [PubMed]
5. Despotovic, A.; Milosevic, B.; Milosevic, I.; Mitrovic, N.; Cirkovic, A.; Jovanovic, S.; Stevanovic, G. Hospital-acquired infections in the adult intensive care unit—Epidemiology, antimicrobial resistance patterns, and risk factors for acquisition and mortality. *Am. J. Infect. Control* **2020**, *48*, 1211–1215. [CrossRef]
6. Raoofi, S.; Pashazadeh Kan, F.; Rafiei, S.; Hosseinipalangi, Z.; Noorani Mejareh, Z.; Khani, S.; Abdollahi, B.; Seyghalani Talab, F.; Sanaei, M.; Zarabi, F.; et al. Global prevalence of nosocomial infection: A systematic review and meta-analysis. *PLoS ONE* **2023**, *18*, e0274248. [CrossRef]
7. Murugaiyan, J.; Kumar, P.A.; Rao, G.S.; Iskandar, K.; Hawser, S.; Hays, J.P.; Mohsen, Y.; Adukkadukkam, S.; Awuah, W.A.; Jose, R.A.M.; et al. Progress in alternative strategies to combat antimicrobial resistance: Focus on antibiotics. *Antibiotics* **2022**, *11*, 200. [CrossRef]
8. Zong, T.-X.; Silveira, A.P.; Morais, J.A.V.; Sampaio, M.C.; Muehlmann, L.A.; Zhang, J.; Jiang, C.-S.; Liu, S.-K. Recent advances in antimicrobial nano-drug delivery systems. *Nanomaterials* **2022**, *12*, 1855. [CrossRef] [PubMed]
9. Skwarczynski, M.; Bashiri, S.; Yuan, Y.; Ziora, Z.M.; Nabil, O.; Masuda, K.; Khongkow, M.; Rimsueb, N.; Cabral, H.; Ruktanonchai, U. Antimicrobial activity enhancers: Towards smart delivery of antimicrobial agents. *Antibiotics* **2022**, *11*, 412. [CrossRef]
10. Wang, Y.; Yang, Y.; Shi, Y.; Song, H.; Yu, C. Antibiotic-free antibacterial strategies enabled by nanomaterials: Progress and perspectives. *Adv. Mater.* **2020**, *32*, 1904106. [CrossRef]
11. Materón, E.M.; Miyazaki, C.M.; Carr, O.; Joshi, N.; Picciani, P.H.S.; Dalmaschio, C.J.; Davis, F.; Shimizu, F.M. Magnetic nanoparticles in biomedical applications: A review. *Appl. Surf. Sci. Adv.* **2021**, *6*, 100163. [CrossRef]
12. Chircov, C.; Mincă, M.-A.; Serban, A.B.; Bîrcă, A.C.; Dolete, G.; Ene, V.-L.; Andronescu, E.; Holban, A.-M. Zinc/cerium-substituted magnetite nanoparticles for biomedical applications. *Int. J. Mol. Sci.* **2023**, *24*, 6249. [CrossRef] [PubMed]
13. Chircov, C.; Ștefan, R.-E.; Dolete, G.; Andrei, A.; Holban, A.M.; Oprea, O.-C.; Vasile, B.S.; Neacșu, I.A.; Tihăuan, B. Dextran-coated iron oxide nanoparticles loaded with curcumin for antimicrobial therapies. *Pharmaceutics* **2022**, *14*, 1057. [CrossRef] [PubMed]
14. Chircov, C.; Bejenaru, I.T.; Nicoară, A.I.; Bîrcă, A.C.; Oprea, O.C.; Tihăuan, B. Chitosan-dextran-glycerol hydrogels loaded with iron oxide nanoparticles for wound dressing applications. *Pharmaceutics* **2022**, *14*, 2620. [CrossRef]
15. Chircov, C.; Pîrvulescu, D.-C.; Bîrcă, A.C.; Andronescu, E.; Grumezescu, A.M. Magnetite microspheres for the controlled release of rosmarinic acid. *Pharmaceutics* **2022**, *14*, 2292. [CrossRef] [PubMed]
16. Dolete, G.; Chircov, C.; Motelica, L.; Ficai, D.; Oprea, O.-C.; Gheorghe, M.; Ficai, A.; Andronescu, E. Magneto-mechanically triggered thick films for drug delivery micropumps. *Nanomaterials* **2022**, *12*, 3598. [CrossRef]

17. Chircov, C.; Grumezescu, A.M.; Holban, A.M. Magnetic particles for advanced molecular diagnosis. *Materials* **2019**, *12*, 2158. [CrossRef]
18. Dudchenko, N.; Pawar, S.; Perelshtein, I.; Fixler, D. Magnetite nanoparticles: Synthesis and applications in optics and nanophotonics. *Materials* **2022**, *15*, 2601. [CrossRef]
19. Wallyn, J.; Anton, N.; Vandamme, T.F. Synthesis, principles, and properties of magnetite nanoparticles for in vivo imaging applications-a review. *Pharmaceutics* **2019**, *11*, 601. [CrossRef]
20. Abdullah, N.H.; Shameli, K.; Abdullah, E.C.; Abdullah, L.C. Solid matrices for fabrication of magnetic iron oxide nanocomposites: Synthesis, properties, and application for the adsorption of heavy metal ions and dyes. *Compos. Part B Eng.* **2019**, *162*, 538–568. [CrossRef]
21. Wu, W.; Wu, Z.; Yu, T.; Jiang, C.; Kim, W.S. Recent progress on magnetic iron oxide nanoparticles: Synthesis, surface functional strategies and biomedical applications. *Sci. Technol. Adv. Mater.* **2015**, *16*, 023501. [CrossRef]
22. Ganapathe, L.S.; Mohamed, M.A.; Mohamad Yunus, R.; Berhanuddin, D.D. Magnetite (Fe_3O_4) nanoparticles in biomedical application: From synthesis to surface functionalisation. *Magnetochemistry* **2020**, *6*, 68. [CrossRef]
23. Chircov, C.; Vasile, B.S. New approaches in synthesis and characterization methods of iron oxide nanoparticles. In *Iron Oxide Nanoparticles*; IntechOpen: Rijeka, Croatia, 2022.
24. Deng, H.; Li, X.; Peng, Q.; Wang, X.; Chen, J.; Li, Y. Monodisperse magnetic single-crystal ferrite microspheres. *Angew. Chem. Int. Ed.* **2005**, *44*, 2782–2785. [CrossRef] [PubMed]
25. Sun, X.; Sun, K.; Liang, Y. Hydrothermal synthesis of magnetite: Investigation of influence of aging time and mechanism. *Micro Nano Lett.* **2015**, *10*, 99–104. [CrossRef]
26. Cao, S.-W.; Zhu, Y.-J.; Chang, J. Fe_3O_4 polyhedral nanoparticles with a high magnetization synthesized in mixed solvent ethylene glycol–water system. *New J. Chem.* **2008**, *32*, 1526–1530. [CrossRef]
27. Medinger, J.; Nedyalkova, M.; Lattuada, M. Solvothermal synthesis combined with design of experiments—Optimization approach for magnetite nanocrystal clusters. *Nanomaterials* **2021**, *11*, 360. [CrossRef] [PubMed]
28. Chircov, C.; Matei, M.-F.; Neacșu, I.A.; Vasile, B.S.; Oprea, O.-C.; Croitoru, A.-M.; Trușcă, R.-D.; Andronescu, E.; Sorescu, I.; Bărbuceanu, F. Iron oxide–silica core–shell nanoparticles functionalized with essential oils for antimicrobial therapies. *Antibiotics* **2021**, *10*, 1138. [CrossRef]
29. Chircov, C.; Bîrcă, A.C.; Dănciulescu, L.A.; Neacșu, I.A.; Oprea, O.C.; Trușcă, R.D.; Andronescu, E. Usnic acid-loaded magnetite nanoparticles-a comparative study between synthesis methods. *Molecules* **2023**, *28*, 5198. [CrossRef]
30. Chellappa, M.; Vijayalakshmi, U. Fabrication of Fe_3O_4-silica core-shell magnetic nano-particles and its characterization for biomedical applications. *Mater. Today Proc.* **2019**, *9*, 371–379. [CrossRef]
31. Karimi Pasandideh, E.; Kakavandi, B.; Nasseri, S.; Mahvi, A.H.; Nabizadeh, R.; Esrafili, A.; Rezaei Kalantary, R. Silica-coated magnetite nanoparticles core-shell spheres ($Fe_3O_4@SiO_2$) for natural organic matter removal. *J. Environ. Health Sci. Eng.* **2016**, *14*, 21. [CrossRef]
32. Chircov, C.; Bîrcă, A.C.; Grumezescu, A.M.; Vasile, B.S.; Oprea, O.; Nicoară, A.I.; Yang, C.-H.; Huang, K.-S.; Andronescu, E. Synthesis of magnetite nanoparticles through a lab-on-chip device. *Materials* **2021**, *14*, 5906. [CrossRef] [PubMed]
33. Chircov, C.; Bîrcă, A.C.; Vasile, B.S.; Oprea, O.C.; Huang, K.S.; Grumezescu, A.M. Microfluidic synthesis of -nh(2)- and -cooh-functionalized magnetite nanoparticles. *Nanomaterials* **2022**, *12*, 3160. [CrossRef]
34. Yu, B.; Lee, R.J.; Lee, L.J. Chapter 7—*Microfluidic* methods for production of liposomes. In *Methods in Enzymology*; Academic Press: Cambridge, MA, USA, 2009; Volume 465, pp. 129–141. [CrossRef]
35. Kašpar, O.; Koyuncu, A.H.; Hubatová-Vacková, A.; Balouch, M.; Tokárová, V. Influence of channel height on mixing efficiency and synthesis of iron oxide nanoparticles using droplet-based microfluidics. *RSC Adv.* **2020**, *10*, 15179–15189. [CrossRef]
36. Zhang, H.; Yang, J.; Sun, R.; Han, S.; Yang, Z.; Teng, L. Microfluidics for nano-drug delivery systems: From fundamentals to industrialization. *Acta Pharm. Sin. B* **2023**, *13*, 3277–3299. [CrossRef]
37. Bendre, A.; Bhat, M.P.; Lee, K.-H.; Altalhi, T.; Alruqi, M.A.; Kurkuri, M. Recent developments in microfluidic technology for synthesis and toxicity-efficiency studies of biomedical nanomaterials. *Mater. Today Adv.* **2022**, *13*, 100205. [CrossRef]
38. Niculescu, A.G.; Chircov, C.; Bîrcă, A.C.; Grumezescu, A.M. Nanomaterials synthesis through microfluidic methods: An updated overview. *Nanomaterials* **2021**, *11*, 864. [CrossRef] [PubMed]
39. Liu, Y.; Yang, G.; Hui, Y.; Ranaweera, S.; Zhao, C.-X. Microfluidic nanoparticles for drug delivery. *Small* **2022**, *18*, 2106580. [CrossRef] [PubMed]
40. Neacsu, I.A.; Leau, S.-A.; Marin, S.; Holban, A.M.; Vasile, B.-S.; Nicoara, A.-I.; Ene, V.L.; Bleotu, C.; Albu Kaya, M.G.; Ficai, A. Collagen-carboxymethylcellulose biocomposite wound-dressings with antimicrobial activity. *Materials* **2021**, *14*, 1153. [CrossRef]
41. Caciandone, M.; Niculescu, A.-G.; Roșu, A.R.; Grumezescu, V.; Negut, I.; Holban, A.M.; Oprea, O.; Vasile, B.Ș.; Bîrcă, A.C.; Grumezescu, A.M. Peg-functionalized magnetite nanoparticles for modulation of microbial biofilms on voice prosthesis. *Antibiotics* **2022**, *11*, 39. [CrossRef] [PubMed]
42. European Committee for Antimicrobial Susceptibility Testing (EUCAST) of the European Society of Clinical Microbiology and Infectious Diseases. Determination of minimum inhibitory concentrations (mics) of antibacterial agents by agar dilution. *Clin. Microbiol. Infect.* **2000**, *6*, 509–515. [CrossRef]

43. Rattanachueskul, N.; Dokkathin, O.; Dechtrirat, D.; Panpranot, J.; Watcharin, W.; Kaowphong, S.; Chuenchom, L. Sugarcane bagasse ash as a catalyst support for facile and highly scalable preparation of magnetic fenton catalysts for ultra-highly efficient removal of tetracycline. *Catalysts* **2022**, *12*, 446. [CrossRef]
44. Mukhopadhyay, P.; Kundu, P.P. Chitosan-graft-pamam–alginate core–shell nanoparticles: A safe and promising oral insulin carrier in an animal model. *RSC Adv.* **2015**, *5*, 93995–94007. [CrossRef]
45. Ficai, D.; Ficai, A.; Vasile, B.; Ficai, M.; Oprea, O.; Guran, C.; Andronescu, E. Synthesis of rod-like magnetite by using low magnetic field. *Dig. J. Nanomater. Biostructures* **2011**, *6*, 943–951.
46. Mohammed, H.B.; Rayyif, S.M.I.; Curutiu, C.; Birca, A.C.; Oprea, O.-C.; Grumezescu, A.M.; Ditu, L.-M.; Gheorghe, I.; Chifiriuc, M.C.; Mihaescu, G.; et al. Eugenol-functionalized magnetite nanoparticles modulate virulence and persistence in pseudomonas aeruginosa clinical strains. *Molecules* **2021**, *26*, 2189. [CrossRef]
47. Gherasim, O.; Popescu, R.C.; Grumezescu, V.; Mogoșanu, G.D.; Mogoantă, L.; Iordache, F.; Holban, A.M.; Vasile, B.S.; Bîrcă, A.C.; Oprea, O.-C.; et al. Maple coatings embedded with essential oil-conjugated magnetite for anti-biofilm applications. *Materials* **2021**, *14*, 1612. [CrossRef] [PubMed]
48. Zhang, X.; Zhou, R.; Rao, W.; Shanghai 201800 P.R. China. Influence of precipitator agents naoh and NH$_4$OH on the preparation of Fe$_3$O$_4$ nano-particles synthesized by electron beam irradiation. *J. Radioanal. Nucl. Chem.* **2006**, *270*, 285–289. [CrossRef]
49. Mascolo, M.C.; Pei, Y.; Ring, T.A. Room temperature co-precipitation synthesis of magnetite nanoparticles in a large ph window with different bases. *Materials* **2013**, *6*, 5549–5567. [CrossRef]
50. Zou, L.; Huang, B.; Zheng, X.; Pan, H.; Zhang, Q.; Xie, W.; Zhao, Z.; Li, X. Microfluidic synthesis of magnetic nanoparticles in droplet-based microreactors. *Mater. Chem. Phys.* **2022**, *276*, 125384. [CrossRef]
51. Bemetz, J.; Wegemann, A.; Saatchi, K.; Haase, A.; Häfeli, U.O.; Niessner, R.; Gleich, B.; Seidel, M. Microfluidic-based synthesis of magnetic nanoparticles coupled with miniaturized nmr for online relaxation studies. *Anal. Chem.* **2018**, *90*, 9975–9982. [CrossRef]
52. Baby, T.; Liu, Y.; Yang, G.; Chen, D.; Zhao, C.-X. Microfluidic synthesis of curcumin loaded polymer nanoparticles with tunable drug loading and ph-triggered release. *J. Colloid Interface Sci.* **2021**, *594*, 474–484. [CrossRef] [PubMed]
53. Elsana, H.; Olusanya, T.O.B.; Carr-wilkinson, J.; Darby, S.; Faheem, A.; Elkordy, A.A. Evaluation of novel cationic gene based liposomes with cyclodextrin prepared by thin film hydration and microfluidic systems. *Sci. Rep.* **2019**, *9*, 15120. [CrossRef] [PubMed]
54. Damiati, S.A.; Damiati, S. Microfluidic synthesis of indomethacin-loaded plga microparticles optimized by machine learning. *Front. Mol. Biosci.* **2021**, *8*, 67754. [CrossRef] [PubMed]
55. Xu, J.; Zhang, S.; Machado, A.; Lecommandoux, S.; Sandre, O.; Gu, F.; Colin, A. Controllable microfluidic production of drug-loaded plga nanoparticles using partially water-miscible mixed solvent microdroplets as a precursor. *Sci. Rep.* **2017**, *7*, 4794. [CrossRef] [PubMed]
56. Gdowski, A.; Johnson, K.; Shah, S.; Gryczynski, I.; Vishwanatha, J.; Ranjan, A. Optimization and scale up of microfluidic nanolipomer production method for preclinical and potential clinical trials. *J. Nanobiotechnology* **2018**, *16*, 12. [CrossRef] [PubMed]
57. Zamani, M.H.; Khatibi, A.; Tavana, B.; Zahedi, P.; Aghamohammadi, S. Characterization of drug-loaded alginate-chitosan polyelectrolyte nanoparticles synthesized by microfluidics. *J. Polym. Res.* **2023**, *30*, 86. [CrossRef]

Disclaimer/Publisher's Note: The statements, opinions and data contained in all publications are solely those of the individual author(s) and contributor(s) and not of MDPI and/or the editor(s). MDPI and/or the editor(s) disclaim responsibility for any injury to people or property resulting from any ideas, methods, instructions or products referred to in the content.

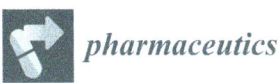

Article

High Efficacy on the Death of Breast Cancer Cells Using SPMHT with Magnetite Cyclodextrins Nanobioconjugates

Costica Caizer [1], Isabela Simona Caizer-Gaitan [1,2,3], Claudia Geanina Watz [4,5,*], Cristina Adriana Dehelean [5,6], Tiberiu Bratu [2] and Codruța Soica [5,7]

[1] Department of Physics, Faculty of Physics, West University of Timisoara, 300223 Timisoara, Romania
[2] Department of Plastic and Reconstructive Surgery, Faculty of Medicine, "Victor Babes" University of Medicine and Pharmacy of Timisoara, 300041 Timisoara, Romania
[3] Department of Clinical Practical Skills, Faculty of Medicine, "Victor Babes" University of Medicine and Pharmacy of Timisoara, 300041 Timisoara, Romania
[4] Department of Pharmaceutical Physics, Faculty of Pharmacy, "Victor Babes" University of Medicine and Pharmacy of Timisoara, 300041 Timisoara, Romania
[5] Research Centre for Pharmaco-Toxicological Evaluation, "Victor Babes" University of Medicine and Pharmacy of Timisoara, 300041 Timisoara, Romania
[6] Department of Toxicology and Drug Industry, Faculty of Pharmacy, "Victor Babes" University of Medicine and Pharmacy Timisoara, 300041 Timisoara, Romania
[7] Department of Pharmaceutical Chemistry, Faculty of Pharmacy, "Victor Babes" University of Medicine and Pharmacy of Timisoara, 300041 Timisoara, Romania
* Correspondence: farcas.claudia@umft.ro

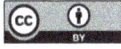

Citation: Caizer, C.; Caizer-Gaitan, I.S.; Watz, C.G.; Dehelean, C.A.; Bratu, T.; Soica, C. High Efficacy on the Death of Breast Cancer Cells Using SPMHT with Magnetite Cyclodextrins Nanobioconjugates. *Pharmaceutics* 2023, 15, 1145. https://doi.org/10.3390/pharmaceutics15041145

Academic Editor: Natalia L. Klyachko

Received: 28 February 2023
Revised: 27 March 2023
Accepted: 31 March 2023
Published: 4 April 2023

Copyright: © 2023 by the authors. Licensee MDPI, Basel, Switzerland. This article is an open access article distributed under the terms and conditions of the Creative Commons Attribution (CC BY) license (https://creativecommons.org/licenses/by/4.0/).

Abstract: In this study, we present the experimental results obtained in vitro on the human breast adenocarcinoma cell line (MCF-7) by applying superparamagnetic hyperthermia (SPMHT) using novel Fe_3O_4-PAA-(HP-γ-CDs) (PAA is polyacrylic acid and HP-γ-CDs is hydroxypropyl gamma-cyclodextrins) nanobioconjugates previously obtained by us. In the in vitro SPMHT experiments, we used concentrations of 1, 5 and 10 mg/mL of Fe_3O_4 ferrimagnetic nanoparticles from Fe_3O_4-PAA-(HP-γ-CDs) nanobioconjugates suspended in culture media containing 1×10^5 MCF-7 human breast adenocarcinoma cells. The harmonic alternating magnetic field used in the in vitro experiments that did not affect cell viability was found to be optimal in the range of 160–378 Gs and at a frequency of 312.2 kHz. The appropriate duration of the therapy was 30 min. After applying SPMHT with these nanobioconjugates under the above conditions, MCF-7 cancer cells died out in a very high percentage, of until 95.11%. Moreover, we studied the field up to which magnetic hyperthermia can be safely applied without cellular toxicity, and found a new upper biological limit $H \times f \sim 9.5 \times 10^9$ A/m·Hz (H is the amplitude and f is the frequency of the alternating magnetic field) to safely apply the magnetic field in vitro in the case of MCF-7 cells; the value was twice as high compared to the currently known value. This is a major advantage for magnetic hyperthermia in vitro and in vivo, because it allows one to achieve a therapy temperature of 43 °C safely in a much shorter time without affecting healthy cells. At the same time, using the new biological limit for a magnetic field, the concentration of magnetic nanoparticles in magnetic hyperthermia can be greatly reduced, obtaining the same hyperthermic effect, while at the same time, reducing cellular toxicity. This new limit of the magnetic field was tested by us in vitro with very good results, without the cell viability decreasing below ~90%.

Keywords: in vitro SPMHT; ferrimagnetic nanobioconjugates; MCF-7 human breast adenocarcinoma cells; Alamar Blue analysis; cell viability

1. Introduction

Magnetic hyperthermia (MHT) of cancer is one of the most promising alternative methods in cancer therapy [1–9], aiming at the total destruction of the malignant tumor with minimal or even no toxicity on the healthy tissue. This non-invasive technique uses biocompatible magnetic nanoparticles and an alternating magnetic field with a small amplitude (kA/m—several tens of kA/m) and a frequency in the range of hundreds of kHz, which leads to the heating of the nanoparticles in the tumor to a temperature of ~43–45 °C [1,8,10]. Thus, at this temperature, tumor cells are thermally destroyed by apoptosis and/or necrosis. Therefore, the therapeutic effect is natural, without radiation and chemical drugs that have a high degree of toxicity on the living organism.

Kandasamy et al. [11], by applying magnetic hyperthermia in vitro, reported the death of MCF-7 tumor cells at a percentage of approximately 90%, using superparamagnetic Fe_3O_4 nanoparticles of 9 nm diameter covered with dual surfactants of TA–ATA (terephthalic acid–aminoterephthalic acid). The concentration used in the experiment was 1 mg/mL of magnetic nanoparticles in suspension, and the frequency of the magnetic field was 751.5 kHz in the admissible biological range.

A similar result on MCF-7 tumor cells was reported by Bhadwaj et al. [12], using magnetic hyperthermia with nanoparticles of $Mn_{0.9}Zn_{0.1}Fe_2O_4$ having a size of 11.3 nm and covered with lauric acid.

Magnetic hyperthermia in vivo also leads to very promising results for cancer therapy. Thus, Alphadery et al. [13] applied magnetic hyperthermia on breast tumors xenografted under the skin of mice using magnetosome chains in suspension until a 10 mg/mL concentration of iron oxide nanoparticles was reached. After applying the therapy several times for 20 min. with a field of 40 mT and frequency of 198 kHz, using doses of 0.1 mL injected each time in the center of the ~100 mm^3 tumor, the tumors in several mice were completely reduced.

Furthermore, Wang et al. [14] used in vivo magnetic hyperthermia with $HPMC/Fe_3O_4$ nanoparticles (HPMC is hydroxyl-propyl methyl cellulose) with 10–50 nm Fe_3O_4 nanoparticles, by intratumoral injection, for the therapy of tumor-bearing mice. After 14 days of treatment by exposure to the magnetic field with a frequency of 626 kHz, a high-efficiency ablation of tumors was obtained.

Currently, MagForce AG [15] uses magnetic hyperthermia with Fe_3O_4 nanoparticles of 12 nm covered with aminosilanes, for the treatment of glioblastoma and prostate cancers in preclinical trials, with good results.

Although in principle, the magnetic hyperthermia technique seems easy to approach, it raises very complex aspects that must be well-clarified and overcome before being safely applied in clinical trials, such as the following: (i) finding the most suitable magnetic nanoparticles (NPs) for this type of therapy; (ii) their high biocompatibility with the biological tissue (lack of cellular toxicity), but also (iii) finding the parameters of the alternating magnetic field; (iv) the most suitable conditions for the practical implementation of magnetic hyperthermia; and (v) the most suitable therapeutic plan. All of these aspects are necessary to obtain the maximum effectiveness on the death of tumor cells, and to minimize the toxicity on normal cells. Until now, there are many studies that have been conducted in this direction to maximize one or more of the aspects listed above (i)–(v) [1,2,9], but they did not establish which are the most suitable to be used in magnetic hyperthermia for in vivo and clinical trials [1,16].

Considering the above aspects, we previously proposed the use of Fe_3O_4 nanoparticles coated with gamma cyclodextrins (γ-CDs) [17,18] to increase the effectiveness and reduce cellular toxicity to a minimum. We also found the optimal conditions [19] in which superparamagnetic hyperthermia (SPMHT) can be applied for maximum effectiveness on tumors. These aspects were studied by us both theoretically [17,19] and experimentally [18], and the recent experimental results showed the possible successful application of nanobioconjugates of Fe_3O_4-PAA–(HP-γ-CDs) (PAA is polyacrylic acid, HP-γ-CDs is hydroxypropyl gamma cyclodextrin) on the destruction of tumors through SPMHT [18], which is more effective than MHT [20]. We used γ-CDs for the bioconjugation of Fe_3O_4 magnetic nanoparticles, due to their advantages for magnetic hyperthermia. Cyclodextrins are very suitable for coating nanoparticles, in terms of stability over time and their biocompatibility with magnetic hyperthermia and drug delivery [21]; they are natural cyclic oligosaccharides without toxicity that are used in pharmaceutics, cosmetic products and biomedicine [22]. Moreover, due to their very reduced thickness on the surface of magnetic nanoparticles, an increase in efficiency in magnetic hyperthermia was obtained by increasing the concentration of nanoparticles in an injectable dispersion targeting tumors. Moreover, cyclodextrins make inclusion complexes possible by encapsulating anticancer drugs in their poorly hydrophilic central cavities (as encapsulated doxorubicin), which in the future would also allow the realization of a double therapy: magnetic hyperthermia followed by the release of the local drug in the tumor, thereby increasing the effectiveness of therapy on tumors.

Using the optimal conditions previously established by us [17–19] for the efficient implementation of SPMHT, in this study we present the experimental results that we obtained in vitro by applying SPMHT using Fe_3O_4-PAA–(HP-γ-CDs) nanobioconjugates on MCF-7 human breast adenocarcinoma cells. We chose this cancer for in vitro testing due to its high incidence in women and high mortality rate, according to the World Health Organization [23]. We mainly present three innovative experimental results that are very important for the advancement of the field of application of superparamagnetic hyperthermia in MCF-7 breast cancer therapy. The following results pertain to the increase in its efficacy on the destruction of tumors and the reduction in toxicity:

(i) The use in superparamagnetic hyperthermia experiments in vitro of biocompatible Fe_3O_4-PAA–(HP-γ-CDs) magnetic nanobioconjugates previously obtained by us, which have not been used so far in the superparamagnetic hyperthermia of tumors;

(ii) Experimental demonstration of the high efficacy of SPMHT using Fe_3O_4-PAA–(HP-γ-CDs) nanobioconjugates via testing in vitro on the MCF-7 breast cancer cell line, with very good results regarding the death of tumor cells at a very high percentage (up to approximately 95%);

(iii) Based on our experimental results on MCF-7 cells, we established a new upper biological limit for the magnetic field without cellular damage for which magnetic hyperthermia can be safely applied on MCF-7 cells: we found that the maximum admissible biological limit can be extended to a double value compared to the previously known one, with superior advantages in the practical implementation of SPMHT for tumors to increase its efficacy and reduce cellular toxicity.

2. Materials and Methods

2.1. Magnetic Nanobioconjugates Used for Testing SPMHT on MCF-7 Breast Cancer Cells

2.1.1. Synthesis Method of Nanobioconjugates

For in vitro SPMHT on MCF-7 breast tumor cells, we used our previously obtained Fe_3O_4-PAA–(HP-γ-CDs) nanobioconjugates [18]. First, ferrimagnetic Fe_3O_4 nanoparticles were obtained by the chemical co-precipitation method; then, the polyacrylic acid (PAA) adsorbed on their surface [24,25] was used for binding (bioconjugation) with hydroxypropyl-gamma-cyclodextrins (HP-γ-CDs), in the second stage, following the procedure described in detail in reference [18]. We used the branched cyclodextrins HP-γ-CDs because by the molecular docking method, we previously showed that this nanobiostructure is the most stable. At the same time, cyclodextrins ensure a very good biocompatibility of nanoparticles with the biological environment [26].

2.1.2. Characterization Techniques of Nanobioconjugates

For the characterization of nanobioconjugates, we used X-ray diffraction (XRD), Fourier transform infrared spectroscopy (FT-IR), high-resolution transmission electron microscopy (HR-TEM) and dynamic light scattering (DLS) techniques, presented in detail in our previous reference [18].

XRD was used to determine the crystalline phases and the average size of the nanocrystallites. A Rigaku UltimaIV Diffractometer with Cu Kα radiation was used for this.

FT-IR was used for the study of ferrite formation and the determination of specific Me–O bonds (Me: metal, O: oxygen) in the magnetite structure. A Shimadzu IR Affinity-1S spectrophotometer was used in the 400–4000 cm^{-1} range.

The morphology of the sample, and the size and distribution of the nanoparticles was studied via HR-TEM, using a Hitachi TEM system (HT7700) with 0.2 nm resolution.

Using the Vasco Particle Size Analyzer, the average hydrodynamic diameter of the nanobioconjugates in dispersion and their distribution was determined using DLS.

2.2. Magnetization of the Fe_3O_4-PAA–(HP-γ-CDs) Nanobioconjugates

The magnetization of the Fe_3O_4-PAA–(HP-γ-CDs) nanobioconjugates and their magnetic behavior in the external magnetic field was carried out with the equipment described in reference [27]. The sample was in the form of nanobioconjugate powder, with a mass of 299.4 mg and a packing volume fraction of 0.62; the applied field was ~1900 Oe (~151 kA/m in SI units). The applied magnetic field was much higher than the one used in the magnetic hyperthermia experiments. The magnetization was determined as a specific value, in emu/g unit. The magnetic behavior in the field of nanobioconjugates was determined from the magnetization curve recorded towards magnetic saturation.

2.3. In Vitro Magnetic Hyperthermia Experiment

2.3.1. MCF-7 Cancer Cell Line

The MCF-7 cell line was acquired from the American Type Culture Collection (ATCC, Manassas, VA, USA) as a frozen vial. The cell line was grown in Eagle's Minimum Essential Medium (EMEM) enriched with 15% FCS (Fetal Calf Serum), and supplemented with an antibiotic mixture of penicillin/streptomycin (100 U/mL penicillin and 100 μg/mL streptomycin) to avoid possible microbial contamination. The cells were passaged every two to three days using trypsin/EDTA until the confluence of the cells reached approximately 80–85%. The cell cultures were maintained under standard conditions: a humidified atmosphere enriched with 5% CO_2 and a temperature of 37 °C, using a Steri-Cycle i160 incubator (Thermo Fisher Scientific, Inc., Waltham, MA, USA).

2.3.2. In Vitro Magnetic Hyperthermia Protocol

To evaluate the cytotoxic effect induced by the Fe_3O_4-PAA–(HP-γ-CDs) suspension under magnetically induced hyperthermia, a slightly modified protocol of Quinto et al. was employed [28]. Briefly, when the MCF-7 cells reached a confluence higher than 80%, the cells were split using trypsin/EDTA solution. Afterwards, the cells were counted using the trypan blue exclusion technique. Based on this step, a cell suspension of 1×10^5 cells/mL was obtained by dilution of the cell pellet in cell medium. The sample-free cell suspension and cell suspensions containing Fe_3O_4-PAA–(HP-γ-CDs) of different concentrations (1, 5, 10 mg/mL) were inserted in 2 mL vials, and were further exposed to alternating magnetic fields (AMF) (312.2 kHz and different fields 160, 200 and 378 Gs).

2.3.3. Alamar Blue Testing

To quantify the effect induced by the AMF on sample-free cell suspensions, and to evaluate the cytotoxic potential of the Fe_3O_4-PAA–(HP-γ-CDs) suspension at three different concentrations (1, 5 and 10 mg/mL) on the human adenocarcinoma MCF-7 cell suspension, the Alamar Blue colorimetric test was employed. In brief, after AMF exposure of the cell suspension ended, 2×10^4 cells/well were seeded in 96-well plates and were furter maintained in a humidified atmosphere at 37 °C and 5% CO_2 until an interval of 24 h was reached. Afterwards, the cells were rinsed three times with phosphate buffer saline (PBS) to avoid possible interference with the Alamar Blue reagent, as previously described [18]. This washing step was followed by the addition of 200 μL of culture medium in each well. The control cells were exposed only to culture media under standard conditions (37 °C). Afterwards, Alamar Blue reagent was added into each well to a final concentration of 0.01%. The cell viability percentage was quantified at 3 h post-addition of the Alamar Blue reagent by measuring the absorbance of the wells at two different wavelengths (570 nm and 600 nm) with a microplate reader (xMark^{TM} Microplate, Bio-Rad Laboratories, Hercules, CA, USA), as previously described [29].

2.3.4. Magnetic Hyperthermia Experiment

The magnetic hyperthermia experiments were carried out using specialized equipment (F3 Driver, nB, Zaragoza, Spain) for this type of experiment, with 3 kW of power and a varying frequency (f) and magnetic field amplitude (H). In our experiments, we used a frequency of 312.2 kHz, and fields of 160 (12.73), 200 (15.92) and 378 Gs (30.08 kA/m in S.I. units), depending on the concentrations of Fe_3O_4 nanoparticles from Fe_3O_4-PAA–(HP-γ-CDs) nanobioconjugates suspended in the cell culture medium, which allowed us to obtain a magnetic hyperthermia therapy temperature of 42.9 °C, without affecting the cells (see Section 3.3.1). The samples used for the magnetic hyperthermia experiments were in fact MCF-7 cell suspensions (density of 1×10^5 cells/mL) that contained Fe_3O_4-PAA–(HP-γ-CDs) nanobioconjugates at concentrations of 1, 5 and 10 mg/mL equivalents in F_3O_4 NPs. These samples were pipetted into different vials of 2 mL capacity, and were furthermore individually exposed to a magnetically induced hyperthermia for a period of 30 min using adiabatic conditions, and employing the specialized inductor coil of the equipment. The temperature of the samples obtained under magnetic hyperthermia was measured using a precision fiber optic sensor.

2.3.5. Data Representation and Statistical Analysis

GraphPad Prism 9 version 9.3 (GraphPad Software, San Diego, CA, USA) was used for data representation and statistical analysis. The results are presented as mean values ± standard deviations (SDs). One-way ANOVA was performed to obtain the statistical differences, followed by Tukey's multiple comparison test.

3. Results and Discussion

3.1. The Fe_3O_4-PAA–(HP-γ-CDs) Nanobioconjugates Data

The Fe_3O_4-PAA–(HP-γ-CDs) nanobioconjugates obtained by us [18] were formed by ferrimagnetic nanoparticles of Fe_3O_4 (magnetite), as determined with X-ray diffraction (XRD) and high-resolution transmission electron microscopy (HR-TEM). They were approximately spherical, with a size (average diameter) of ~16 nm, and covered by bioconjugation with hydroxypropyl gamma-cyclodextrins (HP-γ-CDs) by means of the polyacrylic acid (PAA) biopolymer [24,25]; these were evidenced by Fourier transform infrared spectroscopy (FT-IR), which formed nontoxic nanobioconjugates of ~20 nm in mean diameter, as determined by dynamic light scattering (DLS) [18]. These nanobioconjugates were very suitable for increasing the efficacy of SPMHT in the destruction of tumor cells, due to the optimal size of the magnetic nanoparticles of magnetite, and the existence of the thin organic layer with which they were covered. This allowed for increasing the concentration of nanobioconjugates of Fe_3O_4-PAA–(HP-γ-CDs) in the suspension to be injected into the tumor, thus increasing the hyperthermic effect. At the same time, using the organic layer with cyclodextrins of the HP-γ-CDs type that formed polyacrylate functionalized complexes of Fe_3O_4-PAA–(HP-γ-CDs), the nanobioconjugates obtained by us and used in the in vitro experiments for magnetic hyperthermia of tumors were nontoxic for healthy cells, as cyclodextrins are natural oligosaccharides [26].

3.2. Magnetic Behavior of Fe_3O_4-PAA–(HP-γ-CDs) Nanobioconjugates

The experimental specific magnetization curves towards saturation and a low magnetic field in the case of Fe_3O_4 nanoparticles from the Fe_3O_4-PAA–(HP-γ-CDs) nanobioconjugates powder sample are shown in Figure 1.

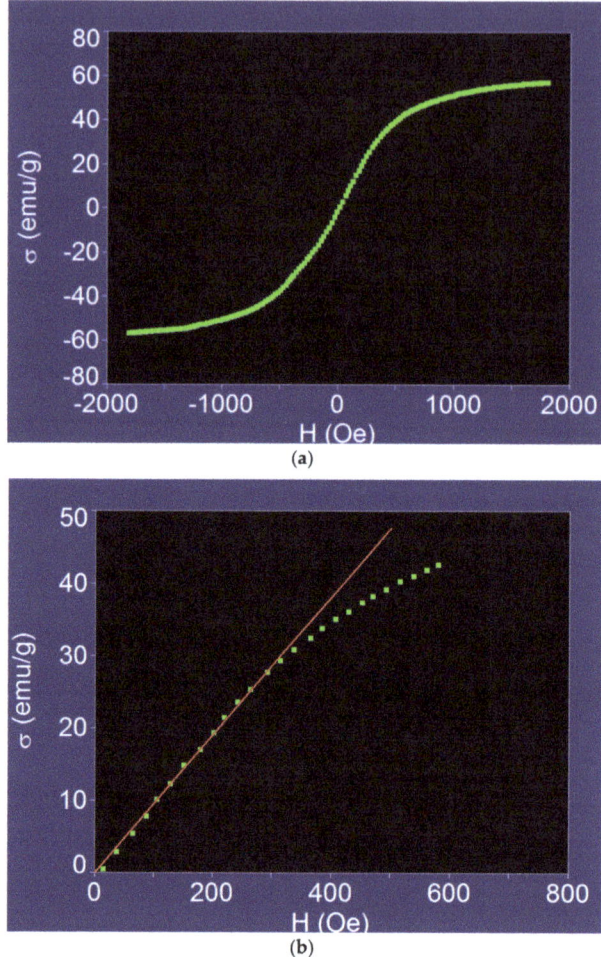

Figure 1. Specific magnetization (σ) loop to (**a**) magnetic saturation and (**b**) low magnetic field (H) of Fe_3O_4 nanoparticles from Fe_3O_4-PAA–(HP-γ-CDs) nanobioconjugates; the green points are experimental data, and the red line is the linear fit function ($r^2 = 0.997$).

The shape of the magnetization curve from Figure 1a shows a very important aspect, namely, that the magnetic behavior in the external magnetic field of the Fe_3O_4-PAA–(HP-γ-CDs) nanobioconjugates, having a ferrimagnetic Fe_3O_4 nanoparticle size (average diameter) of ~16 nm, and an average hydrodynamic diameter of ~20 nm of the superparamagnetic type: the magnetization curve was without hysteresis, and the coercive field was zero. The lack of hysteresis in such a magnetic field, which was much higher than the one used in the magnetic hyperthermia experiments, confirms the fact that the hyperthermic effect was obtained in this case as a result of superparamagnetic hyperthermia (SPMHT), as we presented theoretically in references [17,19]. This result was very important for the practical implementation of magnetic hyperthermia because the loss power, including the heating temperature obtained in superparamagnetic hyperthermia (SPMHT), was higher than that in magnetic hyperthermia (MHT) [30].

Moreover, the specific saturation magnetization (σ) of Fe_3O_4 nanoparticles from Fe_3O_4-PAA–(HP-γ-CDs) nanobioconjugates was in this case quite high, being 56.95 emu/g, compared to that of bulk Fe_3O_4, which is 92 emu/g [31], despite the sample being in a powder state (the magnetization of powders is significantly lower). At the same time, the Fe_3O_4 nanoparticles, whose saturation magnetization was lower due to surface effects [32,33], were additionally covered with the PAA–(HP-γ-CDs) organic layer, which further reduced the saturation magnetization. The high value of the specific saturation magnetization in this case was due to the reduced thickness of the organic layer of PAA–(HP-γ-CDs) on the surface of the nanoparticles, which was only ~3.2 nm; this determined a volume packaging fraction [34] that was significantly higher than in the case of other larger biostructures (e.g., liposomes, which have much larger sizes of tens or hundreds of nm) [26].

The experimental specific initial magnetic susceptibility (mass susceptibility) evaluated from the magnetization curve registered at low magnetic fields (Figure 1b) had a value of 95.4×10^{-3} emu/g Oe (or 6.28 in SI units for initial magnetic susceptibility (volume susceptibility), considering the density of Fe_3O_4 nanoparticles). This value was determined by fitting a linear function (red line in Figure 1b) with the experimental data (green points) obtained for low fields, and then determining the slope of fit line. The value found for the initial magnetic susceptibility is very good for magnetic hyperthermia.

Thus, the high value of the magnetization and magnetic susceptibility of magnetic nanoparticles from the nanobioconjugates allowed us to obtain a high hyperthermic effect in a short time, with the specific loss power [17] leading to the heating of the nanoparticles in proportion to this observables [19].

These results, in the case of our nanobioconjugates indicated (a) superparamagnetic behavior of Fe_3O_4-PAA–(HP-γ-CDs) nanobioconjugates with Fe_3O_4 nanoparticles of ~16 nm, and (b) a high saturation magnetization and initial magnetic susceptibility of nanoparticles that was very important for the in vitro experiments (which are presented in Section 3.3.2) to efficiently obtain the hyperthermic effect (reaching a temperature of ~43 °C) in the shortest possible time, so that healthy cells are not affected.

3.3. In Vitro Testing on Breast Cancer Cells of SPMHT with Fe_3O_4-PAA–(HP-CDs) Nanobioconjugates

For the in vitro testing of SPMHT on MCF-7 breast cancer cells, we used three suspensions of Fe_3O_4-PAA–(HP-γ-CDs) nanobioconjugates suspended in the culture medium, with concentrations of Fe_3O_4 magnetic nanoparticles of 1, 5 and 10 mg/mL. The establishment of these concentrations was based on our previous results [18], which showed that at these concentrations, the viability of healthy cells was not affected. The values used for the magnetic field parameters (amplitude H and frequency f) are those shown in Sections 3.3.1 and 3.3.2 However, in our in vitro SPMHT experiments, we used automatic (electronic) tuning of the amplitude of the magnetic field without exceeding the admissible biological limit, in order to obtain a temperature of 42.9 °C required for hyperthermia; hence, we maintained this temperature throughout the duration of the experiments (see Section 3.3.2). The duration of each in vitro SPMHT experiment was 30 minment.

3.3.1. The Effect of Magnetic Field on Cell Viability of MCF-7 Breast Cancer Cells

An initial experiment we performed was to see if the amplitude of the magnetic field that was going to be used in our in vitro SPMHT experiments could affect MCF-7 breast cancer cells. For this experiment, the frequency of the magnetic field was established at 312.2 kHz, and a cell suspension of MCF-7 cells to a density of 1×10^5 cells/mL was used under standard conditions (37 °C). We also used the case of cellular distribution in suspension, putting the cell culture in the culture medium in 2 mL vial bottles, which is more realistic than the cultures in plates (2D) because this is closer to the in vivo experiments for the tumor animal model [35]. Magnetic fields of 160, 200 and 378 Gs were applied to the samples with MCF-7 cancer cells (three identical samples). These values of the magnetic field were used later in the SPMHT experiments with Fe_3O_4-PAA–(HP-γ-CDs) nanobioconjugates on MCF-7 cancer cells (see Section 3.3.2). We set these values for the magnetic field because they reached the 42.9 °C temperature required for magnetic hyperthermia for the 1, 5 and 10 mg/mL nanobioconjugate preparations (mass of Fe_3O_4

ferrite nanoparticles from Fe$_3$O$_4$-PAA–(HP-γ-CDs)) nanobioconjugates dispersed in 1 mL of PBS).

The experimental curves that show the amplitude of the applied magnetic field and the temperatures of the cell culture recorded for the three samples are in Figure 2.

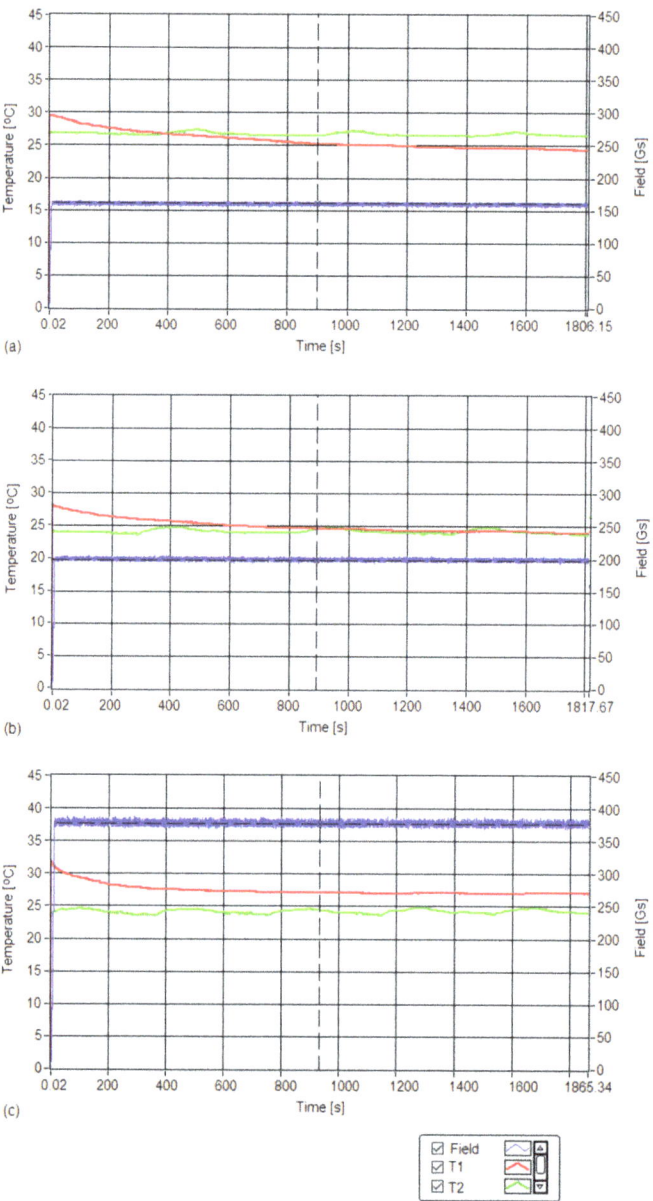

Figure 2. Time diagrams for the temperature of the cell culture (red curve) recorded for 30 min at magnetic field (blue curve) amplitudes of (**a**) 160, (**b**) 200 and (**c**) 378 Gs. The green curve shows the room's temperature.

The obtained experimental results showed the following:

(i) No hyperthermic effect (>40 °C) was obtained; the temperatures of cell cultures T1 (red curve) in all three cases remained close to room temperature T2 (green curve) for all three magnetic fields throughout the 30 min. experiment. Thus, in the absence of magnetic nanoparticles in samples with MCF-7 cancer cells, the alternating magnetic field with a frequency of 312.2 kHz and amplitudes in the range of 160–378 Gs did not lead to an increase in the temperature of the cells;

(ii) For all three values of the magnetic field (160, 200 and 378 Gs), the cell viabilities (Figure 3) of sample-free MCF-7 cancer cells exposed to magnetic fields for 30 min. were practically unaffected, the value of viabilities (Table 1) remaining in the acceptable range of ISO 10993-5 (the International Organization for Standardization) (ISO 10993-5:2009, reviewed and confirmed in 2017) (with a possible viability decrease of 30%) [36].

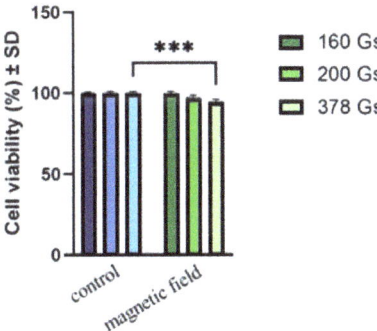

Figure 3. Cell viability of MCF-7 cell line post-exposure to magnetic field for a period of 30 min, at a frequency of 312.2 kHz and different amplitudes (160, 200 and 378 Gs). The viability percentages were normalized to control cells (cells treated only with culture medium and maintained under standard conditions (37 °C)). Data are represented as mean values ± standard deviations (SDs). One-way ANOVA analysis was applied to determine the statistical differences followed by Tukey's post-test (*** $p < 0.001$).

The results obtained following the Implementation of the Alamar Blue test revealed that the viability of the MCF-7 breast cancer line was only slightly affected by exposure to the magnetic field for values greater than 200 Gs. Even after applying the highest field of 378 Gs, the viability of MCF-7 cells remained high, showing a rate of 94.50 ± 1.42%. Increasing the magnetic field from 160 to 378 Gs only led to a very small decrease in cell viability, namely, ~3% for the 200 Gs field, and ~5% for the 378 Gs field. For the smallest field, 160 Gs, the cell viability remained at practically 100%, within the limits of experimental error.

Table 1. Cell viability of the MCF-7 human adenocarcinoma cell line following the application of the magnetic field for a period of 30 min, at a frequency of 312.2 kHz with different amplitudes, after a time interval of 24 h.

	Magnetic Field Amplitude (Gs)	160	200	378
Cell viability (%)	Standard conditions (37 °C)	100 ± 0.61	100 ± 0.83	100 ± 0.76
	After applying the magnetic field	99.63 ± 1.20	96.89 ± 1.64	94.50 ± 1.42

According to ISO 10993-5 [36], related to the biological evaluation of medical devices, a sample is considered cytotoxic if the viability of the cells exposed to the sample is decreased by 30%. Hence, the results obtained showed a viability above 90%, revealing that the magnetic field applied to amplitudes in the range of 160–378 Gs did not induce a cytotoxic effect on MCF-7 cells, and could be safely used for in vitro magnetic hyperthermia experiments on human breast cancer cells. These results were also confirmed by the cellular morphological analyses presented in Figure 4.

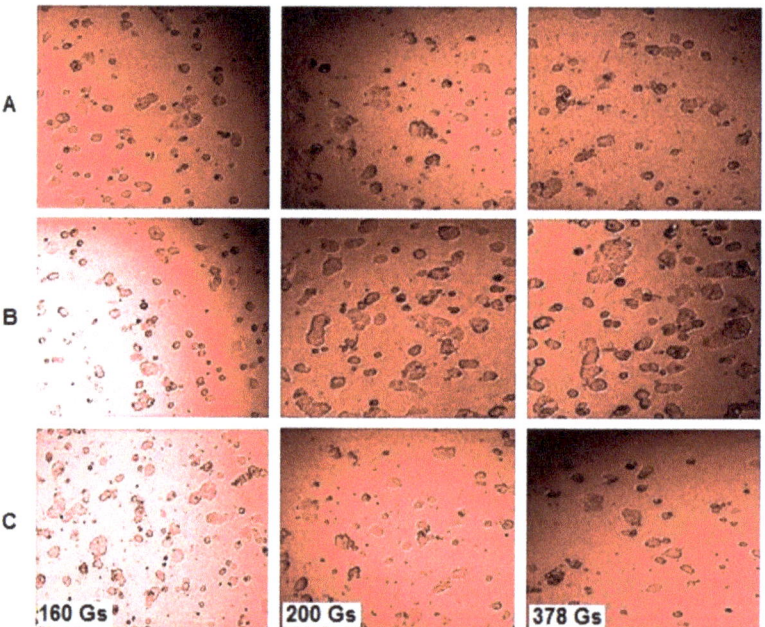

Figure 4. Morphological aspects (nucleus and cytoskeleton) of the MCF-7 human breast adenocarcinoma cell line in the cases of (**A**) standard conditions (37 °C), (**B**) laboratory conditions (24 °C), and (**C**) exposure to magnetic fields (30 min, frequency 312.2 kHz) at different amplitudes (160, 200 and 378 Gs).

Figure 4 presents the morphological aspects observed for the MCF-7 cell line subjected to different experimental conditions: (A) standard conditions (37 °C); (B) laboratory conditions (at room temperature of ~25–27 °C); (C) exposure to a magnetic field. In analyzing Figure 4, it can be easily stated by comparison with the cells maintained in standard conditions that (A), the cells exposed to the magnetic field (C) did not show significant alterations at the morphological level, as cells did at room temperature (laboratory conditions).

In magnetic hyperthermia the admissible upper biological limit of $H \times f = 5 \times 10^9$ A/mHz [37], where H is the amplitude of the magnetic field and f is its frequency, was previously reported. However, in our case and under the conditions established by us, this limit was far exceeded for MCF-7 breast cancer cells, reaching a value of over $\sim 9.5 \times 10^9$ $Am^{-1}Hz$, approximately double the value as in the case of the 378 field Gs. This is a very important experimental result obtained in our case because the field can be increased above the previously known limit ($H \times f = 5 \times 10^9$ $Am^{-1}Hz$); this leads to the increase in the effectiveness of magnetic hyperthermia in this case, and to a reduction in the therapy duration (to avoid possible cytotoxicity), with overall beneficial effects for this therapy.

Furthermore, an increase in the magnetic field to a value that is twice as high as the value given by the admissible biological limit known until now, is very important for magnetic hyperthermia because it can lead to a significant decrease in the concentration of magnetic nanoparticles used to obtain the same hyperthermic effect on cell tumors (reaching a temperature of 43 °C that is necessary in magnetic hyperthermia). At the same time, a significant decrease in the concentration of nanoparticles in magnetic hyperthermia has a very beneficial effect on reducing or even eliminating cytotoxicity at low concentrations.

In summary, we can say that the use of the magnetic field with a frequency of 312.2 kHz and an amplitude in the range of 160–378 Gs in magnetic hyperthermia experiments in vitro is not cytotoxic for MCF-7 tumor cells.

3.3.2. SPMHT with Fe_3O_4-PAA–(HP-γ-CDs) Nanobioconjugates on MCF-7 Cancer Cells

SPMHT on MCF-7 tumor cells using Fe_3O_4-PAA–(HP-γ-CDs) nanobioconjugates was tested in vitro for the concentrations of 1, 5 and 10 mg/mL (mass (in mg) of Fe_3O_4 ferrite nanoparticles from Fe_3O_4-PAA–(HP-γ-CDs) nanobioconjugates dispersed in 1 mL of culture medium), using the specialized professional equipment for magnetic hyperthermia from Figure 5, in adiabatic conditions. The cell culture in this case was very well thermally isolated from the external environment. Thus, the cell culture could be maintained at a constant temperature of 42.9 °C for the entire 30 min. of the magnetic hyperthermia experiment.

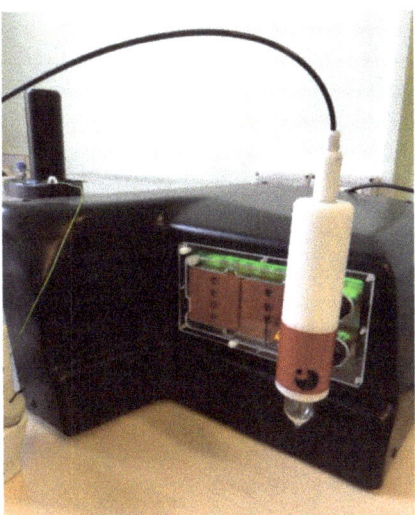

Figure 5. The experimental equipment for testing SPMHT in adiabatic conditions.

Furthermore, performing the experiment in cell suspension and not on 2D surface culture plates may have provided features that were closer to simulating real conditions encountered under in vivo experiments, such us animal models. Thus, the results of the experiments may provide more reliable data [35].

The experimental curves recorded during the SPMHT experiments for the three concentrations are shown in Figure 6.

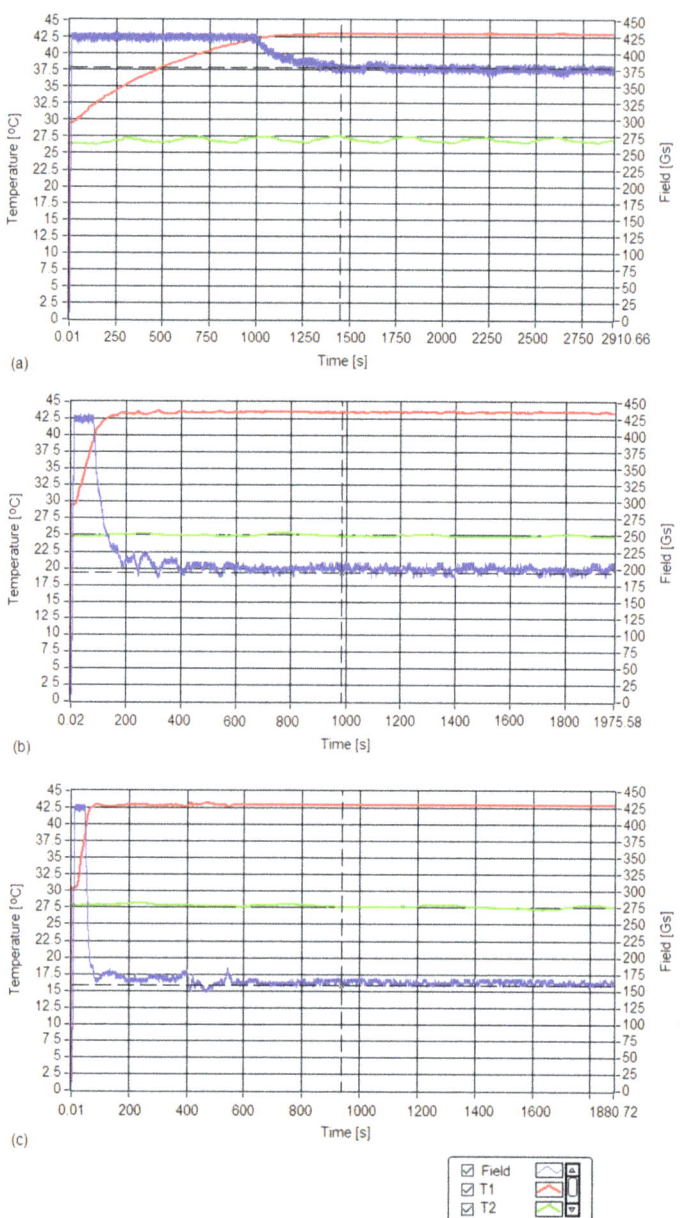

Figure 6. Curves for magnetic field amplitude (blue), therapy temperature T1 (red) and room temperature T2 (green) for concentrations of (**a**) 1, (**b**) 5 and (**c**) 10 mg/mL.

The red curve shows the temperature obtained in magnetic hyperthermia, which was constant at 42.9 ± 0.1 °C throughout the duration of the 30 min. experiments for concentrations of 1 (Figure 6a), 5 (Figure 6b) and 10 mg/mL (Figure 6c). The green curve shows the room temperature during the experiments. The blue curve shows the magnetic fields during the three experiments, electronically maintained during the 30 min. of therapy so that the therapy temperature (42.9 °C) did not change (red curves in

Figure 6). At the beginning, the magnetic field had a higher value that initiated a rapid increase in temperature, after which it quickly dropped to the corresponding value from the experiment, and then remained approximately constant throughout the therapy.

The experimental curves in Figure 6 demonstrate that in all three cases, the temperature required for therapy T1 (red curves) was kept constant at the treatment value of 42.9 ± 0.1 °C for the entire 30 min. therapy, through rigorous and precise (electronic) control of the amplitude of the applied magnetic field (blue curves).

At the same time, the temperature of the environment T2 (green curves) around the inductor coil where the cells were subjected to magnetic hyperthermia remained unchanged, and at a level much lower than the therapy temperature for the entire duration in the experiment; this showed that hyperthermia could effectively be applied to the cells.

The values of the magnetic field in the experiments depended on the concentrations of the magnetic nanoparticles used (1 mg/mL, 5 mg/mL and 10 mg/mL). Thus, the amplitude of the magnetic field increased when the concentration decreased. Its values are given in Table 2.

Table 2. The values of the magnetic field used in therapy depending on the concentration of ferrimagnetic nanoparticles in the samples.

Concentration of Fe_3O_4 nanoparticles (mg/mL)	1	5	10
Magnetic field amplitude (Gs)	378	200	160

However, the speed required to increase the therapy temperature (red curve) to the value corresponding to SPMHT used in our experiments varied, depending on the concentration of the magnetic nanoparticles in the nanobioconjugates (Figure 7). Thus, in the case of the more diluted sample of 1 mg/mL, the temperature reached that corresponding to magnetic hyperthermia in a longer time (20 min.) compared to the more concentrated samples, where the times were much reduced (80 s) (Table 3).

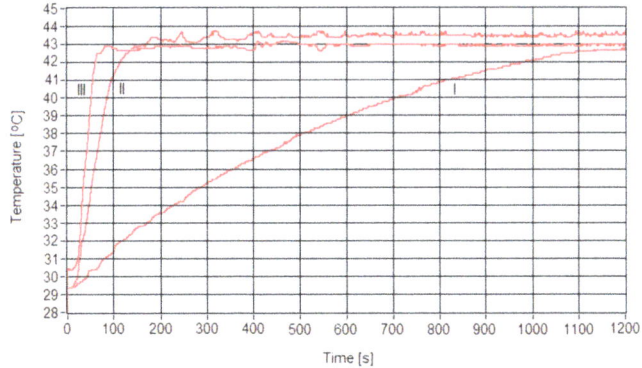

Figure 7. Temperature increase over time from room temperature to that corresponding to SPMHT in the cases of magnetic nanoparticle concentrations of (I) 1, (II) 5 and (III) 10 mg/mL.

Table 3. Times necessary to reach the therapy temperature of 42.9 °C, depending on the concentrations of samples.

Sample concentration (mg/mL)	1	5	10
Duration to reach the therapy temperature 42.9 °C (s)	1200	150	80

All samples with different concentrations were maintained for 30 min. (therapy duration) under identical conditions in the alternating magnetic field with a frequency of

312.2 kHz and amplitudes of 160 (12.73), 200 (15.92) and 378 Gs (30.08 kA/m) (Figure 6 and Table 2), in adiabatic conditions (Figure 5). Then, they were analyzed from the point of view of cell viability to see the hyperthermic effect obtained by SPMHT on MCF-7 breast cancer cells. This assessment was performed using the Alamar Blue calorimetric test (see next section).

3.4. Cell Viability Assessment of MCF-7 Cells after SPMHT Therapy via Alamar Blue Test

A summary of the experimental results obtained after the application of SPMHT with Fe_3O_4-PAA–(HP-γ-CDs) nanobioconjugates in vitro on MCF-7 breast cancer cells is shown in Figure 8. The results obtained regarding the viability of breast cancer cells after hyperthermic therapy (temperature of 42.9 °C for 30 min.) show an important decrease in MCF-7 cell populations for all three test concentrations (1, 5 and 10 mg/mL); the viability of the cells showed percentages between ~5–10%, when compared to the control value (100%) recorded under standard conditions. The highest decrease in cell viability was obtained when the higher concentration of magnetic nanoparticles (10 mg/mL) was applied, revealing that a more intense effect of MCF-7 cell death could be obtained when high concentrations of magnetic nanoparticles are used. Moreover, the IC_{50} parameter showed a good value of 0.06288 mg/mL for the magnetic nanoparticles (Figure S1).

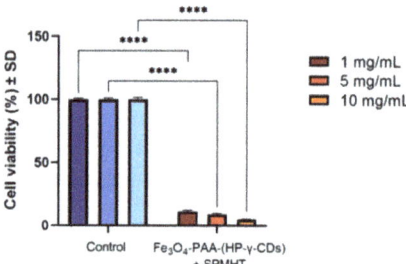

Figure 8. Cell viability percentages of MCF-7 human adenocarcinoma cell lines exposed to different concentrations of Fe_3O_4-PAA–(HP-γ-CDs) nanobioconjugates under SPMHT conditions (temperature of 42.9 °C for 30 min.) at 24 h post-stimulation. The viability percentages were normalized to control cells (cells treated only with culture medium and maintained under standard conditions (37 °C)). Data are represented as mean values ± standard deviations (SDs). One-way ANOVA analysis was applied to determine the statistical differences followed by Tukey's post-test (**** $p < 0.0001$).

The values of the viability percentages of MCF-7 human adenocarcinoma cells treated with Fe_3O_4-PAA–(HP-γ-CDs) nanobioconjugates under SPMHT for 30 min. are presented in Table 4.

Table 4. Data of the cell viability percentages induced by magnetic suspensions under standard conditions (ST) and superparamagnetic hyperthermia (SPMHT) on the human breast adenocarcinoma cell line (MCF-7).

Sample/ Concentration	Cell Viability (%) of MCF-7 Cells under Standard Conditions (ST: 37 °C)	Cell Viability (%) of MCF-7 Cells after SPMHT (42.9 °C, 30 min)
Fe_3O_4-PAA–(HP–γ-CDs)/ 1 mg/mL	100 ± 0.80	11.32 ± 0.91
Fe_3O_4-PAA–(HP–γ-CDs)/ 5 mg/mL	100 ± 1.02	9.09 ± 0.68
Fe_3O_4-PAA–(HP–γ-CDs)/ 10 mg/mL	100 ± 1.40	4.89 ± 0.45

As presented in Table 4, the viability of the MCF-7 cell population was significantly affected after exposure to SPMHT for all three concentrations (1, 5 and 10 mg/mL) of the Fe_3O_4-PAA–(HP-γ-CDs) nanobioconjugates. The data revealed that the Fe_3O_4-PAA–(HP-γ-CDs) sample induced by SPMHT had a viability of only 4.89 ± 0.45% when a concentration of 10 mg/mL was applied.

The results obtained in the current study are more promising compared to those recently obtained by Salimi et al. [38], which revealed that post-magnetic hyperthermia (magnetic field parameters: f = 300 kHz and H = 12 kA/m), the cell viability of MCF-7 breast cancer cells was 36.7% after 24 h. However, Salimi et al. used G4@IONPs nanoparticles (fourth generation of polyamidoamine dendrimer-coated iron oxide nanoparticles) ranging in size between 10 ± 4 nm. Moreover, the concentration of nanoparticles used in the culture medium in this case was 0.5 mg/mL, and the therapy duration was 120 min.

Another result obtained on the MCF-7 breast cancer cells that may be comparable to the ones obtained by us in the current study when referring to the concentration of magnetic nanoparticles of 1 mg/mL, was recently reported by Bhardwaj et al. [12]; the study revealed that nanoparticles of $Mn_{0.9}Zn_{0.1}Fe_2O_4$ ferrites of size 11.3 nm covered with lauric acid, induced a cell viability of 10% after 24 h when the concentration of nanoparticles was 0.35 mg/mL and the treatment duration was 30 min. for magnetic field parameters of f = 330 kHz and H = 15.3 kA/m.

All the above results show that the viability of MCF-7 cells after magnetic hyperthermia depends on a plethora of factors, such as the type, size and concentration of nanoparticles, the duration of treatment, and the parameters of the applied magnetic field. Therefore, finding all of the optimal conditions for the successful application of magnetic hyperthermia for the complete death of tumor cells with minimal side effects is an essential issue, and is of high interest in the field of alternative cancer therapy.

When applying the external alternating magnetic field, the Fe_3O_4 magnetic nanoparticles in the Fe_3O_4-PAA–(HP-γ-CDs) nanobioconjugates heat up. The possible mechanisms that leads to the heating of magnetic nanoparticles under magnetic field action are, in this case, Néel–Brown magnetic relaxation [17], the nanobioconjugates being in suspension (culture medium). However, having in view the size of the nanoparticles of ~16 nm and the presence of the organic layer on the surface of nanoparticles [18], the rotation of the nanobioconjugates (Brown relaxation), which also interacts with the cells in the culture medium, is very limited or even blocked [17]. Thus, in this case, the Néel magnetic relaxation mechanism prevails (the rotation of the magnetic moments inside the magnetic nanoparticles), which leads to the heating of the nanoparticles (Figure 6). The required heating temperature in magnetic hyperthermia (42.9 °C) depends on the concentration of nanobioconjugates and the magnetic field applied at the frequency of 312.2 kHz. Once the nanoparticles are heated, the MCF-7 tumor cells located in the culture medium near them or in contact with them, or even containing the nanoparticles, are also heated through the thermal conduction mechanism, as a result of the good thermal conductivity of the medium. Thus, the tumor cells become heated to the temperature of 42.9 °C used in magnetic hyperthermia, which leads to cell death by apoptosis.

Regarding the possible mechanism of action of the nanoparticles within MCF-7 cells, according to Jacob et al. [39], reactive oxygen species (ROS)-based reactions may play a key role in apoptotic processes, which may be further correlated with mitochondrial membrane potential impairment and caspase-3 up-regulation. Furthermore, it is also well-known that the majority of the iron oxide nanoparticles interfere with lysosomal-related signaling pathways [40,41].

According to the results obtained in vitro by us following the application of SPMHT with Fe_3O_4-PAA–(HP-γ-CDs) nanobioconjugates on MCF-7 human breast adenocarcinoma cells, the following aspects can be concluded:

(i) The magnetic field parameters implemented in the present study are not cytotoxic on the cell line (MCF-7), as the viability of this line did not decrease below 70%, the limit imposed by ISO standards (70%) [36]; the cellular viability in our case was very high, even at the highest field of 378 Gs (30.08 kA/m in SI units), this being 88.68%;

(ii) The concentrations of magnetic nanoparticles used in the SPMHT experiments and the duration of the therapy are suitable for the effective destruction of MCF-7 tumor cells;

(iii) The Fe_3O_4-PAA–(HP-γCDs) sample at a concentration of 10 mg/mL can be considered the sample with the highest in vitro impact, as this concentration induced the most intense cytotoxic effect through SPMHT on MCF-7 human breast adenocarcinoma cells.

The concentrations used by us in the experiment are applicable in magnetic hyperthermia [11,13,15,30,42–47]. Furthermore, we previously showed that concentrations up to 10 mg/mL did not produce toxicity on healthy HaCaT human keratinocytes cells [18]; therefore, we used in this in vitro at concentrations of 1, 5 and 10 mg/mL. These concentrations are feasible for the future in vivo application of superparamagnetic hyperthermia, where the concentrations of magnetite nanoparticles in dispersion with very good biocompatibility can even reach 10–20 mg/mL [13,42,44,46,47]. Recently, an even higher concentration value was reported, namely 112 mg/mL, of 12 nm superparamagnetic iron oxide nanoparticles aminosilane-coated in suspension for the therapy of glioblastoma tumors, using a dose of 0.3 mL of magnetic liquid per cubic centimeter of tumor volume [15].

Regarding the bioaccumulation issue of nanoparticles in organs when SPMHT will be tested in vivo, taking into account the approval of the use of the concentration of iron oxide nanoparticles of 12 nm (biocompatible by aminosilane) until approximately 30 mg/mL in clinical trials for MHT [15] (three times higher than the highest dose used by us (10 mg/mL)), we can consider that there will be no major risk of bioaccumulation of nanoparticles in important organs above acceptable toxicity limits.

However, for safety we will consider such evaluations in the future (bioaccumulation of nanoparticles in different organs after nanoparticles injection and superparamagnetic hyperthermia (hepatotoxicity, nephrotoxicity, etc.)) when we conduct in vivo studies.

In summary, by applying SPMHT with Fe_3O_4-PAA–(HP-γ-CDs) nanobioconjugates with a concentration of 1, 5 and 10 mg/mL, a high efficacy on the death of MCF-7 breast cancer cells was obtained; the percentages of cancer cells dying were very high in these cases, 88.68, 90.91 and 95.11%, respectively, obtaining an IC_{50} value of 62.88 ± 1 µg/mL.

Considering the efficacy obtained for the destruction of tumor cells, after the application of SPMHT with Fe_3O_4-PAA–(HP-γ-CDs) nanobioconjugates, it is important to know what the efficiency is for magnetic hyperthermia with this nanobiomaterial, by determining the intrinsic loss power (ILP) indicator for our nanoparticles, independent of the applied magnetic field. Thus, using the specific loss power (SLP) presented in reference [18], we numerically evaluated its value in the case of our 10 mg/mL sample for the value of a magnetic field amplitude H of 12.73 kA/m and a frequency f of 312.2 kHz, used in the in vitro SPMHT experiment, and found a SLP of 72.2 W/g. By normalizing SLP ($SLP/H^2 f$), we determined the value of the ILP indicator of 1.43 nH·m^2/kg, which indicates that our sample is a very good thermal mediator to efficiently obtain superparamagnetic hyperthermia under the given conditions.

Comparatively, for the bionized nanoferrite (BNF®) commercial nanoparticles prepared via the core-shell method with a core of Fe_3O_4 and a shell of dextran or hydroxyethyl starch, having a nanoparticle size of 14 nm (close to that of our sample (16 nm)), and for a magnetic field of 9.5 kA/m and a frequency of 614.4 kHz, an ILP of 0.25 nH·m^2/kg was obtained [48]. This value is significantly lower than the one obtained in the case of our sample (1.43 nH·m^2/kg).

However, in the same magnetic field conditions (9.5 kA/m and 614.4 kHz), Darwish et al. [48] reported for ILP a value of 3.8 nH·m^2/kg for core-shell nanoparticles of magnesium iron oxide@tetramethyl ammonium hydroxide (MgIONPs@TMAH), having a size of 15 nm. Moreover, Nishimoto et al. [49] reported an ILP value of ~2 and ~4 for commercial Resovist® and MEADM-033-02 nanoparticles, which are γ-Fe_2O_3 nanoparticles coated with carboxydextran and carboxymethyl-diethylaminoethyl dextran, respectively, having a size of 5-6 nm and a concentration of 2 mg-Fe/mL, for a magnetic field of 4 kA/m and 100 kHz.

However, Kandasamy et al. [50] recently showed that in the case of 10 nm nanoparticles of 34DABA-coated SPIOs dispersed in aqueous medium (SPIOs is Fe_3O_4, and 34DABA is 3,4-diaminobenzoic acid), there is a dependence of ILP on the concentration of nanoparticles and the applied magnetic field (H and f). The authors showed that the ILP decreased when the concentration increased in the range of 0.5–8 mg/mL, this being attributed to the formation of nanoparticle agglomerates that influenced the magnetic relaxation and decreased the thermal effect; e.g., for 8 mg/mL, the ILP was 0.9 nH m^2/kg, and for 1 mg/mL, the ILP was 1.7 nH m^2/kg, under the same magnetic field conditions (10.39 kA/m and 330.3 kHz).

4. Conclusions

The use of SPMHT therapy with Fe_3O_4-PAA–(HP-γ-CDs) nanobioconjugates, having a mean Fe_3O_4 nanoparticle diameter of ~16 nm and a mean nanobioconjugate hydrodynamic diameter of ~20 nm, led to the death of MCF-7 breast cancer cells at a high percentage of 95.11% (cell viability of 4.89%) compared to standard conditions 24 h after treatment. The therapy was carried out for 30 min. at a temperature of 42.9 °C in a harmonic alternating magnetic field with a frequency of 312.2 kHz and an amplitude of 160 Gs (12.73 kA/m), at a concentration of 10 mg/mL of magnetic nanoparticles from nanobioconjugates of Fe_3O_4-PAA–(HP-γ-CDs) suspended in the culture medium.

The very good results obtained in our therapy are due to the optimal experimental conditions used for SPMHT and established by us: the optimal size of the Fe_3O_4 nanoparticles; the concentration of magnetic nanoparticles; the use of HP-γ-CDs without toxicity to cover the Fe_3O_4 magnetic nanoparticles and with a very small thickness; the amplitude and frequency of the magnetic field; and the optimal duration of therapy (without damage to healthy cells).

The percentage of dead cancer cells decreased slightly with a decrease in the concentration of magnetic nanoparticles from nanobioconjugates at 5 mg/mL and 1 mg/mL, namely 90.91 (viability of 9.09%) and 88.68% (viability of 11.32%), respectively, with the percentages remaining at high levels. However, in these two cases, the anticancer therapy remained as effective as with the concentration of 10 mg/mL by repeating the therapy session, or even increasing the duration of the therapy to more than 30 min..

Furthermore, through our in vitro study regarding the safe use of the magnetic field on MCF-7 cells, we showed that the maximum admissible biological limit could be extended to a significantly higher value of ~9.5×10^9 A/m Hz, that is approximately double the value than the one known until now (5×10^9 A/m Hz). This result is very important for the safe practical implementation of SPMHT in vitro and in vivo, which allows the concentration of nanoparticles used to be greatly reduced in magnetic hyperthermia, with a beneficial effect on reducing cytotoxicity.

Supplementary Materials: The following supporting information can be downloaded at: https://www.mdpi.com/article/10.3390/pharmaceutics15041145/s1, Figure S1: Schematic representation of IC_{50} parameter using GraphPad Prism software, version 9.3.

Author Contributions: Conceptualization, C.C., C.S., C.A.D. and T.B.; methodology, C.C., I.S.C.-G. and C.G.W.; data analysis, I.S.C.-G. and C.G.W.; explanation, I.S.C.-G. and C.G.W.; manuscript writing, I.S.C.-G. and C.G.W.; manuscript revisions, C.C., I.S.C.-G. and C.G.W.; supervision, C.C., T.B., C.S. and C.A.D. All authors have read and agreed to the published version of the manuscript.

Funding: This research was supported by a grant from the Ministry of Research, Innovation, and Digitization, CNCS/CCCDI—UEFISCDI, project number PN-III-P2-2.1-PED-2019-3067, within PNCDI III, the West University of Timisoara from the CNFIS-FDI-2020-0253 project, and the "Victor Babes" University of Medicine and Pharmacy of Timisoara from its research funds. The authors wish to express their thanks for this support.

Institutional Review Board Statement: Not applicable.

Informed Consent Statement: Not applicable.

Data Availability Statement: Not applicable.

Acknowledgments: The authors thank Roxana Racoviceanu from the Research Centre for Pharmaco-Toxicological Evaluation, "Victor Babes" University of Medicine and Pharmacy of Timisoara for the support in sample preparation.

Conflicts of Interest: The authors declare no conflict of interest.

References

1. Caizer, C. Magnetic/Superparamagnetic hyperthermia as an effective noninvasive alternative method for therapy of malignant tumors. In *Nanotheranostics: Applications and Limitations*; Rai, M., Jamil, B., Eds.; Springer: Berlin/Heidelberg, Germany, 2019; pp. 297–335.
2. Gazeau, F.; Lévy, M.; Wilhelm, C. Optimizing magnetic nanoparticle design for nanothermotherapy. *Nanomedicine* **2008**, *3*, 831–844. [CrossRef] [PubMed]
3. Di Corato, R.; Béalle, G.; Kolosnjaj-Tabi, J.; Espinosa, A.; Clément, O.; Silva, A.; Ménager, C.; Wilhelm, C. Combining magnetic hyperthermia and photodynamic therapy for tumor ablation with photoresponsive magnetic liposomes. *ACS Nano* **2015**, *9*, 2904–2916. [CrossRef]
4. Yan, H.; Shang, W.; Sun, X.; Zhao, L.; Wang, J.; Xiong, Z.; Yuan, J.; Zhang, R.; Huang, Q.; Wang, K.; et al. "All-in-One"Nanoparticles for trimodality imaging-guided intracellular photo-magnetic hyperthermia therapy under intravenous administration. *Adv. Funct. Mater.* **2018**, *28*, 1705710. [CrossRef]
5. Almaki, J.H.; Nasiri, R.; Idris, A.; Majid, F.A.A.; Salouti, M.; Wong, T.S.; Dabagh, S.; Marvibaigi, M.; Amini, N. Synthesis, characterization and in vitro evaluation of exquisite targeting SPIONs–PEG–HER in HER2+ human breast cancer cells. *Nanotechnology* **2016**, *27*, 105601. [CrossRef] [PubMed]
6. Liu, X.L.; Ng, C.T.; Chandrasekharan, P.; Yang, H.T.; Zhao, L.Y.; Peng, E.; Lv, Y.B.; Xiao, W.; Fang, J.; Yi, J.B.; et al. Synthesis of ferromagnetic Fe0.6Mn0.4O nanoflowers as a new class of magnetic theranostic platform for in vivo T1-T2 Dual-Mode magnetic resonance imaging and magnetic hyperthermia therapy. *Adv. Healthc. Mater.* **2016**, *5*, 2092–2104. [CrossRef]
7. Xie, L.; Jin, W.; Zuo, X.; Ji, S.; Nan, W.; Chen, H.; Gao, S.; Zhang, Q. Construction of small-sized superparamagnetic Janus nanoparticles and their application in cancer combined chemotherapy and magnetic hyperthermia. *Biomater. Sci.* **2020**, *8*, 1431–1441. [CrossRef] [PubMed]
8. Liu, X.; Zhang, Y.; Wang, Y.; Zhu, W.; Li, G.; Ma, X.; Zhang, Y.; Chen, S.; Tiwari, S.; Shi, K.; et al. Comprehensive understanding of magnetic hyperthermia for improving antitumor therapeutic efficacy. *Theranostics* **2020**, *10*, 3793–3815. [CrossRef]
9. Caizer, C.; Rai, M. *Magnetic Nanoparticles in Human Health and Medicine: Current Medical Applications and Alternative Therapy of Cancer; Part. II: Magnetic nanoparticles in Alternative Cancer Therapy*; Wiley: Oxford, UK, 2022.
10. Rajan, A.; Sahu, N.K. Review on magnetic nanoparticle-mediated hyperthermia for cancer therapy. *J. Nanoparticle Res.* **2020**, *22*, 1–25. [CrossRef]
11. Kandasamy, G.; Sudame, A.; Bhati, P.; Chakrabarty, A.; Maity, D. Systematic investigations on heating effects of carboxyl-amine functionalized superparamagnetic iron oxide nanoparticles (SPIONs) based ferrofluids for in vitro cancer hyperthermia therapy. *J. Mol. Liq.* **2018**, *256*, 224–237. [CrossRef]
12. Bhardwaj, A.; Parekh, K.; Jain, N. In vitro hyperthermic effect of magnetic fluid on cervical and breast cancer cells. *Sci. Rep.* **2020**, *10*, 15249. [CrossRef]
13. Alphandéry, E.; Chebbi, I.; Guyot, F.; Durand-Dubief, M. Use of bacterial magnetosomes in the magnetic hyperthermia treatment of tumours: A review. *Int J Hyperth.* **2013**, *29*, 801–809. [CrossRef] [PubMed]
14. Wang, F.; Yang, Y.; Ling, Y.; Liu, J.; Cai, X.; Zhou, X.; Tang, X.; Liang, B.; Chen, Y.; Chen, H.; et al. Injectable and thermally contractible hydroxypropyl methyl cellulose/Fe$_3$O$_4$ for magnetic hyperthermia ablation of tumors. *Biomaterials* **2017**, *128*, 84e93. [CrossRef] [PubMed]
15. NanoTherm®Therapy, MagForce Nanomedicine, Germany. Available online: https://magforce.com/en/home/for_physicians/ (accessed on 29 December 2022).
16. Caizer, C. Magnetic/Superparamagnetic Hyperthermia in Clinical Trials for noninvasive Alternative cancer Therapy. In *Magnetic Nanoparticles in Human Health and Medicine: Current Medical Applications and Alternative Therapy of Cancer*; Caizer, C., Rai, M., Eds.; Wiley: Oxford, UK, 2022.
17. Caizer, C.; Caizer, I.S. Study on maximum specific loss power in Fe$_3$O$_4$ nanoparticles decorated with biocompatible gamma-cyclodextrins for cancer therapy with superparamagnetic hyperthermia. *Int. J. Molec. Sci.* **2021**, *22*, 10071. [CrossRef] [PubMed]
18. Caizer, C.; Caizer, I.S.; Racoviceanu, R.; Watz, C.G.; Mioc, M.; Dehelean, C.A.; Bratu, T.; Soica, C. Fe$_3$O$_4$-PAA−(HP-γ-CDs) Biocompatible Ferrimagnetic Nanoparticles for Increasing the Efficacy in Superparamagnetic Hyperthermia. *Nanomaterials* **2022**, *12*, 2577. [CrossRef]
19. Caizer, C. Optimization study on specific loss power in superparamagnetic hyperthermia with magnetite nanoparticles for high efficiency in alternative cancer therapy. *Nanomaterials* **2021**, *11*, 40. [CrossRef]

20. Caizer, C. Magnetic hyperthermia-using magnetic metal/oxide nanoparticles with potential in cancer therapy. In *Metal Nanoparticles in Pharma*; Rai, M., Shegokar, R., Eds.; Springer: Berlin/Heidelberg, Germany, 2017.
21. Caldera, F.; Nisticò, R.; Magnacca, G.; Matencio, A.; Yousef Khazaei Monfared, Y.K.; Trotta, F. Magnetic composites of dextrin-based carbonate nanosponges and iron oxide nanoparticles with potential application in targeted drug delivery. *Nanomaterials* **2022**, *12*, 754. [CrossRef]
22. Duchêne, D. Cyclodextrins and Their Inclusion Complexes. In *Cyclodextrins in Pharmaceutics, Cosmetics, and Biomedicine*; John Wiley & Sons Inc.: Hoboken, NJ, USA, 2011; pp. 1–18.
23. World Health Organization, Cancer—Key Facts. 2022. Available online: https://www.who.int/news-room/fact-sheets/detail/cancer (accessed on 28 December 2022).
24. Hamidreza, S. Synthesis of Nanocomposition of Poly Acrylic Acid/Chitosan Coated-Magnetite Nanoparticles to Investigation of Interaction with BSA and IGG Proteins. *Int. J. Nanomater. Nanotechnol. Nanomed.* **2017**, *3*, 27–33. [CrossRef]
25. Kim, K.D.; Sung, S.K.; Yong-ho, C.; Hee, T.K. Formation and Surface Modification of Fe3O4 Nanoparticles by Co-Precipitation and Sol-Gel Method. *J. Ind. Eng. Chem.* **2007**, *13*, 1137–1141.
26. Caizer, C.; Dehelean, C.; Soica, C. Classical magnetoliposomes vs current magnetocyclodextrins with ferrimagnetic nanoparticle for high efficiency and low toxicity in alternative therapy of cancer by magnetic/superparamagnetic hyperthermia. In *Magnetic Nanoparticles in Human Health and Medicine: Current Medical Applications and Alternative Therapy of Cancer*; Caizer, C., Rai, M., Eds.; Wiley: Oxford, UK, 2022.
27. Caizer, C. T^2 law for magnetite-based ferrofluids. *J. Phys.: Condens. Matter* **2003**, *15*, 765–776.
28. Quinto, C.A.; Mohindra, P.; Tong, S.; Bao, G. Multifunctional superparamagnetic iron oxide nanoparticles for combined chemotherapy and hyperthermia cancer treatment. *Nanoscale* **2015**, *7*, 12728–12736. [CrossRef]
29. Pop, D.; Buzatu, R.; Moaca, E.A.; Watz, C.G.; Cînta-Pînzaru, S.; Barbu Tudoran, L.; Nekvapil, F.; Avram, S.; Dehelean, C.A.; Cretu, M.O.; et al. Development and Characterization of Fe_3O_4@Carbon Nanoparticles and Their Biological Screening Related to Oral Administration. *Materials* **2021**, *14*, 3556. [CrossRef]
30. Pankhurst, Q.A.; Connolly, J.; Jones, S.K.; Dobson, J. Applications of magnetic nanoparticles in biomedicine. *J. Phys. D Appl. Phys.* **2003**, *36*, R167–R181. [CrossRef]
31. Smit, J.; Wijin, H.P.J. *Les Ferites*; Biblioteque Technique Philips: Paris, France, 1961.
32. Coey, J.M.D. Noncollinear spin arrangement in ultrafine ferrimagnetic crystallites. *Phys. Rev. Lett.* **1971**, *27*, 1140. [CrossRef]
33. Berkowitz, A.E.; Kodama, R.H.; Makhlouf, S.A.; Parker, F.T.; Spada, F.E.; McNiff, E.J., Jr.; Foner, S. Anomalous properties of magnetic nanoparticles. *J. Magn. Magn. Mater.* **1999**, *196–197*, 591. [CrossRef]
34. Caizer, C. Nanoparticle size effect on some magnetic properties. In *Handbook of Nanoparticles*; Aliofkhazraei, M., Ed.; Springer International Publishing: Cham, Switzerland, 2016.
35. Vilas-Boas, V.; Carvalho, F.; Espiña, B. Magnetic hyperthermia for cancer treatment: Main parameters affecting the outcome of in vitro and in vivo studies. *Molecules* **2020**, *25*, 2874. [CrossRef] [PubMed]
36. *ISO 10993-5:2009; Reviewed and Confirmed in 2017, Biological Evaluation of Medical Devices—Part 5: Tests for In Vitro Cytotoxicity*. ISO Catalogue, Edition 3; International Standard Organization: Geneva, Switzerland, 2009; Available online: https://www.iso.org/standard/36406.html (accessed on 28 December 2022).
37. Hergt, R.; Dutz, S. Magnetic particle hyperthermia—Biophysical limitations of a visionary tumour therapy. *J. Magn. Magn. Mater.* **2007**, *311*, 187–192. [CrossRef]
38. Salimi, M.; Sarkar, S.; Saber, R.; Delavari, H.; Alizadeh, A.M.; Mulder, H.T. Magnetic hyperthermia of breast cancer cells and MRI relaxometry with dendrimer-coated iron-oxide nanoparticles. *Cancer Nano.* **2018**, *9*, 1–19. [CrossRef] [PubMed]
39. Jacob, J.A.; Salmani, J.M.M.; Chen, B. Magnetic nanoparticles: Mechanistic studies on the cancer cell interaction. *Nanotechnol. Rev.* **2016**, *5*, 481–488. [CrossRef]
40. Portilla, Y.; Mulens-Arias, V.; Paradela, A.; Ramos-Fernández, A.; Pérez-Yagüe, S.; Morales, M.P.; Barber, D.F. The surface coating of iron oxide nanoparticles drives their intracellular trafficking and degradation in endolysosomes differently depending on the cell type. *Biomaterials.* **2022**, *281*, 121365. [CrossRef]
41. Frtús, A.; Smolková, B.; Uzhytchak, M.; Lunova, M.; Jirsa, M.; Kubinová, Š.; Dejneka, A.; Lunov, O. Analyzing the mechanisms of iron oxide nanoparticles interactions with cells: A road from failure to success in clinical applications. *J Control Release.* **2020**, *328*, 59–77. [CrossRef] [PubMed]
42. Ito, A.; Tanaka, K.; Honda, H.; Abe, S.; Yamaguchi, H.; Kobayashi, T. Complete regression of mouse mammary carcinoma with a size greater than 15 mm by frequent repeated hyperthermia using magnetite nanoparticles. *J. Biosci. Bioeng.* **2003**, *96*, 364–369. [CrossRef]
43. Tanaka, K.; Ito, A.; Kobayashi, T.; Kawamura, T.; Shimada, S.; Matsumoto, K.; Saida, T.; Honda, H. Intratumoral injection of immature dendritic cells enhances antitumor effect of hyperthermia using magnetic nanoparticles. *Int. J. Cancer* **2005**, *116*, 624–633. [CrossRef]
44. Kawai, N.; Ito, A.; Nakahara, Y.; Honda, H.; Kobayashi, T.; Futakuchi, M.; Shirai, T.; Tozawa, K.; Kohri, K. Complete regression of experimental prostate cancer in nude mice by repeated hyperthermia using magnetite cationic liposomes and a newly developed solenoid containing a ferrite core. *Prostate* **2006**, *66*, 718–727. [CrossRef]
45. Fortin, J.P.; Gazeau, F.; Wilhelm, C. Intracellular heating of living cells through Néel relaxation of magnetic nanoparticles. *Eur. Biophys. J.* **2008**, *37*, 223–228. [CrossRef] [PubMed]

46. Alphandéry, E.; Faure, S.; Seksek, O.; Guyot, F.; Chebbi, I. Chains of magnetosomes extracted from AMB-1 magnetotactic bacteria for application in alternative magnetic field cancer therapy. *ACS Nano* **2011**, *5*, 6279–6296. [CrossRef] [PubMed]
47. Hu, R.; Zhang, X.; Liu, X.; Xu, B.; Yang, H.; Xia, Q.; Li, L.; Chen, C.; Tang, J. Higher temperature improves the efficacy of magnetic fluid hyperthermia for Lewis lung cancer in a mouse model. *Thorac. Cancer* **2012**, *3*, 34–39. [CrossRef] [PubMed]
48. Darwish, M.; Kim, H.; Bui, M.P.; Le, T.-A.; Lee, H.; Ryu, C.; Lee, J.Y.; Yoon, J. The heating efficiency and imaging performance of magnesium iron oxide@tetramethyl ammonium hydroxide nanoparticles for biomedical applications. *Nanomaterials* **2021**, *11*, 1096. [CrossRef]
49. Nishimoto, K.; Ota, S.; Shi, G.; Takeda, R.; Trisnanto, S.B.; Yamada, T.; Takemura, Y. High intrinsic loss power of multicore magnetic nanoparticles with blood-pooling property for hyperthermia. *AIP Advances* **2019**, *9*, 035347. [CrossRef]
50. Kandasamy, G.; Sudame, A.; Luthra, T.; Saini, K.; Maity, D. Functionalized hydrophilic superparamagnetic iron oxide nanoparticles for magnetic fluid hyperthermia application in liver cancer treatment. *ACS Omega* **2018**, *3*, 3991–4005. [CrossRef] [PubMed]

Disclaimer/Publisher's Note: The statements, opinions and data contained in all publications are solely those of the individual author(s) and contributor(s) and not of MDPI and/or the editor(s). MDPI and/or the editor(s) disclaim responsibility for any injury to people or property resulting from any ideas, methods, instructions or products referred to in the content.

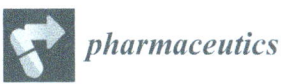

Article

Multimodal Radiobioconjugates of Magnetic Nanoparticles Labeled with [44]Sc and [47]Sc for Theranostic Application

Perihan Ünak [1,*], Volkan Yasakçı [1], Elif Tutun [1], K. Buşra Karatay [1], Rafał Walczak [2], Kamil Wawrowicz [2], Kinga Żelechowska-Matysiak [2], Agnieszka Majkowska-Pilip [2] and Aleksander Bilewicz [2,*]

[1] Department of Nuclear Applications, Institute of Nuclear Sciences, Ege University, Izmir 35100, Turkey
[2] Centre of Radiochemistry and Nuclear Chemistry, Institute of Nuclear Chemistry and Technology, Dorodna 16 St., 03-195 Warsaw, Poland
* Correspondence: perihan.unak@gmail.com (P.Ü.); a.bilewicz@ichtj.waw.pl (A.B.)

Abstract: This study was performed to synthesize multimodal radiopharmaceutical designed for the diagnosis and treatment of prostate cancer. To achieve this goal, superparamagnetic iron oxide (SPIO) nanoparticles were used as a platform for targeting molecule (PSMA-617) and for complexation of two scandium radionuclides, [44]Sc for PET imaging and [47]Sc for radionuclide therapy. TEM and XPS images showed that the Fe_3O_4 NPs have a uniform cubic shape and a size from 38 to 50 nm. The Fe_3O_4 core are surrounded by SiO_2 and an organic layer. The saturation magnetization of the SPION core was 60 emu/g. However, coating the SPIONs with silica and polyglycerol reduces the magnetization significantly. The obtained bioconjugates were labeled with [44]Sc and [47]Sc, with a yield higher than 97%. The radiobioconjugate exhibited high affinity and cytotoxicity toward the human prostate cancer LNCaP (PSMA+) cell line, much higher than for PC-3 (PSMA-) cells. High cytotoxicity of the radiobioconjugate was confirmed by radiotoxicity studies on LNCaP 3D spheroids. In addition, the magnetic properties of the radiobioconjugate should allow for its use in guide drug delivery driven by magnetic field gradient.

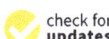

Keywords: SPION; multimodal nanoparticles; PET diagnosis; MRI; [44/47]Sc; PSMA-617; prostate cancer

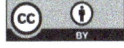

1. Introduction

In nuclear medicine, nanoparticles (NPs) with magnetic properties can be used for imaging, diagnosis, treatment, and separation of biological materials [1]. Initial studies on patients with magnetically controlled drug targeting were reported by Lübbe et al. The authors stated that 0.5–0.8 T magnetic field intensity is sufficient to direct iron nanoparticles to tumors near the surface [2]. It is also possible to target drugs to diseased tissue by loading drug molecules on magnetic particles. Magnetic nanoparticles (MNPs) can also be labeled with radionuclides, which enables them to be used in radiopharmacy. MNPs may be advantageous in alpha radionuclide therapy to retain [225]Ac and its daughter products at a target site. Cedrowska et al. reported that radiolabeled iron oxide nanoparticles with Ac-225 and modified with CEPA-Tmab were proposed for a combination of magnetic hyperthermia and radionuclide therapy [3]. In another publication [223]Ra-doped BaFe nanoparticles were presented as candidates for multimodal drug combining localized magnetic hyperthermia with internal α-therapy [4]. Magnetic nanoparticles labeled also with β[−] emitters ([188]Re, [198]Au, ^{90}Y, and ^{131}I) and Auger electron emitters (^{111}In and ^{125}I) were also investigated, some of them in preclinical studies [5–9].

MNPs in medicine can be classified as therapeutic (hyperthermia and drug targeting) and diagnostic (NMR imaging) agents. Shape and size, biocompatibility, and stability of nanoparticles are parameters to be considered. Silica coating prevents magnetic nanoparticles from aggregating uncontrollably and oxidizing over time. TEOS (tetraethyl orthosilicate) is one of the most commonly used methods although there are different coating methods [10]. The silica layer stabilizes the MNP core by sustaining magnetic dipole interactions. In medical applications, MNPs can be coated with a biocompatible polymer to increase stability and bioavailability [11] or coated with antibody for biomarker immobilization [12]. Among others, MNPs modified with hyperbranched polyglycerol (HPG) have attracted much attention for years [1–11,13–15]. Having three-dimensional structures and numerous internal and external functional groups, these compounds can serve as remarkable hosts for metal complexes, enzymes, and biomaterials. HPG has many reactive functional groups that can be converted to other functional groups. In addition, HPG-modified MNPs have been used in various applications such as magnetic resonance imaging (MRI), drug delivery, and catalysis [16].

In our work, we designed a multifunctional agent combining PET and MRI imaging and radionuclide therapy using SPION nanoparticles as a platform [12]. A prostate-specific membrane antigen (PSMA) molecule is implemented for targeting, while a DOTA chelator incorporated into the PSMA-617 structure is used to complex two scandium radionuclides ^{44}Sc for PET diagnosis and ^{47}Sc for therapy.

The PSMA small molecule is an antagonist with a very high affinity to specific membrane antigens expressed in aggressive prostate cancer. Due to the high resistance of this tumor, it is recommended to use several therapeutic methods, e.g., chemo- and radiotherapy during treatment. The second therapeutic method planned for use is magnetic hyperthermia. The therapeutic effect obtained results from the impact of β-radiation emitted by ^{47}Sc radiation, as well as from local hyperthermia—heating of cancer cells to a temperature above 42 °C, induced by fast oscillations of SPIONs in an external alternating magnetic field. Covalent binding of vector molecules (PSMA) for further radiolabeling in the final step of synthetic processes to the SPIONs provides a precise, targeted delivery of obtained radiobioconjugate only to the selected tumor cells overexpressing PSMA receptors, while the external alternating magnetic field causing an increase temperature multiplies the therapeutic effect.

It is well known that prostate cancer can spread to any part of the body, but metastatic sites are most commonly directed to the bones [17]. Nuclear medicine aims to treat bone metastases with [^{153}Sm]Sm-EDTMP or [^{177}Lu]Lu-EDTMP, while [^{99m}Tc]Tc-MDP is mainly used in the imaging of bone metastases [18]. Phosphate derivatives such as EDTMP and DPAPA may be suitable targeting agents for theragnostics, where imaging and treatment with the same agent are used together. In this work, we added to HPG-modified MNPs two phosphonate derivatives, EDTMP or DPAPA, for targeting of prostate cancer and its metastases. With PSMA-617, we present a compound that, in addition to a PSMA inhibitor as a target vector, also contains a bisphosphonate that is established as a bone tracer and, thus, combines the advantages of PSMA targeting and bone targeting.

Additionally, due to their superparamagnetic behavior, radionuclide labeled SPIONs bioconjugates can be guided and retained exclusively in the tumor tissue with help of an external constant magnetic field. Their accumulation in this tissue can be followed by functional NMR and positron emission tomography (PET). Thus, we proposed a promising radionuclide therapy and imaging tool as an "all-in-one" approach.

2. Materials and Methods

2.1. Reagents and Instruments

Iron(III) acetylacetonate [Fe(acac)$_3$; Fe(C$_5$H$_7$O$_2$)$_3$; 97%], decanoic acid [CH$_3$(CH$_2$)$_8$COOH; 98%], benzyl ether [(C$_6$H$_5$CH$_2$)$_2$O; 98%], tetraethyl orthosilicate [TEOS; (C$_2$H$_5$O)$_4$Si; for synthesis], potassium methylate (CH$_3$OK; for synthesis), anhydrous methanol (CH$_3$OH; 99.8%), glycidol (C$_3$H$_6$O$_2$; 96%), ethylenediamine (NH$_2$CH$_2$CH$_2$NH$_2$; absolute, ≥99.5%), sodium cyanoborohydride (NaBH$_3$CN; reagent grade, 95%), N-ethyl-N'-(3-dimethylaminopropyl) carbodiimide hydrochloride [E.D.C.; C$_8$H$_{17}$N$_3$ hydrochloric acid (HCl) Bio extra], N-hydroxy succinimide (C$_4$H$_5$NO$_3$; 98%), 3-(4,5-dimethylthiazol-2-yl)-2-5-diphenyltetrazolium bromide (MTT; 98%), dimethyl sulfoxide (DMSO), and trifluoroacetic acid [TFA; CF$_3$COOH; high-performance liquid chromatography (HPLC), 99%] were obtained from Sigma-Aldrich

(Taufkirchen, Germany). Acetonitrile (HPLC grade) was purchased from Carlo Erba Reagents (Barcelona, Spain). Dulbecco's modified Eagle's medium (DMEM), fetal bovine serum (FBS), penicillin/streptomycin solution, RPMI-1640, L-glutamine, trypsin-EDTA, nonessential amino acids, sodium pyruvate, and phosphate-buffered saline (PBS) were acquired from Biowest (Nuaillé, France). Muse® Annexin V and Dead Cell Kit and Instrument Cleaning Fluid were purchased from Luminex (Northbrook, IL, USA). HCl (37%), phosphoric acid, and sodium hydroxide were supplied by Merck KGaA (Darmstadt, Germany). Deionized water was processed in a Milli-Q water purification system.

PC-3 [PSMA (−) human prostate derived from the metastatic part of the bone] and LNCaP [PSMA (+) prostate derived from the metastatic site left supraclavicular lymph node] cells were supplied by the American Type Culture Collection (ATCC; Manassas, VA, USA). These cells were obtained from the ATCC using the authors' previous project resources for academic studies in the cell culture laboratory of the Ege University Institute of Nuclear Sciences.

The following reagents were also used: hydrochloric acid 35–38%, analytical pure, Chempur, Poland; ammonium acetate, analytical pure, Chempur, Poland; ammonia solution 25%, analytical pure, Chempur, Poland; human serum, Sigma-Aldrich, USA; Dulbecco's PBS, Biological Industries, Israel; calcium carbonate 4.3% ^{46}Ca, Isoflex, USA; calcium carbonate, 99.999%, Alfa Aesar, USA; syringe filter 0.2 µm, PTFE Whatman, Great Britain; cation-exchange resin Dowex 50WX4, mesh 100–200, H+, Fluka Analytical, USA.

The following materials were used: growing media—DMEM (PC-3) and RPMI 1640 (LNCaP); trypsin EDTA solution C; water, cell culture grade; phosphate-buffered saline (PBS); fetal calf serum from Biological Industries (Beth Haemek, Israel). For cytotoxicity evaluation, CellTiter96® AQueous One Solution Reagent (MTS compound) from Promega (Mannheim, Germany) was used. LNCaP and PC-3 cells were obtained from the American Type Tissue Culture Collection (ATCC, Rockville, MD, USA) and cultured according to the ATCC protocol. For experimental applications, over 80% confluent cells were used. Blocking the PSMA receptors was accomplished with PSMA-617, obtained from Selleck Chemicals L.L.C., Houston, TX USA.

The following equipment was used: HPLC SPD-10AV ultraviolet–visible (UV–vis) and AD2 detector systems with an LC-10Atvp pump (Shimadzu, Kyoto, Japan), Inertsil ODS-3 C-18 4.6 × 250 mm HPLC 5 µm column (G.L. Sciences, Inc., Tokyo, Japan), SIL-20A HT automatic sampler (Shimadzu, Varioskan Flash multimode microplate reader (Thermo Fisher Scientific, Darmstadt, Germany), AR-2000 radioTLC (thin-layer radiochromatography) imaging scanner (Eckert & Ziegler, Berlin, Germany), Packard Tricorb-1200 liquid scintillation counter (Meriden, CT, USA), Malvern Zetasizer Nano ZS dynamic light scattering (D.L.S.; Malvern Panalytical, Malvern, U.K.), Millipore Muse Dead Cell Analyzer Flow Cytometry inverted microscope (Leica Microsystems, Wetzlar, Germany), and Spectrum Two I.R. spectrophotometer (attenuated total reflection; Perkin-Elmer, Boston, MA, USA). The Ege University Central Research Laboratory supplied the following analyses: X-ray photoelectron spectroscopy (XPS) analysis was conducted with the K-Alpha XPS System (Thermo Fisher Scientific, U.K.). The scanning probe microscopy (S.P.M.) image was taken using a Bruker Dimension Edge with ScanAsyst System (Billerica, MA, USA). Scanning electron microscopy (SEM) images were taken with a Thermo Scientific Apreo S device at the Ege University Central Research Laboratory and the SEM Zeiss EVO LS10 (Carl Zeiss Microscopy GmbH, Germany) at the Konya Selçuk University Advanced Research Center (Iltek). ^{1}H-NMR, ^{13}C-NMR, and ^{31}P-NMR spectra of DPAPA were performed with the 400 MHz operating frequency liquid MERCURY plus-AS 400 model NMR spectrometer in the Nuclear Magnetic Resonance Laboratory of Ege University Faculty of Science. Transmission electron microscopy (TEM) measurements were made with a JEOL-2100 Multipurpose 200 kV TEM (Tokyo, Japan) at the Advanced Research and Application Center of Konya Selçuk University (Konya, Turkey). Vibrating sample magnetometer (V.S.M.) measurements were conducted at the Dokuz Eylül University Center for Fabrication and Application of Electronic Materials using Dexing Magnet VSM 550 devices, ICP-MS analyses were performed the Agilent Technologies 7800 Series device, C.A., United States in Izmir Katip Çelebi University Central Research Laboratory (MERLAB).

2.2. Cubic Fe_3O_4 (C-Fe_3O_4) NP Synthesis

Fe_3O_4 nanocubes were prepared according to the procedure described by Martinez-Boubeta et al. [19] involving heating a solution of $Fe(acac)_3$, decanoic acid, and dibenzyl ether. This method is performed by the discriminant separation of nucleation and growth stages caused by the intermediate formation of the iron(III) decanoate complex, as discussed previously [19].

2.3. Silica and HPG Coating of C-Fe_3O_4 NPs and Ethylenediamine Coupling

Silica coating of C-Fe_3O_4 NPs was performed using the procedure described previously [20]. The HPG coating was applied according to the method proposed by Sadri et al. [21]. The synthesis path of ethylenediamine coupling with Fe_3O_4–SiO_2–HPG in the literature was realized with modifications [22].

2.4. Synthesis of DPAPA and Conjugation with Fe_3O_4–SiO_2–HPG–NH_2

DPAPA was synthesized using a modified Mannich-type reaction according to the method given in the literature described for EDTMP [23] (Figure 1). Synthesized cubic MNPs were conjugated with DPAPA using the EDC/(N-(3-dimethyl aminopropyl)-N'-ethyl carbodiimide hydrochloride/N-hydroxy succinimide (NHS) conjugation method [20].

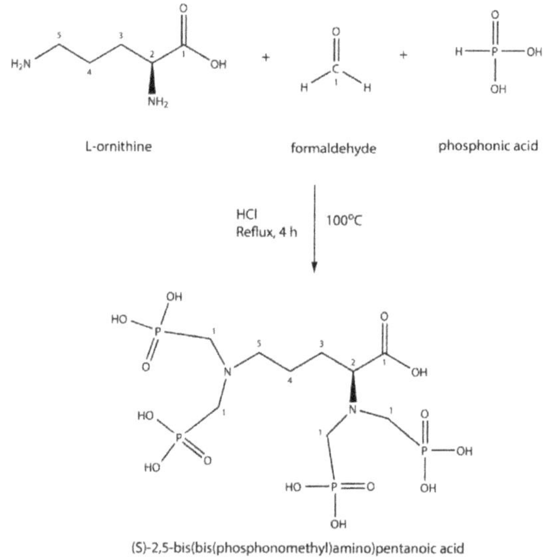

Figure 1. DPAPA synthesis reactions (Mannich-type reaction).

2.5. Production of $^{44/47}Sc$

^{44}Sc: $CaCO_3$ (88.87 mg, 99.999% purity) target material was pressed into a 6 mm disc, supported on graphite. The target was irradiated by 16 MeV proton with 14 µA current on GE-PET trace 840 cyclotron at Heavy Ions Laboratory, Warsaw University. The irradiation was carried out for 100 min.

^{47}Sc: ^{47}Sc was produced in $^{46}Ca(n,\gamma)^{47}Ca \rightarrow {}^{47}Sc$ reaction in Nuclear Reactor—Maria in Świerk (Otwock, Poland). Then, 5 mg of $CaCO_3$ (4.3% ^{46}Ca) was irradiated for 120 h with 10^{14} n/cm^{2}s thermal neutron flux. After irradiation, the target was cooled for 5 days to reach the maximum activity of ^{47}Sc produced from ^{47}Ca decay. Then, 5 days after the irradiation, 90 MBq of ^{47}Sc was produced from ^{47}Ca decay.

2.6. Separation Procedure

For the separation of $^{44/47}$Sc from the target material, a two-step method based on microfiltration [24] and cation exchange on Dowex resin was used [25]. First, the irradiated target was dissolved in 1 M HCl, and then the solution was alkalized with the ammonia solution (25%) to pH ~11. In these conditions, Sc compounds were trapped on 0.22 μm porous microfilters. The loss of radionuclides after this process was no higher than 10%. For the removal of Ca tracers, the microfilter was washed with 5 mL of deionized water. After that, scandium cations were removed from filters with 2 mL of 1 M HCl with an efficiency of 84.6% ± 0.75% and a 200 mg load of Dowex 50WX4 cation exchange resin. The bed was washed with 5 mL of water for removal of residual HCl with almost no loss of the activity. Elution of Sc from DOWEX resin was performed with 0.4 M ammonium acetate buffer, pH 4.5, 0.5 mL/min flow and the eluent was collected with 0.5 mL fractions.

2.7. Radiolabeling with $^{44/47}$Sc

After the separation process, $^{44/47}$Sc was in 0.4 M ammonium acetate buffer, pH 4.5, which is a suitable environment for labeling of DOTA chelator. Then, 1 mL of nanoparticles (41 mg of NP) were centrifuged 4500 rpm for 5 min. After that, supernatants were removed and replaced with 100 μL of 1 M ammonium acetate buffer. Next, 30 MBq of ^{44}Sc or ^{47}Sc in ammonium acetate buffer were added to EDTMP-PSMA NCs or DPAPA-PSMA NCs and incubated for 30 min at 95 °C. After incubation, the samples were centrifuged to remove the unbound $^{44/47}$Sc from the nanoparticles and their activities were measured. In every case, the efficiency of labeling was higher than 97%.

2.8. Stability Tests of $^{44/47}$Sc

Stability tests were performed for EDTMP PSMA NPs and EDTMP PSMA NPs labeled with ^{44}Sc. After labeling, NPs were purified from nonattached scandium and divided onto two parts. Stability of bonding between Sc and NPs was checked in 500 μL of human serum (HS) or phosphate-buffered saline (PBS). Samples were incubated at 37 °C, and the stability was checked after 1, 2, 3, 4, and 24 h. After incubation at 37 °C nanoparticles were centrifuged, and the activity was measured.

2.9. In Vitro Studies

The PC-3 (PSMA−) and LNCaP (PSMA+) prostate cancer cell lines were used for cell culture studies. These cells were obtained from the American Type Culture Collection (ATCC) (USA) using our previous project resources for academic studies at Ege University Institute of Nuclear Sciences Cell culture laboratory. PC-3 was grown in medium consisting of Dulbecco's modified Eagle's medium (DMEM) and 10% fetal bovine serum (FBS). LNCaP was grown in medium consisting of Roswell Park Memorial Institute RPMI-1640 medium and 10% fetal bovine serum (FBS). Cells were incubated in 5% CO_2 and 37 °C. The medium was changed every 2 days, and fresh medium was added. After the cells proliferated to cover 80% of the flasks, they were separated from the flask with 0.25% (W/V) trypsin-EDTA solution and planted in 96-well plates for cytotoxicity studies. Cells not used in the study were placed in media containing 5% DMSO, first frozen at −80 °C, and then stored in liquid nitrogen at below 198 °C, where they were stockpiled for further studies. All cell culture studies were performed in 6 replicates (n = 6).

2.9.1. Cell Binding of ^{44}Sc-Labeled Bioconjugates

^{44}Sc: Receptor binding affinity of synthesized bioconjugates was determined with LNCaP cells overexpressing PSMA receptors, as well as with PC-3 cells (PSMA-negative) used as control. Two days before the experiment, cells (8×10^5 LNCaP and 5×10^5 PC-3 cells, respectively) were seeded into six-well plates and incubated in 37 °C with 5% CO_2 atmosphere. Subsequently, prior tested compounds were added, and the cells were washed once with PBS. Next, 1 mL of various concentrations (0.06–2.0 nM) of bioconjugates labeled with ^{44}Sc (25–30 MBq) suspended in a growing medium were added and incubated for 2 h with slight shaking. Then, the medium was aspirated, and cells were rinsed with PBS twice to remove unbound fraction. In the last step, the cells (bound fraction) were lysed twice with 1 M NaOH, and all fractions were measured using a Wizard2 Detector Gamma Counter (Perkin Elmer, Waltham, MA, USA). For evaluation of nonspecific binding, PSMA receptors were blocked with 2000 M excess of nonconjugated PSMA. To calculate the specific binding, the difference between total and nonspecific binding was quantified. Presented results (mean with SD) contain the data from two individual experiments, wherein each sample was repeated twice.

2.9.2. MTT Assay

Cytotoxicity tests were performed using the MTT (3-[4,5-dimethylthiazol-2-yl]-2,5 diphenyl tetrazolium bromide) method. The MTT test is based on the conversion of MTT into formazan crystals by living cells, which determines mitochondrial activity [18]. Because total mitochondrial activity correlates with the number of viable cells for most cell populations, this assay is widely used to measure the in vitro cytotoxic effects of drugs on cell lines or primary patient cells. Cells were prepared from cell suspensions at 5×10^4 cells/mL per well of 96-well plates. Then, 100 µL of cell suspension was added to each well created, and a solution containing the sterile substance at six different (1, 3, 10, 30, 100, and 300 µg/mL) concentrations was added to the wells except the control. Cells and the reagent-free medium were used as a negative control. In the study, each parameter was studied with n = 5 repetitions. The plate with the cells was incubated at 37 °C in 5% CO_2. At the 24th, 48th and 72nd hours of cell incubation (PC-3 or LNCaP), 10 µL of MTT solution was added to each well and incubated for 4 h. Next, after 4 h of incubation, instead of removing MTT, 100 µL of SDS (sodium dodecyl sulfate) was added and incubated at 37 °C for 24 h in a 5% CO_2 environment. Cells were read using a spectrophotometer for the absorbance value of each well at a wavelength of 540 nm and a reference range of 690 nm.

2.9.3. MTS Assay

Cytotoxicity studies with ^{47}Sc were performed with MTS assay according to the previously reported protocol [5]. LNCaP (10×10^3) and PC-3 (7.5×10^3) cells were seeded into 96-well plates 48 h before treatment and incubated in 37 °C with 5% CO_2-supplemented atmosphere. Subsequently, the medium was replaced with tested compounds labeled with ^{47}Sc and suspended in a growing medium. Cells were incubated with nanoparticles for 48 h and 72 h. Following incubation, the medium was removed, and fresh medium was added. Lastly, 20 µL of CellTiter96®AQueous One Solution Reagent (Promega, MDN, USA) was added for 2 h incubation. Absorbance was measured at 490 nm to calculate the percentage of metabolically active cells. IC50 was calculated using GraphPad Prism v.8 Software (GraphPad Software, San Diego, CA, USA).

2.9.4. 3D Cell Culture Studies

The "Hanging Drop Model" was used for 3D cell culture using with the LNCaP (PSMA+) and PC-3 (PSMA−) prostate cancer cell lines. LNCaP cells were amplified in a medium consisting of Roswell Park Memorial Institute RPMI-1640 medium and 10% fetal bovine serum (FBS), while PC-3 cells were derived from Dulbecco's modified Eagle's medium (DMEM) and 10% fetal bovine serum (FBS). Cells were incubated in 5% CO_2 and 37 °C. The medium was changed every 2 days, and fresh medium was added. After the cells proliferated to cover 80% of the flasks, they were separated from the flask with 0.25% (W/V) trypsin-EDTA solution, and the confluent cell lines were first removed from the surface for 3D cell culture. After being removed and taken into the relevant medium, the total droplet volume was prepared as 50 µL and 50,000 cells, and 3D cell culture models were created in the "hanging drop plate". The medium of the drops containing the cell population was changed every day, and spheroid formation was completed at the end of the 48th hour. After the spheroid was formed, fixation was performed to obtain a 3D cell image.

The formed spheroids were transferred into the chamber slide through the relevant medium. Then, it was washed with 200 µL of PBS, before adding 200 µL of paraformaldehyde and incubating at 4 °C for 30 min. At the end of the incubation, three washes were performed with 200 µL of PBS at 5 min incubation intervals. Then, 200 µL of Triton X-100 was added to the cell lines and incubated for 30 min at room temperature. After this stage, 100 µL (29 µg) of DPAPA and PSMA-DPAPA NCs, and 100 µL (4.5 µg) of EDTMP and PSMA-EDTMP NCs were added separately for each cell line chamber; the cells were incubated for 2 h in 5% CO_2 and 37 °C. After 2 h, the applied substances were removed from the medium and washed three times with PBS. Lastly, 2 µL/mL DAPI was added, and the related cell images were taken using a fluorescent microscope with a fluorescent microscope (Olympus BX53) 10× green filter. At the same time, cell images were taken using "confocal microscopy 3D fluorescent imaging (Zeiss LSM880, Cambridge, UK)".

2.9.5. MRI of PC-3 and LNCaP Cells with Nanoconjugates

MR imaging of PC-3 and LNCaP cells incorporated with C-Fe_3O_4 nanoconjugates was conducted at T2 phase using a Siemens Verio 3T MRI Scanner (GmbH, Ettlingen, Germany) equipped with a 640 mT/m ID 115 mm gradient. Nanoparticles and nanoconjugates encoded with 1, 2, 3, and 4* were added to the LNCaP (PSMA+) and PC-3 (PSMA−) prostate cancer cell lines.

2.10. Statistical Analysis

Statistical analyses were performed using GraphPad Prism software version 8.0 for Windows (GraphPad Software, San Diego, CA, USA). To evaluate whether the collected numerical data are normally distributed to compare four unpaired groups, Kolmogorov–Smirnov normality tests were applied. The comparison of means between separate groups of numerical variables was performed using a one-way analysis of variance (ANOVA). Nonlinear regression analysis was performed with the GraphPad statistical program using the cytotoxicity (%) values. With this analysis, the IC50 (dose leading to death of 50% of the current cell population) values on the cell lines of all applied substances were determined.

3. Results and Discussion

3.1. Synthesis and Characterization of the Nanoparticles and Nanoconjugates

PSMA-DPAPA/EDTMP NC as a magnetite base nanoconjugate was synthesized to develop a multifunctional theranostic agent for imaging and therapy. First, cubic Fe_3O_4 covered with a layer of silica was synthesized. The silica coating was applied to increase the colloidal stability and biocompatibility of core Fe_3O_4 NPs. HPG, as a biocompatible, multifunctional, hyperbranched dendrimer polymer, was added to the structure to increase the biocompatibility and stability of the nanoconjugate [16]. The obtained samples were characterized by SEM and TEM microscopy. According to SEM and TEM images, C-Fe_3O_4 NPs (Figure 2a) were uniform homogeneous cubic crystal shaped with a particle size of about 38–50 nm similar to previously reported images of cubic NPs [19]. According to SEM images (Figure 2b) the shapes of C-Fe_3O_4-SiO_2 NPs differ comparing to C-Fe_3O_4. This may depend on the result of the silica coating. In addition, SEM images of C-Fe_3O_4-SiO_2-HPG samples show a polymeric structure related to HPG modification (Figure 2c).

Figure 2 shows SEM images of (a) C-Fe_3O_4 nanoparticles, (b) C-Fe_3O_4-SiO_2, (c) C-Fe_3O_4-SiO_2-HPG, and (d) DPAPA NCs. SEM images of C-Fe_3O_4 NPs showed that the cubic NPs agreed with previous reports (Figure 2a) [19]. High-density hydroxyl (–OH) groups on the outer surface of core Fe_3O_4 NPs represent the main source of reactive groups for the subsequent chemical surface. These hydroxyl groups on the surface of the nanoparticle core are combined with the silicic acid which are formed directly from sodium silicate, which polymerizes with the decrease in pH during the silication step. As a result, the resulting silanol groups (Si–OH) are condensed into covalent siloxane bonds (Si–O–Si), leading to the formation of the silica coating layer surrounding the particle core [26]. Moreover, silicated C-Fe$_3$O$_4$ nanoparticles do not aggregate easily as they exhibit higher stability compared to uncoated nanospheres. Therefore, the surface of C-Fe$_3$O$_4$-SiO$_2$ NPs differs from that of C-Fe$_3$O$_4$ NPs according to SEM images (Figure 2b). SEM images of C-Fe$_3$O$_4$-SiO$_2$-HPG also show the polymeric structure of HPG on the surface (Figure 2c) since HPG is a glycerol-derived polymer with a large molecular structure. HPG-coated NPs had wrinkled and folded structures with polymers covering the NP surfaces in the SEM image. Similar SEM images were obtained in studies with HPG [27]. The DPAPA NC SEM image (Figure 2d) shows that DPAPA binds to C-Fe$_3$O$_4$-SiO$_2$-HPG, forming a less porous and more planar morphology. However, in closer images, the porous structure formed on the polymer surface could be seen due to the structural properties of DPAPA.

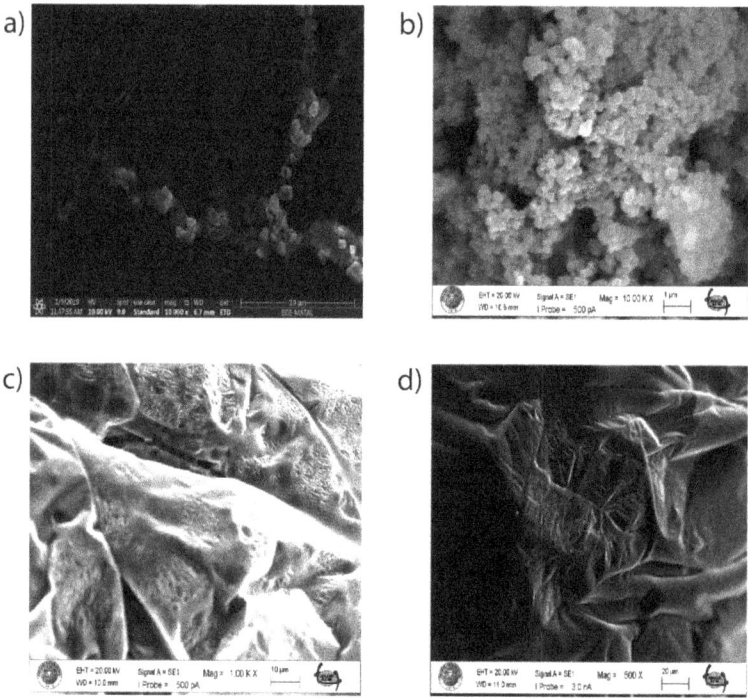

Figure 2. SEM image of obtained nanoparticles and nanoconjugates: (**a**) C-Fe$_3$O$_4$ SEM image, (**b**) C-Fe$_3$O$_4$-SiO$_2$ SEM image, (**c**) C-Fe$_3$O$_4$-SiO$_2$-HPG SEM image, and (**d**) DPAPA NC SEM image.

Figure 3 shows the TEM images of C-Fe$_3$O$_4$ (A), C-Fe$_3$O$_4$-SiO$_2$ (B), and C-Fe$_3$O$_4$-SiO$_2$-HPG (C), which are compatible with cubic Fe$_3$O$_4$ images in the literature [19]. Dark areas or black spots seen in TEM images belong to the Fe$_3$O$_4$ core, whereas the colorless parts belong to silica and HPG polymer due to their lower electron density. Iron gives a more intense appearance compared to other phases. In addition, Fe$_3$O$_4$ NPs are uniformly cubic-shaped with a size from 38 to 50 nm. TEM images showed that the Fe$_3$O$_4$ core is surrounded by SiO$_2$ and the organic phase.

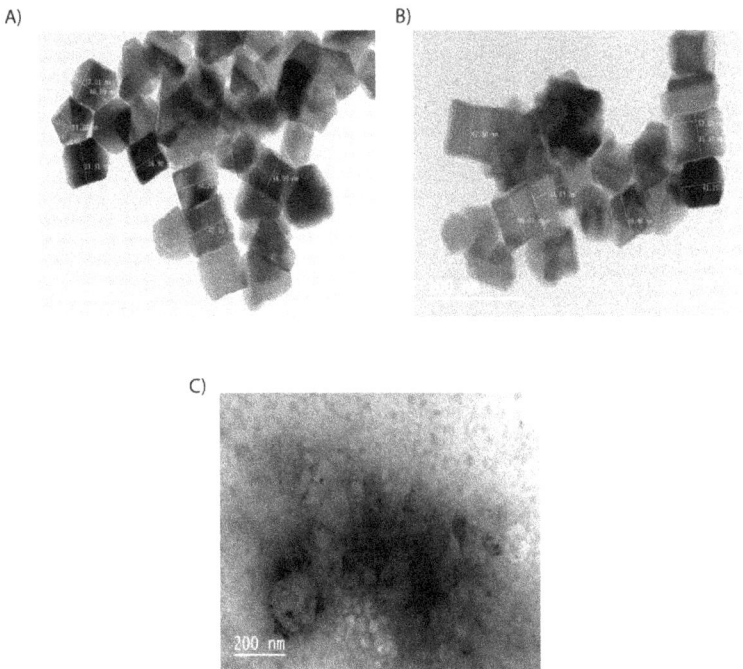

Figure 3. TEM images of NPs and nanoconjugates: (**A**) C-Fe$_3$O$_4$ NPs, (**B**) cubic silica-coated Fe$_3$O$_4$ NPs, and (**C**) cubic HPG-modified and silica-coated Fe$_3$O$_4$ NPs.

The hydrodynamic diameters, zeta potentials and PDI values of the nanoconjugates are given in Table 1. The hydrodynamic sizes of C-Fe$_3$O$_4$ NPs were found to be 116 nm, in accordance with other reports [28], and they increased when the nanoparticles were covered with layers of SiO$_2$, HPG, and DPAPA. Hydrodynamic sizes involving the solvent molecules around the nanoparticles are, therefore, usually measured larger than the dimensions measured by SEM and TEM images. The size distribution of the samples is expressed by the PDI value, where the PDI value and the size homogenization are inversely proportional [29]. The data presented in Table 1 are consistent with the literature [30], indicating a homogenous population of nanoconjugates.

Table 1. Hydrodynamic sizes and zeta potentials of C-Fe$_3$O$_4$ NPs and nanoconjugates (n = 6).

Nanoconjugate	Hydrodynamic Size (d.nm) (n = 3)	Zeta Potential (mV) (n = 3) (pH = 7)	PDI
C-Fe$_3$O$_4$	116 ± 7.90	−18.6 ± 0.60	0.13
C-Fe$_3$O$_4$-SiO$_2$	122 ± 0.20	−21.5 ± 0.01	0.22
C-Fe$_3$O$_4$-SiO$_2$-HPG	145.8 ± 3.50	−18.5 ± 0.20	0.15
DPAPA NC	221.9 ± 16.00	−24.2 ± 0.30	0.06

Zeta potentials (ζ) provide information about the charge distribution on the surface of the nanoconjugates. In general, absolute zeta potential values above 30 mV provide good stability and about 20 mV provide only short-term stability, which is generally considered as a threshold value for the electrostatic stabilization; values in the range −5 mV to +5 mV indicate fast aggregation [31,32]. We performed zeta potential measurements at three various pH (pH = 2, pH = 7, and pH = 12), where, at pH 2 and 12 the hydrodynamic diameter of the NPs did not show any significant changes. According to the literature data, zeta potential values become increasingly negative as the pH value increases [33–35]. At physiological pH (pH = 7.0), the zeta potential value of the DPAPA NC was −24.2 ± 0.30 mV, indicating threshold colloidal stability. At pH = 2, colloidal stability was lost, and zeta potential values of nanoconjugates were +3.20 ± 0.40 mV and +5.40 ± 0.50 mV for C-Fe$_3$O$_4$-SiO$_2$-HPG and DPAPA NC, respectively. In addition, the C-Fe$_3$O$_4$-SiO$_2$-HPG and DPAPA NCs had a zeta potential of −29.10 ± 4.10 and −38.80 ± 3.40 mV at pH = 12, which can be attributed to the –OH groups of HPG molecule. The obtained zeta potential values as a function of pH confirm the presence of amine-decorated HPG on the MNP surface. For aminated HPG-coated MNPs, the particles had higher potential because the introduction of aminated HPG changed the interfacial properties of the particles in the solution. The long molecule chains increased the "water solubility" of particles and protected the particles from congregating [36].

The obtained samples were also characterized by FTIR (Figure 4). The peak observed at wave number 550 cm^{-1} for C-Fe$_3$O$_4$ was related to Fe–O bond [37]. The peak at 1071 cm^{-1} belongs to the Si–O stretch band. FTIR spectra of C-Fe$_3$O$_4$-SiO$_2$-HPG and C-Fe$_3$O$_4$-SiO$_2$-HPG-NH$_2$ showed Fe–O bonds in the 530 cm^{-1} band. Si–O bonds at 1023 cm^{-1}, N–H stretch at 1455 cm^{-1}, C=C tension at 1635 cm^{-1}, C–H tension at 2874 cm^{-1}, and the –OH peak at 3338 cm^{-1} confirm the HPG molecular structure [38]. P–O and P=O stresses were seen at 975 cm^{-1} and 1123 cm^{-1} in the FTIR spectra of C-Fe$_3$O$_4$-SiO$_2$-HPG-NH$_2$ and DPAPA conjugated NPs. The N–H stretch at 1458 cm^{-1} and C=O stretch at 1628 cm^{-1} of –COOH groups were observed, which is consistent with the literature [39]. Thus, FTIR studies confirmed the coating of magnetite nanoparticles with a layer of silica, HPG polymers, and DPAPA molecules.

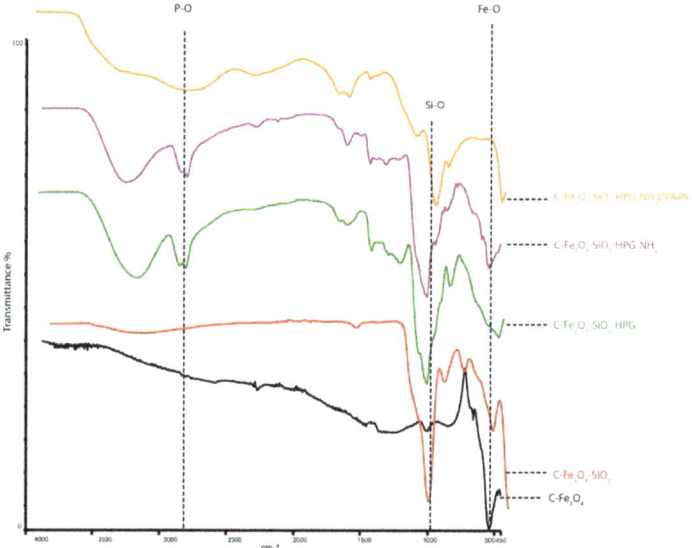

Figure 4. FTIR spectra of NPs and nanoconjugates.

The magnetic properties of nanoparticles and bioconjugates were measured by an applied magnetic field between −3000 and +3000 Gauss. The saturation magnetization of the SPION core was 60 emu/g; however, the coating of the SPIONs with silica and polyglycerol reduced the magnetization significantly. The saturation magnetizations were 25 and 0.1 emu/g for silica-coated magnetite nanospheres and HPG-coated nanoconjugates, respectively. NPs exhibited ferrimagnetic characteristics with a small coercivity value [28,33,40]. A similar value 25 emu/g was reported previously [41] for silica-coated magnetite NPs. Xu et al. pointed out that coating with nonmagnetic materials affected the magnitude of magnetization of the coated magnetic materials due to the quenching of surface moments [42]. Because, in our studies, magnetite NPs were coated with non-magnetic silica and HPG polymer, a similar mechanism could be considered to decrease saturation magnetization after silica and HPG coating [28,32]. Unfortunately, the low values of saturation magnetization do not allow the use of synthesized bioconjugates in magnetic hyperthermia therapy.

3.2. ^{44}Sc Radiolabeling of Nanoconjugates

The scandium radiolabeling yield was measured using a cyclotron producing ^{44}Sc. First, 17.76 MBq ^{44}Sc for EDTMP-PSMA and 17.76 MBq ^{44}Sc for DPAPA-PSMA were added to NP's and incubated for 30 min at 95 °C. After incubation, the samples were centrifuged to remove the unbound ^{44}Sc from the nanoparticles, and their activities were measured. The radiolabeling efficiency for EDTMP-PSMA was found to be almost 98%. For DPAPA-PSMA, the radiolabeling efficiency was found to be almost 97%.

3.3. Stability of the Obtained Radiobioconjugates

For stability studies, human serum (HS) and PBS solutions was used. The samples labeled with ^{44}Sc were incubated at 37 °C. After 1, 2, 3, 4, and 20 h of incubation, samples were measured and centrifuged, and then the supernatant was removed from NPs. NPs without supernatant were measured once more, and the stability of the connection between NP and Sc was determined. As expected, due to the strong complexation of ^{44}Sc by the DOTA ligand, the stability of the radiobioconjugates was high (Table 2).

Table 2. Stability of the ^{44}Sc labeled C-Fe$_3$O$_4$ NC (n = 6).

	1 h	2 h	3 h	4 h	24 h
EDTMP (HS)	93.0	89.7	89.6	90.0	91.7
EDTMP (PBS)	98.9	97.4	97.3	98.3	96.0
DPAPA (HS)	95.3	94.3	92.1	92.2	84.0
DPAPA (PBS)	98.4	96.8	97.4	97.4	92.3

As expected, due to the high thermodynamic and kinetic stability of the DOTA complexes, the stability of the radiobioconjugates was also high.

3.4. Cell Studies

3.4.1. Cell Binding of ^{44}Sc-Labeled Bioconjugates

As presented in Figure 5, both tested compounds bound specifically to PSMA receptors. The significant ($p < 0.05$) decrease in bound fraction confirmed this during the receptor blocking with excess PSMA. The EDTMP- and DPAPA-based conjugates showed a similar percentage of total bound fraction, calculated as 6.6% (EDTMP) and 5.1% (DPAPA), while the specifically bound fraction was 4.6% and 3.1%, respectively. No binding was observed for PSMA-negative PC-3 cells, which directly shows that synthesized conjugates were successfully conjugated with PSMA, and their biological activity was maintained. PSMA-617-DPAPA/EDTMP NCs are PSMA receptor-specific. Loveless et al. showed that PSMA receptors on LNCaP cells were specifically targeted by using [$^{44/47}$Sc]-PSMA-617 at a molar activity of 10 MBq/nmol [43].

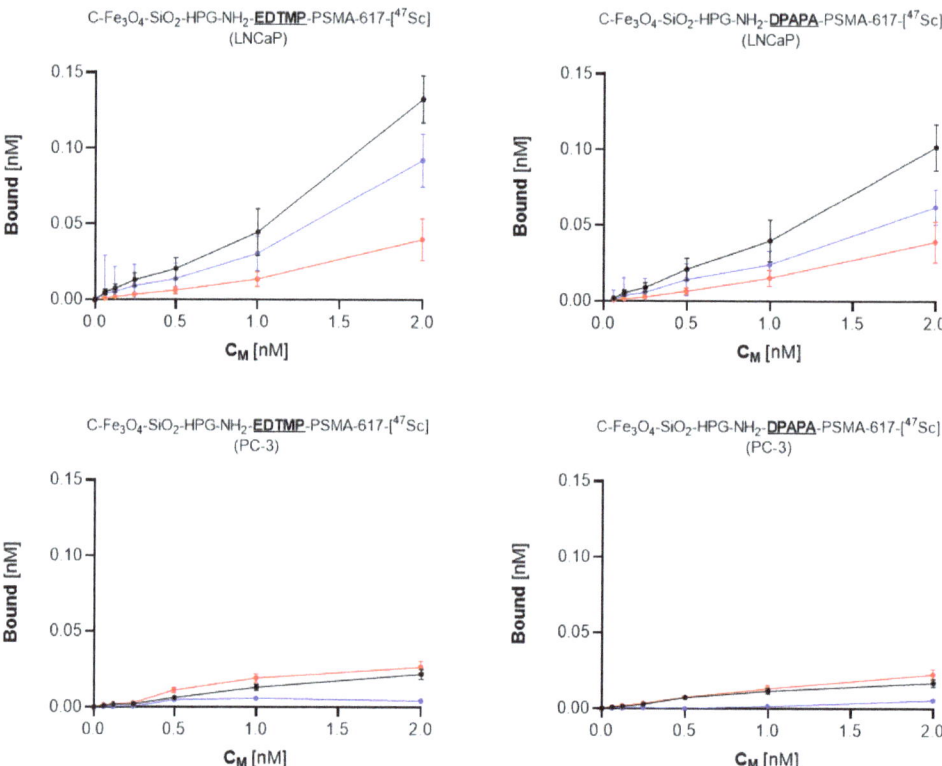

Figure 5. Receptor binding affinity studies of ^{44}Sc labeled EDTMP- and DPAPA-based radiobioconjugates. Upper graphs show data for LNCaP cells; bottom graphs show data for PC-3 cells.

3.4.2. MTT Assay

The percentage viabilities decreased with time in PC-3 and LNCaP cell lines (Figure 6). PSMA-617 conjugated nanoconjugates had a less toxic effect on cells. The affinities of PSMA and PSMA conjugated nanoparticles to LNCaP cells were relatively higher since LNCaP cells are PSMA+ prostate cancer cells [44].

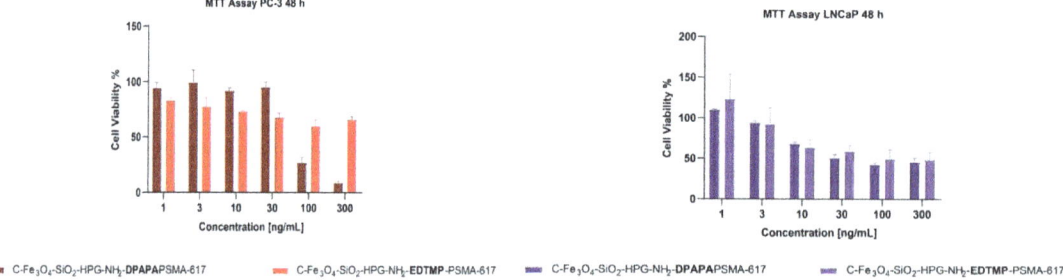

Figure 6. Cell viability of PC-3 and LNCaP cells treated with nanoconjugates after 48 h of incubation.

3.4.3. MTS Assay

Neither EDTMP nor DPAPA conjugates affected the mitochondrial activity of LNCaP and PC-3 cells (Figure 7). This agrees with our expectations, because PSMA function is limited to effective targeting without any therapeutic demands due to its low concentration in bioconjugates. We chose nontoxic nanoconjugates concentration, according to the data shown in Figure 5 (1 ng/mL). A significant decrease in survival fraction was found after 48 and 72 h incubation of ^{47}Sc labeled radiobioconjugates in LNCaP cells (Figure 7). After 48 h, both EDTMP and DPAPA induced a ~40% decrease in metabolically active cells regardless of the activity concentration ($p \leq 0.01$). Subsequently, we found dose-dependent cytotoxicity progression after 72 h. The EDTMP-based radiobioconjugate efficacy was variable from 64.14% ± 5.2% ($p \leq 0.001$) survived fraction (1.25 MBq/mL) to 35.75% ± 3.2% (20 MBq/mL; $p \leq 0.0001$). DPAPA-based radiobioconjugates were slightly more cytotoxic, and 31.22% ± 1.9% of cells remained unaffected after 72 h incubation with 20 MBq/mL of ^{47}Sc ($p \leq 0.0001$). The calculated half maximal inhibitory concentration (IC50) also showed that DPAPA-based conjugates were more effective (IC50 = 5.3 MBq/mL) when compared to EDTMP (IC50 = 7.1 MBq/mL). Any impact of nonradioactive and radioactive conjugates was found for PC-3 cell line, additionally proving specific anticancer activity only against PSMA(+) cells.

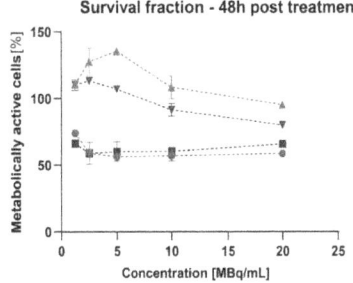

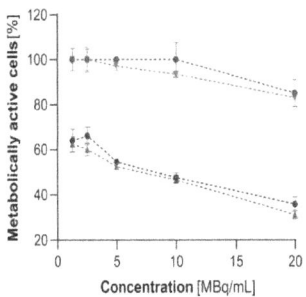

Figure 7. Cell viability of LNCaP and PC-3 cells treated with radiobioconjugates.

3.4.4. Three-Dimensional (3D) Cell Culture Studies

According to data obtained during MTS assay (Figure 7) we found a slight advantage of DPAPA-based NC over EDTMP-based NC. Taking into account the stronger effect (lower IC_{50} and lower cell viability after 72 h), we decided to investigate DPAPA-based NC against 3D cell cultures. In terms of fluorescence spectra, DPAPA and DPAPA NC nanoconjugates presented fluorescence at 290 nm excitation and 420 nm emission wavelengths. Taking advantage of their green fluorescence properties, these nanoconjugates were applied to the prepared PC-3 and LNCaP 3D spheroids, and fluorescence images were obtained (Figure 8).

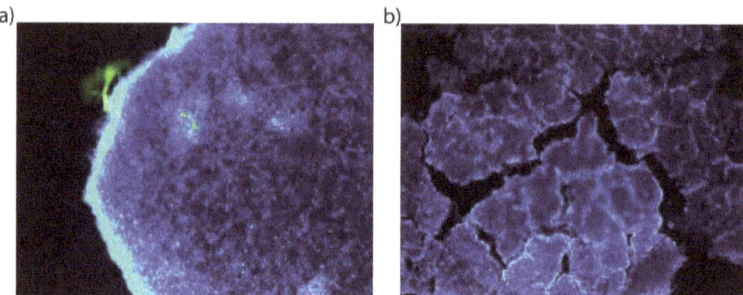

Figure 8. Three-dimensional fluorescence microscope images of (**a**) PC-3 cells (10× objective magnification, green filter) and (**b**) LNCaP cells (10× objective magnification, blue filter). The image of the nanoconjugates applied to the PC-3 cell line in the green filter can be seen. While cell nuclei are seen with DAPI, the intensely glowing region on the cell wall is thought to be the fluorescence feature from our nanoconjugates.

Confocal microscopic images of PSMA-617-DPAPA NC and DPAPA NC applied to the PC-3 cells are shown in Figures 9 and 10. In these images, PSMA-617-DPAPA NC and DPAPA NC are green-colored because of the fluorescence property of DPAPA, while DAPI-stained cell nuclei are seen as blue in the cell nucleus. Images are given with an overlapping blue and red filter.

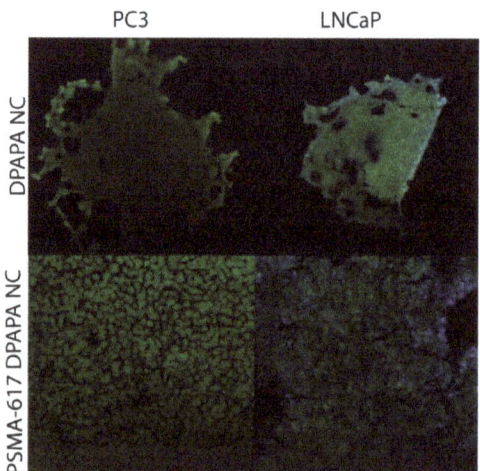

Figure 9. Images of C-Fe$_3$O$_4$-SiO$_2$-HPG-NH$_2$-DPAPA and C-Fe$_3$O$_4$-SiO$_2$-HPG-NH$_2$-DPAPA-PSMA-617 applied to PC-3 and LNCaP three-dimensional cell lines (10× objective magnification taken with blue and red filter).

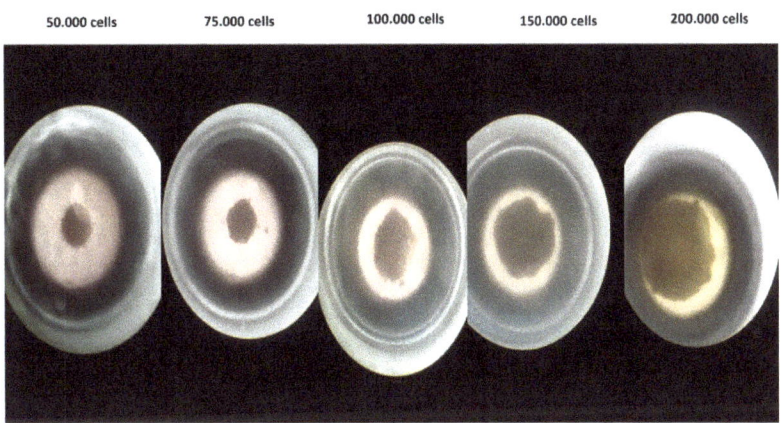

Figure 10. Spheroid images of 3D PC-3 cells (LEICA-DFC280 inverter microscope, 100×).

Confocal microscope images were acquired at 500 nm low-resolution and suggested a maximum cell "thickness" of 9.5 μm. which was in excellent quantitative agreement with S.P.M. measurements in the cell nucleus region. These images also showed that the nanoconjugates were homogeneously distributed in the cell cytoplasm and that DPAPA retained its fluorescence (Figures 9 and 10). DPAPA (similarly to EDTMP) shows the fluorescence properties, and a report with lanthanide complexes showed that it can be used in cell imaging by taking advantage of this property [45].

3.4.5. MRI

MR contrast measurement revealed that the iron contrast could be seen in cell media, although limits were much more significant compared to the PET and SPECT methods (Figure 11). Both SPECT and PET have contrast measurement limits in the picomolar range, while MRI and CT have contrast measurement limits at much higher nmol concentrations [46]. The superior spatial resolution of PET (4–5 mm) makes it more attractive than SPECT (10–15 mm). However, the spatial and temporal resolution of both methods is significantly less than that achieved with MRI or CT. The high sensitivity of nuclear methods combined with the favorable resolution of CT and MRI is the driving force behind hybrid imaging systems such as PET/CT and PET/MRI now available.

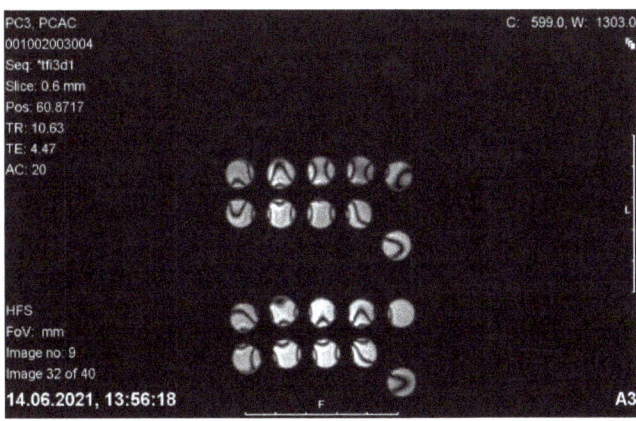

Figure 11. Relaxivity (R2): 0.421/3 T nanoconjugates applied on C-Fe_3O_4 and PC-3 LNCaP) (n = 6).

The MRI imaging potential of Fe_3O_4 nanoconjugates in vivo is essential in terms of adding PET/MRI imaging to the theranostic property of these nanoparticles. In our previous studies, MRI images were taken of prostate tumor-bearing mice given FDG-linked Fe_3O_4 nanoparticles (FDG-MNP), and FDG-MNPs were concentrated in the prostate tumor. At the same time, relatively small amounts were found in organs of other tissues, particularly the spleen and liver, and FDG-MNP concentrations decreased over time in all tissues [47]. In vivo animal MRI images containing Fe_3O_4 and showing the Fe contrast of different conjugate nanoparticles are available in the literature [48,49].

Metastases of prostate cancer cells usually move to the bones. The pelvis and spinal bones are some of the most common areas where prostate cancer spreads. However, radionuclide-labeled phosphonate derivatives are effective for imaging bone metastases and in radionuclide bone pain therapy. While [^{99m}Tc]Tc-diphosphonate imaging is used for imaging, ^{153}Sm- or ^{177}Lu-radiolabeled EDTMP was applied for radionuclide bone pain therapy. Combining both imaging and treatment with the same agent may be advantageous regarding theranostic potential. Therefore, in this study, a phosphate derivative EDTMP conjugate was added to the nanoconjugate enabling imaging of bone metastases with MR and PET techniques. Another advantage of this approach is to increase the hydrophilicity and solubility of the nanoconjugate.

4. Conclusions

In our work, we proposed a new solution that involves the use of multimodal superparamagnetic iron oxide-based nanoparticles (SPIONs), labeled with two scandium radionuclides, ^{44}Sc and ^{47}Sc, that allow for visualization of the cancer tissue and simultaneous direct irradiation of the tumor. The synthesized nanoparticles were conjugated with biologically active PSMA-617 molecules directing to and recognizing the targeted tumor tissue. The proposed multimodal SPIONs are advantageous because they can provide successful diagnosis and therapy even for chemo- and radioresistant tumor cells.

Prostate cancer bone metastases are common at the advanced stage of disease. This issue deserves particular attention due to its huge impact on patient management and the recent introduction of many new therapeutic options. Imaging of bone metastases is essential to localize lesions, determine their size and number, and examine features and changes during treatment. Therefore, in the present study, the phosphonates EDTMP and DPAPA were added to the nanoconjugate, which enabled MR and PET imaging of bone metastases and palliative therapy with β^- radiation emitted by ^{47}Sc.

We think that a practical application of our proposal is a stable magnetic PSMA radiobioconjugate labeled with ^{44}Sc and ^{47}Sc, which according to the in vivo studies, can be used for aggressive prostate cancer. We also expect that our results can be helpful in designing other multimodal magnetic radiopharmaceuticals applied in simultaneous PET and NMR diagnosis and radionuclide therapy.

Author Contributions: Conceptualization, P.Ü.; methodology, P.Ü., V.Y., E.T., K.B.K., R.W., K.W., K.Ż.-M. and A.M.-P.; software, V.Y., E.T. and K.B.K.; formal analysis, P.Ü., V.Y., E.T., K.B.K., R.W., K.W., K.Ż.-M. and A.M-P.; investigation, P.Ü., V.Y., E.T., K.B.K., R.W., K.W., K.Ż.-M. and A.M.-P.; resources, A.B. and P.Ü.; data curation, V.Y., E.T., K.B.K., R.W. and K.W.; writing P.Ü., V.Y., E.T., K.B.K., R.W., K.W., K.Ż-M., A.M.-P. and A.B.; original draft preparation, P.Ü., V.Y., E.T., K.B.K., R.W., K.W., K.Ż.-M., A.M.-P. and A.B.; writing—review and editing, P.Ü., V.Y., E.T., K.B.K., R.W., K.W., K.Ż.-M., A.M.-P. and A.B.; visualization, V.Y.; supervision, P.Ü. and A.B.; project administration, P.Ü. and A.B.; funding acquisition, P.Ü. and A.B. All authors have read and agreed to the published version of the manuscript.

Funding: This research was funded by TUBİTAK Grant 218S749 by The Scientific And Technological Research Council of Türkiye and POLTUR3/Nanotheran/3/2020 grant funded by the National Center for Research and Development (NCBR), Poland.

Data Availability Statement: Data are available on request.

Conflicts of Interest: The authors declare no conflict of interest.

References

1. Jahandar, M.; Zarrabi, A.; Shokrgozar, M.A.; Mousavi, H. Synthesis, Characterization and Application of Polyglycerol Coated Fe$_3$O$_4$ Nanoparticles as a Nano-Theranostics Agent. *Mater. Res. Express* **2015**, *2*, 125002. [CrossRef]
2. Lübbe, A.S.; Alexiou, C.; Bergemann, C. Clinical Applications of Magnetic Drug Targeting. *J. Surg. Res.* **2001**, *95*, 200–206. [CrossRef]
3. Cędrowska, E.; Pruszyński, M.; Gawęda, W.; Żuk, M.; Krysiński, P.; Bruchertseifer, F.; Morgenstern, A.; Karageorgou, M.-A.; Bouziotis, P.; Bilewicz, A. Trastuzumab Conjugated Superparamagnetic Iron Oxide Nanoparticles Labeled with 225Ac as a Perspective Tool for Combined α-Radioimmunotherapy and Magnetic Hyperthermia of HER2-Positive Breast Cancer. *Molecules* **2020**, *25*, 1025. [CrossRef]
4. Gawęda, W.; Pruszyński, M.; Cędrowska, E.; Rodak, M.; Majkowska-Pilip, A.; Gaweł, D.; Bruchertseifer, F.; Morgenstern, A.; Bilewicz, A. Trastuzumab Modified Barium Ferrite Magnetic Nanoparticles Labeled with Radium-223: A New Potential Radiobioconjugate for Alpha Radioimmunotherapy. *Nanomaterials* **2020**, *10*, 2067. [CrossRef] [PubMed]
5. Żuk, M.; Podgórski, R.; Ruszczyńska, A.; Ciach, T.; Majkowska-Pilip, A.; Bilewicz, A.; Krysiński, P. Multifunctional Nanoparticles Based on Iron Oxide and Gold-198 Designed for Magnetic Hyperthermia and Radionuclide Therapy as a Potential Tool for Combined HER2-Positive Cancer Treatment. *Pharmaceutics* **2022**, *14*, 1680. [CrossRef] [PubMed]
6. Chen, J.; Zhu, S.; Tong, L.; Li, J.; Chen, F.; Han, Y.; Zhao, M.; Xiong, W. Superparamagnetic Iron Oxide Nanoparticles Mediated 131I-HVEGF SiRNA Inhibits Hepatocellular Carcinoma Tumor Growth in Nude Mice. *BMC Cancer* **2014**, *14*, 114. [CrossRef]
7. Patel, N.; Duffy, B.A.; Badar, A.; Lythgoe, M.F.; Årstad, E. Bimodal Imaging of Inflammation with SPECT/CT and MRI Using Iodine-125 Labeled VCAM-1 Targeting Microparticle Conjugates. *Bioconjug. Chem.* **2015**, *26*, 1542–1549. [CrossRef] [PubMed]
8. Wang, H.; Kumar, R.; Nagesha, D.; Duclos, R.I.; Sridhar, S.; Gatley, S.J. Integrity of 111In-Radiolabeled Superparamagnetic Iron Oxide Nanoparticles in the Mouse. *Nucl. Med. Biol.* **2015**, *42*, 65–70. [CrossRef]
9. Azadbakht, B.; Afarideh, H.; Ghannadi-Maragheh, M.; Bahrami-Samani, A.; Yousefnia, H. Absorbed Doses in Humans from 188 Re-Rituximab in the Free Form and Bound to Superparamagnetic Iron Oxide Nanoparticles: Biodistribution Study in Mice. *Appl. Radiat. Isot.* **2018**, *131*, 96–102. [CrossRef] [PubMed]
10. Turrina, C.; Oppelt, A.; Mitzkus, M.; Berensmeier, S.; Schwaminger, S.P. Silica-Coated Superparamagnetic Iron Oxide Nanoparticles: New Insights into the Influence of Coating Thickness on the Particle Properties and Lasioglossin Binding. *MRS Commun.* **2022**, *12*, 632–639. [CrossRef]
11. Khan, A.; Malik, S.; Bilal, M.; Ali, N.; Ni, L.; Gao, X.; Hong, K. Polymer-Coated Magnetic Nanoparticles. In *Biopolymeric Nanomaterials*; Elsevier: Amsterdam, The Netherlands, 2021; pp. 275–292.
12. Chapa Gonzalez, C.; Martínez Pérez, C.A.; Martínez Martínez, A.; Olivas Armendáriz, I.; Zavala Tapia, O.; Martel-Estrada, A.; García-Casillas, P.E. Development of Antibody-Coated Magnetite Nanoparticles for Biomarker Immobilization. *J. Nanomater.* **2014**, *2014*, 978284. [CrossRef]
13. Li, M.; Neoh, K.-G.; Wang, R.; Zong, B.-Y.; Tan, J.Y.; Kang, E.-T. Methotrexate-Conjugated and Hyperbranched Polyglycerol-Grafted Fe3O4 Magnetic Nanoparticles for Targeted Anticancer Effects. *Eur. J. Pharm. Sci.* **2013**, *48*, 111–120. [CrossRef] [PubMed]
14. Zhao, S.; Yu, X.; Qian, Y.; Chen, W.; Shen, J. Multifunctional Magnetic Iron Oxide Nanoparticles: An Advanced Platform for Cancer Theranostics. *Theranostics* **2020**, *10*, 6278–6309. [CrossRef] [PubMed]
15. Mostaghasi, E.; Zarepour, A.; Zarrabi, A. Folic Acid Armed Fe3O4-HPG Nanoparticles as a Safe Nano Vehicle for Biomedical Theranostics. *J. Taiwan Inst. Chem. Eng.* **2018**, *82*, 33–41. [CrossRef]
16. Heydari Sheikh Hossein, H.; Jabbari, I.; Zarepour, A.; Zarrabi, A.; Ashrafizadeh, M.; Taherian, A.; Makvandi, P. Functionalization of Magnetic Nanoparticles by Folate as Potential MRI Contrast Agent for Breast Cancer Diagnostics. *Molecules* **2020**, *25*, 4053. [CrossRef] [PubMed]
17. Dendy, P.P. Further Studies on the Uptake of Synkavit and a Radioactive Analogue into Tumour Cells in Tissue Culture. *Br. J. Cancer* **1970**, *24*, 817–825. [CrossRef]
18. Lorente, J.A.; Morote, J.; Raventos, C.; Encabo, G.; Valenzuela, H. Clinical Efficacy of Bone Alkaline Phosphatase and Prostate Specific Antigen in the Diagnosis of Bone Metastasis in Prostate Cancer. *J. Urol.* **1996**, *155*, 1348–1351. [CrossRef]
19. Martinez-Boubeta, C.; Simeonidis, K.; Makridis, A.; Angelakeris, M.; Iglesias, O.; Guardia, P.; Cabot, A.; Yedra, L.; Estradé, S.; Peiró, F.; et al. Learning from Nature to Improve the Heat Generation of Iron-Oxide Nanoparticles for Magnetic Hyperthermia Applications. *Sci. Rep.* **2013**, *3*, 1652. [CrossRef]
20. Heister, E.; Neves, V.; Tîlmaciu, C.; Lipert, K.; Beltrán, V.S.; Coley, H.M.; Silva, S.R.P.; McFadden, J. Triple Functionalisation of Single-Walled Carbon Nanotubes with Doxorubicin, a Monoclonal Antibody, and a Fluorescent Marker for Targeted Cancer Therapy. *Carbon* **2009**, *47*, 2152–2160. [CrossRef]

21. Sadri, N.; Moghadam, M.; Abbasi, A. MoO$_2$(Acac)$_2$@Fe$_3$O$_4$/SiO$_2$/HPG/COSH Nanostructures: Novel Synthesis, Characterization and Catalyst Activity for Oxidation of Olefins and Sulfides. *J. Mater. Sci. Mater. Electron.* **2018**, *29*, 11991–12000. [CrossRef]
22. Babu, P.; Sinha, S.; Surolia, A. Sugar−Quantum Dot Conjugates for a Selective and Sensitive Detection of Lectins. *Bioconjug. Chem.* **2007**, *18*, 146–151. [CrossRef]
23. Bahrami Samani, A.; Ghannadi-Maragheh, M.; Jalilian, A.; Meftahi, M.; Shirvani, S.; Moradkhani, S. Production, Quality Control and Biological Evaluation of 153Sm-EDTMP in Wild-Type Rodents. *Iran. J. Nucl. Med.* **2009**, *7*, 12–19.
24. Minegishi, K.; Nagatsu, K.; Fukada, M.; Suzuki, H.; Ohya, T.; Zhang, M.-R. Production of Scandium-43 and -47 from a Powdery Calcium Oxide Target via the Nat/44Ca(α,x)-Channel. *Appl. Radiat. Isot.* **2016**, *116*, 8–12. [CrossRef]
25. Pruszyński, M.; Majkowska-Pilip, A.; Loktionova, N.S.; Eppard, E.; Roesch, F. Radiolabeling of DOTATOC with the Long-Lived Positron Emitter 44Sc. *Appl. Radiat. Isot.* **2012**, *70*, 974–979. [CrossRef] [PubMed]
26. White, L.D.; Tripp, C.P. Reaction of (3-Aminopropyl)Dimethylethoxysilane with Amine Catalysts on Silica Surfaces. *J. Colloid Interface Sci.* **2000**, *232*, 400–407. [CrossRef]
27. Zhang, P.; Li, Y.; Tang, W.; Zhao, J.; Jing, L.; McHugh, K.J. Theranostic Nanoparticles with Disease-Specific Administration Strategies. *Nano Today* **2022**, *42*, 101335. [CrossRef]
28. Pourmiri, S.; Tzitzios, V.; Hadjipanayis, G.C.; Meneses Brassea, B.P.; El-Gendy, A.A. Magnetic Properties and Hyperthermia Behavior of Iron Oxide Nanoparticle Clusters. *AIP Adv.* **2019**, *9*, 125033. [CrossRef]
29. Vasić, K.; Knez, Ž.; Konstantinova, E.A.; Kokorin, A.I.; Gyergyek, S.; Leitgeb, M. Structural and Magnetic Characteristics of Carboxymethyl Dextran Coated Magnetic Nanoparticles: From Characterization to Immobilization Application. *React. Funct. Polym.* **2020**, *148*, 104481. [CrossRef]
30. Feuser, P.E.; dos Santos Bubniak, L.; dos Santos Silva, M.C.; da Cas Viegas, A.; Fernandes, A.C.; Ricci-Junior, E.; Nele, M.; Tedesco, A.C.; Sayer, C.; de Araújo, P.H.H. Encapsulation of Magnetic Nanoparticles in Poly(Methyl Methacrylate) by Miniemulsion and Evaluation of Hyperthermia in U87MG Cells. *Eur. Polym. J.* **2015**, *68*, 355–365. [CrossRef]
31. Honary, S.; Zahir, F. Effect of Zeta Potential on the Properties of Nano-Drug Delivery Systems—A Review (Part 1). *Trop. J. Pharm. Res.* **2013**, *12*, 255–264. [CrossRef]
32. Çitoğlu, S.; Coşkun, Ö.D.; Tung, L.D.; Onur, M.A.; Thanh, N.T.K. DMSA-Coated Cubic Iron Oxide Nanoparticles as Potential Therapeutic Agents. *Nanomedicine* **2021**, *16*, 925–941. [CrossRef]
33. Wang, J.; Zheng, S.; Shao, Y.; Liu, J.; Xu, Z.; Zhu, D. Amino-Functionalized Fe$_3$O$_4$@SiO$_2$ Core–Shell Magnetic Nanomaterial as a Novel Adsorbent for Aqueous Heavy Metals Removal. *J. Colloid Interface Sci.* **2010**, *349*, 293–299. [CrossRef]
34. Shapiro, E.M.; Skrtic, S.; Koretsky, A.P. Sizing It up: Cellular MRI Using Micron-Sized Iron Oxide Particles. *Magn. Reason. Med.* **2005**, *53*, 329–338. [CrossRef]
35. Tang, F.; Li, L.; Chen, D. Mesoporous Silica Nanoparticles: Synthesis, Biocompatibility and Drug Delivery. *Adv. Mat.* **2012**, *24*, 1504–1534. [CrossRef] [PubMed]
36. Wang, S.-Y.; Chen, X.-X.; Li, Y.; Zhang, Y.-Y. Application of Multimodality Imaging Fusion Technology in Diagnosis and Treatment of Malignant Tumors under the Precision Medicine Plan. *Chin. Med. J.* **2016**, *129*, 2991–2997. [CrossRef]
37. Yasakci, V.; Tekin, V.; Guldu, O.K.; Evren, V.; Unak, P. Hyaluronic Acid-Modified [19F]FDG-Conjugated Magnetite Nanoparticles: In Vitro Bioaffinities and HPLC Analyses in Organs. *J. Radioanal. Nucl. Chem.* **2018**, *318*, 1973–1989. [CrossRef]
38. Sigma-Aldrich IR Spectrum Table & Chart. Available online: https://www.sigmaaldrich.com/PL/pl/technical-documents/technical-article/analytical-chemistry/photometry-and-reflectometry/ir-spectrum-table (accessed on 15 February 2023).
39. Hampton, C.; Demoin, D. Vibrational Spectroscopy Tutorial: Sulfur and Phosphorus; Fall 2010 Organic Spectroscopy Dr. Rainer E. Glaser; University of Missouri: Columbia, MO, USA, 2010.
40. Bekiş, R.; Medine, İ.; Dağdeviren, K.; Ertay, T.; Ünak, P. A New Agent for Sentinel Lymph Node Detection: Preliminary Results. *J. Radioanal. Nucl. Chem.* **2011**, *290*, 277–282. [CrossRef]
41. Medine, E.I.; Ünak, P.; Sakarya, S.; Özkaya, F. Investigation of in Vitro Efficiency of Magnetic Nanoparticle-Conjugated 125I-Uracil Glucuronides in Adenocarcinoma Cells. *J. Nanopart. Res.* **2011**, *13*, 4703–4715. [CrossRef]
42. Xu, Y.H.; Bai, J.; Wang, J.-P. High-Magnetic-Moment Multifunctional Nanoparticles for Nanomedicine Applications. *J. Magn. Magn. Mater.* **2007**, *311*, 131–134. [CrossRef]
43. Loveless, C.S.; Blanco, J.R.; Diehl, G.L.; Elbahrawi, R.T.; Carzaniga, T.S.; Braccini, S.; Lapi, S.E. Cyclotron Production and Separation of Scandium Radionuclides from Natural Titanium Metal and Titanium Dioxide Targets. *J. Nucl. Med.* **2021**, *62*, 131–136. [CrossRef] [PubMed]
44. Xing, Y.; Xu, K.; Li, S.; Cao, L.; Nan, Y.; Li, Q.; Li, W.; Hong, Z. A Single-Domain Antibody-Based Anti-PSMA Recombinant Immunotoxin Exhibits Specificity and Efficacy for Prostate Cancer Therapy. *Int. J. Mol. Sci.* **2021**, *22*, 5501. [CrossRef] [PubMed]
45. Li, R.; Ji, Z.; Dong, J.; Chang, C.H.; Wang, X.; Sun, B.; Wang, M.; Liao, Y.-P.; Zink, J.I.; Nel, A.E.; et al. Enhancing the Imaging and Biosafety of Upconversion Nanoparticles through Phosphonate Coating. *ACS Nano* **2015**, *9*, 3293–3306. [CrossRef] [PubMed]
46. Sadeghi, M.M.; Glover, D.K.; Lanza, G.M.; Fayad, Z.A.; Johnson, L.L. Imaging Atherosclerosis and Vulnerable Plaque. *J. Nucl. Med.* **2010**, *51*, 51S–65S. [CrossRef]
47. Aras, O.; Pearce, G.; Watkins, A.J.; Nurili, F.; Medine, E.I.; Guldu, O.K.; Tekin, V.; Wong, J.; Ma, X.; Ting, R.; et al. An In-Vivo Pilot Study into the Effects of FDG-MNP in Cancer in Mice. *PLoS ONE* **2018**, *13*, e0202482. [CrossRef]

48. Kim, B.M.; Lee, D.R.; Park, J.S.; Bae, I.; Lee, Y. Liquid Crystal Nanoparticle Formulation as an Oral Drug Delivery System for Liver-Specific Distribution. *Int. J. Nanomed.* **2016**, *11*, 853. [CrossRef] [PubMed]
49. Arias-Ramos, N.; Ibarra, L.E.; Serrano-Torres, M.; Yagüe, B.; Caverzán, M.D.; Chesta, C.A.; Palacios, R.E.; López-Larrubia, P. Iron Oxide Incorporated Conjugated Polymer Nanoparticles for Simultaneous Use in Magnetic Resonance and Fluorescent Imaging of Brain Tumors. *Pharmaceutics* **2021**, *13*, 1258. [CrossRef] [PubMed]

Disclaimer/Publisher's Note: The statements, opinions and data contained in all publications are solely those of the individual author(s) and contributor(s) and not of MDPI and/or the editor(s). MDPI and/or the editor(s) disclaim responsibility for any injury to people or property resulting from any ideas, methods, instructions or products referred to in the content.

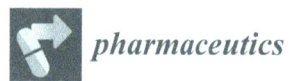

Article

Paclitaxel-Loaded Lipid-Coated Magnetic Nanoparticles for Dual Chemo-Magnetic Hyperthermia Therapy of Melanoma

Relton R. Oliveira [1], Emílio R. Cintra [1], Ailton A. Sousa-Junior [1], Larissa C. Moreira [2], Artur C. G. da Silva [2], Ana Luiza R. de Souza [1], Marize C. Valadares [2], Marcus S. Carrião [3], Andris F. Bakuzis [3,4] and Eliana M. Lima [1,4,*]

[1] FarmaTec—Laboratory of Pharmaceutical Technology, School of Pharmacy, Federal University of Goiás, Alameda Flamboyant, Qd. K, Ed. LIFE, Parque Tecnológico Samambaia, Goiânia 74690-631, Brazil
[2] ToxIn—Laboratory of Education and Research in In Vitro Toxicology, Federal University of Goiás, Alameda Flamboyant, Qd. K, Ed. LIFE, Parque Tecnológico Samambaia, Goiânia 74690-631, Brazil
[3] Physics Institute, Federal University of Goiás, Avenida Esperança, s/n, Campus Samambaia, Goiânia 74690-900, Brazil
[4] CNanoMed—Nanomedicine Integrated Research Center, Federal University of Goiás, Alameda Flamboyant, Qd. K, Ed. LIFE, Parque Tecnológico Samambaia, Goiânia 74690-631, Brazil
* Correspondence: emlima@ufg.br

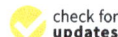

Citation: Oliveira, R.R.; Cintra, E.R.; Sousa-Junior, A.A.; Moreira, L.C.; da Silva, A.C.G.; de Souza, A.L.R.; Valadares, M.C.; Carrião, M.S.; Bakuzis, A.F.; Lima, E.M. Paclitaxel-Loaded Lipid-Coated Magnetic Nanoparticles for Dual Chemo-Magnetic Hyperthermia Therapy of Melanoma. *Pharmaceutics* **2023**, *15*, 818. https://doi.org/10.3390/pharmaceutics15030818

Academic Editors: Xiangyang Shi and Constantin Mihai Lucaciu

Received: 30 December 2022
Revised: 17 February 2023
Accepted: 1 March 2023
Published: 2 March 2023

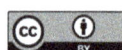

Copyright: © 2023 by the authors. Licensee MDPI, Basel, Switzerland. This article is an open access article distributed under the terms and conditions of the Creative Commons Attribution (CC BY) license (https://creativecommons.org/licenses/by/4.0/).

Abstract: Melanoma is the most aggressive and metastasis-prone form of skin cancer. Conventional therapies include chemotherapeutic agents, either as small molecules or carried by FDA-approved nanostructures. However, systemic toxicity and side effects still remain as major drawbacks. With the advancement of nanomedicine, new delivery strategies emerge at a regular pace, aiming to overcome these challenges. Stimulus-responsive drug delivery systems might considerably reduce systemic toxicity and side-effects by limiting drug release to the affected area. Herein, we report the development of paclitaxel-loaded lipid-coated manganese ferrite magnetic nanoparticles (PTX-LMNP) as magnetosomes synthetic analogs, envisaging the combined chemo-magnetic hyperthermia treatment of melanoma. PTX-LMNP physicochemical properties were verified, including their shape, size, crystallinity, FTIR spectrum, magnetization profile, and temperature profile under magnetic hyperthermia (MHT). Their diffusion in porcine ear skin (a model for human skin) was investigated after intradermal administration via fluorescence microscopy. Cumulative PTX release kinetics under different temperatures, either preceded or not by MHT, were assessed. Intrinsic cytotoxicity against B16F10 cells was determined via neutral red uptake assay after 48 h of incubation (long-term assay), as well as B16F10 cells viability after 1 h of incubation (short-term assay), followed by MHT. PTX-LMNP-mediated MHT triggers PTX release, allowing its thermal-modulated local delivery to diseased sites, within short timeframes. Moreover, half-maximal PTX inhibitory concentration (IC_{50}) could be significantly reduced relatively to free PTX (142,500×) and Taxol® (340×). Therefore, the dual chemo-MHT therapy mediated by intratumorally injected PTX-LMNP stands out as a promising alternative to efficiently deliver PTX to melanoma cells, consequently reducing systemic side effects commonly associated with conventional chemotherapies.

Keywords: paclitaxel; magnetosomes; triggered release; magnetic hyperthermia; B16F10 cells

1. Introduction

Skin cancers are usually classified as either non-melanoma or melanoma. In global cancer statistics, non-melanoma skin cancers are often not reported since their incidence is extremely frequent worldwide relative to all the other cancer types. Additionally, since instances of non-melanoma skin cancers are frequently treated by primary care clinicians, the risks posed by such cancers tend to be underreported [1,2]. In contrast, melanoma is the 17th most common cancer worldwide [2]. It represents almost half of the cases among white populations. Of all skin cancers, melanoma is the most aggressive form, affecting deeper layers of the skin and having greater potential for metastasis [3].

Anti-melanoma therapies based on conventional chemotherapy are frequently ineffective. Therefore, alternatives to improve the prognostics have been explored. Some studies have demonstrated the efficacy of paclitaxel (PTX), a triterpene drug extracted from *Taxus brevifolia*, as a single agent or in combination with carboplatin to treat metastatic melanoma [4–7]. PTX inhibits cell growth by interacting with the microtubules through a non-covalent bond with tubulins, thus blocking mitosis [8,9].

Despite its potent antiproliferative effects, PTX presents major drawbacks, including systemic toxicity, due to its non-selective distribution to normal cells, and low water solubility. Hence, encapsulation of PTX into drug delivery systems, such as liposomes [10–12], magnetic nanoparticles [13–15], polymeric nanoparticles [16,17], solid lipid nanoparticles [18–20], as well as micelles [21,22], has been extensively investigated as an alternative to commercial formulations available in the market (Abraxane® and Taxol®). Additionally, strategies comprising the combination of chemotherapeutic agents with other therapeutic modalities, such as photoinduced (e.g., photodynamic therapy) and heat-mediated therapies (e.g., photothermal therapy and magnetic hyperthermia) have been assessed, aiming to enhance treatment efficacy, while reducing chemotherapy side effects [23–28].

In particular, magnetic hyperthermia (MHT) emerges as a promising technique to treat cancers, based on its selective heat delivery to tumor cells, leading to cell death, either as a monotherapy, with the magnetothermal converting agents intratumorally injected so as to optimize the thermal dose, or in combination with chemotherapy or radiation therapy [27]. In MHT, an alternating magnetic field (AMF) is applied to the tumor region, where magnetic nanoparticles were previously injected [27,29]. Systemic administration is a major challenge, since interactions of nanoparticles with non-targeted tissues, particularly along the bloodstream, lead to nonspecific and inefficient delivery, consequently hindering the induction of thermal doses within therapeutic ranges at biologically safe regimes [30–33].

Excited by the AMF, the magnetic nanoparticles dissipate heat as a result of the interaction of their magnetic moments with the AMF, inducing a biological response. This response can range from a change in transport processes across the cell membranes to a modulation in the expression of specific molecules, eventually culminating with cell death by apoptosis or necrosis, depending on the thermal dose [27,29,34–36]. Clinical use of MHT, however, depends on a relatively homogeneous distribution of magnetic nanoparticles with improved SLP (specific loss power) within a significant volume of the tumor tissue [32]. Moreover, the range of field amplitudes and frequencies allowed for biologically safe conditions is limited, so as to prevent nonspecific heating (induced by eddy currents), as well as peripheral nerve stimulation and even cardiac muscle stimulation [32,33]. Thereby, MHT is currently being used in the clinic in combination with other therapies. Particularly, researchers have combined chemotherapy agents and magnetic nanoparticles aiming to enhance the pharmacological efficacy of the former against various types of cancer via dual chemo-MHT therapy [37–41].

Nevertheless, to fulfill these purposes, magnetic nanoparticles must exhibit specific properties, which are dependent on their size, shape, composition, collective organization, as well as on the frequency and amplitude of the AMF to which they are submitted [25,27,28,42]. An interesting approach, which has received increasing attention, is the use of magnetosomes in MHT [43–47]. Magnetosomes are magnetic nanoparticles (especially magnetite, Fe_3O_4) coated by a phospholipid bilayer, a product of magnetotactic bacteria [48]. Due to their biological nature, they are considered biocompatible and safe when used as a delivery framework [49]. However, the industrial-scale biosynthesis of magnetosomes would be a challenging task, justifying the search for synthetic analogs.

Herein, we report the development and characterization of thermoresponsive PTX-loaded lipid-coated magnetic nanoparticles (PTX-LMNP) that are conceptually synthetic analogs of magnetosomes. Their distribution in a skin model after intradermal injection was investigated. The influence of MHT both on their PTX release profiles and on their cytotoxicity against B16F10 melanoma cells were assessed. Our two initial hypotheses were: (1) PTX release from PTX-LMNP can be modulated by temperature (hence, by MHT) and (2) the combination of chemotherapy and MHT will result in an enhanced cytotoxicity against B16F10 melanoma cells.

2. Materials and Methods

2.1. Materials

Methylamine, manganese II chloride ($MnCl_2 \cdot 4H_2O$), iron III chloride ($FeCl_3 \cdot 6H_2O$), iron III nitrate ($Fe(NO_3)_3 \cdot 9H_2O$), sodium oleate (SO), rhodamine, Dulbecco's Modified Eagle Medium (DMEM), fetal bovine serum (FBS), trypsin-EDTA, Hoechst stain solution, and neutral red were purchased from Sigma Aldrich® (St, Louis, MO, USA). Soy phosphatidylcholine (PC) was bought from Lipoid® (Ludwigshafen, Germany). Paclitaxel (PTX) was acquired from LC Laboratories (United States). Penicillin/streptomycin was obtained from Gibco™ (Waltham, MA, USA). HPLC grade solvents were purchased from J.T. Baker (Radnor, PA, USA). B16F10 murine melanoma cells were provided by Banco de Células do Rio de Janeiro (BCRJ, Rio de Janeiro, Brazil). Ultrapure Milli-Q water was used throughout the experiments. All other reagents and solvents used were of analytical grade of superior.

2.2. Synthesis of Manganese Ferrite ($MnFe_2O_4$) Magnetic Nanoparticles (MNP)

Manganese ferrite ($MnFe_2O_4$) magnetic nanoparticles (MNP) were prepared by coprecipitation in methylamine, as previously reported [50]. Briefly, 90 mL of methylamine were first diluted in 400 mL of ultrapure water. Continuous magnetic stirring and heating were applied until boiling. Then, 50 mL of $MnCl_2$ (0.5 M) and 50 mL of $FeCl_3$ (1 M) aqueous solutions were poured in. Upon boiling, the mixture remained under stirring and heating for 30 min, during which a dark precipitate gradually formed. The ensemble was then left for cooling at room temperature for additional 30 min, at the end of which the precipitate containing $MnFe_2O_4$ MNP was magnetically separated and washed three times in water.

To protect the MNP surfaces from corrosion and oxidation, passivation with $Fe(NO_3)_3$ was performed, as previously described [50,51]. Briefly, 50 mL of HNO_3 (0.5 M) and 50 mL of $Fe(NO_3)_3$ (0.5 M) aqueous solutions were poured on the MNP precipitate, followed by magnetic stirring and heating until boiling. Upon boiling, the mixture was left under stirring and heating for 30 min, at the end of which the ensemble was allowed to cool down. The passivated MNP were then magnetically separated and washed three times in acetone. Most of the MNP were stored in the fridge for later use, still in acetone. For characterization purposes, however, part of the synthesized MNP were further coated with citrate ions and resuspended in water, as previously reported [50].

2.3. Characterization of $MnFe_2O_4$ MNP

$MnFe_2O_4$ MNP aliquots were submitted to transmission electron microscopy (TEM, Jeol, JEM-2100, Thermo Scientific, Waltham, MA, USA), so that their shape and size distribution could be verified. Additionally, their crystallinity and size were assessed via X-ray diffraction (XRD, XRD-6000, Shimadzu, Kyoto, Japan). Mean diameters were then calculated via Scherrer's equation:

$$D = \frac{k\lambda}{\beta \cos \theta} \quad (1)$$

where k is the Scherrer's constant (0.89), λ is the wavelength of the X-ray beam (0.154 nm), β is the full width at half-maximum (in rad) of the diffractogram peak under analysis, and θ is its corresponding Bragg's angle [52].

Magnetization profiles of both powder and fluid samples were obtained by vibrating sample magnetometry (VSM, EV9 Magnetometer, ADE Magnetics). Specific saturation magnetizations of these samples were then used to determine the MNP colloid concentration, as previously reported [50]. The behavior of powder samples under magnetic hyperthermia (MHT) was observed for different alternating magnetic field (AMF) amplitudes (100–342 Oe) at 310 kHz (MagneTherm, NanoTherics®). Temperature measurements were performed using a fiber optic temperature sensor (Luxtron®).

Specific loss power (SLP) values were obtained (in W/g) as follows:

$$\text{SLP} = \frac{\rho c}{x}\left(\frac{dT}{dt}\right)_{t\to 0} \qquad (2)$$

where ρ and c represent, respectively, the density (g/mL) and the specific heat capacity ($Jg^{-1}\,°C^{-1}$) of the sample (both assumed to be approximately equal to those of the dispersant, for colloidal dispersions), whereas x denotes the concentration of magnetic material in the sample (g/mL), and $(dT/dt)_{t\to 0}$ is the rate at which temperature T (°C) changes right at the beginning of the experiment (in practice, the first 30 s of MHT).

2.4. Preparation of PTX-Loaded Lipid-Coated Magnetic Nanoparticles (PTX-LMNP)

PTX-loaded lipid-coated magnetic nanoparticles (PTX-LMNP) were prepared by lipid film hydration followed by probe sonication—an adaption of a previously reported method, originally designed to prepare magnetic solid lipid nanoparticles [15].

First, 0.5 mL of the previously stored suspension of $MnFe_2O_4$ MNP in acetone was added to 0.5 mL of chloroform containing 200 mg of phosphatidylcholine (PC) and 5 mg of paclitaxel (PTX). The mixture was then probe-sonicated (40 Hz, 5 min) to produce a homogeneous dispersion. The amount of MNP in this suspension was found to be 50 mg.

Then, the dispersion was transferred to a round bottom flask and the organic solvents were removed at room temperature and low pressure via rotary evaporation (IKA). After complete solvent evaporation, the MNP/PC/PTX film was left to dry under vacuum conditions overnight.

Next, the film was hydrated with 4 mL of an aqueous dispersion of sodium oleate (SO, 5 mg/mL) and probe-sonicated intermittently (40 Hz, 5 min) in an ice bath to form a homogeneous dispersion of PTX-LMNP. The resulting PTX-LMNP colloid was then filtered through a 0.22-µm syringe filter and centrifuged to remove traces of water-insoluble reagents.

For fluorescence microscopy experiments, about 1% (w/w) of rhodamine was incorporated to the PTX-LMNP, by adding 2 mg of this fluorophore to the MNP/PC/PTX mixture in acetone/chloroform whilst preparing the lipid film, as described here above.

For the preparation of freeze-dried (lyophilized) samples, microcrystalline trehalose was used as cryoprotectant, initially at 1:1 up to 1:6 (trehalose:PC, w/w). The freeze-dryer MicroModulyo (ThermoFisher) was used for the lyophilization procedures.

2.5. Characterization of PTX-LMNP

PTX-LMNP mean hydrodynamic sizes and polydispersity indexes were determined via dynamic light scattering (DLS, Zetasizer Nano S, Malvern, UK).

PTX quantitation was carried out by a high performance liquid chromatography equipment (HPLC Varian Pro Star) coupled to an automated sampler and to an UV detector, following a previously reported protocol [15]. The chromatographic runs were performed through a Zorbax Eclipse XDB-C18 column (particle size: 3.5 µm; length × internal diameter: 150 mm × 4.6 mm). The mobile phase consisted of acetonitrile, methanol, and water (50/10/40, $v/v/v$). The flow rate was 1 mL/min, and the column was kept at 25 °C during the runs. Detection was set at a wavelength of 227 nm. The injection volume was 20 µL. This analytical method was validated, showing selectivity, linearity within 0.5–50 µg/mL ($r^2 > 0.99$), precision (relative standard deviation, RSD < 5%), and accuracy (>95%).

For PTX extraction, prior to HPLC quantitation, 100 µL of PTX-LMNP were poured into 1 mL of methanol, followed by sonication (10 min) and centrifugation (14,500 rpm, 10 min). The supernatant was filtered through a 0.45 µm and then submitted to HPLC. PTX entrapment efficiency (EE) and drug loading (DL) were determined as follows:

$$\text{EE (\%)} = 100 \times \frac{\text{PTX mass entrapped}}{\text{initial (total) PTX mass}} \qquad (3)$$

$$\text{DL (\%)} = 100 \times \frac{\text{PTX mass entrapped}}{\text{total mass of structural lipids (PC)}} \tag{4}$$

To evaluate PTX-LMNP stability, lyophilized samples were stored at 4 °C for 30 days, whereas fluid samples were stored at 25 °C for 60 days. Then, mean hydrodynamic size, polydispersity index, and EE were determined. Lyophilized samples were reconstituted with ultrapure water.

To attest the success of PTX-LMNP assembly, Fourier Transform Infrared spectroscopy analyses (FTIR, Varian 640-IR) were carried out both for PTX-LMNP and each of its constituents (PTX, MNP, PC, and SO).

Magnetization profiles for both freeze-dried (lyophilized) and colloidally dispersed (fluid) samples were obtained by VSM.

The behavior of PTX-LMNP samples (1 mL at 3.5 mg/mL, in terms of MNP contents) under MHT was observed for different AMF amplitudes (100–305 Oe) at 310 kHz. Whenever needed, PC liposomes were used as non-magnetic controls.

2.6. PTX-LMNP Distribution in Porcine Ear Skin

To evaluate the distribution of PTX-LMNP in skin, 0.5 µL of PTX-LMNP labeled with rhodamine (about 1%) was injected intradermally. Porcine ear skin, an in vitro model for human skin [53], was placed on the top of a vertical diffusion cell. The receptor medium consisted of saline 0.9%, kept at 32 °C. After 2 h, an area of 50 mm^2 of skin was harvested. The tissue was embedded in Tissue-Tek® gel and frozen in N$_2$ liquid. Next, 5-µm thick cryostat transversal sections were obtained using a Leica CM1850 cryomicrotome and mounted directly on microscope slides. The sections were stained with Hoechst (1 ng/mL) for 5 min. Then, samples were observed on a Leica DMI4000 B fluorescence microscope.

2.7. PTX-LMNP In Vitro Drug Release Profile

In vitro drug release profiles were obtained via diffusion through dialysis membrane. PTX quantitation was performed via HPLC. Briefly, 1 mL of PTX-LMNP (comprising approximately 1 mg of PTX and 3.5 mg of MNP) was placed in a dialysis bag (MWCO:14 kDa). Then, the bag was placed in a flask containing 20 mL of receptor medium, consisting of isopropanol:saline 0.9% (30:70, v/v). The flask was kept in a temperature-controlled orbital shaker incubator at 25 °C, 37 °C, or 43 °C for 96 h. Aliquots of 500 µL were withdrawn for PTX quantitation via HPLC at scheduled times—the withdrawn volume being replenished each time with fresh receptor medium.

Additionally, to assess the influence of MHT on PTX release, firstly, an AMF (310 kHz, 305 Oe) was applied to samples for about 40 min. After this single session of MHT, samples were then placed in dialysis bags, which were in turn placed in flasks containing the receptor medium and kept under orbital shaking at 25 °C for 96 h, as described here above. Similarly, aliquots were withdrawn for PTX quantitation at scheduled times with replenishment of the receptor medium after each withdrawal. No additional sessions of MHT were applied to the samples prior to PTX quantitation via HPLC.

All experiments were performed in quintuplicate. Cumulative PTX release profiles were expressed in terms of percentages of the total entrapped PTX. Data were then fit to Baker–Lonsdale, Peppas, Hixson–Crowell, Higuchi, and first-order models. The adjusted coefficient of determination (R^2) was calculated for each case, and the best fits were used as predictive models of the corresponding drug release profiles.

2.8. PTX-LMNP Cytotoxicity against B16F10 Melanoma Cells

B16F10 cells (4 × 10^4 cells/mL) were seeded on 96-well plates (100 µL/well) and incubated for 24 h at 37 °C under 5% CO$_2$ atmosphere and controlled humidity. Next, cells were treated with liposomes, LMNP, or PTX-LMNP at concentrations ranging from 1:10 down to 1:10^8 (v/v) relatively to the volume of culture medium (DMEM supplemented with 2% FBS), enabling the determination of the half-maximal inhibitory concentration (IC$_{50}$) for each formulation. Cells were incubated for additional 48 h and then submitted to neutral red uptake assay [54]. Cells incubated only with culture medium were used as control samples and served as a reference for 100% of cell viability. Results were averaged over three independent experiments, each performed in sextuplicate.

The influence of MHT on PTX-LMNP cytotoxicity against B16F10 melanoma cells was assessed via trypan blue assay. First, cells were cultured in DMEM supplemented with 2% FBS and 1% penicillin/streptomycin. Culture flasks were incubated for 24 h at 37 °C under 5% CO_2 atmosphere and controlled humidity. Next, cells were detached from the flask bottom using trypsin-EDTA (0.25–0.03%), resuspended in DMEM supplemented with 2% FBS, and divided into four aliquots (4×10^7 cells/mL each). Aliquots labeled PTX-LMNP+ were treated with 10% PTX-LMNP (v/v), up to a final volume of 10 mL. About 1 h after incubation, which allowed sample homogenization and some PTX-LMNP internalization by the B16F10 cells, aliquots labeled MHT+ were submitted to an AMF (310 kHz, 305 Oe) for 25 min. Cell suspensions were then homogenized, and 10% trypan blue (v/v) was added to each aliquot to allow viable/non-viable cell counting in a Neubauer chamber.

2.9. Statistical Analyses

Unless otherwise stated, measurements were expressed as mean ± standard deviation (SD), and statistical analyses were performed by analysis of variance (ANOVA) followed by Tukey's Post-Hoc test in GraphPad Prism 6. Statistically significant differences were assumed for $p < 5\%$.

3. Results

3.1. Characterization of $MnFe_2O_4$ MNP

Manganese ferrite ($MnFe_2O_4$) magnetic nanoparticles (MNP) comprise the core of our paclitaxel-loaded lipid-coated magnetic nanoparticles (PTX-LMNP). Therefore, they were fully characterized (Figure 1). Unless otherwise stated, they will be referred to simply as MNP in the following.

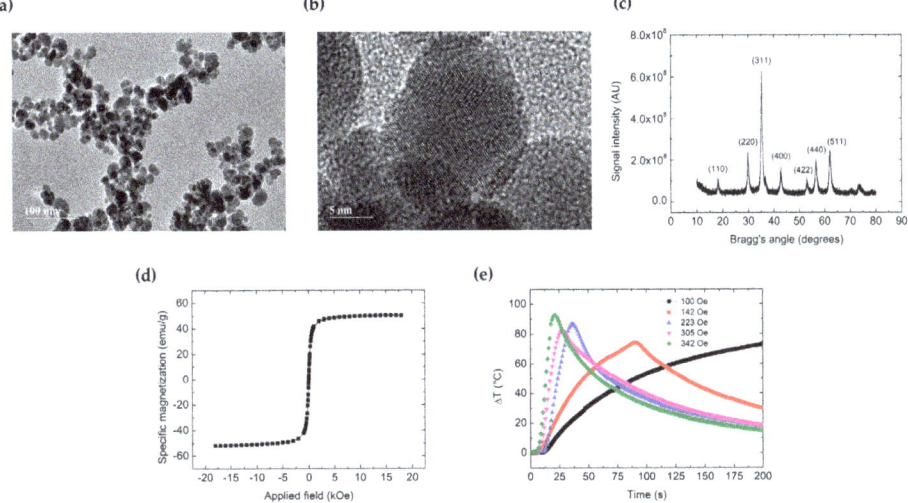

Figure 1. $MnFe_2O_4$ MNP characterization. (**a**,**b**) Representative transmission electron microscopy (TEM) and high-resolution (HR) TEM images, respectively, of the passivated manganese ferrite ($MnFe_2O_4$) magnetic nanoparticles (MNP). (**c**) X-ray diffraction (XRD) pattern and (**d**) specific magnetization profile of powder (dried) MNP samples. (**e**) Temperature profiles (relatively to room temperature, 25 °C) of MNP submitted to magnetic hyperthermia (MHT), with alternating magnetic field (AMF) frequency fixed at 310 kHz and varying amplitude (100–342 Oe).

Figure 1a,b are representative transmission electron microscopy (TEM) images of the MNP. In terms of their shape, MNP synthesized via co-precipitation as in the described protocol are roughly spherical, measuring about 15 nm in diameter, as previously reported [50].

Figure 1c shows the X-ray diffraction (XRD) pattern of a typical powder (dried) sample of the original colloidal aqueous dispersion of MNP. The crystallite mean diameter, as calculated via Equation (1), was found to be 13.5 nm, in accordance with previous reports of our group for similarly synthesized MNP [50].

Figure 1d brings a representative magnetization profile of a powder sample of MNP, obtained via vibrating sample magnetometry (VSM). Specific saturation magnetization (about 50 emu/g) served as a reference for calculating the concentration (in terms of magnetic contents) of the corresponding MNP colloidal dispersions, as previously reported [50].

Figure 1e shows the behavior of a powder sample of MNP submitted to magnetic hyperthermia (MHT). Alternating magnetic field (AMF) amplitudes were varied within 100–342 Oe, with the field frequency fixed at 310 kHz. The initial slope ($t \to 0$) of the temperature profiles is proportional to the specific loss power (SLP, given in W/g) of the sample [27,50], a measure of its magnetothermal conversion efficiency under a given MHT setup. To be noted that higher temperatures could be attained in shorter timeframes (higher SLP) for higher field amplitudes. The exciting field was turned off as the temperature approached 100 °C to avoid damaging the temperature sensor.

For comparison purposes, Figure S1 brings Fe_3O_4 (magnetite) MNP characterization: XRD diffractogram, specific magnetization profile, as well as MHT temperature profiles.

3.2. Characterization of PTX-LMNP

PTX-LMNP hydrodynamic size distributions for samples with and without SO are shown in Figure 2a. Their mean hydrodynamic diameter (D_H) and polydispersity index (PdI) are summarized in Table 1. D_H was two-fold lower for samples with SO. Moreover, PTX-LMNP with SO were less polydispersed. Therefore, as depicted in Figure 2b, our optimal PTX-LMNP consisted of a core of magnetic MNP coated by a layer of phosphatidylcholine (PC), with SO as surfactant. Due to its lipophilic nature and relatively low solubility in water, PTX is expected to be found amidst the hydrophobic tails of the PC coating. Optimal mass proportions were, thus, set to 50:200:20:5 (MNP:PC:SO:PTX), as described in Section 2.4.

Table 1. PTX-LMNP size and polydispersity × SO contents.

Sample	D_H (nm)	PdI
without SO	186 ± 1	0.50 ± 0.15
with SO	90 ± 1	0.26 ± 0.03

D_H = mean hydrodynamic diameter, PdI = polydispersity index, SO = sodium oleate.

PTX entrapment efficiency (EE) and drug loading efficiency (DL) were calculated on the basis of HPLC results via Equations (3) and (4), respectively. The EE was found to be 81.2 ± 0.3%, whereas the DL amounted to 2.2 ± 0.6%.

No increase in D_H or PdI was observed for PTX-LMNP, neither for the colloidal dispersion stored at 4 °C for 30 days nor for the freeze-dried PTX-LMNP stored at 25 °C and reconstituted after 60 days (Table S1). In terms of the PTX cargo, a reduction of 8% was observed for the colloidal dispersion after 30 days, whereas no significant losses were observed for the freeze-dried PTX-LMNP reconstituted in water after 60 days (Figure S2).

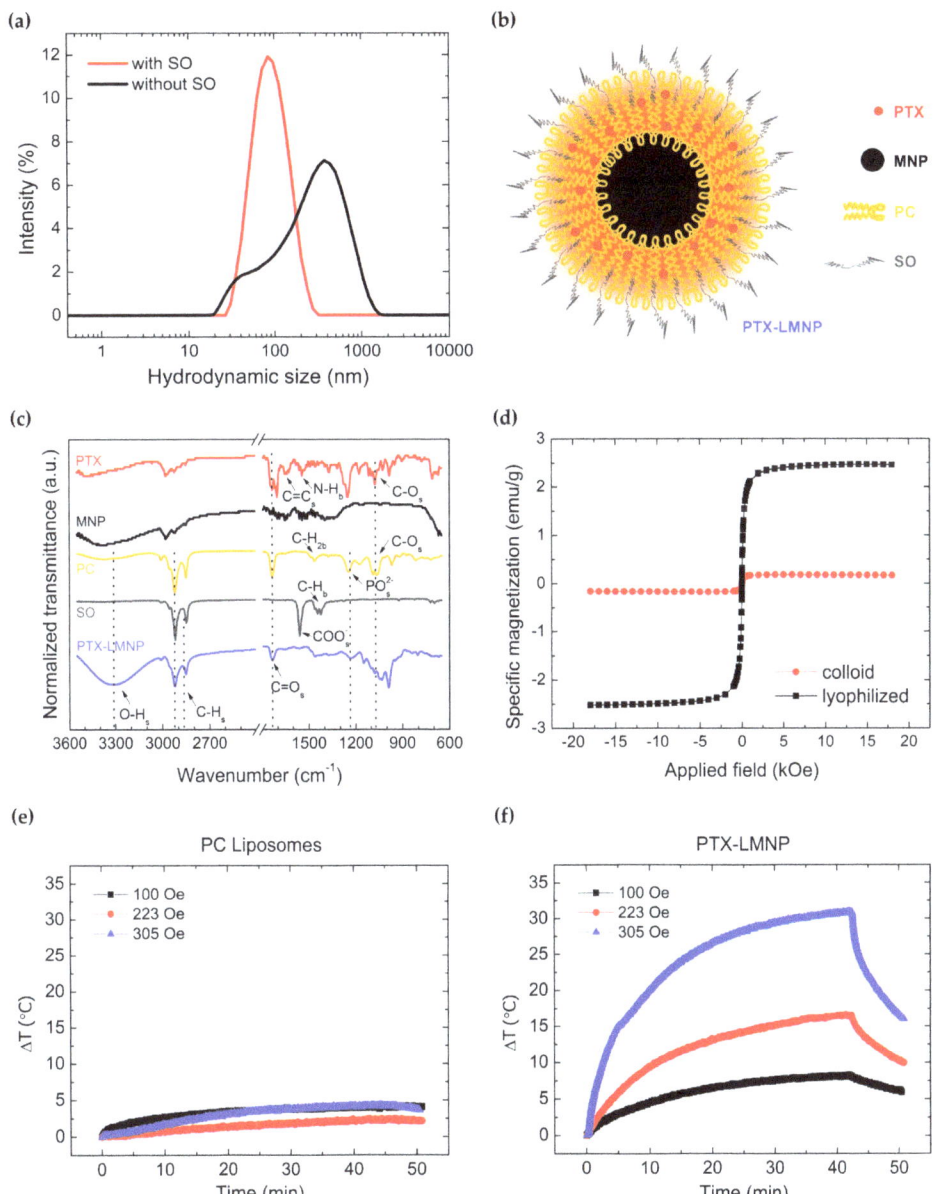

Figure 2. Characterization of PTX-LMNP. (**a**) Hydrodynamic size distributions obtained via DLS for samples with and without SO. (**b**) Schematic view of a paclitaxel-loaded lipid-coated magnetic nanoparticle (PTX-LMNP). PTX: paclitaxel; MNP: the core of manganese ferrite ($MnFe_2O_4$) magnetic nanoparticles (MNP); PC: the phosphatidylcholine coating; and SO: the sodium oleate surfactant molecules. (**c**) Normalized FTIR transmittance spectra for PTX-LMNP and its different components. (**d**) Specific magnetization profiles both for colloidally dispersed (fluid) and freeze-dried (lyophilized) PTX-LMNP samples. (**e**,**f**) Temperature profiles (relatively to room temperature, 25 °C) of PC liposomes (non-magnetic control sample) and PTX-LMNP, respectively, once submitted to magnetic hyperthermia (MHT), with alternating magnetic field (AMF) frequency fixed at 310 kHz and varying amplitude (100–305 Oe).

Figure 2c shows the results of the Fourier Transform Infrared spectroscopy (FTIR) analyses carried out for PTX-LMNP and each of its components (PTX, MNP, PC, and SO) for wavenumbers at 650–3600 cm^{-1}. To be noted that the transmittance spectra were normalized, and a break at 1800–2400 cm^{-1} was performed to highlight the most prominent absorption bands for each sample. Noteworthy, all prominent bands arising from the transmittance spectra of PTX, MNP, PC, and SO are also present in PTX-LMNP signal, which suggests that the nanocarrier was successfully assembled, as originally designed. Non-normalized FTIR spectra for PTX-LMNP and its components are provided in Figure S3.

The concentration of MNP in PTX-LMNP was obtained on the basis of specific magnetization profiles determine via vibrating sample magnetometry (VSM). Figure 2d shows the specific magnetization profiles of both aqueous-dispersed (fluid) and freeze-dried (lyophilized) PTX-LMNP samples. Similarly to the MNP magnetization profile (Figure 1d), the curves do not exhibit quasi-static hysteresis at room temperature, suggesting that the typical quasi-static superparamagnetic behavior of MNP [55] was preserved in PTX-LMNP. See Figure S4 for a zoomed view of Figure 2d around the origin for further details.

Figure 2e,f bring the temperature profiles of PC liposomes (non-magnetic control sample) and PTX-LMNP, respectively, when submitted to MHT. Temperatures were registered relatively to room temperature (25 °C). Devoid of magnetic constituents, PC liposomes are not excited by the AMF, and the observed temperature increase (less than 5 °C for all field amplitudes) is mostly due to heat release via eddy current losses (Figure 2e) [56]. In contrast, temperature variations within about 7.5 °C up to 30 °C were obtained as a result of dynamic (AC) hysteresis losses [57], due to the interaction between the AMF and PTX-LMNP magnetic core (Figure 2f).

3.3. PTX-LMNP Distribution in Porcine Ear Skin

Fluorescence images of PTX-LMNP biodistribution in porcine ear skin are shown in Figure 3. Hoechst-stained epithelial cells appear in blue, whereas rhodamine-labeled PTX-LMNP appear in red. Right after intradermal injection, some PTX-LMNP could be found within the interface between the epidermis and the dermis (Figure 3, 0 h). In contrast, 2 h after injection, PTX-LMNP were no longer found in the epidermis or in its interface with the dermis, but only in deeper layers of the dermis (Figure 3, 2 h).

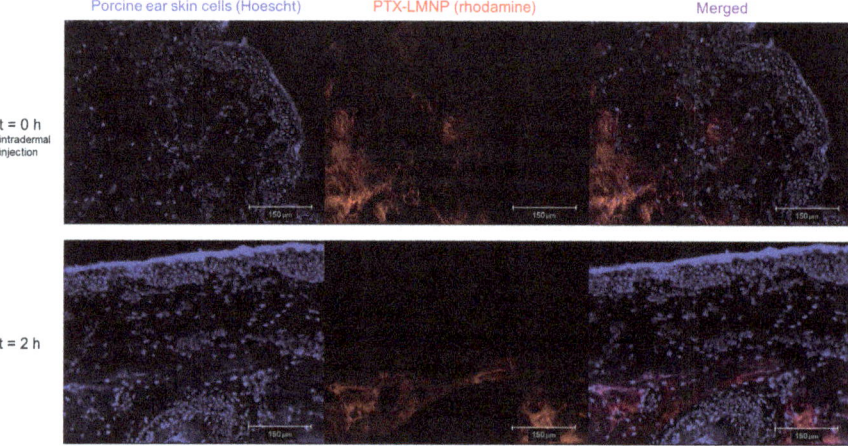

Figure 3. PTX-LMNP biodistribution in porcine ear skin. Representative fluorescence images of Hoechst-stained (blue fluorescence) porcine ear skin cells immediately after intradermal administration of rhodamine-labeled (red fluorescence) PTX-LMNP (0 h) and two hours later (2 h). Initially, at the interface between the epidermis and the dermis, PTX-LMNP diffuses to deeper layers of the dermis.

3.4. PTX-LMNP In Vitro Drug Release Profile

Figure 4a shows the in vitro cumulative PTX release profiles for PTX-LMNP samples submitted to dialysis at 25, 37, and 43 °C for 96 h (4 days), as well as for PTX-LMNP samples that first underwent MHT, and then were submitted to dialysis at 25 °C for 96 h for PTX release assessment at scheduled times. Free PTX was used as a control sample at 1 mg/mL—the same concentration carried by a typical PTX-LMNP.

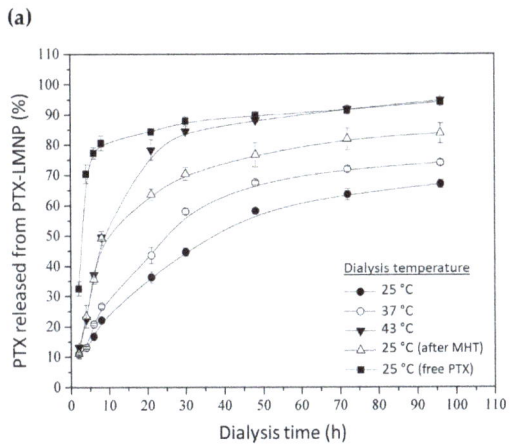

(a)

(b)

Kinetic model	Parameter	25 °C	37 °C	43 °C	25 °C (after MHT)
Baker-Lonsdale	R^2	0.982	0.963	0.938	0.917
Peppas	R^2	0.977	0.949	0.876	0.899
	n	0.466	0.442	0.347	0.334
Hixon-Crowell	R^2	0.793	0.797	0.879	0.692
Higuchi	R^2	0.974	0.938	0.770	0.763
1st order	R^2	0.866	0.883	0.973	0.802

Figure 4. PTX release kinetics from PTX-LMNP. (**a**) PTX release profiles for different temperatures (25, 37, and 43 °C), as well as for a sample first submitted to MHT, and then left for dialysis at room temperature (25 °C). Free PTX was adopted as a control sample. (**b**) Coefficients of determination (R^2) for different models of drug release kinetics after fitting the corresponding model equations to the experimental data. The parameter n represents the exponent of release (related to the release mechanism) of Peppas' model [58]. R^2 coefficients closest to unit are highlighted in blue.

About 70% of the free PTX control sample reaches the receptor chamber within the first 4 h of experiment, and about 95% within 96 h. PTX percentual release from PTX-LMNP after 8 h of experiment could be doubled, relatively to the sample kept at 25 °C, either by (1) increasing the incubation temperature up to 43 °C or (2) applying MHT (310 kHz, 305 Oe) prior to the drug release assay.

Figure 4b summarizes the different attempts to fit the cumulative drug release data to five distinct models of drug release kinetics. Considering the coefficients of determination associated to the different fittings, Baker and Lonsdale's model seems to be the best option to predict PTX release from PTX-LMNP over time for all five experimental setups, although first-order kinetics better models PTX release from PTX-LMNP at 43 °C.

3.5. PTX-LMNP Cytotoxicity against B16F10 Melanoma Cells

Figure 5a shows the results of the cytotoxicity assay (neutral red uptake, formulations incubated for 48 h with B16F10 cells). No significant decrease on cell viability was observed for PC liposomes (control samples, without PTX). Similarly, LMNP were cytotoxic only at high concentrations ($IC_{50} \approx 1:230\ v/v$, corresponding to about 14,000 ng/mL of MNP). In contrast, significant cell death was observed for PTX-LMNP, even at low concentrations ($IC_{50} \approx 1:10^6\ v/v$, equivalent to approximately 0.4 ng/mL of PTX or 3.2 ng/mL of MNP).

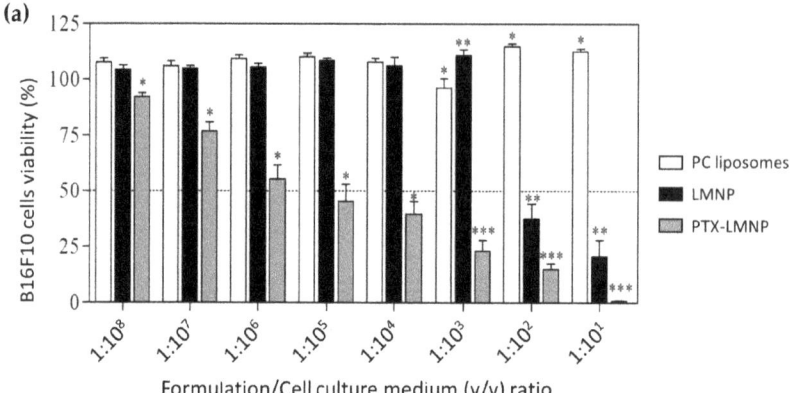

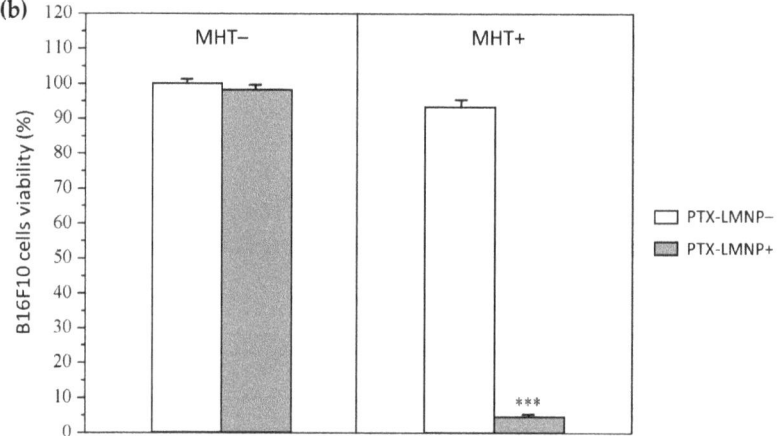

Figure 5. PTX-LMNP against B16F10 melanoma cells. (**a**) Cell viability 48 h after incubation with PC liposomes, LMNP, or PTX-LMNP samples. (**b**) Cell viability 1 h after incubation with or without PTX-LMNP (PTX-LMNP+ or PTX-LMNP− samples, respectively), followed or not by MHT (MHT+ or MHT− samples, respectively). * $p < 0.05$, ** $p < 0.01$, *** $p < 0.001$.

Figure 5b summarizes the results of the experiment designed to verify the influence of MHT on PTX-LMNP cytotoxicity against B16F10 cells. Cell viability decreased to less than 5% for aliquot MHT+ PTX-LMNP+, whereas no significant differences in cell viability were observed for the other aliquots within the short timeframe of the experiment, i.e., 1 h of incubation followed or not by 25 min of MHT (Figure 5b).

4. Discussion

In previous works, we have already explored the controlled release of model drugs from nanostructures eventually triggered by magnetic hyperthermia (MHT). For instance, rapamycin was successfully encapsulated with Fe_3O_4 (magnetite) magnetic nanoparticles (MNP) within poly(lactic-co-glycolic acid) (PLGA) polymeric nanocapsules and nanospheres [59]. Additionally, paclitaxel (PTX) was incorporated to solid lipid nanoparticles composed by glyceryl monostearate (GMS) and phosphatidylcholine (PC) with magnetite cores and further stabilized by Pluronic F-68 [15]. Herein, we report the development of PTX-loaded lipid-coated magnetic nanoparticles (PTX-LMNP) to explore the potential of MHT-triggered release on treating skin cancer (B16F10 melanoma) by dual chemo-MHT therapy.

The delivery strategy herein reported was designed as a bioinspired synthetic analog of the naturally occurring magnetosomes [43–45]. This strategy has also captured the attention of other authors. For instance, magnetite MNP were embedded within a glyceryl trimyristate solid matrix as a platform for treating colon cancer via MHT [60]. Magnetite MNP embedding near infrared (NIR) fluorophores have also been coated with galactosyl and targeting moieties to enable dual-modal (fluorescence/magnetic resonance) imaging of hepatocellular carcinomas [61]. Moreover, 1,2-dipalmitoyl-sn-glycero-3-phosphocholine (DPPC) and L-α-dipalmitoylphosphatidyl glycerol (DPPG) were used as the lipidic coating of magnetite MNP envisaging the MHT-induced thermo-responsiveness of the resulting delivery system [62]. Magnetite MNP were also coated with PC and cationic lipids, in association with transferrin, for MHT-controlled gene delivery [63]. Oleic acid has also been previously used as the lipidic coating of magnetite MNP for the MHT-triggered release of doxorubicin [64].

PTX-LMNP are schematically depicted in Figure 2b. The presence of Fe^{+3} ions on the surface of the passivated manganese ferrite ($MnFe_2O_4$) MNP enables the interaction with lipid molecules, such as PC. PC predominantly negative polar heads are attracted by the positive Fe ions on the surface of MNP, leading to the assembly of lipid layers around the magnetic cores. Sodium oleate (SO) grafting, with surfactant properties, stabilize the resultant particles, preventing their aggregation. Due to the lipophilic nature of PTX, it is entrapped within PC hydrophobic tails [65,66]. $MnFe_2O_4$ MNP was adopted as an alternative to the ubiquitous Fe_3O_4 MNP. Biocompatible and safe for medical use, $MnFe_2O_4$ MNP has been explored by our group as magnetite MNP surrogates, eventually outperforming magnetite in terms of MHT (Figure S1), and figuring as promising candidates for MRI as contrast agents [67,68].

Figure 2c displays the normalized FTIR spectra for PTX-LMNP and its components (PTX, MNP, PC, and SO). The non-normalized spectra can be found in Figure S3. The C-O stretching band around 1070 cm^{-1} is present in both PTX and PC spectra, as well as amidst a series of adjacent bands in the spectrum for PTX-LMNP in the 900–1200 cm^{-1} range. The phosphate (PO^{-2}) stretching vibration band near 1230 cm^{-1}, which is present in PC spectrum, can also be found in PTX-LMNP spectrum. Notably, the carboxylate (COO$^-$) stretching band, identified in the SO spectrum near 1550 cm^{-1}, correlates to an almost negligible peak in PTX-LMNP spectrum, suggesting that this functional group may be responsible for the attachment of SO to the PTX-LMNP structure. The carbonyl (C=O) stretching band, centered at 1730 cm^{-1}, was identified for PTX, PC, as well as PTX-LMNP. Typical C-H stretching vibrations were also observed for PC, SO, and PTX-LMNP. A broad and relatively strong band in PTX-LMNP spectrum, starting at 3000 cm^{-1} and going up to 3600 cm^{-1}, seemingly correlates to an equally broad (though relatively weaker) band within the PC spectrum, probably indicating that a relatively large amount of PC could be successfully attached to the final PTX-LMNP structure. Since the FTIR data were acquired at 650–4000 cm^{-1}, the typical Fe-O stretching vibrations from $MnFe_2O_4$ octahedral and tetrahedral sites (usually 400–600 cm^{-1}) could not be clearly identified, although they do stand out within the FTIR results of very similar samples produced by our group (e.g., Zn-doped $MnFe_2O_4$), as previously reported [69]. Taken together, these results indicate that the PTX-LMNP nanocarrier was successfully assembled, as designed.

The efficiency of MHT applications depends on several properties of magnetic nanoparticles, including their size, polydispersion, functionalization, spatial arrangement, and concentration [25,28]. Herein, we focused our investigation on the influence of concentration on the heating efficiency. In particular, the heat released by $MnFe_2O_4$ MNP aggregates under MHT seem to depend strongly on the collective magnetic relaxation [57].

The difference in specific saturation magnetization between aqueous-dispersed and freeze-dried PTX-LMNP (Figure 2d) accounts for the fact that the magnetization signal was divided by the whole sample mass—including the mass of water (dispersant) for the fluid sample. The concentration of magnetic material in PTX-LMNP samples can be determined on the basis of the specific saturation magnetization obtained for powdered MNP (50 emu/g, Figure 1d), as previously reported [50]. Freeze-dried PTX-LMNP specific saturation magnetization of 2.6 emu/g, thus, translates to approximately 10.4 mg/mL of MNP, while the 0.6 emu/g obtained for the aqueous-dispersed PTX-LMNP corresponds to about 2.4 mg/mL. Similar results were observed in our previous work [15].

Temperatures as high as 55 °C can be achieved by PTX-LMNP-mediated MHT within about 40 min (Figure 2f). Knowing that skin temperature is about 32 °C, only 4 min are needed to increase it to the hyperthermia range of 43–46 °C, consequently promoting the desired therapeutic effects [36]. Note that the thermal dose can be tuned by controlling both the magnetic field amplitude and frequency, as well as the time of treatment, enabling local MHT-triggered release, while avoiding patient harm in a clinical scenario [36].

PTX-LMNP-facilitated diffusion through the skin (Figure 3) can be explained by their lipid composition. PTX-LMNP structural phospholipids and surfactants ease their diffusion through the different skin layers by enabling interactions with local tissue lipids and proteins [70]. Indeed, once delivered intradermally, we observed that PTX-LMNP migrate from the epidermis-dermis interface to deeper layers of the dermis. Therefore, PTX-LMNP are potentially able to deliver their therapeutic benefits to skin cancers established either within the epidermis, deeply in the dermis, or within both skin layers [71].

PTX-LMNP specific loss power (SLP) was found to be 37.8 W/g (with field frequency and amplitude set to 310 kHz and 305 Oe, respectively, and sample volume of 1 mL at 3.5 mg/mL, Figure 2f). Though higher SLP values can be found in the literature [72], PTX-LMNP SLP was high enough to efficiently trigger PTX release (Figure 4). Indeed, the temperature increase changes the molecular dynamics of the phospholipids in PTX-LMNP, increasing the lipid layer fluidity and permeability [73], thus favoring release of the drug cargo [74]. After fitting the experimental data to five different models, Baker–Lonsdale's model for drug release from spherical matrices reasonably accounted for the release kinetics of all the different experimental setups. Noticeably, MHT-triggered release at 25 °C was comparable to PTX release kinetics at 43 °C, especially within the first 10 h (Figure 4). Note, however, that the release profiles in Figure 4 account both for restricted diffusion, within the dialysis bag, and free diffusion, outside the dialysis bag, where aliquots were then sampled at scheduled times for PTX quantitation via HPLC.

Baker–Lonsdale's model has been most commonly applied to describe drug release from microcapsules and microspheres [58], but it also accounts for slow sustained release from spherical matrices [75]—which is the case depicted in Figure 4a for PTX-LMNP. Hydrophobic PTX molecules tend to be slowly released from the lipidic PC layer coating PTX-LMNP, to which they are attracted through hydrophobic interactions. Solubility and diffusion within the matrix, prior to release, are taken into account by Baker–Lonsdale's model, but not by the first-order model, whose sole assumption is that release rates are proportional to the remaining concentration of the drug in the matrix. Temperature-induced phenomena might corroborate this assumption, since R^2 more closely approached 1 for a first-order fit only when the experiment was carried out at 43 °C (Figure 4b).

Results of the cytotoxicity (neutral red uptake) assay suggest that B16F10 cell death is expected to be predominantly due to the chemotherapeutic action of PTX (Figure 5a). Additionally, although MNP were shown to be non-cytotoxic at concentrations as high as 0.1 mg/mL [76], some toxicity might occur at higher concentrations, as per the observed LMNP cytotoxicity profile. Noteworthy, the half-maximal inhibitory concentration (IC_{50}) value obtained for PTX-LMNP (0.4 ng/mL) was nearly 340 times lower than that reported for the commercial formulation Taxol® (137 ng/mL) [77] and remarkably 142,500 times lower than that of free PTX (57 µg/mL) [78].

Significant cytotoxicity against B16F10 cells was observed for cells treated with both PTX-LMNP and MHT (PTX-LMNP+ MHT+ aliquot, Figure 5b). In contrast, no significant cytotoxicity was observed for cells treated only with PTX-LMNP (PTX-LMNP+ MHT−).

One drawback of this experiment, however, is that the effect of MHT in isolation cannot be determined. An additional control sample would be needed, either MNP or LMNP, at the same concentration of PTX-LMNP, in terms of magnetic contents, submitted to MHT in presence of B16F10 cells. We would then be able to determine whether B16F10 cells are dying exclusively due to the chemotherapeutic effect of PTX, or if cell death is a result of the combined effect of MHT and PTX, eventually in synergy. Nevertheless, in a previous work, we showed that B16F10 cells were resistant to hyperthermia temperatures up to 4 h of incubation [50]. This suggests that, in the current study, cells would be dying because of PTX.

Nevertheless, according to Figure 4a, PTX release from PTX-LMNP is too slow, even under the influence of MHT. Indeed, about 50% of the PTX cargo is released only after approximately 10 h after the beginning of the experiment. However, one might notice that both restricted diffusion (inside the dialysis bag) and free diffusion (outside the dialysis bag) are taken into account in Figure 4a. By contrast, in Figure 5b, there is no dialysis bag in the experimental setup, meaning that the whole PTX cargo released, whether or not under the influence of MHT, is immediately allowed to interact with the B16F10 cells, eventually exerting its cytotoxic action.

Still, according to Figure 5a, a 10% v/v concentration, as employed for the experiment in Figure 5b, seems to be intrinsically cytotoxic. However, the timeframes of both setups must be considered: in Figure 5a cytotoxicity is evaluated for 48 h (long-term assay), in contrast with Figure 5b, for which cytotoxicity is evaluated for no longer than 1 h 30 min (short-term assay). In this short-term assay, Figure 5b clearly shows that PTX-LMNP are not intrinsically cytotoxic, while significant cytotoxicity is observed under MHT.

Additionally, the volume adopted for the experiment of Figure 5b (10 mL) is significantly higher than that of a well in a 96-well plate, where PTX-LMNP are allowed to interact with B16F10 cells for the experiment of Figure 5a. Increased interaction with the formulation, allied to an increased incubation period, might also have contributed to the differences observed between the two experiments.

Moreover, the 10 mL might obscure the effect of temperature during the experiment, since the temperature variation of the ensemble at the macroscopic scale for these conditions is negligible. However, at the microscopic and at the nanoscopic scales, a localized MHT-mediated increase in temperature might have altered the PC-coating fluidity, favoring PTX release within the short timeframe of the experiment in Figure 5b, thus favoring a cytotoxic action. Indeed, 95% of cell death was observed within 1 h of incubation with PTX-LMNP followed by 25 min of MHT, while no significant reduction in cell viability was observed for cells incubated with PTX-LMNP but not submitted to MHT. Similarly, other authors also report a significant improvement in chemotherapy outcomes as a result of its combination with MHT [79–81].

Taken together, our results indicate that PTX-LMNP-mediated combined chemo-MHT therapy stands out as a promising strategy against melanoma. Prospectively, we envisage the elucidation of the mechanisms underlying the cytotoxicity induced by the combination of chemotherapy and MHT [82–85]. In vivo experiments will certainly challenge the in vitro results herein reported, although other authors have already corroborated the benefits of chemo-MHT and radiation-MHT combined therapy in pre-clinical assays using analogous drug-heat delivery systems [50,70,86–88].

5. Conclusions

Paclitaxel-loaded magnetic-lipid nanoparticles (PTX-LMNP) were developed envisaging the combined chemo-magnetic hyperthermia therapy of melanoma. With hydrodynamic diameters around 90 nm, PTX-LMNP consist of manganese ferrite ($MnFe_2O_4$) magnetic nanoparticles (MNP) coated by phosphatidylcholine (PC). With surfactant properties, sodium oleate (SO) successfully endowed PTX-LMNP dispersions with colloidal stability. Due to the hydrophobic nature of PTX, its entrapment efficiency (EE) within PC hydrophobic tails was greater than 80%. PTX-LMNP rapidly diffuse across different skin layers, due to interactions between its lipidic cloak with the epithelial tissue lipids and proteins. In vitro drug release profiles revealed that temperature modulates PTX release, with higher temperatures correlating with higher release rates. Magnetic hyperthermia (MHT) triggers and consequently enhances PTX cumulative release. PTX-LMNP cytotoxicity against B16F10 melanoma cells is concentration-dependent, with an IC_{50} corresponding to 0.4 ng/mL of PTX, significantly lower than the IC_{50} reported for free PTX and for PTX-loaded nanostructured formulations. Cytotoxicity was strikingly higher when PTX-LMNP were submitted to MHT, which suggests that the dual chemo-MHT therapy mediated by intratumorally injected PTX-LMNP stands out as a promising alternative to efficiently deliver PTX to melanoma cells, consequently reducing systemic side effects commonly associated with conventional chemotherapies.

Supplementary Materials: The following supporting information can be downloaded at: https://www.mdpi.com/article/10.3390/pharmaceutics15030818/s1, Figure S1: Fe_3O_4 MNP characterization; Figure S2: PTX-LMNP stability assay; Figure S3: Non-normalized FTIR spectra; Figure S4: PTX-LMNP magnetization within −100 to 100 Oe; Table S1: PTX-LMNP stability assay data.

Author Contributions: Conceptualization, R.R.O., A.F.B. and E.M.L.; data acquisition, R.R.O., E.R.C., L.C.M. and A.C.G.d.S.; data curation, A.A.S.-J., A.L.R.d.S. and M.S.C.; writing—original draft preparation, R.R.O. and A.L.R.d.S.; writing—review and editing, A.A.S.-J., A.F.B. and E.M.L.; supervision, M.C.V. and E.M.L.; funding acquisition, M.C.V., A.F.B., and E.M.L. All authors have read and agreed to the published version of the manuscript.

Funding: This research was partially funded by the Brazilian agencies CNPq (Conselho Nacional de Desenvolvimento Científico e Tecnológico), including INCT NanoFarma (Institutos Nacionais de Ciência e Tecnologia de Nanotecnologia Farmacêutica) and CAPES (Coordenação para Aperfeiçoamento de Pessoal de Nível Superior).

Institutional Review Board Statement: Not applicable.

Informed Consent Statement: Not applicable.

Data Availability Statement: Not applicable.

Acknowledgments: The authors would like to thank Marcus Vinícius-Araújo for kindly providing the representative TEM images of the $MnFe_2O_4$ magnetic nanoparticles used in this work.

Conflicts of Interest: The authors declare no conflict of interest.

References

1. Sung, H.; Ferlay, J.; Siegel, R.L.; Laversanne, M.; Soerjomataram, I.; Jemal, A.; Bray, F. Global Cancer Statistics 2020: GLOBOCAN Estimates of Incidence and Mortality Worldwide for 36 Cancers in 185 Countries. *CA Cancer J. Clin.* **2021**, *71*, 209–249. [CrossRef] [PubMed]
2. International World Cancer Research Fund. Skin Cancer Statistics. Available online: https://www.wcrf.org/cancer-trends/skin-cancer-statistics/ (accessed on 1 March 2023).
3. Lens, M.B.; Dawes, M. Global Perspectives of Contemporary Epidemiological Trends of Cutaneous Malignant Melanoma. *Br. J. Dermatol.* **2004**, *150*, 179–185. [CrossRef] [PubMed]
4. Hersh, E.M.; Del Vecchio, M.; Brown, M.P.; Kefford, R.; Loquai, C.; Testori, A.; Bhatia, S.; Gutzmer, R.; Conry, R.; Haydon, A.; et al. A Randomized, Controlled Phase III Trial of Nab-Paclitaxel versus Dacarbazine in Chemotherapy-Naïve Patients with Metastatic Melanoma. *Ann. Oncol.* **2015**, *26*, 2267–2274. [CrossRef] [PubMed]
5. Pflugfelder, A.; Eigentler, T.K.; Keim, U.; Weide, B.; Leiter, U.; Ikenberg, K.; Berneburg, M.; Garbe, C. Effectiveness of Carboplatin and Paclitaxel as First- and Second-Line Treatment in 61 Patients with Metastatic Melanoma. *PLoS ONE* **2011**, *6*, e16882. [CrossRef] [PubMed]
6. Rao, R.D.; Holtan, S.G.; Ingle, J.N.; Croghan, G.A.; Kottschade, L.A.; Creagan, E.T.; Kaur, J.S.; Pitot, H.C.; Markovic, S.N. Combination of Paclitaxel and Carboplatin as Second-Line Therapy for Patients with Metastatic Melanoma. *Cancer* **2006**, *106*, 375–382. [CrossRef] [PubMed]
7. Bombelli, F.B.; Webster, C.A.; Moncrieff, M.; Sherwood, V. The Scope of Nanoparticle Therapies for Future Metastatic Melanoma Treatment. *Lancet Oncol.* **2014**, *15*, e22–e32. [CrossRef] [PubMed]
8. Schiff, P.B.; Fant, J.; Horwitz, S.B. Promotion of Microtubule Assembly in Vitro by Taxol. *Nature* **1979**, *277*, 665–667. [CrossRef]
9. Altmann, K.H.; Gertsch, J. Anticancer Drugs from Nature-Natural Products as a Unique Source of New Microtubule-Stabilizing Agents. *Nat. Prod. Rep.* **2007**, *24*, 327–357. [CrossRef]

10. Lim, S.-J.; Hong, S.-S.; Choi, J.Y.; Kim, J.O.; Lee, M.-K.; Kim, S.H. Development of Paclitaxel-Loaded Liposomal Nanocarrier Stabilized by Triglyceride Incorporation. *Int. J. Nanomed.* **2016**, *11*, 4465–4477. [CrossRef]
11. Wang, Z.; Ling, L.; Du, Y.; Yao, C.; Li, X. Reduction Responsive Liposomes Based on Paclitaxel-Ss-Lysophospholipid with High Drug Loading for Intracellular Delivery. *Int. J. Pharm.* **2019**, *564*, 244–255. [CrossRef]
12. Jain, S.; Kumar, D.; Swarnakar, N.K.; Thanki, K. Polyelectrolyte Stabilized Multilayered Liposomes for Oral Delivery of Paclitaxel. *Biomaterials* **2012**, *33*, 6758–6768. [CrossRef] [PubMed]
13. Tian, J.; Yan, C.; Liu, K.; Tao, J.; Guo, Z.; Liu, J.; Zhang, Y.; Xiong, F.; Gu, N. Paclitaxel-Loaded Magnetic Nanoparticles: Synthesis, Characterization, and Application in Targeting. *J. Pharm. Sci.* **2017**, *106*, 2115–2122. [CrossRef] [PubMed]
14. Yu, H.; Wang, Y.; Wang, S.; Li, X.; Li, W.; Ding, D.; Gong, X.; Keidar, M.; Zhang, W. Paclitaxel-Loaded Core–Shell Magnetic Nanoparticles and Cold Atmospheric Plasma Inhibit Non-Small Cell Lung Cancer Growth. *ACS Appl. Mater. Interfaces* **2018**, *10*, 43462–43471. [CrossRef] [PubMed]
15. Oliveira, R.R.; Carrião, M.S.; Pacheco, M.T.; Branquinho, L.C.; de Souza, A.L.R.; Bakuzis, A.F.; Lima, E.M. Triggered Release of Paclitaxel from Magnetic Solid Lipid Nanoparticles by Magnetic Hyperthermia. *Mater. Sci. Eng. C* **2018**, *92*, 547–553. [CrossRef] [PubMed]
16. Abriata, J.P.; Turatti, R.C.; Luiz, M.T.; Raspantini, G.L.; Tofani, L.B.; do Amaral, R.L.F.; Swiech, K.; Marcato, P.D.; Marchetti, J.M. Development, Characterization and Biological In Vitro Assays of Paclitaxel-Loaded PCL Polymeric Nanoparticles. *Mater. Sci. Eng. C* **2019**, *96*, 347–355. [CrossRef]
17. Hu, J.; Fu, S.; Peng, Q.; Han, Y.; Xie, J.; Zan, N.; Chen, Y.; Fan, J. Paclitaxel-Loaded Polymeric Nanoparticles Combined with Chronomodulated Chemotherapy on Lung Cancer: In Vitro and In Vivo Evaluation. *Int. J. Pharm.* **2017**, *516*, 313–322. [CrossRef]
18. Baek, J.S.; Kim, J.H.; Park, J.S.; Cho, C.W. Modification of Paclitaxel-Loaded Solid Lipid Nanoparticles with 2-Hydroxypropyl-β-Cyclodextrin Enhances Absorption and Reduces Nephrotoxicity Associated with Intravenous Injection. *Int. J. Nanomed.* **2015**, *10*, 5397–5405. [CrossRef]
19. Banerjee, I.; De, K.; Mukherjee, D.; Dey, G.; Chattopadhyay, S.; Mukherjee, M.; Mandal, M.; Bandyopadhyay, A.K.; Gupta, A.; Ganguly, S.; et al. Paclitaxel-Loaded Solid Lipid Nanoparticles Modified with Tyr-3-Octreotide for Enhanced Anti-Angiogenic and Anti-Glioma Therapy. *Acta Biomater.* **2016**, *38*, 69–81. [CrossRef]
20. Tosta, F.V.; Andrade, L.M.; Mendes, L.P.; Anjos, J.L.V.; Alonso, A.; Marreto, R.N.; Lima, E.M.; Taveira, S.F. Paclitaxel-Loaded Lipid Nanoparticles for Topical Application: The Influence of Oil Content on Lipid Dynamic Behavior, Stability, and Drug Skin Penetration. *J. Nanoparticle Res.* **2014**, *16*, 2782. [CrossRef]
21. Han, L.M.; Guo, J.; Zhang, L.J.; Wang, Q.S.; Fang, X.L. Pharmacokinetics and Biodistribution of Polymeric Micelles of Paclitaxel with Pluronic P123. *Acta Pharmacol. Sin.* **2006**, *27*, 747–753. [CrossRef]
22. Lee, S.C.; Huh, M.; Lee, J.; Cho, Y.W.; Galinsky, R.E.; Park, K. Hydrotropic Polymeric Micelles for Enhanced Paclitaxel Solubility: In Vitro and In Vivo Characterization. *Biomacromolecules* **2007**, *8*, 202–208. [CrossRef] [PubMed]
23. Idris, N.M.; Gnanasammandhan, M.K.; Zhang, J.; Ho, P.C.; Mahendran, R.; Zhang, Y. In Vivo Photodynamic Therapy Using Upconversion Nanoparticles as Remote-Controlled Nanotransducers. *Nat. Med.* **2012**, *18*, 1580–1585. [CrossRef]
24. Busetti, A.; Soncin, M.; Jori, G.; Rodgers, M.A.J. High Efficiency of Benzoporphyrin Derivative in the Photodynamic Therapy of Pigmented Malignant Melanoma. *Br. J. Cancer* **1999**, *79*, 821–824. [CrossRef] [PubMed]
25. Branquinho, L.C.; Carrião, M.S.; Costa, A.S.; Zufelato, N.; Sousa, M.H.; Miotto, R.; Ivkov, R.; Bakuzis, A.F. Effect of Magnetic Dipolar Interactions on Nanoparticle Heating Efficiency: Implications for Cancer Hyperthermia. *Sci. Rep.* **2013**, *3*, 2887. [CrossRef] [PubMed]
26. Balivada, S.; Rachakatla, R.S.; Wang, H.; Samarakoon, T.N.; Dani, R.K.; Pyle, M.; Kroh, F.O.; Walker, B.; Leaym, X.; Koper, O.B.; et al. A/C Magnetic Hyperthermia of Melanoma Mediated by Iron(0)/Iron Oxide Core/Shell Magnetic Nanoparticles: A Mouse Study. *BMC Cancer* **2010**, *10*, 119. [CrossRef]
27. Carrião, M.S.; Bakuzis, A.F. Mean-Field and Linear Regime Approach to Magnetic Hyperthermia of Core–Shell Nanoparticles: Can Tiny Nanostructures Fight Cancer? *Nanoscale* **2016**, *8*, 8363–8377. [CrossRef]
28. Aquino, V.R.R.; Vinícius-Araújo, M.; Shrivastava, N.; Sousa, M.H.; Coaquira, J.A.H.; Bakuzis, A.F. Role of the Fraction of Blocked Nanoparticles on the Hyperthermia Efficiency of Mn-Based Ferrites at Clinically Relevant Conditions. *J. Phys. Chem. C* **2019**, *123*, 27725–27734. [CrossRef]
29. Chang, D.; Lim, M.; Goos, J.A.C.M.; Qiao, R.; Ng, Y.Y.; Mansfeld, F.M.; Jackson, M.; Davis, T.P.; Kavallaris, M. Biologically Targeted Magnetic Hyperthermia: Potential and Limitations. *Front. Pharmacol.* **2018**, *9*, 831. [CrossRef]
30. Wilhelm, S.; Tavares, A.J.; Dai, Q.; Ohta, S.; Audet, J.; Dvorak, H.F.; Chan, W.C.W. Analysis of Nanoparticle Delivery to Tumours. *Nat. Rev. Mater.* **2016**, *1*, 16014. [CrossRef]
31. Safavi-Sohi, R.; Maghari, S.; Raoufi, M.; Jalali, S.A.; Hajipour, M.J.; Ghassempour, A.; Mahmoudi, M. Bypassing Protein Corona Issue on Active Targeting: Zwitterionic Coatings Dictate Specific Interactions of Targeting Moieties and Cell Receptors. *ACS Appl. Mater. Interfaces* **2016**, *8*, 22808–22818. [CrossRef]
32. Pankhurst, Q.A.; Thanh, N.K.T.; Jones, S.K.; Dobson, J. Progress in Applications of Magnetic Nanoparticles in Biomedicine. *J. Phys. D Appl. Phys.* **2009**, *42*, 224001. [CrossRef]
33. Southern, P.; Pankhurst, Q.A. Commentary on the Clinical and Preclinical Dosage Limits of Interstitially Administered Magnetic Fluids for Therapeutic Hyperthermia Based on Current Practice and Efficacy Models. *Int. J. Hyperth.* **2018**, *34*, 671–686. [CrossRef] [PubMed]

34. Jordan, A.; Scholz, R.; Wust, P.; Schirra, H.; Schiestel, T.; Schmidt, H.; Felix, R. Endocytosis of Dextran and Silan-Coated Magnetite Nanoparticles and the Effect of Intracellular Hyperthermia on Human Mammary Carcinoma Cells in Vitro. *J. Magn. Magn. Mater.* **1999**, *194*, 185–196. [CrossRef]
35. Orgill, D.P.; Porter, S.A.; Taylor, H.O. Heat Injury to Cells in Perfused Systems. *Ann. N. Y. Acad. Sci.* **2006**, *1066*, 106–118. [CrossRef]
36. Rodrigues, H.F.; Capistrano, G.; Bakuzis, A.F. In Vivo Magnetic Nanoparticle Hyperthermia: A Review on Preclinical Studies, Low-Field Nano-Heaters, Noninvasive Thermometry and Computer Simulations for Treatment Planning. *Int. J. Hyperth.* **2020**, *37*, 76–99. [CrossRef]
37. Jing, H.; Wang, J.; Yang, P.; Ke, X.; Xia, G.; Chen, B. Magnetic Fe3O4 Nanoparticles and Chemotherapy Agents Interact Synergistically to Induce Apoptosis in Lymphoma Cells. *Int. J. Nanomed.* **2010**, *5*, 999–1004. [CrossRef]
38. Hua, M.-Y.; Liu, H.-L.; Yang, H.-W.; Chen, P.-Y.; Tsai, R.-Y.; Huang, C.-Y.; Tseng, I.-C.; Lyu, L.-A.; Ma, C.-C.; Tang, H.-J.; et al. The Effectiveness of a Magnetic Nanoparticle-Based Delivery System for BCNU in the Treatment of Gliomas. *Biomaterials* **2011**, *32*, 516–527. [CrossRef]
39. Yang, H.-W.; Hua, M.-Y.; Liu, H.-L.; Huang, C.-Y.; Tsai, R.-Y.; Lu, Y.-J.; Chen, J.-Y.; Tang, H.-J.; Hsien, H.-Y.; Chang, Y.-S.; et al. Self-Protecting Core-Shell Magnetic Nanoparticles for Targeted, Traceable, Long Half-Life Delivery of BCNU to Gliomas. *Biomaterials* **2011**, *32*, 6523–6532. [CrossRef]
40. Yang, H.-W.; Hua, M.-Y.; Liu, H.-L.; Tsai, R.-Y.; Chuang, C.-K.; Chu, P.-C.; Wu, P.-Y.; Chang, Y.-H.; Chuang, H.-C.; Yu, K.-J.; et al. Cooperative Dual-Activity Targeted Nanomedicine for Specific and Effective Prostate Cancer Therapy. *ACS Nano* **2012**, *6*, 1795–1805. [CrossRef]
41. Yang, H.-W.; Hua, M.-Y.; Liu, H.-L.; Tsai, R.-Y.; Pang, S.-T.; Hsu, P.-H.; Tang, H.-J.; Yen, T.-C.; Chuang, C.-K. An Epirubicin–Conjugated Nanocarrier with MRI Function to Overcome Lethal Multidrug-Resistant Bladder Cancer. *Biomaterials* **2012**, *33*, 3919–3930. [CrossRef]
42. Yadollahpour, A.; Rashidi, S. Magnetic Nanoparticles: A Review of Chemical and Physical Characteristics Important in Medical Applications. *Orient. J. Chem.* **2015**, *31*, 25–30. [CrossRef]
43. Dai, Q.; Long, R.; Wang, S.; Kankala, R.K.; Wang, J.; Jiang, W.; Liu, Y. Bacterial Magnetosomes as an Efficient Gene Delivery Platform for Cancer Theranostics. *Microb. Cell Factories* **2017**, *16*, 216. [CrossRef]
44. Long, R.; Dai, Q.; Zhou, X.; Cai, D.; Hong, Y.; Wang, S.; Liu, Y. Bacterial Magnetosomes-Based Nanocarriers for Co-Delivery of Cancer Therapeutics in Vitro. *Int. J. Nanomed.* **2018**, *13*, 8269–8279. [CrossRef] [PubMed]
45. Wang, J.; Geng, Y.; Zhang, Y.; Wang, X.; Liu, J.; Basit, A.; Miao, T.; Liu, W.; Jiang, W. Bacterial Magnetosomes Loaded with Doxorubicin and Transferrin Improve Targeted Therapy of Hepatocellular Carcinoma. *Nanotheranostics* **2019**, *3*, 284–298. [CrossRef]
46. Alphandéry, E.; Chebbi, I.; Guyot, F.; Durand-Dubief, M. Use of Bacterial Magnetosomes in the Magnetic Hyperthermia Treatment of Tumours: A Review. *Int. J. Hyperth.* **2013**, *29*, 801–809. [CrossRef] [PubMed]
47. Usov, N.A.; Gubanova, E.M. Application of Magnetosomes in Magnetic Hyperthermia. *Nanomaterials* **2020**, *10*, 1320. [CrossRef] [PubMed]
48. Balkwill, D.L.; Maratea, D.; Blakemore, R.P. Ultrastructure of a Magnetotactic Spirillum. *J. Bacteriol.* **1980**, *141*, 1399–1408. [CrossRef] [PubMed]
49. Sun, J.; Tang, T.; Duan, J.; Xu, P.; Wang, Z.; Zhang, Y.; Wu, L.; Li, Y. Biocompatibility of Bacterial Magnetosomes: Acute Toxicity, Immunotoxicity and Cytotoxicity. *Nanotoxicology* **2010**, *4*, 271–283. [CrossRef]
50. Cintra, E.R.; Hayasaki, T.G.; Sousa-Junior, A.A.; Silva, A.C.G.; Valadares, M.C.; Bakuzis, A.F.; Mendanha, S.A.; Lima, E.M. Folate-Targeted PEGylated Magnetoliposomes for Hyperthermia-Mediated Controlled Release of Doxorubicin. *Front. Pharmacol.* **2022**, *13*, 854430. [CrossRef]
51. Tourinho, F.A.; Franck, R.; Massart, R. Aqueous Ferrofluids Based on Manganese and Cobalt Ferrites. *J. Mater. Sci.* **1990**, *25*, 3249–3254. [CrossRef]
52. Scherrer, P. Bestimmung Der Größe Und Der Inneren Struktur von Kolloidteilchen Mittels Röntgenstrahlen. *Nachr. Ges. Wiss. Göttingen Math. Kl.* **1918**, *1918*, 98–100.
53. Jacobi, U.; Kaiser, M.; Toll, R.; Mangelsdorf, S.; Audring, H.; Otberg, N.; Sterry, W.; Lademann, J. Porcine Ear Skin: An in Vitro Model for Human Skin. *Ski. Res. Technol.* **2007**, *13*, 19–24. [CrossRef] [PubMed]
54. Carpentier, A.; McNichols, R.J.; Stafford, R.J.; Itzcovitz, J.; Guichard, J.P.; Reizine, D.; Delaloge, S.; Vicaut, E.; Payen, D.; Gowda, A.; et al. Real-Time Magnetic Resonance-Guided Laser Thermal Therapy for Focal Metastatic Brain Tumors. *Neurosurgery* **2008**, *63*, 21–29. [CrossRef]
55. Frenkel, J.; Dorfman, J. Spontaneous and Induced Magnetisation in Ferromagnetic Bodies. *Nature* **1930**, *126*, 274–275. [CrossRef]
56. Jiles, D.C. Modelling the Effects of Eddy Current Losses on Frequency Dependent Hysteresis in Electrically Conducting Media. *IEEE Trans. Magn.* **1994**, *30*, 4326–4328. [CrossRef]
57. Zufelato, N.; Aquino, V.R.R.; Shrivastava, N.; Mendanha, S.; Miotto, R.; Bakuzis, A.F. Heat Generation in Magnetic Hyperthermia by Manganese Ferrite-Based Nanoparticles Arises from Néel Collective Magnetic Relaxation. *ACS Appl. Nano Mater.* **2022**, *5*, 7521–7539. [CrossRef]
58. Bruschi, M.L. Mathematical Models of Drug Release. In *Strategies to Modify the Drug Release from Pharmaceutical Systems*; Woodhead Publishing: Cambridge, UK, 2015; pp. 63–86. ISBN 9780081000922.

59. Oliveira, R.R.; Ferreira, F.S.; Cintra, E.R.; Branquinho, L.C.; Bakuzis, A.F.; Lima, E.M. Magnetic Nanoparticles and Rapamycin Encapsulated into Polymeric Nanocarriers. *J. Biomed. Nanotechnol.* **2012**, *8*, 193–201. [CrossRef]
60. Muñoz de Escalona, M.; Sáez-Fernández, E.; Prados, J.C.; Melguizo, C.; Arias, J.L. Magnetic Solid Lipid Nanoparticles in Hyperthermia against Colon Cancer. *Int. J. Pharm.* **2016**, *504*, 11–19. [CrossRef]
61. Liang, J.; Zhang, X.; Miao, Y.; Li, J.; Gan, Y. Lipid-Coated Iron Oxide Nanoparticles for Dual-Modal Imaging of Hepatocellular Carcinoma. *Int. J. Nanomed.* **2017**, *12*, 2033–2044. [CrossRef]
62. Allam, A.A.; Sadat, M.E.; Potter, S.J.; Mast, D.B.; Mohamed, D.F.; Habib, F.S.; Pauletti, G.M. Stability and Magnetically Induced Heating Behavior of Lipid-Coated Fe3O4 Nanoparticles. *Nanoscale Res. Lett.* **2013**, *8*, 426. [CrossRef]
63. Pan, X.; Guan, J.; Yoo, J.-W.; Epstein, A.J.; Lee, L.J.; Lee, R.J. Cationic Lipid-Coated Magnetic Nanoparticles Associated with Transferrin for Gene Delivery. *Int. J. Pharm.* **2008**, *358*, 263–270. [CrossRef] [PubMed]
64. Ying, X.-Y.; Du, Y.-Z.; Hong, L.-H.; Yuan, H.; Hu, F.-Q. Magnetic Lipid Nanoparticles Loading Doxorubicin for Intracellular Delivery: Preparation and Characteristics. *J. Magn. Magn. Mater.* **2011**, *323*, 1088–1093. [CrossRef]
65. Lin, J.; Cai, Q.; Tang, Y.; Xu, Y.; Wang, Q.; Li, T.; Xu, H.; Wang, S.; Fan, K.; Liu, Z.; et al. PEGylated Lipid Bilayer Coated Mesoporous Silica Nanoparticles for Co-Delivery of Paclitaxel and Curcumin: Design, Characterization and Its Cytotoxic Effect. *Int. J. Pharm.* **2018**, *536*, 272–282. [CrossRef] [PubMed]
66. Meng, H.; Wang, M.; Liu, H.; Liu, X.; Situ, A.; Wu, B.; Ji, Z.; Chang, C.H.; Nel, A.E. Use of a Lipid-Coated Mesoporous Silica Nanoparticle Platform for Synergistic Gemcitabine and Paclitaxel Delivery to Human Pancreatic Cancer in Mice. *ACS Nano* **2015**, *9*, 3540–3557. [CrossRef] [PubMed]
67. Islam, K.; Haque, M.; Kumar, A.; Hoq, A.; Hyder, F.; Hoque, S.M. Manganese Ferrite Nanoparticles (MnFe2O4): Size Dependence for Hyperthermia and Negative/Positive Contrast Enhancement in MRI. *Nanomaterials* **2020**, *10*, 2297. [CrossRef]
68. Lu, J.; Ma, S.; Sun, J.; Xia, C.; Liu, C.; Wang, Z.; Zhao, X.; Gao, F.; Gong, Q.; Song, B. Manganese Ferrite Nanoparticle Micellar Nanocomposites as MRI Contrast Agent for Liver Imaging. *Biomaterials* **2009**, *30*, 2919–2928. [CrossRef]
69. Vinícius-Araújo, M.; Shrivastava, N.; Sousa-Junior, A.A.; Mendanha, S.A.; de Santana, R.C.; Bakuzis, A.F. ZnxMn1-XFe2O4@SiO2:ZNd+3 Core-Shell Nanoparticles for Low-Field Magnetic Hyperthermia and Enhanced Photothermal Therapy with the Potential for Nanothermometry. *ACS Appl. Nano Mater.* **2021**, *4*, 2190–2210. [CrossRef]
70. Regenold, M.; Bannigan, P.; Evans, J.C.; Waspe, A.; Temple, M.J.; Allen, C. Turning down the Heat: The Case for Mild Hyperthermia and Thermosensitive Liposomes. *Nanomed. Nanotechnol. Biol. Med.* **2022**, *40*, 102484. [CrossRef]
71. Gray-Schopfer, V.; Wellbrock, C.; Marais, R. Melanoma Biology and New Targeted Therapy. *Nature* **2007**, *445*, 851–857. [CrossRef]
72. Espinosa, A.; Di Corato, R.; Kolosnjaj-Tabi, J.; Flaud, P.; Pellegrino, T.; Wilhelm, C. Duality of Iron Oxide Nanoparticles in Cancer Therapy: Amplification of Heating Efficiency by Magnetic Hyperthermia and Photothermal Bimodal Treatment. *ACS Nano* **2016**, *10*, 2436–2446. [CrossRef]
73. Kong, G.; Dewhirst, M.W. Hyperthermia and Liposomes. *Int. J. Hyperth.* **1999**, *15*, 345–370. [CrossRef]
74. Katagiri, K.; Nakamura, M.; Koumoto, K. Magnetoresponsive Smart Capsules Formed with Polyelectrolytes, Lipid Bilayers and Magnetic Nanoparticles. *ACS Appl. Mater. Interfaces* **2010**, *2*, 768–773. [CrossRef] [PubMed]
75. Ge, M.; Li, X.; Li, Y.; Jahangir Alam, S.M.; Gui, Y.; Huang, Y.; Cao, L.; Liang, G.; Hu, G. Preparation of Magadiite-Sodium Alginate Drug Carrier Composite by Pickering-Emulsion-Templated-Encapsulation Method and Its Properties of Sustained Release Mechanism by Baker–Lonsdale and Korsmeyer–Peppas Model. *J. Polym. Environ.* **2022**, *30*, 3890–3900. [CrossRef]
76. Iacovita, C.; Florea, A.; Scorus, L.; Pall, E.; Dudric, R.; Moldovan, A.I.; Stiufiuc, R.; Tetean, R.; Lucaciu, C.M. Hyperthermia, Cytotoxicity, and Cellular Uptake Properties of Manganese and Zinc Ferrite Magnetic Nanoparticles Synthesized by a Polyol-Mediated Process. *Nanomaterials* **2019**, *9*, 1489. [CrossRef] [PubMed]
77. Joshi, N.; Shirsath, N.; Singh, A.; Joshi, K.S.; Banerjee, R. Endogenous Lung Surfactant Inspired PH Responsive Nanovesicle Aerosols: Pulmonary Compatible and Site-Specific Drug Delivery in Lung Metastases. *Sci. Rep.* **2015**, *4*, 7085. [CrossRef] [PubMed]
78. Huang, Y.; Shi, Y.; Wang, Q.; Qi, T.; Fu, X.; Gu, Z.; Zhang, Y.; Zhai, G.; Zhao, X.; Sun, Q.; et al. Enzyme Responsiveness Enhances the Specificity and Effectiveness of Nanoparticles for the Treatment of B16F10 Melanoma. *J. Control. Release* **2019**, *316*, 208–222. [CrossRef]
79. Asín, L.; Ibarra, M.R.; Tres, A.; Goya, G.F. Controlled Cell Death by Magnetic Hyperthermia: Effects of Exposure Time, Field Amplitude, and Nanoparticle Concentration. *Pharm. Res.* **2012**, *29*, 1319–1327. [CrossRef]
80. Zhang, W.; Shi, Y.; Chen, Y.; Hao, J.; Sha, X.; Fang, X. The Potential of Pluronic Polymeric Micelles Encapsulated with Paclitaxel for the Treatment of Melanoma Using Subcutaneous and Pulmonary Metastatic Mice Models. *Biomaterials* **2011**, *32*, 5934–5944. [CrossRef]
81. Torres-Lugo, M.; Rodriguez, H.L.; Latorre-Esteves, M.; Mendez, J.; Soto, O.; Rodriguez, A.R.; Rinaldi, C. Enhanced Reduction in Cell Viability by Hyperthermia Induced by Magnetic Nanoparticles. *Int. J. Nanomed.* **2011**, *6*, 373–380. [CrossRef]
82. Toraya-Brown, S.; Fiering, S. Local Tumour Hyperthermia as Immunotherapy for Metastatic Cancer. *Int. J. Hyperth.* **2014**, *30*, 531–539. [CrossRef]
83. Toraya-Brown, S.; Sheen, M.R.; Zhang, P.; Chen, L.; Baird, J.R.; Demidenko, E.; Turk, M.J.; Hoopes, P.J.; Conejo-Garcia, J.R.; Fiering, S. Local Hyperthermia Treatment of Tumors Induces CD8+ T Cell-Mediated Resistance against Distal and Secondary Tumors. *Nanomed. Nanotechnol. Biol. Med.* **2014**, *10*, 1273–1285. [CrossRef] [PubMed]

84. Soetaert, F.; Korangath, P.; Serantes, D.; Fiering, S.; Ivkov, R. Cancer Therapy with Iron Oxide Nanoparticles: Agents of Thermal and Immune Therapies. *Adv. Drug Deliv. Rev.* **2020**, *163–164*, 65–83. [CrossRef] [PubMed]
85. Gorbet, M.J.; Singh, A.; Mao, C.; Fiering, S.; Ranjan, A. Using Nanoparticles for in Situ Vaccination against Cancer: Mechanisms and Immunotherapy Benefits. *Int. J. Hyperth.* **2020**, *37*, 18–33. [CrossRef] [PubMed]
86. Sebeke, L.C.; Castillo Gómez, J.D.; Heijman, E.; Rademann, P.; Simon, A.C., Ekdawi, S., Vlachakis, S.; Toker, D.; Mink, B.L.; Schubert-Quecke, C.; et al. Hyperthermia-Induced Doxorubicin Delivery from Thermosensitive Liposomes via MR-HIFU in a Pig Model. *J. Control. Release* **2022**, *343*, 798–812. [CrossRef]
87. Murray, A.A.; Wang, C.; Fiering, S.; Steinmetz, N.F. In Situ Vaccination with Cowpea vs Tobacco Mosaic Virus against Melanoma. *Mol. Pharm.* **2018**, *15*, 3700–3716. [CrossRef]
88. Hoopes, P.J.; Wagner, R.J.; Duval, K.; Kang, K.; Gladstone, D.J.; Moodie, K.L.; Crary-Burney, M.; Ariaspulido, H.; Veliz, F.A.; Steinmetz, N.F.; et al. Treatment of Canine Oral Melanoma with Nanotechnology-Based Immunotherapy and Radiation. *Mol. Pharm.* **2018**, *15*, 3717–3722. [CrossRef]

Disclaimer/Publisher's Note: The statements, opinions and data contained in all publications are solely those of the individual author(s) and contributor(s) and not of MDPI and/or the editor(s). MDPI and/or the editor(s) disclaim responsibility for any injury to people or property resulting from any ideas, methods, instructions or products referred to in the content.

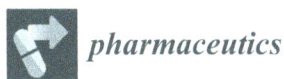

Article

Doxorubicin Loaded Thermosensitive Magneto-Liposomes Obtained by a Gel Hydration Technique: Characterization and In Vitro Magneto-Chemotherapeutic Effect Assessment

Stefan Nitica [1,†], Ionel Fizesan [2,†], Roxana Dudric [3], Felicia Loghin [2], Constantin Mihai Lucaciu [1,*] and Cristian Iacovita [1]

1. Department of Pharmaceutical Physics-Biophysics, Faculty of Pharmacy, "Iuliu Hatieganu" University of Medicine and Pharmacy, 6 Pasteur St., 400349 Cluj-Napoca, Romania
2. Department of Toxicology, Faculty of Pharmacy, "Iuliu Hațieganu" University of Medicine and Pharmacy, 6A Pasteur St., 400349 Cluj-Napoca, Romania
3. Faculty of Physics, "Babes-Bolyai" University, 1 Kogalniceanu St., 400084 Cluj-Napoca, Romania
* Correspondence: clucaciu@umfcluj.ro; Tel.: +40-744-647-854
† These authors contributed equally to this work.

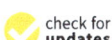

Citation: Nitica, S.; Fizesan, I.; Dudric, R.; Loghin, F.; Lucaciu, C.M.; Iacovita, C. Doxorubicin Loaded Thermosensitive Magneto-Liposomes Obtained by a Gel Hydration Technique: Characterization and In Vitro Magneto-Chemotherapeutic Effect Assessment. *Pharmaceutics* 2022, *14*, 2501. https://doi.org/10.3390/pharmaceutics14112501

Academic Editor: Xiangyang Shi

Received: 25 October 2022
Accepted: 16 November 2022
Published: 18 November 2022

Publisher's Note: MDPI stays neutral with regard to jurisdictional claims in published maps and institutional affiliations.

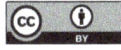

Copyright: © 2022 by the authors. Licensee MDPI, Basel, Switzerland. This article is an open access article distributed under the terms and conditions of the Creative Commons Attribution (CC BY) license (https://creativecommons.org/licenses/by/4.0/).

Abstract: The combination of magnetic hyperthermia with chemotherapy is considered a promising strategy in cancer therapy due to the synergy between the high temperatures and the chemotherapeutic effects, which can be further developed for targeted and remote-controlled drug release. In this paper we report a simple, rapid, and reproducible method for the preparation of thermosensitive magnetoliposomes (TsMLs) loaded with doxorubicin (DOX), consisting of a lipidic gel formation from a previously obtained water-in-oil microemulsion with fine aqueous droplets containing magnetic nanoparticles (MNPs) dispersed in an organic solution of thermosensitive lipids (transition temperature of ~43 °C), followed by the gel hydration with an aqueous solution of DOX. The obtained thermosensitive magnetoliposomes (TsMLs) were around 300 nm in diameter and exhibited 40% DOX incorporation efficiency. The most suitable MNPs to incorporate into the liposomal aqueous lumen were Zn ferrites, with a very low coercive field at 300 K (7 kA/m) close to the superparamagnetic regime, exhibiting a maximum absorption rate (SAR) of 1130 W/gFe when dispersed in water and 635 W/gFe when confined inside TsMLs. No toxicity of Zn ferrite MNPs or of TsMLs was noticed against the A459 cancer cell line after 48 h incubation over the tested concentration range. The passive release of DOX from the TsMLs after 48h incubation induced a toxicity starting with a dosage level of 62.5 ug/cm². Below this threshold, the subsequent exposure to an alternating magnetic field (20–30 kA/m, 355 kHz) for 30 min drastically reduced the viability of the A459 cells due to the release of incorporated DOX. Our results strongly suggest that TsMLs represent a viable strategy for anticancer therapies using the magnetic field-controlled release of DOX.

Keywords: thermosensitive liposomes; doxorubicin; magnetoliposomes; magnetic hyperthermia; zinc ferrite nanoparticles; A459 cells

1. Introduction

One of the biggest challenges now facing chemotherapy, one of the most commonly used anti-tumor therapeutic approaches for cancer treatments, is represented by the controlled release of anti-cancer drugs targeted at a tumor area, as they are highly cytotoxic to healthy tissues [1,2]. Reducing systemic exposure to chemotherapeutic drugs is of paramount importance since it would drastically reduce the hard side effects on healthy tissues and the amount of anti-cancer drugs used during chemotherapy [3,4]. In the last decades, the possibility of using nanocarriers, encapsulating anti-cancer drugs, capable to circulate in the body to target the tumor and release their payload at controllable rates, has been extensively studied [5–7].

Nanocarriers based on magnetic nanoparticles (MNPs) are very promising for such use, as they can firstly be easily guided in the body and concentrated at the desired site by an extracorporeal magnetic field [8–10]. Secondly, the MNPs under the application of an alternating magnetic field (AMF) produce heat which can be exploited to sensitize the cancer cells (mild magnetic hyperthermia (MH)) and, at the same time, to trigger the fast release of the anti-cancer agents. Therefore, the synergistic effects of the simultaneous application of MH and chemotherapy, in the same nanocarrier-based MNPs, are expected to increase the effectiveness of cancer treatment.

A wide range of studies has focused on developing nanocarrier-based MNPs displaying a core-shell architecture, with the core being the MNPs. The shell was usually constituted from an organic polymer loaded with an anti-cancer drug. The organic polymer can be thermo-responsive, which means that it undergoes a conformational change at a specific temperature. Thus, the anti-cancer drug is retained at a physiological temperature within the shell and released as a consequence of MH that locally increase the temperature [11–13]. Often exploited also are pH-responsive polymers, which can release the anti-cancer drug due to the pH difference between blood/healthy tissues and tumors [14,15]. A much more robust shell is given by the mesoporous silica (SiO_2) [16–18] or metal-organic frameworks (MOFs) [19–21], which are highly porous crystalline materials providing high porosity for encapsulating or incorporating anti-cancer drugs.

One of the most attractive and studied nanocarrier systems for drug delivery is represented by liposomes (Ls) [22]. These nanocarriers present a spherical shape consisting of at least one lipid bilayer and an aqueous core, being capable of encapsulating either hydrophilic or hydrophobic anti-cancer drugs [23]. Nanoscale liposomal formulations, considered one of the most advanced delivery systems for cytotoxic drugs [24,25], have been used in clinical cancer therapy for many years, the most known example being the Doxorubicin (DOX)-loaded liposomes (Caelyx®, Schering-Plough; DOXIL®, OrthoBiotech) [26] with an improved pharmacokinetic profile and reduced cardiotoxic side effects as compared with the free drug [27]. Nevertheless, a much higher therapeutic efficacy of liposomal formulations is still needed and a large number of studies were conducted aiming at increasing the drug concentration at the target site by further enhancing their targeting and by localized triggering of the drug release from responsive liposomal formulations [28]. One of the main strategies used recently for reaching this goal is to use heat-activated liposomal drug carriers, lyso-thermosensitive liposomal doxorubicin (Thermodox®) being the first such system that has been evaluated in seven clinical studies [29].

The incorporation of MNPs in the Ls gives rise to the so-called magneto-liposomes (MLs), these structures being capable of controlled movement in the presence of a magnetic field gradient [30,31]. Regarding the aqueous MLs, the distribution of MNPs in the Ls' structure defines three classes, in which MNPs are dispersed in the Ls' aqueous core [32–34], embedded in the lipid bilayer [35,36] or attached to the Ls' surface [37–40]. Recently, by combining MNPs and gold nanoparticles (NPs) inside the Ls' aqueous core or distributed in different Ls compartments, plasmonic MLs have been created, with a great potential to achieve a synergistic effect between multiple treatment methodologies, such as chemotherapy, MH, and phototherapy [41–44].

For a controlled anti-cancer drug release, the MLs have been prepared by employing different formulations of thermo-sensitive lipids, thus resulting in thermo-responsive MLs (TsMLs) [45]. Similar to the case of thermo-responsive polymers, this class of MLs is characterized by a transition temperature (T_m), above which the permeability of the lipid bilayer increases, thus facilitating the release of the anti-cancer drugs in a controlled manner [46,47]. The manufacturing processes of TsMLs are laborious, thus their clinical translation has been slowed down. Conventional preparation methods, such as thin film hydration [48–54], reverse-phase evaporation [55,56], and the double emulsion method [57] give rise to large and multilamellar TsMLs. To reduce their dimension (a few hundred nanometers in diameter) and obtain unilamellar TsMLs, different post-synthesis techniques must be applied, such as sonication, extrusion, and size-exclusion chromatography. The sonication process degrades or contaminates the sample, resulting in poor batch-to-batch reproducibility, while extrusion suffers from great product loss, obtaining a low production yield in the end. Therefore, there is a need to develop new synthesis protocols that allow efficient MNP loading into TsLs and eliminate the use of post-synthesis techniques [58,59].

In this paper, we have developed and optimized a simple and reproducible route for the synthesis of unilamellar TsMLs without the need for post-synthesis techniques. Moreover, the one-pot method allows the loading of the Ls with both the drug and the MNPs simultaneously. The MNPs, successfully entrapped in the liposomal aqueous core, consist of zinc ferrites that were fully investigated using multiple analytical methods such as transmission electron microscopy (TEM), X-ray diffraction (XRD), vibrating sample magnetometer (VSM), and magnetic hyperthermia (MH). The prepared TsMLs were characterized for physicochemical properties such as size, morphology, and DOX entrapment efficiency. Two independent cytotoxicity assays were applied to determine the cytotoxicity of TsMLs loaded with DOX on the human pulmonary carcinoma A549 cancer cell line. The in vitro DOX release and the magneto-chemotherapeutic effect under an alternating magnetic field (AMF) stimulus have also been examined.

2. Materials and Methods

2.1. Materials

The synthesis of Zn ferrites has been done using the following chemicals: iron (III) acetylacetonate ($\geq$98.00%, Merck Schuchardt OHG, Hohenbrunn, Germany), zinc (II) acetylacetonate ($\geq$98.00%, Merck KGaA, Darmstadt, Germany), oleic acid (Sigma-Aldrich, Steinheim, Germany), tetra ethylene glycol (Carl-Roth, Karlsruhe, Germany, $\geq$99%) and benzyl ether (Sigma-Aldrich, Steinheim, Germany). The following lipids have been used in the preparation of TsMLs: 1,2-dipalmitoyl-sn-glycero-3-phosphocholine (DPPC) (Lipoid, Ludwigshafen, Germany), 1,2-distearoyl-sn-glycero-3-phosphocholine (DSPC) (Lipoid, Ludwigshafen, Germany), and cholesterol (Sigma-Aldrich, Steinheim, Germany). Additional chemicals used in the study were ethanol (Chemical, Iasi, Romania), hexane (Honeywell, Seelze, Germany), cyclohexane (Honeywell, Seelze, Germany), sodium periodate (Sigma-Aldrich, Steinheim, Germany), acetonitrile (Sigma-Aldrich, Steinheim, Germany), ethyl acetate (Chemical, Iasi, Romania), chloroform (Chemical, Iasi, Romania), ammonium sulfate (Sigma-Aldrich, Steinheim, Germany), doxorubicin hydrochloride (Sigma-Aldrich, Steinheim, Germany) and Osmium tetroxide (Merck Schuchardt OHG, Hohenbrunn, Germany)

2.2. Synthesis of MNPs and Their Water Transfer

The Zn ferrites have been synthesized by means of the thermal decomposition method. Briefly, a mixture of 1.00 mmol of iron (III) acetylacetonate, 0.1 mmol of zinc (II) acetylacetonate, 2.9 mL of oleic acid, 1 mL of oleylamine, 1 mL of tetra ethylene glycol, and 20 mL benzyl ether were magnetically stirred at 50 °C with 500 rot/min for 1h (MR-HEi-TEC, Heidolph Instruments GmbH&Co.KG, Schwabach, Germany). Upon degassing with a flux of gaseous nitrogen for 5 min, the mixture was sealed in a stainless steel reaction vessel using a Teflon gasket and five screws. The reaction mixture was primely heated to 200 °C with at a rate of 6 °C/min using an oven (Nabertherm GmbH, Lilienthal, Germany) equipped with a temperature controller (JUMO dTron 316, JUMO GmbH & Co.KG, Darmstadt, Germany) and kept at that temperature for 2 h, after which the temperature was raised to 300 °C at a rate of 3 °C/min and kept at that temperature for an additional 1h. The resulting black product was separated with a neodymium magnet and washed several times using a 20 mL mixture of ethanol/hexane through ultrasonication (15 min) and magnetic separation. The purified Zn ferrites were stored in 20 mL cyclohexane for further processing.

Water transfer has been realized through the oxidation of oleic acid by sodium periodate. Briefly, 30 mL of aqueous sodium periodate solution (c = 60 mg/mL) was added with 10 mL of acetonitrile and ethyl acetate mixture (v:v = 1:1) and 10 mL of MNPs dispersed in cyclohexane. The mixture was mechanically stirred (Nahita, Auxilab S.L., Beriain, Spain) for 2 h until all MNPs passed from cyclohexane (top) into the water (bottom) phase. The

MNPs were separated by a neodymium magnet and washed with double distilled water three more times. Finally, the hydrophilized MNPs were dispersed in the necessary volume of double distilled water to achieve a concentration of 4 mg$_{MNPs}$/mL. The obtained aqueous dispersion was stored in a glass container.

2.3. Preparation of Thermosensitive Liposomes Loaded with MNPs and Doxorubicin

A mixture consisting of 30 mg of DPPC, 15 mg of DSPC and 5 mg of cholesterol (6:3:1 weight ratio) has been dissolved in a mixture continning 2 mL of chloroform and 3 mL of hexane, which has a density slightly lower than that of water. 1.5 mL of MNPs dispersion in 1M aqueous ammonium sulfate solution—was added to the lipidic solution. The mixture was then sonicated for 6 min using a Vibra-Cell™ Ultrasonic probe sonicator, model VCX 500 equipped with a tapered microtip of Ø 6 mm (Sonics&Materials, Inc., Newtown, CT, USA). The micro-emulsion formed was further introduced in the round bottom flask of a rotary-evaporator (Heidolph Instruments GmbH&Co.KG, Schwabach, Germany)). The installation parameters were set as follows: the flask rotation speed to 220 rot/min, the installation pressure to 600 mbar, and the water bath temperature to 45 °C. The mixture was kept in the installation for 10 min, resulting in the formation of a gel-like phase. The gel was further hydrated with 18.5 mL of double distilled water or an aqueous solution of doxorubicin hydrochloride—of desired concentration (either 10^{-4} M or 2×10^{-5} M). In the end, the mixture was introduced in the rotary-evaporator and vortexed at 45 °C for 5 min at 60 rot/min and a subsequent 10 min at 150 rot/min, resulting in TsMLs loaded with doxorubicin (DOX).

2.4. Characterization Methods

Transmission electron microscopy (TEM) images were obtained on a JEOL JEM-100CX II (JEOL, Tokyo, Japan) at 80 kV with a MegaView G3 camera (Emsis, Münster, Germany) running with Radius 2.1 software (Emsis). A drop of cyclohexane suspension of MNPs (10 µg$_{MNPs}$/mL) was deposited on a carbon-coated copper grid, and we then waited for the solvent to evaporate. In the particular cases of TsLs and TsMLs, in 1 mL of liposomal aqueous solution (obtained by diluting 20 times the initial liposomal aqueous solution), a volume of 100 µL Osmium tetroxide was added to fix and stain the liposomes. After 30 min, a drop of the liposomal aqueous solution was deposited on a carbon-coated copper grid, and the excess water was removed by filter paper after 10 min.

X-ray diffraction (XRD) patterns of powdered MNPs were collected with a Bruker D8 Advance diffractometer using Cu Kα radiation (Bruker AXS GmbH, Karlsruhe, Germany). The intensities were measured from 20° to 80° in continuous mode with a step size of 0.03° and a counting rate of 5 s per scanning step.

The UV–VIS absorption spectra of all samples were recorded with a T92+ UV–VIS Spectrophotometer PG INSTRUMENTS, using standard quartz cells at room temperature, over a spectral range between 400 nm and 600 nm and a spectral resolution of 2 nm.

Hydrodynamic size and zeta potential measurements of samples (10 µg$_{MNPs}$/mL) were determined using a Zetasizer Nano ZS90 (Malvern Instruments, Worcestershire, UK) in a 90° configuration, at room temperature.

The magnetization curves of the MNPs were measured using a Cryogenic Limited (London, UK) vibrating sample magnetometer (VSM), operating at both 4K and 300K from 0 to ±4 T.

The Specific Absorption Rate (SAR) was measured on a commercially available magnetic hyperthermia system, the Easy Heat 0224 from Ambrell (Scottsville, NY, USA) equipped with an 8-turn heating coil, made of a water-cooled copper tube, and a fiber-optic thermometer, placed in the middle of the sample volume, to measure the temperature value each second. The samples (0.5 mL of MNPs suspended in water, PEG 8K, or incorporated in TsLs at different concentrations) were placed in the center of the heating coil. The environment in close vicinity of samples was held at a physiological temperature of around 37 °C. The heating curves were recorded under a fixed frequency of 355 kHz at different alternating magnetic field (AMF) amplitudes: 10–60 kA/m. Details about the hyperthermia setup are provided elsewhere [60], and SAR calculations are provided in the Supplementary Materials (Section S1).

2.5. Cell Lines

The in vitro studies were conducted on a human pulmonary carcinoma A549 cell line, purchased from the American Type Culture Collection (ATCC, Manassas, VA, USA). Dulbecco's Modified Eagle's Medium (DMEM, Gibco, Paisley, UK) supplemented with 10% Fetal Bovine Serum (FBS, Gibco, Paisley, UK) was used to keep the cells at a temperature of 37 °C and 5% CO_2 supplementation. The cell culture media was changed every other day, and the cells were used in the experiments once confluency of 80–90% was reached.

2.6. In Vitro Cytocompatibility Assays

Two different assays: Alamar Blue (AB) and Neutral Red (NR) assays were employed to assess the cytotoxicity of nanomaterials after 48 h of exposure to A549 cells seeded in 6 well plates. The cytotoxicity evaluation was performed on samples containing MNPs in a concentration of 15.625, 31.25, 62.5, 125, and 250 µg/cm². After the exposure, cells were thoroughly washed with PBS and the AB and NR dyes were added. For the AB assay, cells were incubated for 3 h with a 200 µM resazurin solution, and the fluorescence was measured at an $\lambda_{excitation}$ = 530/25 nm and $\lambda_{emission}$ = 590/35 nm. For the NR assay, cells were exposed for 2 h to a 40 µg/mL filtered NR dye solution, and post-incubation, cells were washed to remove the non-internalized dye. The intra-cellular accumulated dye was further solubilized in a 50% hydroalcoholic solution containing 1% glacial acetic acid, and the fluorescence was measured at a $\lambda_{excitation}$ = 530/25 nm and a $\lambda_{emission}$ = 620/40 nm. For both assays, experiments were done in biological triplicates and the measurement of fluorescence was performed using a Synergy 2 Multi-Mode Microplate Reader.

2.7. Evaluation of Cellular Uptake

The cellular uptake of MNPs and TsMLs was quantitatively evaluated by the Liebig reaction of free Fe^{3+} with thiocyanate as described in the Supplementary Materials (Section S2) after incubation for 48 h. After the exposure, washed and trypsinized cells were centrifuged for 5 min at 4500× g and then processed for the Fe^{3+} quantification.

2.8. In Vitro Magnetic Hyperthermia

TsMLs and DOX-loaded TsMLs, suspended in a cell culture medium, were mixed with A549 cells that were previously seeded in 6-well plates for 24 h. Subsequently, the two aliquots of similar volume resulting from each mixture were centrifuged for 10 min at 100× g to reduce their volume to 0.5 mL. Upon removal of the excess supernatant, one of the aliquots was introduced in a water bath at 37 °C representing the negative control. The twin aliquot was exposed to an alternating magnetic field (AMF) for 30 min, working at a fixed frequency of 355 kHz and variable amplitudes of 10, 20, and 30 kA/m. Immediately after the AMF treatment, the cells from both aliquots were plated in 96-wells as six technical replicates. After 48 h, the cellular viability was measured by using AB and NR assays. Three biological replicates were considered for each experiment, while the data were normalized to the negative control.

2.9. Statistics

One-way Analysis of Variance (ANOVA) equipped with a post-hoc + Dunn's test was used to analyze the data sets, while SigmaPlot 11.0 computer software (Systat) was employed to graphically represent the results, which are average values ± standard deviation (SD). Statistically relevant results were those showing p values < 0.05.

3. Results and Discussion

3.1. Characterization of Zinc Ferrites Nanoparticles and Their Heating Performances

Small-sized magnetite MNPs (10 nm in diameter) have been generally used to fabricate TsMLs. This class of MNPs is mainly in a superparamagnetic state (SP) at room temperature and their heating performances under AMF are rather weak. Moreover, upon the confinement of MNPs inside the TsL, the heating properties are further reduced. Consequently, there is a need for MNPs with larger magnetic moments to enable the release of sufficient heat to destabilize the lipid bilayer membrane [61]. An already proven efficient way to increase the heating performances of magnetite MNPs is doping their structure with Zn cations [62–67]. We have used the well-known thermal decomposition technique to prepare Zn ferrites [65,68], in which the 1,2 hexadecanediol (a very expensive surfactant) has been replaced with tetra-ethylene-glycol (TEG). With 1 mL of TEG in the reaction mixture, the modified synthetic approach enables the formation of magnetite (Fe_3O_4) nanoparticles (NPs) of quasi-spherical shape and average diameter around 9 nm (Figure S3a,b). The addition of zinc (II) acetylacetonate in the reaction mixture produces well-defined spherical Zn ferrites with an average diameter of 16.6 nm, twice the diameter of Fe_3O_4 MNPs (Figure 1a–c). The X-ray diffraction pattern of Zn ferrites under 2θ values ranging from 20 to $80°$ are plotted in Figure 1d. The occurring diffraction peaks were ascribed to crystal planes: (220), (311), (400), (422), (511) and (440), respectively (JCPDS No. 88-0315) being similar to those of pure Fe_3O_4, indicating that Zn ferrites possess the crystal unit of a face-centered cubic spinel crystalline structure [62,63]. The Zn ferrites are single crystals as the average diameter from TEM images is close to the corresponding one given by XRD diffractogram, calculated using Scherrer's formula by Gaussian fit of the peaks (220), (311), and (440). According to the hysteresis loop recorded at 4K (Figure 1e), the saturation magnetization (M_s) is around 106 emu/g, higher than that of pure magnetite, confirming the location of Zn^{2+} ions in tetrahedral sites [69]. The spin canting effects, well-pronounced for MNPs of spherical shape, reduced the M_s at 300K with 26 emu/g. The low field hysteresis loops (Figure 1f) showed the presence of a coercive field (H_c) of 25 mT (20 kA/m) at 4K, which is reduced to 9 mT (7 kA/m) at 300K, suggesting that the Zn ferrites are close to a superparamagnetic type behavior at the above temperature.

The SAR dependence of Zn ferrites on the concentration and amplitude of the magnetic field is presented in Figure 1g for the concentration range 0.25–4.00 mg_{Fe}/mL. The SAR dependence on the amplitude of the alternating magnetic field is sigmoidal and was fitted with a logistic function (Equations (S3) and (S4)), to obtain the SAR_{max} and the hyperthermia coercive field, i.e., the point of highest slope in the SAR = f(H_{max}) curve [70]. The concentration dependence of SAR is nonmonotonic. SAR_{max} increases as the concentration increases in the range of 0.25–1.00 mg_{Fe}/mL and decreases as the concentration further increases. The maximum SAR of 1130 W/g_{Fe} is reached for a concentration of 1 mg_{Fe}/mL (Section S1 Table S1). As explained in our previous paper [66], the increase in the colloidal concentration drives the Zn ferrites from individual behavior to a collective one. In the concentration range of 0.25–1.00 mg_{Fe}/mL, the interparticle interaction enhances their magnetization, while in the concentration range of 1.00–4.00 mg/mL, the dipolar interactions between the MNPs lead to a demagnetizing effect, reducing the magnetization of the colloid and thus the SAR_{max} [71]. As a consequence, the SAR_{max} values increase from 450 W/g_{Fe} at 0.25 mg_{Fe}/mL to 1130 W/g_{Fe} at 1 mg_{Fe}/mL and then decrease again to 810 W/g_{Fe} at 4 mg_{Fe}/mL. Compared with Fe_3O_4 MNPs (Figure S3c), the Zn ferrites display a 3-fold higher SAR value due to the Zn doping. As expected, the random distribution of Zn ferrites in a solid matrix (PEG 8K) led to an important decrease of the SAR values: on average by 70% for 1 mg_{Fe}/mL, 65% for 0.50 mg_{Fe}/mL and 50% for 0.25 mg_{Fe}/mL. For all three concentrations, the SAR values are almost identical in the H range of 10 to 30 kA/m. A small decrease of SAR values with decreasing the concentration can be identified starting with H of 40 kA/m.

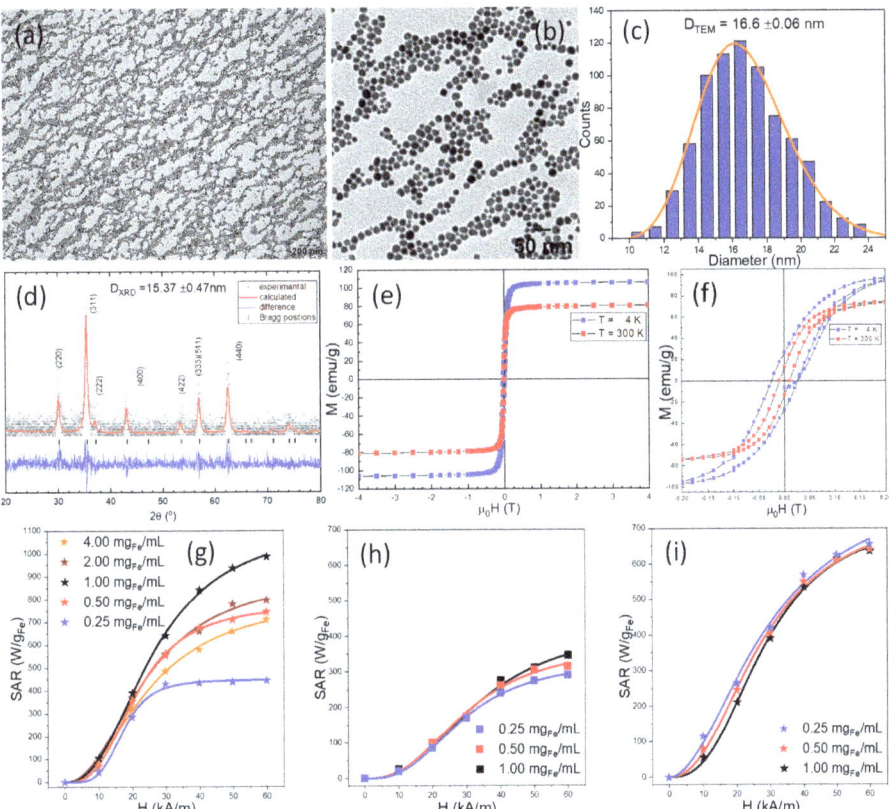

Figure 1. (a) Large scale and (b) zoom-in TEM image of Zn ferrites. (c) Size distribution histograms fitted to a log-normal distribution (orange line). (d) XRD diffraction patterns of Zn ferrites. (e) Hysteresis loops of Zn ferrites. (f) Low-field regime hysteresis loops of Zn ferrites. Specific absorption rate (SAR) dependence on the AMF amplitude (H) for Zn ferrites dispersed in (g) water and (h) PEG 8K at three different concentrations. (i) SAR dependence on H for TsMLs.

3.2. Preparation of Thermosensitive Magneto-Liposomes Loaded with Doxorubicin and Their Heating Performances

Normally, by selecting the phospholipids and adjusting their composition, thermosensitive liposomes (TsL) can be designed to display a leakage temperature range, within which the lipid bilayer membrane undergoes a phase transition from the crystalline form to a liquid one and cause the release of payload. In this work, we adopted the phospholipidic composition used by Anikeeva et al. [57]—with less cholesterol, that enables the formulation of TsL with a phase-transition temperature between 42–43 °C. Instead of the double emulsion method for liposome preparation, we used an osmotic-mediated hydration of the lipid gel method, as described in the Section 2. An ammonium sulfate aqueous phase containing Zn ferrites was transferred into a solution of thermosensitive lipids in a mixture of hydrophobic solvents. After the formation of the micro-emulsion through sonication, the hydrophobic phase was rapidly evaporated. The hydration of the formed gel with an aqueous solution of doxorubicin produced spherical TsMLs with an average diameter of 365 (±170) nm (Figure 2a). Various amounts of Zn ferrite were used in the preparation to achieve a maximum ratio between encapsulated and empty TsLs. We found that an amount of 10 mg_{MNPs} in the microemulsion mixture is adequate to obtain a high number of TsLs containing Zn ferrites, with a small fraction (less than 5%) of empty TsLs. All Zn ferrites were encapsulated inside the TsLs as no free MNPs were observed on the TEM images. However, above this threshold, some Zn ferrites remain outside of TsLs within the supernatant of the liposomal solution. Room temperature TEM analysis clearly shows that the Zn ferrites are homogeneously distributed inside the inner aqueous core of the TsLs (Figure 2b). The Zeta potential of Zn ferrites upon water transfer was found to be −37.28 mV, this negative value being due to the carboxyl groups resulting upon oxidation of oleic acid by sodium periodate [65,72]. The incorporation of Zn ferrites inside the aqueous core of TsLs led to TsMLs exhibiting a less negative Zeta potential of −13.47 mV.

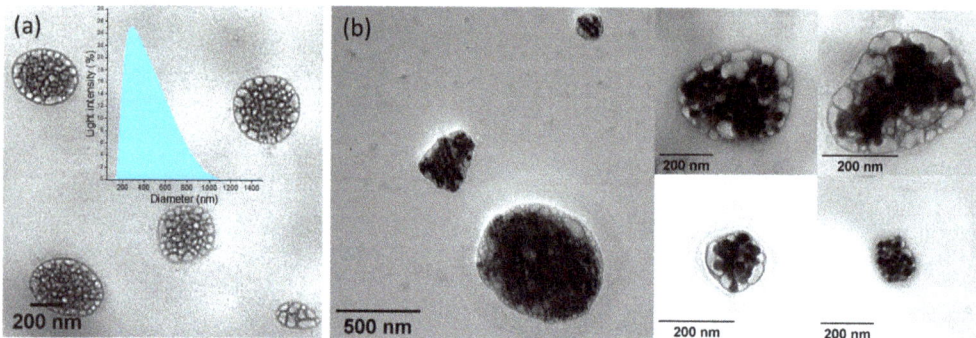

Figure 2. TEM images of (**a**) TsLs and (**b**) TsMLs. The inset represents the DLS spectrum of TsLs.

The preparation method of TsMLs developed herein is very efficient as basically all MNPs, below a certain threshold, are embedded in the liposomal pool, eliminating the need for post-synthesis purification methods. Moreover, the size of TsMLs of a few hundred nanometers directly resulting from synthesis, without the use of downsizing techniques, is adequate for biomedical applications. It is worth mentioning that the concentration of ammonium sulfate from the solution used for emulsion preparation played an important role in the gel hydration efficiency, the optimal value being situated at 1M in our experiments.

To check the suitability of our preparation method, we have extended it to other types of MNPs. The small Fe_3O_4 NPs, presented above are incorporated in the liposomal pool resulting in well-defined TsMLs (Figure S4a). Instead, 27 nm ferromagnetic Zn ferrites with higher SAR (>3000 W/g_{Fe}) [65] tend to form chains and avoid entrapping in the liposomal pool (Figure S4b). Therefore, it appears that the successful preparation of TsMLs is restricted to using SP-MNPs or MNPs close to the superparamagnetic regime. In the third case, we have coated the current Zn ferrites in a silica shell, according to a procedure published previously [65] in small clusters containing few MNPs. According to TEM analysis, there is no embedment in the liposomal pool: the silica-coated Zn ferrites are located either outside the TsLs or are attached to the lipid bilayer (Figure S4c). Both Zn ferrites and Fe_3O_4 NPs exhibit a higher negative Zeta potential as compared to silica-coated ones. It results that negatively charged MNPs are prone to be entrapped in the liposomal pool, probably due to a possible interaction with the positive charges of the zwitterionic lipids (the ammonium group from phosphatidylcholine) occurring during the preparation.

The amount of DOX encapsulated in TsMLs was estimated by UV-Vis spectroscopy based on a calibration curve that exhibits the DOX concentration as a function of the absorbance at 495 nm (Figure S5). Upon preparation of the TsMLs with DOX, the liposomal solution was magnetically decanted, and the supernatant was used to determine the non-encapsulated DOX amount. The difference between the initial DOX amount and that of non-encapsulated DOX gives the amount of encapsulated DOX. Two different starting concentrations of DOX have been used: 10^{-4} M and 2×10^{-5} M corresponding to 930.47 and 178.29 µg of DOX respectively. According to Table 1, for the high initial DOX concentration, the amount of encapsulated DOX was 392 µg, resulting in an encapsulation efficiency (EE = DOX$_{encapsulated}$/DOX$_{inital}$ × 100) of 42%. The EE decreases to 39% for low initial DOX concentration, the encapsulated DOX amount being 70 µg, representing an amount 5.6 times lower than the first case.

Table 1. Loading capacity of TsMLs with doxorubicin.

Liposomes	Initial DOX Concentration	Initial DOX Amount	Non-Encapsulated DOX Amount	Encapsulated DOX Amount	Encapsulation Efficiency
h-DOX-TsMLs	10^{-4} M	930 ± 26 µg	538 ± 36 µg	392 ± 11 µg	42%
l-DOX-TsMLs	2×10^{-5} M	178 ± 19 µg	109 ± 28 µg	70 ± 9 µg	39%

The release of encapsulated doxorubicin from TsMLs crucially depends on the capabilities of Zn ferrites, confined in TsLs, to produce heat under AMF stimulus. Therefore, in the next step of our study, we have examined the heating capabilities of well-designed TsMLs. As presented in Figure 1i, for a concentration of 1.00 mg$_{Fe}$/mL, the SAR values exhibit a sigmoidal increase from 55 W/g$_{Fe}$ to 635 W/g$_{Fe}$ with increasing H from 10 to 60 kA/m. For the entire H range, the decrease in concentration led to only a very slight increase in SAR values (Figure 1i), contrary to previous cases for unconfined or immobilized Zn ferrites (Figure 1g,h) for which the concentration dependence of SAR is much more pronounced. This situation is similar to the case of Zn ferrites coated in an SiO$_2$ layer in relatively small clusters [65], which also present a very slight dependence of SAR on concentration. In both cases, with the MNPs confined in the liposomes or clustered in a silica shell, the SAR values are smaller as compared to the water dispersion case. This is explained by the strong dipolar interaction between the MNPs within the TLs or the cluster. However, the fact that increasing the number of clusters and thus reducing the main distance between them has very small or no influence on SAR is a clear indication that inter-cluster or inter-liposomal interactions are negligible [66] and either the lipidic bilayer or the silica shell avoids the confined Zn ferrites to come into contact and form bigger aggregates as the concentration increases. Thus, the inter-TsMLs interaction energy is negligible and the increase in the number of TsMLs in a given volume will not affect the SAR. Compared with the case where the Zn ferrites are dispersed in water, their confinement in the aqueous lumen of TsLs led to a reduction of SAR values. As mentioned above, this decrease can be explained by an increase in the dipolar interaction between the MNPs confined inside the TsMLs. As can be seen from Table S1, the SAR values for the water dispersions decrease from 1130 W/g$_{Fe}$ at 1mg$_{Fe}$/mL to 810 W/g$_{Fe}$ at 4 mg$_{Fe}$/mL. Based on the initial concentrations of MNPs and the final volumes obtained, the actual concentration of MNPs inside a TsLs is 6–7 mg$_{Fe}$/mL or higher, and this concentration increase is a reasonable explanation for SAR$_{max}$ values of 700 W/g$_{Fe}$ for the TsMLs.

With respect to immobilized Zn ferrites, the SAR values of Zn ferrites confined in TsMLs are higher for all H (Tables S1 and S2). This can be due to a certain mobility of TsMLs generating heat through physical rotation. We checked if this partial mobility allows the MNPs to align themselves in a static DC field aiming at increasing the SAR. In our recent paper, we have shown that a direct current bias magnetic field (H$_{DC}$) applied parallel or perpendicular to AFM lines enhances the SAR mainly at higher H for water-dispersed MNPs [66]. Therefore, an H$_{DC}$ of 10 kA/m has been applied parallel to AMF lines during MH experiments in the second set of experiments performed on TsMLs. According to Figure S6, for all three concentrations and all H$_{max}$ values, the SAR values are smaller than those recorded without H$_{DC}$, while the H$_{cHyp}$ values are shifted toward higher H (Table S2). This type of behavior is similar to that recorded for immobilized Zn ferrites [66]. Thus, by confinement inside the aqueous lumen of TsLs, the Zn ferrites are partially immobilized, being restricted to organize in chains under the influence of either field.

3.3. Cellular Viability of Doxorubicin-Loaded TsMLs

Before evaluating the synergistic effect of DOX-loaded TsMLs upon MH treatment, in our study, we have determined the anti-tumoral effect (IC_{50}) of doxorubicin (DOX) on the A549 cell line. Cellular viability of A549 cells was measured by Alamar Blue (AB) and Neutral Red (NR) assays after exposure to various concentrations of DOX (ranging from 0.0145 to 0.870 µg/mL) for 24 and 48 h. The AB assay shows that the DOX presents a cytotoxic effect, after 24 h, starting with a concentration of 0.03 µg/mL. The cell viability decreases with increasing the DOX concentration, reaching a plateau of around 36% for the last three tested concentrations (Figure 3a) with an IC_{50} of 0.3 µg/mL, similar to other reports in the literature for A459 cells [70]. By doubling the incubation time to 48 h, the cell viability continued to decrease for all concentrations (Figure 3b). The drop in cell viability was more pronounced at higher tested concentrations. The IC_{50} was shifted from 0.3 µg/mL at 24 h to 0.18 µg/mL at 48 h. The NR assay, which is less sensitive than the AB assay, also indicated a pronounced cytotoxic effect of DOX on A549 cells at 48h. Since DOX presents a relevant anti-tumoral effect towards A549 cells at 48 h, the safe working concentrations of the three Zn ferrites, TsMLs and DOX-loaded TsMLs were established at this incubation interval time.

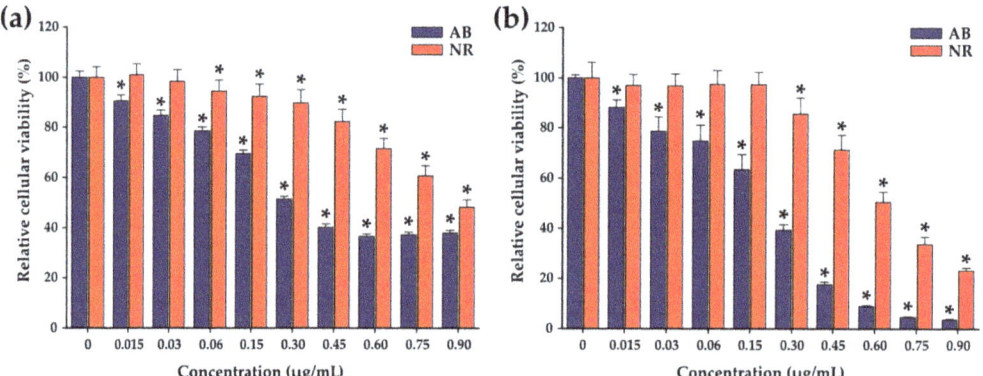

Figure 3. Cytocompatibility of doxorubicin on A549 cell line after (**a**) 24 h and (**b**) 48 h exposure. Data are presented as relative values to the negative control (100%), as mean ± SD of three biological replicates. The significant differences compared to the negative control (ANOVA + Dunn's; $p < 0.05$) are noted with asterisks (*).

As Figure 4a,b show, the lack of cytotoxic effects after 48 h of exposure of A549 cell lines to the Zn ferrites and TsMLs over the entire concentrations range (15.625 to 250 µg/cm^2) can be noted. The lack of cytotoxic effect can be explained by the poor internalization of both Zn ferrites and TsMLs (Figure S7). After 48 h, the relative internalization of Zn ferrites was low: ranging between 2.7% and 25% for Zn ferrites alone and between 2.3–18% for Zn ferrites entrapped in TsLs (Figure S7). For both cases, the relative internalization decreased by increasing the exposure dose (Figure S7). These small percentages of relative internalization mean a very low amount of internalized MNPs. In each case, the highest internalized amount was 20 µg$_{Fe}$ per well (around 20 pg$_{Fe}$ per cell), which is well below the toxicity threshold of MNPs. The lack of internalization can be explained by the negative surface charge of Zn ferrites and TsMLs which are hardly endocytosed by A549 cells, as their membrane displays extensive negatively charged domains.

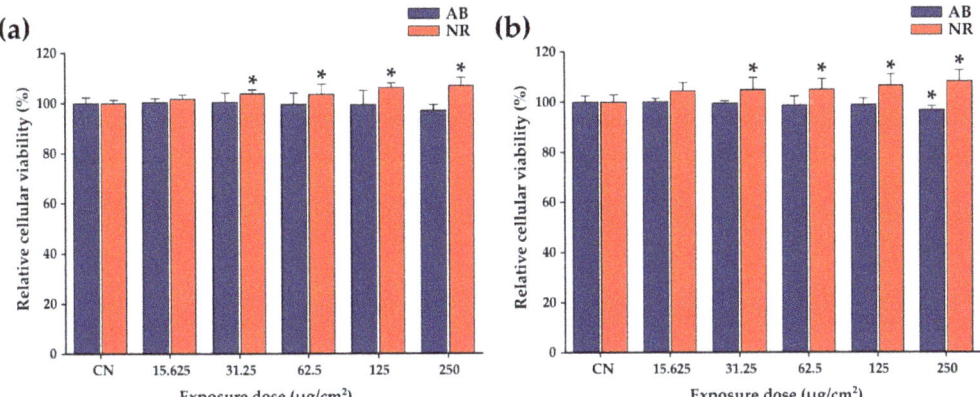

Figure 4. Cytocompatibility of (**a**) Zn ferrites and (**b**) TsMLs on A549 cell line after 48h exposure. Data are presented as relative values to the negative control (100%), as mean ± SD of three biological replicates. The significant differences compared to the negative control (ANOVA + Dunn's; $p < 0.05$) are noted with asterisks (*).

In contrast to previous observations obtained for Zn ferrites either alone or entrapped in TsLs, the exposure of A549 cells to the TsMLs loaded with DOX caused a decrease in the cell viability of A549 cells (Figure 5). After 48h of exposure to l-DOX-TsMLs (TsMLs loaded with a small amount of DOX), the NR assay showed no toxicity over the entire concentration range (Figure 5a). Based on the fact that the concentration of the tested nanomaterial can be described as non-toxic if the cells' viability is above 80%, the AB assay indicated a concentration threshold of 250 µg/cm^2, where a drop in the cell viability to 65% was recorded (Figure 5b). In the case of h-DOX-TsMLs (TsMLs loaded with a high amount of DOX), the NR assay indicated toxicity at a concentration of 250 µg/cm^2 (Figure 5b). Instead, the AB assay showed a more pronounced toxicity effect, starting with a concentration of 62.5 µg/cm^2, where a cell viability of 69% was reached (Figure 5b). By increasing the concentration of h-DOX-TsMLs, the cell viability decreased considerably, reaching 19% at the highest tested concentration (250 µg/cm^2). Since the TsMLs without DOX are not toxic over the tested concentration range, the decrease in the cell viability may suggest that the DOX was released from the TsMLs during the incubation with A549 cells through a passive flux. Samples containing the same amount of h-DOX-TsMLs have been incubated without cells for 48 h to quantify the amount of DOX passively released from TsMLs. By applying the second protocol for DOX concentration determination (Section S5), we were able to detect a DOX concentration of 1.8–2.1 µg/mL in the samples containing the highest amount of h-DOX-TsMLs (dosage of 250 µg/cm^2), which represent roughly 10% of the encapsulated DOX concentration. For the other samples, the amount of DOX passively released was under the detection limit of the employed spectroscopic method, which is around 1.5 µg/mL.

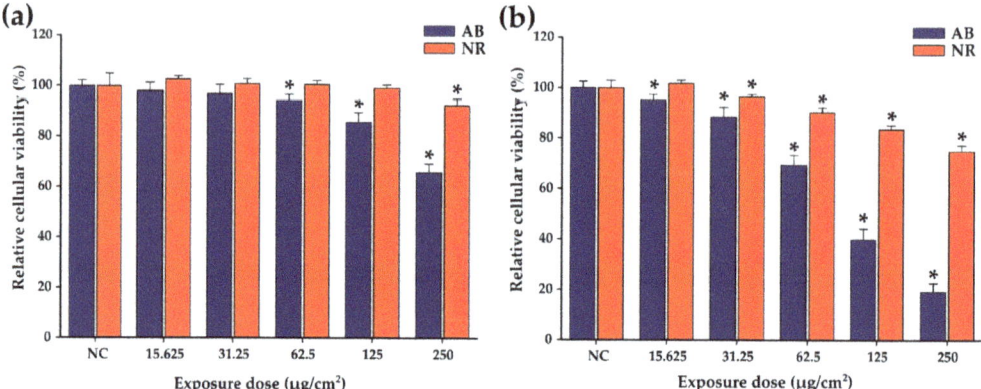

Figure 5. Cytocompatibility of (**a**) l-DOX-TsMLs and (**b**) h-DOX-TsMLs on A549 cell line after 48h exposure. Data are presented as relative values to the negative control (100%), as mean ± SD of three biological replicates. The significant differences compared to the negative control (ANOVA + Dunn's; $p < 0.05$) are noted with asterisks (*).

3.4. In Vitro Magnetic Hyperthermia

According to the cytotoxicity studies, the threshold concentration of h-DOX-TsMLs below which there is no induced toxicity by the passively released DOX is 31.25 μg/cm². This dosage corresponds to 0.2 mg_{Fe}/mL. In the first step of in vitro MH experiments, the A549 cells were mixed with TsMLs in a concentration of 0.2 mg_{Fe}/mL and exposed for 30 min to AMF of 10, 20, and 30 kA/m, to check whether or not the heat released by the encapsulated MNPs will affect the cell integrity. As can be seen in Figure 6a,b, both assays indicated no toxicity when exposing the mixture (A549cells+TsMLs) to an AFM of 10 and 20 kA/m. This is in accordance with the small values of saturation temperature reached upon AFM exposure: 39.6 ± 0.3 °C for 10 kA/m and 42.4 ± 0.2 °C for 20 kA/m (Figure 7). A statistical decrease in the A549 cell viability is observed with both assays (38% for AB and 58% for NR) upon exposure to 30 kA/m (Figure 6a,b). The saturation temperature reached during AMF exposure was 44.2 ± 0.2 °C (Figure 7), which is above the temperature at which the A549 cells, exposed for 30 min to MH treatment, received a 50% lethal dose (LD50%) [65].

The same experiments were repeated with l- and h-DOX-TsMLs in the mixture. At 10 kA/m the l-DOX-TsMLs did not induce any toxicity to A549 cells (Figure 6a,b). A comparison between the groups based on the AB data indicated a statistical difference between h-DOX-TsMLs and the other two treatments (l-DOX-TsMLs and TsMLs) (Figure 6a), while no difference was observed based on the NR data (Figure 6b). By increasing the AMF amplitude to 20 kA/m, lower cellular viability was measured in all three conditions, with a more prominent decrease being observed in the case of DOX-loaded TsMLs (Figure 6a,b). Similar to the previous observation, the AB assay indicated stronger toxicity than the NR assay. At this amplitude, the recorded viabilities were 87, 47, and 9% for the TsMLs, l- and h-DOX-TsMLs, respectively, with significant differences being observed between all groups (pairwise comparisons). As the recorded temperatures were almost identical, these values indicate that the release of DOX from the TsMLs is responsible for the higher cytotoxicity observed in the case of DOX-loaded TsMLs, the toxicity being also dependent on the DOX loading of the TsMLs. A statistically significant difference between the groups was also observed using the NR assay; however, the recorded viabilities were slightly higher (Figure 6b). By further increasing the amplitude of the AMF to 30 kA/m, the recorded viabilities decreased in all three cases. Similar to the results observed at 20 kA/m, significant differences were observed between the DOX-loaded and unloaded TsMLs, the recorded viabilities being less than 10% from the control values in both assays for the DOX-loaded TsMLs (Figure 6a,b). The Two-Way ANOVA test having as variables, the type of TsMLs and the AMF amplitude, indicated that both factors influence the measured viability resulted from both AB and NR assays.

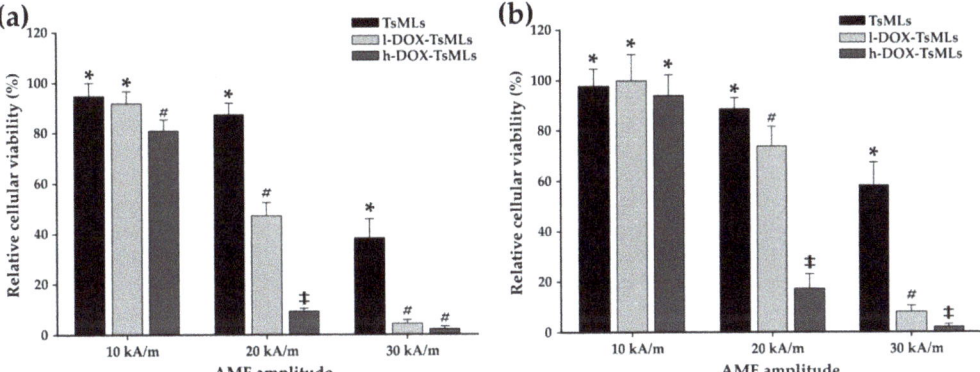

Figure 6. Cytotoxic effects of TsMLs with and without DOX, mixed with A549 cells were evaluated after a 30 min exposure to AMF of 355 kHz and amplitudes of 10, 20, and 30 kA/m. Cellular viability was measured using Alamar Blue (**a**) and Neutral Red (**b**) assays and presented as the mean ± SD of three biological replicates. Data are presented as relative values to their negative control (100%). Different symbols(*,#,‡) indicate a statistically significant difference between the groups (ANOVA + Holm-Sidak; $p < 0.05$).

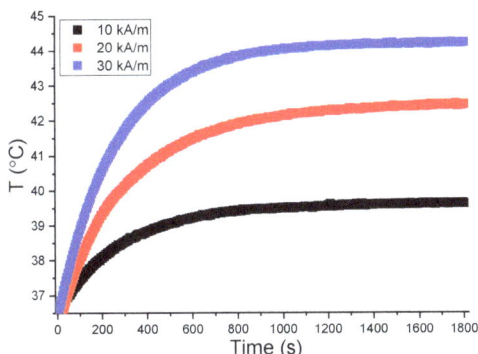

Figure 7. Typical heating curves of TsMLs mixed with A549 cells at a concentration of 0.2 mg$_{Fe}$/mL in a volume of 500 µL at different H$_{max}$ values: 10, 20, and 30 kA/m at a constant frequency of 355 kHz.

Overall, the performed experiments indicate that the decreased cellular viability can only be caused by the DOX flux released from TsMLs structure under the oscillating magnetic field. Moreover, as the negative control of each sample was represented by the same number of cells exposed to the loaded or unloaded TsMLs, but not to the AMF, the current results are not the result of a passive flux of DOX from the TsMLs during the 48 h incubation period.

For a more straightforward explanation of the biological effects observed, we attempted to quantify the release of DOX from the l- and h-DOX-TsMLs under the influence of the AMF. In the case of h-DOX-TsMLs, the amount of encapsulated DOX was 8.1 µg/mL per sample, allowing the quantification of the released DOX from TsMLs after the MH treatment. Upon 30 min MH exposure of h-DOX-TsMLs to 30 kA/m, 55% of the DOX load was released (4.4 ± 0.3 µg/mL). For 20 kA/m, the released DOX amount was 2.8 ± 0.3 µg/mL, representing 35% of the DOX load, while for 10 kA/m no DOX released was measured.

These results support the cytotoxicity observed after AMF treatment, as at these concentrations the cytotoxic effects of doxorubicin are present (Figure 3). Since the amount of encapsulated DOX in the l-DOX-TsMLs at a concentration of 0.2 mg$_{Fe}$/mL was 1.4 µg/mL, close to the detection limit of the employed spectroscopic method, the amount of released DOX could not be quantified. However, taking into consideration the releases observed from h-DOX-TsMLs, a high enough quantity of DOX (0.8 µg/mL and 0.5 µg/mL at a 55% and 35% release) would be attained to induce cytotoxic effects on the cancerous cells, thus explaining the current results, and the difference between the more potent cytotoxic effects of l-DOX-TsMLs in comparison with TsMLs upon MH treatment.

Since both high-frequency and high-amplitude AMF produce eddy currents in conducting media that can lead to damage to the human body, human exposure to AMF sets a safety limit on the frequency and amplitude of the AC magnetic field, the product between these two parameters should be 5×10^9 Am^{-1}s^{-1} [73]. It was demonstrated recently that this safety limit can be extended to a product of 9.59×10^9 Am^{-1}s^{-1} [74]. Our AFM parameters of 20–30 kA/m and 355 kHz, which led to an A549 cell survival reduction by more than 90% upon 30 min exposure, fall in the new safety limit, indicating that the MH applicability of our DOX-TsMLs might be extended to in vivo experiments. DOX release from TsMLs reaching a cell death rate as high as 83% was also recently demonstrated by Forte Brolo et al. [40]. Although their AMF parameters defined an Hf product of 4.85×10^9 Am^{-1}s^{-1}, which is smaller than ours (Hf = $7-10.65 \times 10^9$ Am^{-1}s^{-1}), the AMF was applied for 1h. A similar time interval has been applied by Pradhan et al. [75] in their study on HeLa cells targeted by folate-DOX-TsMLs, resulting in less than 7% cell viability with an Hf product of 3.5×10^9 Am^{-1}s^{-1}; however, the DOX concentration was twice that in our case. Complete elimination of HeLa cells by combined MH and chemotherapy has also been realized by Shah et al. [76], with an Hf product of 5×10^9 Am^{-1}s^{-1} and an exposure time of 30 min; the amount of DOX-TsMLs in the samples being 10 times higher than in our case.

A key parameter for the successful application of DOX-TsMLs in both in vitro and in vivo experiments is the heating capabilities of MNPs. For a Hf product satisfying the safety limit, the MNPs should deliver sufficient heat in a short time to reach the T_m of TsMLs for releasing the DOX. Our Zn ferrites have excellent heating performances, individually dispersed in water or even confined in the liposomal pool, which enable us to reach T_m at a very low concentration (0.2 mg$_{Fe}$/mL) in 15 min (Figure 7). It is worth mentioning that we were able to induce an A549 cell death rate of 45% and 85% by exposing samples containing h-DOX-TsMLs and A549 cells for 15 min to 20 and 30 kA/m, respectively. In addition, compared to previous studies, the preparation protocol developed herein is very simple and quite fast, and the amount of resulting DOX-TsMLs is larger due to the high Zn ferrites' entrapping efficiency. Since the TsMLs have a short lifetime (three-four days), all of these issues are of paramount importance for subsequent in vivo studies and clinical trials, which require large quantities of DOX-TsMLs.

4. Conclusions

In summary, the presented results prove the successful obtaining of thermosensitive magneto-liposomes capable of drug encapsulation and release under the influence of an alternating magnetic field. The employed synthetic procedure was fast, cost-effective, and reproducible, and consisted of two main steps: (1) lipid gel formation; and (2) osmotic-driven lipid gel hydration plus ammonium gradient-driven drug incorporation. The obtained thermo-sensitive magneto-liposomes were nano-sized, of spherical shape, homogeneous, and presented a high MNP$_S$ entrapping efficiency. Thus, no further post-treatment was needed for improving the liposomal system's physical characteristics. The effect of the formulation parameters such as the solvents used for dissolving lipids, the ratio between lipds, Zn ferrites and $(NH_4)_2SO_4$ concentrations of the aqueous dispersion used for water-in-oil emulsion preparation, solvent temperature, pressure, and vortex speed employed in the gel formation step, were investigated and optimized.

The SAR values of Zn ferrites exhibited a sigmoidal increase with H and strongly depend on the colloidal concentration, the maximum SAR of 1130 W/g_{Fe} being achieved for a concentration of 1 mg_{Fe}/mL. The MH experiments of TsMLs showed that the SAR values of Zn ferrites decreased for each H, exhibiting a similar sigmoidal dependence on H, and did not vary within the colloidal concentration. These experimental observations represent further proof of the Zn ferrites confinement as small clusters within the liposomal core.

Due to the poor internalization in A549 cells, both Zn ferrites and TsMLs are not toxic upon 48 h incubation time over the studied concentration range (15.625 to 250 µg/cm^2). In the absence of an AMF, the TsMLs loaded with doxorubicin exhibited a toxic effect due to the passive release of small drug amounts during the 48 h incubation time. When exposed to AMF, the doxorubicin-loaded TsMLs exhibited enhanced toxicity due to the release of higher drug amounts compared to the previous ones.

The synthesis procedure described in this paper may be extended to incorporate multiple classes of MNPs and drugs, either hydrophilic or hydrophobic, and may present a practical interest due to its simplicity, effectiveness and high yield.

Supplementary Materials: The following supporting information can be downloaded at: https://www.mdpi.com/article/10.3390/pharmaceutics14112501/s1, Section S1: Details regarding hyperthermia setup, SAR calculation, and fitting the SAR = f(H$_{max}$) curves; Figure S1: Heating curves for Zn ferrite MNPs dispersed in water and their fit with the Box-Lucas eq.; Table S1: Fitting parameters for SAR evolution with H$_{max}$ for samples dispersed in water and immobilized in PEG 8K; Section S2: Iron concentration determination; Figure S2: Calibration curve for the iron concentration determination; Figure S3: TEM image, size distribution and SAR dependence on AMF amplitude of iron oxide MNPs; Figure S4: TEM images of TsMLs loaded with small superparamagnetic iron oxide MNPs, high coercivity Zn ferrite MNPs and silica-coated Zn ferrite MNPs; Section S5: Calculations for the determination of the doxorubicin concentrations in liposomes; Figure S5: UV-Vis absorption spectrum of doxorubicin and calibration curve for the concentration determination; Figure S6: SAR dependence on the AMF amplitude for the TsMLs with and without a superposed 10 kA/m static magnetic field; Table S2: Fitting parameters of the SAR evolution with H for TsMLs with and without the static DC magnetic field; Figure S7: Cellular internalization of the Zn ferrite MNPS in A459 cells after 48 h exposure.

Author Contributions: Conceptualization, S.N. and C.I.; methodology, S.N., I.F. and C.I.; software, S.N., I.F. and C.I.; validation, F.L., C.M.L., and C.I.; formal analysis, S.N., I.F., R.D., C.M.L., and C.I.; investigation, S.N., I.F., R.D. and C.I.; resources, C.I.; data curation, S.N., I.F., C.M.L., and C.I.; writing—original draft preparation, S.N., I.F., C.M.L. and C.I. writing—review and editing, C.M.L. and C.I.; visualization, C.I.; supervision, F.L., C.M.L., and C.I.; project administration, I.F., and C.I.; funding acquisition, I.F., and C.I. All authors have read and agreed to the published version of the manuscript.

Funding: This research was funded by two grants from the Romanian Ministry of Education and Research, CNCS—UEFISCDI, project number PN-III-P1-1.1-TE-2019-1392, and PN-III-P1-1.1-PD-2019-0804, within PNCDI III.

Institutional Review Board Statement: Not applicable.

Informed Consent Statement: Not applicable.

Data Availability Statement: Not applicable.

Conflicts of Interest: The authors declare that they have no conflicts of interest. The funders had no role in the design of the study and the published results.

References

1. Lee, P.Y.; Wong, K.K.Y. Nanomedicine: A new frontier in cancer therapeutics. *Curr. Drug Deliv.* **2011**, *8*, 245–253. [CrossRef]
2. Almohammadi, A.; Alqarni, A.; Alraddadi, R.; Alzahrani, F. Assessment of Patients' Knowledge in Managing Side Effects of Chemotherapy: Case of King Abdul-Aziz University Hospital. *J. Cancer Educ.* **2020**, *35*, 334–338. [CrossRef]
3. Gerber, E.D. Targeted therapies: A new generation of cancer treatments. *Am. Fam. Physician* **2008**, *77*, 311–319.
4. Singh, R.; Lillard, J.W., Jr. Nanoparticle-based targeted drug delivery. *Exp. Mol. Pathol.* **2009**, *86*, 215–223. [CrossRef]

5. Peng, Y.; Bariwal, J.; Kumar, V.; Tan, C.; Mahato, R.I. Organic Nanocarriers for Delivery and Targeting of Therapeutic Agents for Cancer Treatment. *Adv. Ther.* **2020**, *3*, 1900136. [CrossRef]
6. Edis, Z.; Wang, J.; Waqas, M.K.; Ijaz, M.; Ijaz, M. Nanocarriers-Mediated Drug Delivery Systems for Anticancer Agents: An Overview and Perspectives. *Int. J. Nanomed.* **2021**, *16*, 1313–1330. [CrossRef] [PubMed]
7. Sabit, H.; Abdel-Hakeem, M.; Shoala, T.; Abdel-Ghany, S.; Abdel-Latif, M.M.; Almulhim, J.; Mansy, M. Nanocarriers: A Reliable Tool for the Delivery of Anticancer Drugs. *Pharmaceutics* **2022**, *14*, 1566. [CrossRef]
8. Farzin, A.; Etesami, S.A.; Quint, J.; Memic, A.; Tamayol, A. Magnetic Nanoparticles in Cancer Therapy and Diagnosis. *Adv. Healthc. Mater.* **2022**, *9*, 1901058. [CrossRef] [PubMed]
9. Eslami, P.; Albino, M.; Scavone, F.; Chiellini, F.; Morelli, A.; Baldi, G.; Cappiello, L.; Doumett, S.; Lorenzi, G.; Ravagli, C.; et al. Smart Magnetic Nanocarriers for Multi-Stimuli On-Demand Drug Delivery. *Nanomaterials* **2022**, *12*, 303. [CrossRef]
10. Nogueira, J.; Soares, S.F.; Amorim, C.O.; Amaral, J.S.; Silva, C.; Martel, F.; Trindade, T.; Daniel-da-Silva, A.L. Magnetic Driven Nanocarriers for pH-Responsive Doxorubicin Release in Cancer Therapy. *Molecules* **2020**, *25*, 333. [CrossRef]
11. Chen, L.; Li, L.; Zhang, H.; Liu, W.; Yang, Y.; Liu, X.; Xu, B. Magnetic thermosensitive core/shell microspheres: Synthesis, characterization and performance in hyperthermia and drug delivery. *RSC Adv.* **2014**, *4*, 46806–46812. [CrossRef]
12. Reyes-Ortega, F.; Delgado, A.V.; Schneider, E.K.; Checa Fernandez, B.L.; Iglesias, G.R. Magnetic Nanoparticles Coated with a Thermosensitive Polymer with Hyperthermia Properties. *Polymers* **2018**, *10*, 10. [CrossRef]
13. Mai, B.T.; Balakrishnan, P.B.; Barthel, M.J.; Piccardi, F.; Niculaes, D.; Marinaro, F.; Fernandes, S.; Curcio, A.; Kakwere, H.; Autret, G.; et al. Thermoresponsive Iron Oxide Nanocubes for an Effective Clinical Translation of Magnetic Hyperthermia and Heat-Mediated Chemotherapy. *ACS Appl. Mater. Interfaces* **2019**, *11*, 5727–5739. [CrossRef]
14. Mai, B.T.; Fernandes, S.; Balakrishnan, P.B.; Pellegrino, T. Nanosystems Based on Magnetic Nanoparticles and Thermo- or pH-Responsive Polymers: An Update and Future Perspectives. *Acc. Chem. Res.* **2018**, *51*, 999–1013. [CrossRef] [PubMed]
15. Sahoo, B.; Devi, K.S.P.; Banerjee, R.; Maiti, T.K.; Pramanik, P.; Dhara, D. Thermal and pH Responsive Polymer-Tethered Multifunctional Magnetic Nanoparticles for Targeted Delivery of Anticancer Drug. *ACS Appl. Mater. Interfaces* **2013**, *5*, 3884–3893. [CrossRef] [PubMed]
16. Gao, Y.; Gao, D.; Shen, J.; Wang, Q. A review of mesoporous silica nanoparticle delivery systems in chemo-based combination cancer therapies. *Front. Chem.* **2020**, *8*, 598722. [CrossRef]
17. Adam, A.; Parkhomenko, K.; Duenas-Ramirez, P.; Nadal, C.; Cotin, G.; Zorn, P.-E.; Choquet, P.; Begin-Colin, S.; Mertz, D. Orienting the Pore Morphology of Core-Shell Magnetic Mesoporous Silica with the Sol-Gel Temperature. Influence on MRI and Magnetic Hyperthermia Properties. *Molecules* **2021**, *26*, 971. [CrossRef]
18. Perez-Garnes, M.; Morales, V.; Sanz, R.; Garcia-Munoz, R.A. Cytostatic and Cytotoxic Effects of Hollow-Shell Mesoporous Silica Nanoparticles Containing Magnetic Iron Oxide. *Nanomaterials* **2021**, *11*, 2455. [CrossRef] [PubMed]
19. Matlou, G.G.; Abrahamse, H. Nanoscale metal–organic frameworks as photosensitizers and nanocarriers in photodynamic therapy. *Front. Chem.* **2022**, *10*, 971747. [CrossRef] [PubMed]
20. Chen, J.; Liu, J.; Hu, Y.; Tian, Z.; Zhu, Y. Metal-organic framework-coated magnetite nanoparticles for synergistic magnetic hyperthermia and chemotherapy with pH-triggered drug release. *Sci. Technol. Adv. Mater.* **2019**, *20*, 1043–1054. [CrossRef]
21. Chen, G.; Yu, B.; Lu, C.; Zhang, H.; Shena, Y.; Cong, H. Controlled synthesis of Fe_3O_4@ZIF-8 nanoparticles for drug delivery. *CrystEngComm* **2018**, *20*, 7486–7491. [CrossRef]
22. Liu, P.; Chen, G.; Zhang, J. A Review of Liposomes as a Drug Delivery System: Current Status of Approved Products, Regulatory Environments, and Future Perspectives. *Molecules* **2022**, *27*, 1372. [CrossRef] [PubMed]
23. Beltran-Gracia, E.; Lopez-Camacho, A.; Higuera-Ciapara, I.; Velazquez-Fernandez, J.B.; Vallejo-Cardona, A.A. Nanomedicine review: Clinical developments in liposomal applications. *Cancer Nanotechnol.* **2019**, *10*, 11. [CrossRef]
24. Allen, T.M.; Cullis, P.R. Liposomal drug delivery systems: From concept to clinical applications. *Adv. Drug Deliv. Rev.* **2013**, *65*, 36–48. [CrossRef]
25. Tahover, E.; Patil, Y.P.; Gabizon, A.A. Emerging delivery systems to reduce doxorubicin cardiotoxicity and improve therapeutic index: Focus on liposomes. *Anti-Cancer Drugs* **2015**, *26*, 241–258. [CrossRef]
26. Duggan, S.T.; Keating, G.M. Pegylated liposomal doxorubicin. *Drugs* **2011**, *71*, 2531–2558. [CrossRef]
27. Du, B.; Han, S.; Li, H.; Zhao, F.; Su, X.; Cao, X.; Zhang, Z. Multi-functional liposomes showing radiofrequency-triggered release and magnetic resonance imaging for tumor multi-mechanism therapy. *Nanoscale* **2015**, *7*, 5411–5426. [CrossRef]
28. May, J.P.; Li, S.D. Hyperthermia-induced drug targeting. *Expert Opin. Drug Deliv.* **2013**, *10*, 511–527. [CrossRef]
29. Borys, N.; Dewhirst, M.W. Drug development of lyso-thermosensitive liposomal doxorubicin: Combining hyperthermia and thermosensitive drug delivery. *Adv. Drug Deliv. Rev.* **2021**, *178*, 113985. [CrossRef]
30. Veloso, S.R.S.; Andrade, R.G.D.; Castanheira, E.M.S. Magnetoliposomes: Recent advances in the field of controlled drug delivery. *Expert Opin. Drug Deliv.* **2021**, *18*, 1323–1334. [CrossRef]
31. Kostevsek, N.; Cheung, C.C.L.; Sersa, I.; Kreft, M.E.; Monaco, I.; Comes Franchini, M.; Vidmar, J.; Al-Jamal, W.T. Magneto-Liposomes as MRI Contrast Agents: A Systematic Study of Different Liposomal Formulations. *Nanomaterials* **2020**, *10*, 889. [CrossRef] [PubMed]
32. Rodrigues, A.R.O.; Ramos, J.M.F.; Gomes, I.T.; Almeida, B.G.; Araujo, J.P.; Queiroz, M.J.R.P.; Coutinho, P.J.G.; Castanheira, E.M.S. Magnetoliposomes based on manganese ferrite nanoparticles as nanocarriers for antitumor drugs. *RSC Adv.* **2016**, *6*, 17302–17313. [CrossRef]

33. Pereira, D.S.M.; Cardoso, B.D.; Rodrigues, A.R.O.; Amorim, C.O.; Amaral, V.S.; Almeida, B.G.; Queiroz, M.-J.R.P.; Martinho, O.; Baltazar, F.; Calhelha, R.C.; et al. Magnetoliposomes Containing Calcium Ferrite Nanoparticles for Applications in Breast Cancer Therapy. *Pharmaceutics* **2019**, *11*, 477. [CrossRef]
34. Lopes, F.A.C.; Fernandes, A.V.F.; Rodrigues, J.M.; Queiroz, M.-J.R.P.; Almeida, B.G.; Pires, A.; Pereira, A.M.; Araujo, J.P.; Castanheira, E.M.S.; Rodrigues, A.R.O.; et al. Magnetoliposomes Containing Multicore Nanoparticles and a New Antitumor Thienopyridine Compound with Potential Application in Chemo/Thermotherapy. *Biomedicines* **2022**, *10*, 1547. [CrossRef]
35. Chen, Y.; Bose, A.; Bothun, G. Controlled release from bilayer-decorated magnetoliposomes via electromagnetic heating. *ACS Nano.* **2010**, *4*, 3215–3221. [CrossRef]
36. Amstad, E.; Kohlbrecher, J.; Müller, E. Triggered release from liposomes through magnetic actuation of iron oxide nanoparticle containing membranes. *Nano Lett.* **2011**, *11*, 1664–1670. [CrossRef]
37. Choi, W.I.; Sahu, A.; Wurm, F.R.; Jo, S.M. Magnetoliposomes with size controllable insertion of magnetic nanoparticles for efficient targeting of cancer cells. *RSC Adv.* **2019**, *9*, 15053–15060. [CrossRef]
38. Salvatore, A.; Montis, C.; Berti, D.; Baglioni, P. Multifunctional magnetoliposomes for sequential controlled release. *ACS Nano* **2016**, *10*, 7749–7760. [CrossRef]
39. Hasa, J.; Hanus, J.; Stepanek, F. Magnetically controlled liposome aggregates for on-demand release of reactive payloads. *ACS Appl. Mater. Interfaces* **2018**, *10*, 20306–20314. [CrossRef]
40. Forte Brolo, M.E.; Dominguez-Bajo, A.; Tabero, A.; Dominguez Arca, V.; Gisbert, V.; Prieto, G.; Johansson, C.; Garcia, R.; Villanueva, A.; Serrano, M.C.; et al. Combined Magnetoliposome Formation and Drug Loading in One Step for Efficient AC-Magnetic Field Remote Controlled Drug Release. *ACS Appl. Mater. Interfaces* **2020**, *12*, 4295–4307. [CrossRef] [PubMed]
41. Stiufiuc, G.F.; Nitica, S.; Toma, V.; Iacovita, C.; Zahn, D.; Tetean, R.; Burzo, E.; Lucaciu, C.M.; Stiufiuc, R.I. Synergistical Use of Electrostatic and Hydrophobic Interactions for the Synthesis of a New Class of Multifunctional Nanohybrids: Plasmonic Magneto-Liposomes. *Nanomaterials* **2019**, *9*, 1623. [CrossRef]
42. Acharya, B.; Chikan, V. Pulse Magnetic Fields Induced Drug Release from Gold Coated Magnetic Nanoparticle Decorated Liposomes. *Magnetochemistry* **2020**, *6*, 52. [CrossRef]
43. Rio, I.S.R.; Rodrigues, A.R.O.; Rodrigues, J.M.; Queiroz, M.-J.R.P.; Calhelha, R.C.; Ferreira, I.C.F.R.; Almeida, B.G.; Pires, A.; Pereira, A.M.; Araújo, J.P.; et al. Magnetoliposomes Based on Magnetic/Plasmonic Nanoparticles Loaded with Tricyclic Lactones for Combined Cancer Therapy. *Pharmaceutics* **2021**, *13*, 1905. [CrossRef] [PubMed]
44. Khosroshahi, M.E.; Ghazanfari, L.; Hassannejad, Z.; Lenhert, S. In-vitro Application of Doxorubicin Loaded Magnetoplasmonic Thermosensitive Liposomes for Laser Hyperthermia and Chemotherapy of Breast Cancer. *J. Nanomed. Nanotechnol.* **2015**, *6*, 1–9. [CrossRef]
45. Taa, T.; Porter, T.M. Thermosensitive liposomes for localized delivery and triggered release of chemotherapy. *J. Control. Release* **2013**, *169*, 112–125. [CrossRef] [PubMed]
46. Kulshrestha, P.; Gogoia, M.; Bahadur, D.; Banerjee, R. In vitro application of paclitaxel loaded magnetoliposomes for combined chemotherapy and hyperthermia. *Colloids Surf. B Biointerfaces* **2012**, *96*, 1–7. [CrossRef]
47. Qiu, D.; An, X. Controllable release from magnetoliposomes by magnetic stimulation and thermal stimulation. *Colloids Surf. B Biointerfaces* **2013**, *104*, 326–329. [CrossRef]
48. Tai, L.-A.; Tsai, P.-J.; Wang, Y.-C.; Wang, Y.-J.; Lo, L.-W.; Yang, C.-S. Thermosensitive liposomes entrapping iron oxide nanoparticles for controllable drug release. *Nanotechnology* **2009**, *20*, 135101. [CrossRef] [PubMed]
49. Calle, D.; Negri, V.; Ballesteros, p.; Cerdan, s. Magnetoliposomes Loaded with Poly-Unsaturared Fatty Acids as Novel Theranostic Anti-Inflammatory Formulations. *Theranostic* **2015**, *5*, 489–503. [CrossRef] [PubMed]
50. Ferreira, R.V.; da Mata Martins, T.M.; Goes, A.M.; Fabris, J.D.; Cavalcante, L.C.D.; Outon, L.E.F.; Domingues, R.Z. Thermosensitive gemcitabine-magnetoliposomes for combined hyperthermia and chemotherapy. *Nanotechnology* **2016**, *27*, 085105. [CrossRef] [PubMed]
51. Ray, S.; Cheng, C.-A.; Chen, W.; Li, Z.; Zink, J.I.; Lin, Y.-Y. Magnetic Heating Stimulated Cargo Release with Dose Control using Multifunctional MR and Thermosensitive Liposome. *Nanotheranostics* **2019**, *3*, 16–178. [CrossRef] [PubMed]
52. Theodosiou, M.; Sakellis, E.; Boukos, N.; Kusigerski, V.; Kalska-Szostko, B.; Efthimiadou, E. Iron oxide nanoflowers encapsulated in thermosensitive fluorescent liposomes for hyperthermia treatment of lung adenocarcinoma. *Sci. Rep.* **2022**, *12*, 8697. [CrossRef] [PubMed]
53. Bealle, G.; DiCorato, R.; Kolosnjaj-Tabi, J.; Dupuis, V.; Clement, O.; Gazeau, F.; Wilhelm, C.; Menager, C. Ultra magnetic liposomes for MR imaging, targeting, and hyperthermia. *Langmuir* **2012**, *28*, 11834–11842. [CrossRef] [PubMed]
54. Redolfi Riva, E.; Sinibaldi, E.; Grillone, A.F.; Del Turco, S.; Mondini, A.; Li, T.; Takeoka, S.; Mattoli, V. Enhanced In Vitro Magnetic Cell Targeting of Doxorubicin-Loaded Magnetic Liposomes for Localized Cancer Therapy. *Nanomaterials* **2020**, *10*, 2104. [CrossRef] [PubMed]
55. Corato, R.D.; Bealle, G.; Kolosnjaj-Tabi, J.; Espinosa, A.; Clement, O.; Silva, A.K.A.; Menager, C.; Wilhelm, C. Combining magnetic hyperthermia and photodynamic therapy for tumor ablation with photoresponsive magnetic liposomes. *ACS Nano* **2015**, *9*, 2904–2916. [CrossRef]
56. Al-Ahmady, Z.; Lozano, N.; Mei, K.C.; Al-Jamal, W.T.; Kostarelos, K. Engineering thermosensitive liposome-nanoparticle hybrids loaded with doxorubicin for heat triggered drug release. *Int. J. Pharm.* **2016**, *514*, 133–141. [CrossRef] [PubMed]

57. Rao, S.; Chen, R.; LaRocca, A.A.; Christiansen, M.G.; Senko, A.W.; Shi, C.H.; Chiang, P.-H.; Varnavides, G.; Xue, J.; Zhou, Y.; et al. Remotely controlled chemomagnetic modulation of targeted neural circuits. *Nat. Nanotechnol.* **2019**, *14*, 967–973. [CrossRef] [PubMed]
58. Cheung, C.C.L.; Monaco, I.; Kostevsek, N.; Franchini, M.C.; Al-Jamal, W.T. Nanoprecipitation preparation of low temperature-sensitive magnetoliposomes. *Colloids Surf. B Biointerfaces* **2021**, *198*, 111453. [CrossRef] [PubMed]
59. Cintra, E.R.; Hayasaki, T.G.; Sousa-Junior, A.A.; Silva, A.C.G.; Valadares, M.C.; Bakuzis, A.F.; Mendanha, S.A.; Lima, E.M. Folate-Targeted PEGylated Magnetoliposomes for Hyperthermia-Mediated Controlled Release of Doxorubicin. *Front. Pharmacol.* **2022**, *13*, 854430. [CrossRef] [PubMed]
60. Iacovita, C.; Stiufiuc, R.; Radu, T.; Florea, A.; Stiufiuc, G.; Dutu, A.; Mican, S.; Tetean, R.; Lucaciu, C.M. Polyethylene glycol-mediated synthesis of cubic iron oxide nanoparticles with high heating power. *Nanoscale Res. Lett.* **2015**, *10*, 391. [CrossRef] [PubMed]
61. Arbab, A.; Tufail, S.; Rehmat, U.; Pingfan, Z.; Manlin, G.; Muhammad, O.; Zhiqiang, T.; YuKui, R. Review on Recent Progress in Magnetic Nanoparticles: Synthesis, Characterization, and Diverse Applications. *Front. Chem.* **2021**, *9*, 629054. [CrossRef]
62. Iacovita, C.; Florea, A.; Scorus, L.; Pall, E.; Dudric, R.; Moldovan, A.I.; Stiufiuc, R.; Tetean, R.; Lucaciu, C.M. Hyperthermia, Cytotoxicity, and Cellular Uptake Properties of Manganese and Zinc Ferrite Magnetic Nanoparticles Synthesized by a Polyol-Mediated Process. *Nanomaterials* **2019**, *9*, 1489. [CrossRef] [PubMed]
63. Kerroum, M.A.A.; Iacovita, C.; Baaziz, W.; Ihiawakrim, D.; Rogez, G.; Benaissa, M.; Lucaciu, C.M.; Ersen, O. Quantitative Analysis of the Specific Absorption Rate Dependence on the Magnetic Field Strength in $Zn_xFe_{3-x}O_4$ Nanoparticles. *Int. J. Mol. Sci.* **2020**, *21*, 7775. [CrossRef] [PubMed]
64. Fizesan, I.; Iacovita, C.; Pop, A.; Kiss, B.; Dudric, R.; Stiufiuc, R.; Lucaciu, C.M.; Loghin, F. The Effect of Zn-Substitution on the Morphological, Magnetic, Cytotoxic, and In Vitro Hyperthermia Properties of Polyhedral Ferrite Magnetic Nanoparticles. *Pharmaceutics* **2021**, *13*, 2148. [CrossRef]
65. Nitica, S.; Fizesan, I.; Dudric, R.; Barbu-Tudoran, L.; Pop, A.; Loghin, F.; Vedeanu, N.; Lucaciu, C.M.; Iacovita, C. A Fast, Reliable Oil-In-Water Microemulsion Procedure for Silica Coating of Ferromagnetic Zn Ferrite Nanoparticles Capable of Inducing Cancer Cell Death In Vitro. *Biomedicines* **2022**, *10*, 1647. [CrossRef] [PubMed]
66. Lucaciu, C.M.; Nitica, S.; Fizesan, I.; Filip, L.; Bilteanu, L.; Iacovita, C. Enhanced Magnetic Hyperthermia Performance of Zinc Ferrite Nanoparticles under a Parallel and a Transverse Bias DC Magnetic Field. *Nanomaterials* **2022**, *12*, 3578. [CrossRef]
67. Souca, G.; Dudric, R.; Iacovita, C.; Moldovan, A.; Frentiu, T.; Stiufiuc, R.; Lucaciu, C.M.; Tetean, R.; Burzo, E. Physical properties of Zn doped Fe_3O_4 nanoparticles. *J. Optoelectron. Adv. Mater.* **2020**, *22*, 298–302.
68. Cotin, G.; Kiefer, C.; Perton, F.; Ihiawakrim, D.; Blanco-Andujar, C.; Moldovan, S.; Lefevre, C.; Ersen, O.; Pichon, B.; Mertz, D.; et al. Unravelling the Thermal Decomposition Parameters for The Synthesis of Anisotropic Iron Oxide Nanoparticles. *Nanomaterials* **2018**, *8*, 881. [CrossRef]
69. Lee, J.-H.; Huh, Y.-M.; Jun, Y.-W.; Seo, J.-W.; Jang, J.-T.; Song, H.-T.; Kim, S.; Cho, E.-J.; Yoon, H.-G.; Suh, J.-S.; et al. Artificially engineered magnetic nanoparticles for ultra-sensitive molecular imaging. *Nat. Med.* **2007**, *13*, 95–99. [CrossRef]
70. Castro-Carvalho, B.; Ramos, A.; Prata-Sena, M.; Malhão, F.; Moreira, M.; Gargiulo, D.; Dethoup, T.; Buttachon, S.; Kijjoa, A.; Rocha, E. Marine-derived fungi extracts enhance the cytotoxic activity of doxorubicin in nonsmall cell lung cancer cells A459. *Pharmacogn. Res.* **2017**, *9*, S92–S95. [CrossRef]
71. Conde-Leboran, I.; Baldomir, D.; Martinez-Boubeta, C.; Chubykalo-Fesenko, O.; del Puerto Morales, M.; Salas, G.; Cabrera, D.; Camarero, J.; Teran, F.J.; Serantes, D. A Single Picture Explains Diversity of Hyperthermia Response of Magnetic Nanoparticles. *J. Phys. Chem. C* **2015**, *119*, 15698–15706. [CrossRef]
72. Wang, M.; Peng, M.-L.; Cheng, W.; Cui, Y.-L.; Chen, C. A Novel Approach for Transferring Oleic Acid Capped Iron Oxide Nanoparticles to Water Phase. *J. Nanosci. Nanotechnol.* **2011**, *11*, 3688–3691. [CrossRef] [PubMed]
73. Hergt, R.; Dutz, S. Magnetic Particle Hyperthermia-Biophysical Limitations of a Visionary Tumour Therapy. *J. Magn. Magn. Mater.* **2007**, *311*, 187–192. [CrossRef]
74. Herrero de la Parte, B.; Rodrigo, I.; Gutiérrez-Basoa, J.; Iturrizaga Correcher, S.; Mar Medina, C.; Echevarría-Uraga, J.J.; Garcia, J.A.; Plazaola, F.; García-Alonso, I. Proposal of New Safety Limits for In Vivo Experiments of Magnetic Hyperthermia Antitumor Therapy. *Cancers* **2022**, *14*, 3084. [CrossRef] [PubMed]
75. Pradhan, P.; Giri, J.; Rieken, F.; Koch, C.; Mykhaylyk, O.; Döblinger, M.; Banerjee, R.; Bahadur, D.; Plank, C. Targeted temperature sensitive magnetic liposomes for thermo-chemotherapy. *J. Control. Release* **2010**, *142*, 108–121. [CrossRef] [PubMed]
76. Shah, S.A.; Aslam Khan, M.U.; Arshad, M.; Awan, S.U.; Hashmi, M.U.; Ahmad, N. Doxorubicin-loaded photosensitive magnetic liposomes for multi-modal cancer therapy. *Colloids Surf. B Biointerfaces* **2016**, *148*, 157–164. [CrossRef] [PubMed]

Article

The Anti-Obesity Potential of Superparamagnetic Iron Oxide Nanoparticles against High-Fat Diet-Induced Obesity in Rats: Possible Involvement of Mitochondrial Biogenesis in the Adipose Tissues

Aisha H. A. Alsenousy [1,*], Rasha A. El-Tahan [1], Nesma A. Ghazal [1], Rafael Piñol [2], Angel Millán [2], Lamiaa M. A. Ali [1,3] and Maher A. Kamel [1,*]

[1] Department of Biochemistry, Medical Research Institute, Alexandria University, 165 El-Horeya Rd, Alexandria 21561, Egypt
[2] Instituto de Nanociencia y Materiales de Aragón (INMA), CSIC-Universidad de Zaragoza, 50009 Zaragoza, Spain
[3] IBMM, University Montpellier, CNRS, ENSCM, 34093 Montpellier, France
* Correspondence: aisha.ali@alexu.edu.eg (A.H.A.A.); maher.kamel@alexu.edu.eg (M.A.K.)

Abstract: Background: Obesity is a pandemic disease that is rapidly growing into a serious health problem and has economic impact on healthcare systems. This bleak image has elicited creative responses, and nanotechnology is a promising approach in obesity treatment. This study aimed to investigate the anti-obesity effect of superparamagnetic iron oxide nanoparticles (SPIONs) on a high-fat-diet rat model of obesity and compared their effect to a traditional anti-obesity drug (orlistat). Methods: The obese rats were treated daily with orlistat and/or SPIONs once per week for 8 weeks. At the end of the experiment, blood samples were collected for biochemical assays. Then, the animals were sacrificed to obtain white adipose tissues (WAT) and brown adipose tissues (BAT) for assessment of the expression of thermogenic genes and mitochondrial DNA copy number (mtDNA-CN). Results: For the first time, we reported promising ameliorating effects of SPIONs treatments against weight gain, hyperglycemia, adiponectin, leptin, and dyslipidemia in obese rats. At the molecular level, surprisingly, SPIONs treatments markedly corrected the disturbed expression and protein content of inflammatory markers and parameters controlling mitochondrial biogenesis and functions in BAT and WAT. Conclusions: SPIONs have a powerful anti-obesity effect by acting as an inducer of WAT browning and activator of BAT functions.

Keywords: obesity; superparamagnetic iron oxide nanoparticles; white adipose tissue browning; mitochondrial biogenesis; mitochondrial DNA copy number

1. Introduction

Obesity is an increasingly spreading pandemic that is a global health issue and has a direct economic effect on healthcare services. Its prevalence has tripled globally since 1975, according to the WHO. More than 1.9 billion (39%) adults were estimated to be overweight, with 650 million obese, accounting for nearly 13% of the world's adult population [1]. Obesity is caused by a variety of factors, including, but not limited to, genetic, epigenetic, biochemical, hormonal, microbial, sociocultural, and environmental influences that disrupt the balance between calorie intake and energy expenditure [2]. Frequently, it is associated with several disorders such as type 2 diabetes (T2D), insulin resistance (IR), cardiovascular disorders, and cancers [3]. It is characterized by a state of chronic low-level inflammation due to the increased expression level of tumor necrosis factor alpha (TNF-α) from adipose tissue, which participates in the simulation of lipolysis in adipocytes and in insulin resistance development [4,5].

Adipose tissue is one of the most essential organs affected by obesity. It is divided into white adipose tissue (WAT) and brown adipose tissue (BAT). The WAT is composed of large lipid droplets and participates in energy storage as triglycerides (TG), whereas BAT has high mitochondrial content and involves energy consumption via non-shivering thermogenesis, mostly through tissue-specific uncoupling protein-1 (UCP-1) [6]. Mitochondria are key organelles that control the physiological roles of adipocytes such as regulation of whole-body energy homeostasis, adipocyte differentiation, lipid homeostasis, insulin sensitivity, oxidative capacity, and browning of WAT into beige adipose tissue through the transcriptional control of the brown fat gene program (e.g., UCP-1) [7]. Beige adipocytes are characterized by possessing more mitochondria than WAT, with enhanced gene expression of proteins involved in lipolysis and thermogenesis. So, WAT browning and/or BAT activation constitute a possible clinical target for the treatment of obesity [8].

Mitochondrial biogenesis is controlled by the transcription factor peroxisome proliferator-activated receptor-gamma coactivator-1alpha (PGC-1α) [9]. Sirtuin-1 (SIRT-1) is an important regulator of adipocyte differentiation and adipogenesis, and it is downregulated by a high-fat diet (HFD) in adipose tissue [10,11]. SIRT-1 induces mitochondrial biogenesis by activating PGC-1α [12]. Sterol regulatory element-binding protein 1c (SREBP-1c), a master regulator of fatty acid (FA) biosynthesis, is upregulated in WAT metabolic dysfunction in obesity [13]. The mitochondrial DNA copy number (mtDNA-CN) reflects the level of mtDNA in a cell relative to the nuclear DNA (nDNA) and is linked to mitochondrial enzyme activity and ATP level, all of which are considered indicators of mitochondrial biogenesis and function [14].

Currently, anti-obesity or weight loss treatments decrease or regulate weight by modifying calorie absorption or appetite; for example, orlistat serves as an antagonist of the lipase enzyme, which inhibits TG from being digested, thus inhibiting TG absorption and hydrolysis. These therapies are only prescribed for short-term consumption, making them ineffective for chronically obese patients who will need to lose weight over months. As a result, researchers are looking for new approaches to increase thermogenesis and treat obesity and its associated health risks [15]. Nanotechnology is a branch of science that involves design and synthesis of nano-sized materials (1 to 100 nm) for application in various fields such as medicine, and it is regarded as a promising approach in obesity treatment [16].

Superparamagnetic iron oxide nanoparticles (SPIONs) are inorganic nanomaterials that show special properties such as superparamagnetism and low toxicity. SPIONs are used in a variety of biomedical applications either as a therapeutic, diagnostic, or theranostic tool for hyperthermia, drug delivery, magnetic resonance imaging, and cell separation [17]. Over several years, we have been developing SPIONs for biomedical applications, and they showed a non-specific anticoagulant effect with no hemolytic effect on blood, low cytotoxicity, and powerful diagnostic ability in magnetic resonance imaging in vivo [18,19].

Recently, our lab indicated that SPIONs have an anti-diabetic effect on the diabetic rat model, with a low toxic effect recorded for the dose (22 μmol Fe/kg) [20]. Sharifi et al. showed the involvement of SPIONs in the regulation of genes involved in lipid and glucose metabolism, suggesting that they could be used as therapeutics for diabetes and obesity [21].

Therefore, our study aims to explore the anti-obesogenic potential of SPIONs compared to the commercial orlistat in the rat model of obesity. In this study, the effect of SPIONs coating will be evaluated by using two different types of SPIONs coated with different molecular weights of the polyethylene glycol (PEG) (550 and 2000 Da). The SPIONs will be used alone or combined with orlistat. Finally, we will explore the possible molecular mechanisms of SPIONs' effects including inflammation, lipogenesis, IR, mitochondrial biogenesis, and WAT browning.

2. Materials and Methods

2.1. Synthesis of Ferrofluids and Characterization

The synthesis was performed in two steps: (a) coating preparation and (b) synthesis of SPIONs coated with PEG (Mw: 550) (SPION-PEG-550) or with PEG (Mw: 2000) (SPION-PEG-2000), as previously described in [20]. The prepared ferrofluids were purified by filtration through 0.45 and 0.22 μm nitrocellulose membrane filters (Merck Millipore Ltd., Carrigtwohill, County Cork, Ireland)) followed by magnetic separation using MidiMACS™ separator and LS column (Miltenyi Biotec GmbH, Bergisch Gladbach, Germany). The collected nanoparticles were dispersed in MilliQ water, and the pH was adjusted to physiological pH. Samples were sterilized by filtration through Millex®-GP sterile syringe filters (Merck Millipore Ltd., Carrigtwohill, County Cork, Ireland) with a 0.22 μm pore size and hydrophilic polyethersulfone (PES) membrane in a laminar flow hood and stored at room temperature till the moment of animal injection. It is worth mentioning that the nanoparticle samples used in this work are the same used in [20]. A detailed and full description of the samples was included in this reference.

In order to determine the iron content, inductively coupled plasma optical emission spectrometry (ICP-OES) in a plasma 40 ICP Perkin-Elmer spectrometer was used. Hydrodynamic diameter was determined by dynamic light scattering (DLS) measurements performed using a Malvern Zetasizer NS (Malvern Instruments Ltd., Worcestershire, UK) equipped with a HeNe laser (633 nm). Zeta-potential measurements were performed using a folded capillary cell, DTS 1060 (Malvern Instruments Ltd. Worcestershire, UK). The aqueous colloidal suspension stability was verified using DLS. Transmission electron microscopy (TEM) and high-resolution (HR) TEM images were obtained in an aberration-corrected transmission electron microscope Tecnai Titan.

Structural characterization by attenuated total reflectance Fourier transform infrared spectroscopy (ATR-FTIR) and thermal analysis (TA) to confirm the attachment of bis (phophonic) end-capped PEG chains to the iron oxide nanoparticles was performed on lyophilized samples. ATR-FTIR spectra of SPIONs and SPION-PEG-NPs were recorded with a Perkin Elmer Spectrum 100 FTIR spectrophotometer equipped with a UATR sampling accessory in the range 4000–380 cm^{-1}. Thermogravimetric (TGA) analysis was conducted on a TA Instruments SDT 2960 simultaneous DTA-TGA. Samples were heated from 25 to 700 °C at a heating rate of 10 °C·min^{-1} under air flow. The mass remaining at 700 °C was taken as the fraction of maghemite present in the nanoparticles.

2.2. Experimental Animals

A total number of 56 albino Sprague-Dawley male rats, 2 months old (80–90 g), was used. The animals were obtained from the animal house of Medical Research Institute, Alexandria University, Egypt. Rats were housed in standard cages in a well-ventilated room (25 ± 2 °C), with a relative humidity of (43 ± 3), with free access to water and food and 12 h light/dark cycle before experimentation.

2.3. Ethical Statement

All experiments pursued the standards of the National Institutes of Health's *Guide for the Care and Use of Laboratory Animals* (NIH, Bethesda, MD, USA, publications no. 8023, revised 1978) and were performed after the approval of the Institutional Animal Care and Use Committee (IACUC), Alexandria University, Egypt (approval no. AU01219101613). The study also followed ARRIVE guidelines and complied with the National Research Council's guide for the care and use of laboratory animals.

2.4. Obesity Induction

Obesity was induced in rats by feeding them with an obesogenic diet for 2–3 months. Rats that became 20% heavier than control rats of the same age were considered obese. The composition of the obesogenic diet used in this experiment (per 100 g diet) was 30 g protein

(300 cal), 26.5 g fat (195 cal lard, 70 cal corn oil), 36.5 g carbohydrate (105 cal dextran, 106 cal corn starch, 140 cal sucrose), 3 g vitamin mix (30 cal), and 4 g mineral mix (40 cal) [22].

2.5. Experimental Design

Animals were classified into the following groups: (1) healthy control group that consisted of 8 healthy male rats, after the establishment of obesity, with the 48 obese male rats being divided into six groups (8 rats each) according to the treatment; (2) untreated obese group, (3) orlistat-treated obese group that was orally treated with orlistat (Orly^R from EVA PHARMA Product Code: 11659) dissolved in dimethyl sulfoxide at a dose of 30 mg/kg daily [23]; (4) SPION-PEG-550-treated obese group, in which obese rats were intravenously injected with SPION-PEG-550 at a dose of 22 µmol Fe/kg once a week [20,23]; (5) SPION-PEG-550 + orlistat-treated obese group, in which obese rats were intravenously injected with SPION-PEG-550 at a dose of 22 µmol Fe/kg once a week and were orally treated with orlistat at a dose of 30 mg/kg daily; (6) SPION-PEG-2000-treated obese group, in which obese rats were intravenously injected with SPION-PEG-2000 at a dose of 22 µmol Fe/kg once a week [20,23]; (7) SPION-PEG-2000 + orlistat-treated obese group, in which obese rats were intravenously injected with SPION-PEG-2000 at a dose of 22 µmol Fe/kg once a week and were orally treated with orlistat at a dose of 30 mg/kg daily.

All treatments were continued for 8 weeks, and all obese rats were maintained under the obesogenic diet during the experimental period.

2.6. Collection of Samples

After the end of the treatment period, overnight fasting rats were weighed and fasting blood glucose (FBG) was determined in the fasted animals with an automatic glucose meter (Accu-Chek, Roche Diagnostics, Mannheim, Germany) using blood samples from the tail tip. Afterwards, rats were anesthetized by intraperitoneal injection of ketamine (75 mg/kg) and xylazine (10 mg/kg) and then sacrificed. The serum samples were prepared by collecting the blood from the retroorbital vein in anticoagulant free tubes, followed by centrifugation at $3000 \times g$ for 10 min. The serum samples were used for the determination of insulin, lipid profile (TG, total cholesterol (TC), high-density lipoprotein cholesterol (HDL-C), low-density lipoprotein cholesterol (LDL-C)), alanine aminotransferase (ALT) activity, aspartate aminotransferase (AST) activity, urea, creatinine, leptin, adiponectin, and non-esterified fatty acid (NEFA) levels. The WAT and BAT were obtained and divided into three aliquots: (i) for the extraction of total RNA for quantitative real-time-polymerase chain reaction (qRT-PCR) analysis, in order to assess the gene expression of TNF-α, PGC-1α, SIRT-1, SREBP-1c, and UCP-1, (ii) for the extraction of total DNA for the determination of mtDNA-CN, and (iii) for protein assays.

2.7. Serum Parameters Measurements

Serum insulin concentration was determined following the instructions of the Insulin rat ELISA kit (EMD Millipore, Burlington, MA, USA), absorbance was measured at 450 nm, and the homeostasis model assessment index for insulin resistance (HOMA-IR) was then calculated using the following formula [24]:

$$\text{HOMA} - \text{IR} = \frac{\text{Fasting insulin}((\mu \text{IU})/\text{mL}) \times \text{Fasting glucose}(\text{mg}/\text{dL})}{22.5 \times 18}$$

Serum TG, TC, and HDL–C levels were determined by the enzymatic colorimetric method using reagents obtained from BioMed Diagnostics, Inc. (White City, OR, USA), and absorbance was measured at 546 nm. Serum LDL-C was calculated from TG, TC, and HDL-C concentrations using the following equation [25]:

$$\text{LDL-C (mg/dL)} = \text{TC} - (\text{HDL-C}) - \text{TG}/5$$

Serum ALT and AST activities were determined using reagents obtained from BioMed Diagnostics, Inc. (USA), and absorbance was measured at 340 nm. Urea and creatinine were determined using reagents obtained from BioMed Diagnostics, Inc. (USA), and absorbance was measured at 570 nm and 510 nm, respectively. Serum leptin was assayed using rat ELISA kit (eBioscience, San Diego, CA, USA), adiponectin and NEFA were assayed using rat ELISA kit (Elabscience, Houston, TX, USA), and serum lipase activity was assayed using colorimetric kit (Spectrum, Alexandria, Egypt). All procedures were performed according to the manufacturer's instructions.

2.8. Mitochondrial DNA Copy Number Determination

The qRT-PCR assay was used for the determination of mtDNA number relative to nDNA. First, the total DNA was extracted from WAT and BAT using DNeasy Mini Kit (Qiagen, Hilden, Germany) according to the manufacturer's instructions, and then the PCR reaction was performed using a specific primer pair for mtDNA sequence and a primer pair specific for nuclear sequence (PGC-1α) to perform the same number of PCR cycles and calculate the threshold cycle (Ct) of both mtDNA and nDNA sequences. The nuclear gene was used to quantify nDNA and therefore normalization of the mtDNA amount per the nDNA of the diploid cells using the equation:

$$R = 2^{-\Delta Ct} \text{ where } \Delta Ct = Ct_{mtDNA} - Ct_{nuclear}$$

A specific primer pair for mtDNA (forward: 5'-ACACCAAAAGGACGAACCTG-3'; reverse: 5'-ATGGGGAAGAAGCCCTAGAA-3') and a primer pair for the nuclear PGC-1α gene (forward: 5'-ATGAATGCAGCGGTCTTAGC-3'; reverse: 5'-AACAATGGCAGG GTTTGTTC-3') were used. PCR reactions were carried out using Rotor Gene SYBR Green PCR Kit (Qiagen®, Germantown, MA, USA), 0.5 µM forward and reverse primer, and 50 ng of extracted DNA under the following conditions: 95 °C for 10 min followed by 40 cycles of 95 °C for 15 s, 60 °C for 30 s, and 72 °C for 30 s [26].

2.9. Gene Expression Detection of TNF-α, PGC-1α, UCP-1, SIRT-1, and SREBP-1c

Total RNA was isolated from WAT and BAT using RNeasy Mini Kit (Qiagen®, Germany) according to the manufacturer's instructions, and the concentration and integrity of extracted RNA were checked using nanodrop. Reverse transcription was conducted using miScript II RT Kit according to the manufacturer's instructions. The tissue expression of TNF-α, PGC-1α, SIRT-1, SREBP-1c, and UCP-1 was quantified in the cDNA using Rotor Gene SYBR Green PCR Kit (Qiagen®, USA). Quantitative PCR amplification conditions were adjusted as an initial denaturation at 95 °C for 10 min and then 45 cycles of PCR for amplification as follows: denaturation at 95 °C for 20 s, annealing at 55 °C for 20 s, and extension at 70 °C for 15 s. The housekeeping gene glyceraldehyde 3-phosphate dehydrogenase (GAPDH) was used as a reference gene for normalization. The primers used for the determination of rat genes are presented in Table 1. The relative change in mRNA expression in samples was estimated using the $2^{-\Delta\Delta Ct}$ method [27].

Table 1. Primer sets of the gene expression of PGC-1α, SIRT-1, UCP-1, SREBP-1c, TNF-α, and GAPDH.

Gene	Accession Number		Primer Sequence
PGC-1α	NM_031347.1	F:	GTGCAGCCAAGACTCTGTATGG
		R:	GTCCAGGTCATTCACATCAAGTTC
SIRT-1	NM_001372090.1	F:	TGGCAAAGGAGCAGATTAGTAGG
		R:	CTGCCACAAGAACTAGAGGATAAGA
UCP-1	NM_012682.2	F:	AGAGGTGGTCAAGGTCAG
		R:	ATTCTGTAAGCATTGTAAGTCC
SREBP-1c	NM_001276708.1	F:	GACGACGGAGCCATGGATT
		R:	GGGAAGTCACTGTCTTGGTTGTT

Table 1. Cont.

Gene	Accession Number		Primer Sequence
TNF-α	NM_012675.3	F:	GGGCTCCCTCTCATCAGTTC
		R:	TCCGCTTGGTGGTTTGCTAC
GAPDH	NM_017008.4	F:	GGGTGTGAACCACGAGAAATA
		R:	AGTTGTCATGGATGACCTTGG

2.10. Protein Levels Determination of PGC-1α, SREBP-1c, and TNF-α by ELISA

The excised WAT and BAT were homogenized in bicinchoninic acid (BCA) using BCA protein assay kit (Chongqing Biospes Co., Ltd., Chongqing, China, catalog no. BWR1023) according to the instructions of the manufacturer. The supernatants were used for determination of PGC-1α using specific rat ELISA kits (MyBioSource, San Diego, CA, USA, catalog no. MBS27063799) according to the instructions of the manufacturer. Moreover, SREBP-1c and TNF-α were assayed using specific rat ELISA kits (Chongqing Biospes Co., Ltd., catalog no. BYEK3082 and BEK1214) according to the manufacturer's instructions.

2.11. Statistical Analysis

Data were analyzed using SPSS software package version 18.0 (SPSS Chicago, IL, USA). The data were expressed as mean ± standard deviation (SD) and analyzed using one-way analysis of variance (ANOVA) to compare between different groups. The p-value was assumed to be significant at $p < 0.05$. The correlation coefficients (r) between different assayed parameters were evaluated using the Pearson correlation coefficient; $p < 0.05$ was considered as the significance limit for all comparisons.

3. Results

3.1. Ferrofluids Characterization

A detailed and full description of samples characterization is included in reference [20]. The DLS measurements showed that the hydrodynamic size values of SPION-PEG-550 and SPION-PEG-2000 were 30.1 ± 9.1 nm and 34.2 ± 10.4 nm with polydispersity index (PDI) values of 0.158 and 0.143, respectively. The aqueous colloidal suspension of ferrofluids showed great stability over time, up to several years, without any appreciable change in the stability, as was confirmed by DLS (Figure 1). After 2 years, the hydrodynamic size values of SPION-PEG-550 and SPION-PEG-2000 were 30.2 ± 8.9 nm and 35.9 ± 10.6 nm with PDI values of 0.154 and 0.130, respectively.

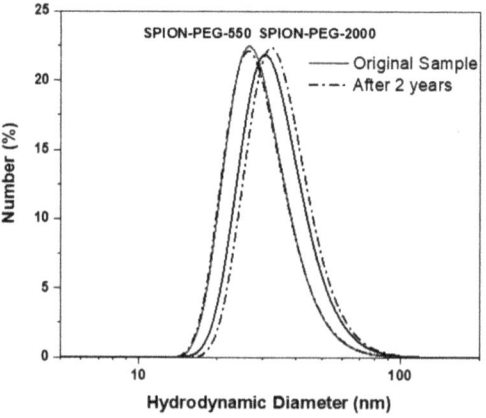

Figure 1. Particle size distribution in water determined by dynamic light scattering (DLS) measurements after being synthesized and after two years of storage.

The TEM images (Figure 2) showed the polynuclear character of the maghemite (γ-Fe_2O_3) nuclei, formed by clusters with a discrete number of maghemite nanoparticles, with a spherical shape and a mean diameter of DTEM(SD) = 11.2 (2.4) nm.

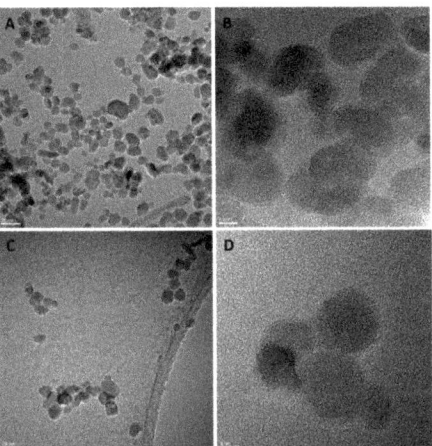

Figure 2. TEM and HR-TEM images of nanoparticles coated with PEG (Mw: 550), (**A,B**), and PEG (Mw: 2000), (**C,D**), respectively.

The FTIR spectra confirmed the presence of the maghemite SPIONs and the PEG polymer layer around the magnetic core present in both samples (SPION-PEG-550 and SPION-PEG-2000), as shown Figure 3. The infrared spectrum of sample SPION-PEG-2000 showed a higher intensity of the characteristic band of PEG at 1105 cm^{-1} attributed to the C-O-C stretching vibration band of PEG. These data are consistent with the presence of polymer chains of higher molecular weight and a higher content in organic polymer in the SPION-PEG-2000 sample and are in concordance with the data obtained by TGA. According to the thermograms obtained, the calculated mass of PEG present in the samples was 13% for sample SPION-PEG-2000 and 6% for sample SPION-PEG-550.

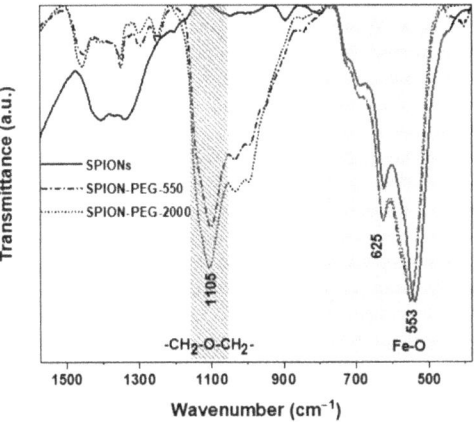

Figure 3. Fourier transform infrared (FTIR) spectra of SPIONs, SPION-PEG-550 and SPION-PEG-2000. The characteristic C-O-C ether stretching vibration band of PEG (1105 cm^{-1}) and the bands associated with the Fe-O vibrational modes in γ-Fe_2O_3 (625 cm^{-1} and 553 cm^{-1}) are highlighted in grey stripped pattern and grey, respectively.

3.2. Weight Change

Before the start of treatments, all the obese rats were significantly heavier than the control rats, with no significant difference between the obese groups. After the treatments, all the obese groups were still significantly heavier than the healthy control group; however, their body weight was significantly lower than the untreated obese rats (Table 2). The untreated obese rats and orlistat-treated rats had significantly higher weight gain compared with the healthy control rats, while the other treated obese rats had significantly lower weight gain compared with untreated obese rats. The obese rats treated with a combination of SPION-PEG-550 and orlistat showed the best lowering effect on weight gain, as shown in Table 2.

Table 2. Statistical analysis of initial and final body weights and weight gain in the different studied groups.

	Groups	Initial Weight (g)	Final Weight (g)	Weight Gain (g)
	Healthy control	229 ± 10 [b]	250 ± 11 [d]	21 ± 5 [c]
Obese rats	Untreated	370 ± 20 [a]	439 ± 29 [a]	69 ± 9 [a]
	Orlistat	355 ± 24 [a]	411 ± 27 [ab]	56 ± 13 [ab]
	SPION-PEG-550	352 ± 24 [a]	393 ± 29 [b]	41 ± 9 [be]
	SPION-PEG-550 +orlistat	357 ± 16 [a]	363 ± 15 [c]	6 ± 4 [cd]
	SPION-PEG-2000	357 ± 22 [a]	389 ± 29 [b]	32 ± 17 [ce]
	SPION-PEG-2000 +orlistat	354 ± 19 [a]	367 ± 18 [c]	13 ± 6 [c]

Results are expressed as means ± SD of 8 rats for each group. Groups were compared at $p < 0.05$ using one-way ANOVA and Tukey post hoc test, and those which are not assigned with a shared letter (a–e) in the same column are statistically significant.

3.3. Parameters of Glucose Homeostasis

Untreated obese rats had a significant elevation in glucose homeostasis parameters (FBG, insulin, and HOMA-IR) compared with the healthy control group. The orlistat treatment did not significantly affect these parameters, except for HOMA-IR, which showed significant reduction compared with the untreated obese rats. The treatment of obese rats with the two types of SPIONs (SPION-PEG-550 or SPION-PEG-2000) alone or in combination with orlistat significantly reduced these parameters compared with the untreated rats with the exception of insulin which showed no significant changes with SPIONs alone. Better effects were observed in the obese rats treated with SPION-PEG-2000 combined with orlistat (Table 3).

Table 3. Statistical analysis of glucose homeostasis parameters in the different studied groups.

	Groups	FBG (mg/dL)	Insulin (µIU/mL)	HOMA-IR
	Healthy control	104.5 ± 10.6 [e]	6.8 ± 0.76 [c]	1.7 ± 0.14 [e]
Obese rats	Untreated	214.3 ± 38.7 [a]	10.2 ± 1.2 [a]	5.4 ± 1.4 [a]
	Orlistat	189.3 ± 17.4 [ab]	9.08 ± 0.58 [a]	4.2 ± 0.54 [b]
	SPION-PEG-550	180.5 ± 4.2 [b]	9.5 ± 0.62 [a]	4.2 ± 0.21 [b]
	SPION-PEG-550 +orlistat	155.6 ± 18.2 [c]	8.3 ± 0.38 [b]	3.2 ± 0.28 [c]
	SPION-PEG-2000	169.5 ± 7.3 [bc]	9.1 ± 0.69 [a]	3.8 ± 0.33 [b]
	SPION-PEG-2000 +orlistat	123 ± 20.3 [de]	8.08 ± 0.64 [b]	2.4 ± 0.32 [de]

Results are expressed as means ± SD of 8 rats for each group. Groups were compared at $p < 0.05$ using one-way ANOVA and Tukey post hoc test, and those which are not assigned with a shared letter (a–e) in the same column are statistically significant.

3.4. Liver and Kidney Function Tests

The untreated obese rats showed significantly higher ALT and AST activities compared with healthy control rats. Orlistat-treated rats had a significant decline in both ALT and AST activities compared with the untreated rats. Moreover, the obese rats treated with both types of SPIONs showed significantly lower activities compared with obese untreated rats, especially in the rats treated with a combination of SPIONs and orlistat (Table 4).

Table 4. Statistical analysis of parameters of liver and kidney function tests in the different studied groups.

	Groups	ALT (IU/L)	AST (IU/L)	Urea (mg/dL)	Creatinine (mg/dL)
	Healthy control	36.7 ± 4.3 [c]	122 ± 12 [c]	18 ± 3 [b]	0.66 ± 0.1 [b]
Obese rats	Untreated	56 ± 6.2 [a]	173.1 ± 14.1 [a]	24 ± 3.6 [a]	0.78 ± 0.05 [a]
	Orlistat	48 ± 3.1 [b]	154 ± 5.8 [b]	22 ± 3.2 [ab]	0.73 ± 0.04 [a]
	SPION-PEG-550	51.2 ± 3.6 [a]	149.3 ± 5 [b]	25 ± 3.2 [a]	0.76 ± 0.07 [a]
	SPION-PEG-550 +orlistat	45.2 ± 4.7 [bc]	142.7 ± 5.3 [b]	21 ± 2 [ab]	0.75 ± 0.04 [a]
	SPION-PEG-2000	48.5 ± 4.5 [b]	155.1 ± 6.4 [b]	27 ± 2.6 [a]	0.72 ± 0.05 [ab]
	SPION-PEG-2000 +orlistat	42.7 ± 3.5 [bc]	147.3 ± 4.7 [b]	25 ± 2.4 [a]	0.77 ± 0.07 [a]

Results are expressed as means ± SD of 8 rats for each group. Groups were compared at $p < 0.05$ using one-way ANOVA and Tukey post hoc test, and those which are not assigned with a shared letter (a–c) in the same column are statistically significant.

Untreated obese rats had a mild but significant increase in urea and creatinine levels compared with healthy control rats. The group that was treated with orlistat, treated with the two different coatings of SPIONs alone, or in combination with orlistat experienced no significant changes on urea and creatinine levels compared with the untreated group (Table 4).

3.5. Serum of Lipid Profile

The levels of TG and total and LDL cholesterol were significantly higher while HDL cholesterol was significantly lower in the untreated obese rats compared with the healthy control group. The obese rats treated with orlistat showed significantly lower TG and total and LDL cholesterol and significantly higher HDL cholesterol levels compared with the untreated group. Moreover, the obese rats treated with the SPIONs with two different coatings showed significant improvement of lipid profile but to a lesser extent than with orlistat. The rats treated with a combination of SPIONs and orlistat showed better improvements than orlistat alone, especially those treated with SPION-PEG-2000 combined with orlistat. A similar pattern of change was observed in the levels of serum NEFA (Table 5).

Table 5. Statistical analysis of lipid profile parameters and NEFA in the different studied groups.

	Groups	TG (mg/dL)	TC (mg/dL)	HDL-C (mg/dL)	LDL-C (mg/dL)	NEFA (pg/mL)
	Healthy control	37.6 ± 3.1 [f]	121 ± 9.2 [e]	49 ± 2.4 [a]	64.3 ± 9.6 [e]	0.44 ± 0.05 [d]
Obese rats	Untreated	62.2 ± 3.1 [a]	168 ± 8.9 [a]	33 ± 1.3 [d]	122 ± 8.9 [a]	1.2 ± 0.06 [a]
	Orlistat	47 ± 2.9 [c]	145.6 ± 3.1 [c]	45 ± 2.2 [ab]	91 ± 4.5 [c]	0.67 ± 0.03 [c]
	SPION-PEG-550	57.1 ± 2.2 [ab]	156.2 ± 2.4 [b]	36 ± 3.5 [d]	108 ± 4 [b]	0.85 ± 0.04 [b]
	SPION-PEG-550 +orlistat	46.1 ± 4.1 [c]	144 ± 4.7 [c]	44 ± 2.2 [bc]	91 ± 4.8 [c]	0.63 ± 0.03 [c]

Table 5. Cont.

Groups	TG (mg/dL)	TC (mg/dL)	HDL-C (mg/dL)	LDL-C (mg/dL)	NEFA (pg/mL)
SPION-PEG-2000	54±3.4 [bd]	155 ± 3.9 [b]	40 ± 3.3 [c]	103.5 ± 5.3 [b]	0.81 ± 0.05 [b]
SPION-PEG-2000 +orlistat	44 ± 3.7 [ce]	142 ± 4.5 [cd]	44 ± 2.9 [bc]	89.3 ± 2.2 [c]	0.59 ± 0.02 [c]

Results are expressed as means ± SD of 8 rats for each group. Groups were compared at $p < 0.05$ using one-way ANOVA and Tukey post hoc test, and those which are not assigned with a shared letter (a–f) in the same column are statistically significant.

3.6. Serum Leptin and Adiponectin Levels

The untreated obese rats showed significantly higher leptin levels than the healthy control rats. The orlistat treatment did not show significant correction of leptin level; however, the obese rats treated with SPIONs alone or in combination with orlistat showed significantly lower leptin levels compared with untreated rats and orlistat-treated rats. The best leptin-lowering effect was shown in the obese rats treated with SPION-PEG-550 combined with orlistat, but the levels of leptin were still higher than the healthy control value, as presented in Figure 4A.

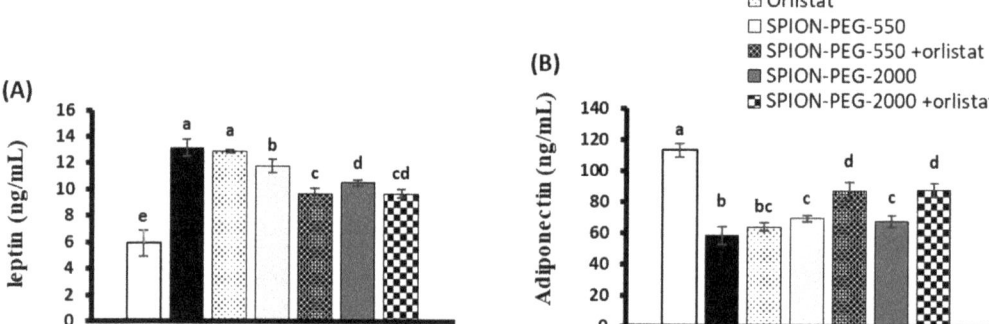

Figure 4. Serum leptin (**A**) and adiponectin (**B**) levels in control rats and obese rats untreated or treated with SPIONs and/or orlistat. Data presented as mean ± SD, and n = 8. Groups were compared at $p < 0.05$ using one-way ANOVA and Tukey post hoc test, and those which are not assigned with a shared letter (a–e) are statistically significant.

The adiponectin levels showed a significant decline in all obese rats compared with healthy control rats. However, the obese rats treated with SPIONs alone or in combination with orlistat showed significantly higher adiponectin levels compared with the untreated rats. The combined treatments have the best amelioration effects on the adiponectin levels, as shown in Figure 4B.

3.7. TNF-α Expression in WAT and BAT

The untreated obese rats had marked upregulation of TNF-α expression at mRNA and protein levels in both WAT and BAT compared with the healthy control group. On the other hand, orlistat-treated rats showed significant downregulation of TNF-α expression at mRNA and protein levels compared with untreated obese rats in the WAT, while in BAT the expression is downregulated only at the protein level. The obese rats treated with SPIONs showed significantly downregulated expression of TNF-α at mRNA and protein in both tissues compared with untreated obese rats. The combined treatment showed more reduction in the expression of TNF-α expression at mRNA and protein levels in both tissues compared with untreated obese rats or with other treated groups (Figure 5A,B).

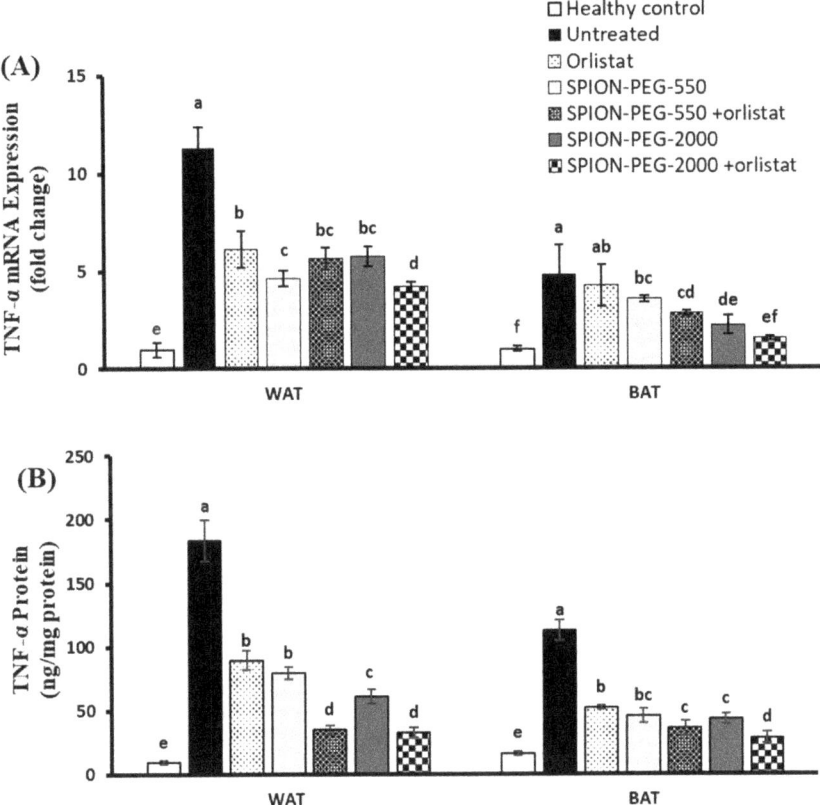

Figure 5. TNF-α expression in white and brown adipose tissues at mRNA (**A**) and protein (**B**) levels in control rats and obese rats untreated or treated with SPIONs and/or orlistat. Data presented as mean ± SD, and n = 8. Groups were compared at $p < 0.05$ using one-way ANOVA and Tukey post hoc test, and those which are not assigned with a shared letter (a–f) are statistically significant.

3.8. PGC-1α Expression in WAT and BAT

The expression of PGC-1α at mRNA and protein levels of untreated obese rats showed significant downregulation in both WAT and BAT compared with healthy control rats. In WAT, only the combined treatment with SPION-PEG-2000 and orlistat showed significant upregulation and completely normalized the expression of PGC-1α. In BAT, all treatments significantly upregulated the expression of PGC-1α at mRNA and protein levels with the best effects observed in the obese rats treated with combined treatment of SPION-PEG-2000 and orlistat (Figure 6A,B).

3.9. SREBP-1c Expression in WAT and BAT

In both WAT and BAT, the untreated obese rats had a significant upregulation of SREBP-1c expression at mRNA and protein levels compared with the healthy control group. In WAT, all treatments significantly downregulated the expression of SREBP-1c compared with the untreated rats; however, the best effects were observed in the rats treated with a combined treatment of SPION-PEG-2000 and orlistat, which completely normalized the expression at mRNA and protein levels. Like WAT, the SREBP-1c expression in BAT was significantly downregulated by all the treatments used compared with the untreated rats, with the best effects observed in the rats treated by the combined treatments SPION-PEG-550 or SPION-PEG-2000 with orlistat (Figure 7A,B).

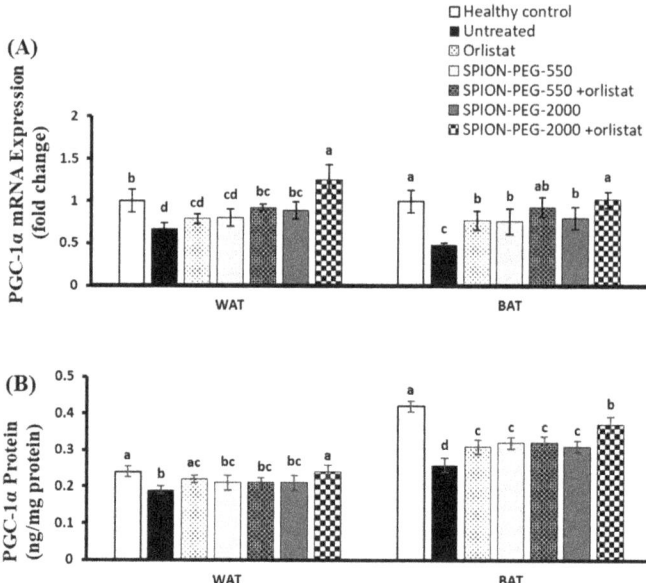

Figure 6. PGC-1α expression in white and brown adipose tissues at mRNA (**A**) and protein (**B**) levels in control rats and obese rats untreated or treated with SPIONs and/or orlistat. Data presented as mean ± SD, and n = 8. Groups were compared at $p < 0.05$ using one-way ANOVA and Tukey post hoc test, and those which are not assigned with a shared letter (a–d) are statistically significant.

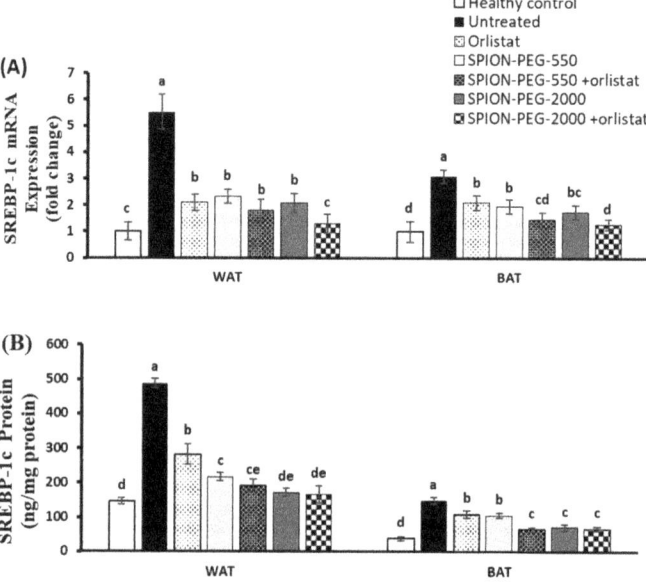

Figure 7. SREBP-1c expression in white and brown adipose tissues at mRNA (**A**) and protein (**B**) levels in control rats and obese rats untreated or treated with SPIONs and/or orlistat. Data presented as mean ± SD, and n = 8. Groups were compared at $p < 0.05$ using one-way ANOVA and Tukey post hoc test, and those which are not assigned with a shared letter (a–e) are statistically significant.

3.10. SIRT-1 Expression in WAT and BAT

The mRNA expression of SIRT-1 was significantly downregulated in both WAT and BAT of the untreated obese rats compared with healthy control rats. The orlistat treatment did not significantly affect the expression of SIRT-1 in WAT or BAT. However, the treatments with the two types of SPIONs alone significantly upregulated the expression of SIRT-1 compared with untreated rats in both tissues. In WAT, the expression of SIRT-1 was significantly upregulated by SPIONs treatment when compared with orlistat. The combined treatment of obese rats with any of SPIONs (SPION-PEG-550 or SPION-PEG-2000) together with the orlistat significantly upregulated the expression compared with the other treatments, with the best effect observed in the rats treated with SPION-PEG-2000 and orlistat, which showed complete normalization, with no significant difference from healthy controls, of SIRT-1 expression in both WAT and BAT (Figure 8).

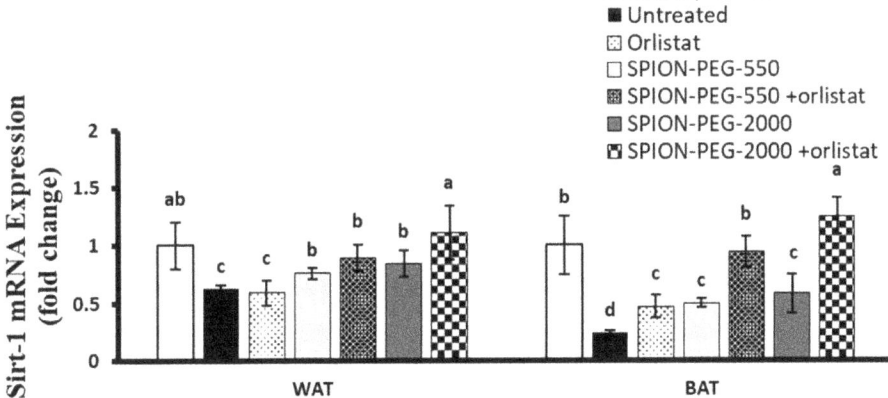

Figure 8. SIRT-1 expression in white and brown adipose tissues at mRNA level in control rats and obese rats untreated or treated with SPIONs and/or orlistat. Data presented as mean ± SD, and n = 8. Groups were compared at $p < 0.05$ using one-way ANOVA and Tukey post hoc test, and those which are not assigned with a shared letter (a–d) are statistically significant.

3.11. UCP-1 Expression in WAT and BAT

The expression of UCP-1 was significantly downregulated in BAT of the untreated obese rats with no significant changes in WAT compared with healthy control rats. The orlistat treatment did not significantly affect the expression of UCP-1 in WAT but significantly upregulated its expression in BAT. In WAT, the treatments with the two types of SPIONs alone significantly upregulated the expression of UCP-1 compared with untreated rats, orlistat-treated obese rats, or healthy control rats. The combined treatment of SPION-PEG-550 or SPION-PEG-2000 together with the orlistat significantly upregulated the expression compared with the other treatments. In BAT, the treatment of obese rats with the SPIONs alone or in combination with orlistat showed a significant upregulation of UCP-1 expression compared with untreated obese rats. The combined treatments completely normalized the expression of UCP-1 with no significant difference observed compared with healthy controls (Figure 9).

3.12. Mitochondrial DNA Copy Number in WAT and BAT

In WAT, no significant difference was observed between the untreated obese rats and healthy control rats regarding the mtDNA-CN, and the treatment with orlistat did not significantly affect it. However, the treatment of obese rats with SPION-PEG-550 or SPION-PEG-2000 alone significantly increased the mtDNA-CN compared with the healthy control, untreated obese, and orlistat-treated groups. The combined treatments showed significantly higher mtDNA-CN compared with all other groups and showed about double the control value (Figure 10).

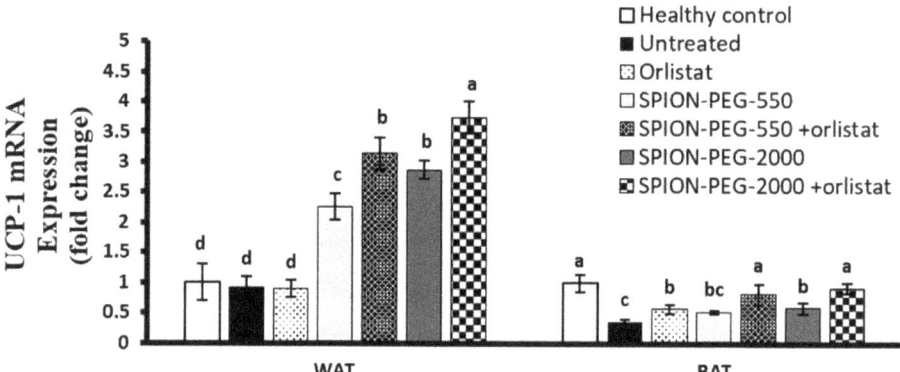

Figure 9. UCP-1 expression in white and brown adipose tissues at mRNA level in control rats and obese rats untreated or treated with SPIONs and/or orlistat. Data presented as mean ± SD, and n = 8. Groups were compared at $p < 0.05$ using one-way ANOVA and Tukey post hoc test, and those which are not assigned with a shared letter (a–d) are statistically significant.

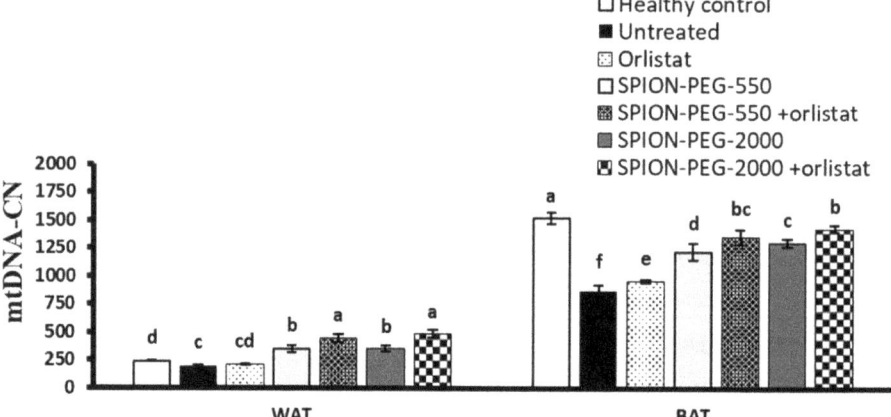

Figure 10. Mitochondrial DNA copy number (mtDNA-CN) in white and brown adipose tissues in control rats and obese rats untreated or treated with SPIONs and/or orlistat. Data presented as mean ± SD, and n = 8. Groups were compared at $p < 0.05$ using one-way ANOVA and Tukey post hoc test, and those which are not assigned with a shared letter (a–f) are statistically significant.

In BAT, the untreated obese rats showed a decline in the mtDNA-CN compared with the healthy control rats. Orlistat-treated rats showed significant elevation of mtDNA-CN compared to untreated obese rats. The treatment with SPIONs alone or in combination with orlistat showed a significantly higher mtDNA-CN compared with untreated obese rats and orlistat-treated rats, with the best effect observed in the combined treatments (Figure 10).

3.13. Correlation Studies

The statistical analysis using Pearson correlation is presented in Table 6, and the analyses showed the following:

- PGC-1α expression was positively correlated with UCP-1 expression in both WAT and BAT. In BAT, PGC-1α expression was positively correlated with SIRT-1 expression and mtDNA-CN. On the other hand, in WAT, PGC-1α expression was negatively correlated with SREBP-1c expression, TNF-α expression, and NEFA level.
- SIRT-1 expression was positively correlated with UCP-1 expression and mtDNA-CN in both tissues. However, it was negatively correlated with SREBP-1c expression and TNF-α expression in WAT and BAT, whereas in BAT, SIRT-1 expression was negatively correlated with NEFA level.
- Serum leptin level was positively correlated with TNF-α expression, SREBP-1c expression, and NEFA level in WAT and BAT. However, it was negatively correlated with UCP-1 expression, SIRT-1 expression, and mtDNA-CN in both organs.
- UCP-1 expression was positively correlated with mtDNA-CN in these tissues but was negatively correlated with TNF-α expression in WAT and BAT and negatively correlated with NEFA level.
- mtDNA-CN was negatively correlated with NEFA level in both WAT and BAT. On the other hand, it was negatively correlated with TNF-α expression in WAT and BAT.

Table 6. Correlation studies.

			Leptin Level	NEFA Level	PGC-1α Expression	SIRT-1 Expression	UCP-1 Expression	mtDNA-CN
Leptin level		r	–	0.658 *	(WAT) ns (BAT) −0.401	(WAT) ns (BAT) −0.358 *	(WAT) −0.446 * (BAT) −0.477 *	(WAT) −0.759 * (BAT) −0.797 *
PGC-1α expression	WAT	r	ns	−0.577 *	–	0.606 *	0.803 *	0.419 *
	BAT	r	−0.401	−0.499 *		0.785 *	0.765 *	0.535 *
SIRT-1 expression	WAT	r	ns	ns	0.606 *	–	0.438 *	ns
	BAT	r	−0.358 *	−0.706 *	0.785 *		0.844 *	0.382 *
UCP-1 expression	WAT	r	−0.446 *	−0.69 *	0.803 *	0.438 *	–	0.51 *
	BAT	r	−0.477 *	−0.692 *	0.765 *	0.844 *		0.546 *
SREBP-1c expression	WAT	r	0.41 *	0.547 *	−0.388 *	−0.331 *	−0.599*	−0.403 *
	BAT	r	0.597 *	0.551 *	ns	−0.428 *	−0.418 *	−0.518 *
TNF-α expression	WAT	r	ns	ns	−0.455 *	−0.533 *	−0.295 *	ns
	BAT	r	0.582 *	0.459 *	−0.343 *	−0.459 *	−0.448 *	−0.562 *
mtDNA-CN	WAT	r	−0.759 *	−0.756 *	0.419 *	ns	0.51 *	–
	BAT	r	−0.797 *	−0.613 *	0.535 *	0.382 *	0.546 *	–

Correlation studies obtained by using Pearson correlation test in which **r** = Pearson correlation coefficient and * = statistically significant ($p < 0.005$); **ns** means not significant.

4. Discussion

The present study showed for the first time the potential anti-obesity properties of SPIONs in an HFD rat model. This effect may be mediated through suppression of WAT expansion, induction of WAT browning, and activation of BAT function.

The HFD-obese rats developed the classical picture of obesity: they were 70% heavier than the control rats, and the weight gains during the experimental period were more than three times the control rats. Moreover, they developed hyperglycemia and insulin resistance, besides elevated liver enzyme activities (AST, ALT) and significantly higher urea and creatinine levels, though within the normal range. The transition from a metabolically stable condition to an obese and insulin-resistant state is characterized by a vicious loop that includes hyperinsulinemia, inflammation, glucose tolerance, dyslipidemia, IR, and adipose tissue expansion. Furthermore, the circulating NEFA levels in the obese rats were markedly higher than the controls, which may be due to the release of NEFA from the enlarged adipose tissue and reduced clearance [28]. The NEFA levels were positively correlated with the leptin level and negatively correlated with mtDNA-CN and with the expression of PGC-1α, SIRT-1, and UCP-1 in BAT and WAT. These patterns of correlations put the elevated NEFA in the core mechanism of obesity pathogenesis. The elevated NEFA levels induce insulin resistance and inhibit insulin's antilipolytic action, which will increase the rate at which NEFA is released into the circulation [29]. Moreover, the elevated NEFA activated the proinflammatory pathways [30] and resulted in increased proinflammatory cytokines expression as TNF-α, IL-1b, and IL-6 [31]. All of these make NEFA the primary link between high-fat feeding and the development of inflammatory alterations [32].

In obesity, WAT expansion leads to a significant decrease of serum adiponectin levels and an increase in leptin levels that are correlated with insulin resistance [13]. Leptin inhibits appetite and food intake, stimulates energy expenditure, and also has proinflammatory effects contributing to the low-grade chronic inflammation by enhancing the TNF-α and IL-6 production [33] and vice versa TNF-α stimulated leptin secretion from adipocytes [34] that induces obesity [35,36]. Our study confirmed the increased levels of serum leptin and TNF-α expression in WAT and BAT, and the correlation studies indicated a positive correlation between the leptin levels and TNF-α expression in BAT, which may explain the impairment of functions of BAT in energy expenditure.

The metabolic and adipocytokine derangements in obese rats are associated with marked activation of the lipogenic protein SREBP-1c and marked suppression of the expression of genes encoding essential proteins implicated in adipose tissue differentiation and activation, as well as mitochondrial biogenesis and function (PGC-1α, UCP-1, and SIRT-1). Mitochondria play an important function in the maintenance of energy homeostasis in metabolic tissues, particularly adipose tissues. Mitochondria play an important role in adipocyte biology and growth, including adipogenesis, lipid metabolism, and thermogenesis [37,38]. Furthermore, adipocyte mitochondria can regulate whole-body energy homeostasis, insulin sensitivity, and glucose metabolism or the crosstalk between muscles and adipose tissues [39,40].

PGC-1α is the key transcription factor that regulates mitochondrial biogenesis and functions by controlling the expression of nuclear respiratory factor 1 (NRF-1), nuclear factor erythroid 2-related factor 2 (NRF-2), and mitochondrial transcription factor A (Tfam) [41,42]. Moreover, PGC-1α has generally been recognized as a master regulator thermogenic gene programmed in differentiated brown and beige adipocytes [43]. So, PGC-1α is essential for thermogenic adipocytes (BAT) to perform their functions, and the observed suppression of PGC-1α expression in BAT impairs their proper functions. PGC-1α is a key regulator of brown adipogenesis by helping peroxisome proliferator-activated receptor gamma (PPAR-γ) induce WAT browning. PGC-1α deficiency can cause the downregulation of UCP-1 and block mitochondria biogenesis [44]. So, the suppressed PGC-1α expression could explain the marked suppressed expression of UCP-1 in BAT found in the obese rats in the present study.

Uncoupling protein 1, a mitochondrial protein, plays a major role in the thermogenic function of BAT [45]. The activity of UCP-1 and thermogenesis in mouse BAT is correlated with body-weight control and energy homeostasis [46]. In line with our data, the UCP-1 expression is reduced in obese subjects, and the metabolic complications are improved with the pharmacological activation of UCP-1 [47]. In human adipose tissues, the expression of UCP-1 was significantly negatively correlated with fasting glucose, and TG was positively correlated with adiponectin. The visceral obesity was aggravated when UCP-1 expression was downregulated [6].

The suppressed expression of PGC-1α in obese rats was associated with a significant decline in mtDNA-CN in adipose tissues, especially BAT, which may indicate impaired mitochondrial biogenesis, while the suppression of UCP-1 in BAT impairs the mitochondrial thermogenesis and functions. The correlation studies indicated a causality relationship between the suppression of PGC-1α and downregulation of UCP-1 expression and the decline in mtDNA-CN in BAT. The impaired mitochondrial function and biogenesis in adipocytes can affect whole-body energy dysregulation and insulin resistance.

The HFD-obese rats showed significant downregulation of SIRT-1 expression and upregulation of expression and protein level of SREBP-1c compared with control rats in both

BAT and WAT. SIRT-1 is known to activate the AMP-activated protein kinase (AMPK) signaling pathway and initiate the lipolysis of adipocytes and activate the thermogenic genes UCP-1 and PGC-1α [48,49]. PGC-1α then upregulates the gene expression of various key enzymes for beta-oxidation and induces fatty acid oxidation. Moreover, SIRT-1-mediated deacetylation of PPAR-γ is necessary for the transcriptional activity [50]. So, SIRT-1, AMPK, PPAR-γ, and PGC-1α cross-regulate each other in energy metabolism [51,52]. The suppressed expression of these machinery genes results in inhibited energy expenditure due to WAT expansion and impaired BAT functions. The inverse association between obesity and active BAT mass was previously confirmed [53,54]. SREBP-1c mediated de novo lipogenesis is an important nutritional regulator in the biosynthesis of FAs and triglyceride, and it also significantly correlated with both HOMA and serum insulin levels and pro-lipogenic factors [55].

The current approaches for obesity treatment include diet control, physical activity, drug therapy, and surgery [56]. However, the applied anti-obesity therapies have shown several limitations. Today, the modulation of mitochondrial biogenesis and activity in adipose tissues and induction of WAT browning has been proposed as a promising approach for the prevention and management of obesity by increasing the energy expenditure strategy [8]. The current study revealed for the first time the promising effects of SPIONs as an anti-obesity treatment that outperforms the commonly prescribed medication orlistat.

SPIONs treatments at the weekly i.p. dose of 22 μmol Fe/kg significantly declined the final body weights and weight gains in the obese rats during the experimental period, irrespective of the coating (PEG-550 or 2000 Da). Moreover, SPIONs treatment significantly ameliorates hyperglycemia, insulin resistance, dyslipidemia, leptin, adiponectin, and NEFA. The weekly dose of SPIONs has similar or even better effects than those observed with the daily orlistat treatment. The combined SPIONs and orlistat treatments showed more pronounced ameliorative effects, with the best outcomes observed in the obese rats treated with the weekly SPION-PEG-2000 and daily orlistat, which nearly normalized most of the studied metabolic and molecular derangement.

SPIONs treatments significantly decreased the elevated levels of leptin and NEFA in obese rats and significantly increased the level of adiponectin. The effect of SPIONs on leptin level and adiponectin level was significantly better than the effect of orlistat, which may imply a leptin-sensitizing effect of SPIONs, especially those coated with PEG-2000. Moreover, the anti-obesity action of SPIONs may be partially mediated through its lipotropic effect, as it significantly ameliorates the lipid profile like orlistat or even better. Considering SPIONs' effect on the lipid components, it can be suggested as a potential hypolipidemic agent, which will be of great advantage for obesity. This effect of SPIONs may be a consequence of the corrected glucose homeostasis and insulin resistance; however, such effect needs further investigation

At the molecular level, surprisingly, SPIONs treatments markedly corrected the disturbed expression of inflammatory genes and genes controlling mitochondrial biogenesis and functions at mRNA and protein levels in BAT and WAT. The observed effects indicated SPIONs as a powerful inducer of WAT browning and activator of BAT functions where the SPIONs treatment significantly suppressed the markedly enhanced expression and protein level of TNF-α in WAT and BAT. This effect may result from declined leptin secretion, which is supported by the correlation studies which indicate a positive correlation between leptin level and the expression of TNF-α. This effect indicates the anti-inflammatory role of SPIONs in the adipose tissues of obese rats.

Obese rats treated with the doses of the two different coatings of SPIONs alone or in combination with orlistat showed a significant upregulation of PGC-1α, UCP-1, and SIRT-1 expression compared with untreated obese rats in WAT and BAT. Orlistat treatment showed a mild but significant effect on the expressions of these genes. Obese rats treated with combined treatment of orlistat and SPIONs coated with PEG-2000 at the dose of 22 μmol Fe/kg have significant upregulation of PGC-1α expression compared with orlistat-treated rats in both WAT and BAT. This dose showed the highest upregulation effect on

PGC-1α expression in WAT, which has a significantly higher expression level compared with control rats. A similar pattern of changes was observed in the mtDNA-CN. Moreover, SPIONs coated with PEG-2000 showed better effects than those coated with PEG-550.

In our present study, the enhanced expression of PGC-1α, which is a central player that regulates the browning program in WAT [57], may cause the enhanced expression of SIRT-1 and UCP-1 in the WAT to be 1.1 and 3.7-fold control values, respectively, and the increased mtDNA-CN in WAT to be higher than the control value. The correlation studies confirm the association between the PGC-1α and WAT browning and BAT activation, as its expression was positively correlated with SIRT-1, UCP-1, and mtDNA-CN and negatively correlated with circulating NEFA. These patterns of gene expression changes may indicate the transformation from WAT into BAT phenotype or browning (or beiging) of the existing WAT. The browning phenomenon has been recognized based on the expression of these specific thermogenic markers that regulate beiging transcription [58].

Sirtuin-1's post-translational modification, such as deacetylation, is a major contributor to the WAT browning [59]. The present data indicated the central role of SIRT-1 in the anti-obesity effects of SPIONs, as it was significantly upregulated in the WAT and BAT of obese rats treated with SPIONs. The correlation studies confirm the critical role of SIRT-1 in the browning of WAT and activation of BAT, as its expression is positively correlated with PGC-1α and UCP-1 expression and negatively correlated with circulating NEFA.

The exact mechanism of the epigenetic effects of SPIONs in vivo is unclear and needs extensive investigations. However, both moieties of SPION-PEG-550 and SPION-PEG-2000 may participate in the observed actions in diabetic rats. PEG moiety facilitates transport across membranes and penetration into intracellular spaces and mitochondria and allows distribution into distant tissues after intraperitoneal injection and exerts significant physiologic effects on the distant organs [60].

The exact molecular mechanism(s) involved in the influence of SPIONs on insulin sensitivity is unclear. A few experiments have been conducted to investigate the metabolic effects of SPIONs. Sharifi et al. recorded a decrease in the expression of genes implicated in the growth of obesity and T2D in human primary adipocytes treated with SPIONs [21]. Interestingly, Ali et al. recently reported the potential anti-diabetic effects of SPIONs mediated through correction of hepatic PGC-1α expression and other components of insulin signaling in hepatic tissues and modulation of lipid metabolism and adipocytokines, leptin, and adiponectin [20]. The last study indicated hepatorenal toxicities as a major concern at high doses of SPIONs (44 μmol Fe/kg and 66 μmol Fe/kg) [20]. So, in the present study, we used the low dose (22 μmol Fe/kg) in combination with orlistat to avoid the possible toxicities of the higher dose (44 μmol Fe/kg and 66 μmol Fe/kg), which showed no significant ameliorative effects on AST and ALT activities and even worsened the parameters of the kidney function, urea and creatinine levels, compared with the untreated rats. On the other hand, the low dose alone or in combination with orlistat significantly ameliorates serum activities of AST and ALT compared with the untreated obese rats with no worsened effects on urea and creatinine levels.

Study Limitations

Nanoparticles biodistribution study is one of the limitations in our study. A systematic study should be performed with the aim to identify their blood circulation half-life time, biodistribution, and clearance. Another limitation is the determination of the principal component in the nanoparticles responsible for this effect and finally determination of the mechanism of action.

5. Conclusions

From the results of the present study and the above discussion, for the first time, a promising effect of SPIONs as an anti-obesity agent that is superior to the conventionally used drug orlistat in the HFD rat model has been reported. It was demonstrated that SPIONs influence the expression of genes involved in lipid and glucose metabolism and therefore may be used as therapeutics for the treatment of diabetes and obesity. These effects may be mediated through suppression of WAT expansion, induction of WAT browning, and activation of BAT. The mechanism of action of SPIONs could be mediated through inducing the expression of the thermogenic genes PGC-1α, SIRT-1, and UCP-1 and mitochondria biogenesis in BAT and WAT. SPIONs coated with PEG-2000 are more efficient anti-obesity agents than those coated with PEG-550. The combination of the low dose of SPION-PEG-2000 (22 µmol Fe/kg/week) with daily orlistat has the best efficiency for the treatment of obesity.

Author Contributions: Formal analysis, M.A.K. and L.M.A.A.; investigation, A.H.A.A. and M.A.K.; methodology, A.H.A.A., R.A.E.-T., N.A.G., R.P., A.M., L.M.A.A. and M.A.K.; supervision, R.A.E.-T., N.A.G. and M.A.K.; visualization, N.A.G. and R.A.E.-T.; writing—original draft, A.H.A.A.; writing—review and editing, R.A.E.-T., R.P., A.M., L.M.A.A. and M.A.K. All authors have read and agreed to the published version of the manuscript.

Funding: This paper is based upon work supported by Science, Technology and Innovation Funding Authority (STDF) under the call 1 of post-graduate support grant (PGSG) with ID number 44406. The Spanish Ministry of Science Innovation and Universities (Grant No: PGC2018_095795_B_I00 (MCIU/AEI/FEDER, UE)) and Diputación General de Aragón (LMP220_21).

Institutional Review Board Statement: All experiments pursued the standards of the National Institutes of Health's *Guide for the Care and Use of Laboratory Animals* (NIH Publications no. 8023, revised 1978) and were performed after the approval of the Institutional Animal Care and Use Committee (IACUC), Alexandria University, Egypt (approval no. AU01219101613). The study also followed ARRIVE guidelines and complied with the National Research Council's guide for the care and use of laboratory animals.

Informed Consent Statement: Not applicable.

Data Availability Statement: Data will be available by request to the corresponding authors.

Acknowledgments: Authors acknowledge the support and funding of the Science, Technology and Innovation Funding Authority (STDF) that has funded this project. R Piñol and A. Millan would like to acknowledgethe use of Servicio General de Apoyo a la Investigación-SAI, Universidad de Zaragoza.

Conflicts of Interest: The authors declare no conflict of interest.

References

1. Di Rosa, C.; Lattanzi, G.; Taylor, S.F.; Manfrini, S.; Khazrai, Y.M. Very low calorie ketogenic diets in overweight and obesity treatment: Effects on anthropometric parameters, body composition, satiety, lipid profile and microbiota. *Obes. Res. Clin. Pr.* **2020**, *14*, 491–503. [CrossRef]
2. Pilitsi, E.; Farr, O.M.; Polyzos, S.A.; Perakakis, N.; Nolen-Doerr, E.; Papathanasiou, A.-E.; Mantzoros, C.S. Pharmacotherapy of obesity: Available medications and drugs under investigation. *Metabolism* **2019**, *92*, 170–192. [CrossRef] [PubMed]
3. Moreno-Indias, I.; Tinahones, F.J. Impaired Adipose Tissue Expandability and Lipogenic Capacities as Ones of the Main Causes of Metabolic Disorders. *J. Diabetes Res.* **2015**, *2015*, 1–12. [CrossRef]
4. Bulló, M.; Garcia-Lorda, P.; Peinado-Onsurbe, J.; Hernández, M.; Del Castillo, D.; Argiles, J.M.; Salas-Salvadó, J. TNFα expression of subcutaneous adipose tissue in obese and morbid obese females: Relationship to adipocyte LPL activity and leptin synthesis. *Int. J. Obes.* **2002**, *26*, 652–658. [CrossRef]
5. Stolarczyk, E. Adipose tissue inflammation in obesity: A metabolic or immune response? *Curr. Opin. Pharmacol.* **2017**, *37*, 35–40. [CrossRef]
6. Lim, J.; Park, H.S.; Kim, J.; Jang, Y.J.; Kim, J.-H.; Lee, Y.; Heo, Y. Depot-specific UCP1 expression in human white adipose tissue and its association with obesity-related markers. *Int. J. Obes.* **2020**, *44*, 697–706. [CrossRef]
7. Lee, J.H.; Park, A.; Oh, K.-J.; Kim, W.K.; Bae, K.-H. The Role of Adipose Tissue Mitochondria: Regulation of Mitochondrial Function for the Treatment of Metabolic Diseases. *Int. J. Mol. Sci.* **2019**, *20*, 4924. [CrossRef]
8. Kuryłowicz, A.; Puzianowska-Kuźnicka, M. Induction of Adipose Tissue Browning as a Strategy to Combat Obesity. *Int. J. Mol. Sci.* **2020**, *21*, 6241. [CrossRef]
9. Stotland, A.; Gottlieb, R.A. Mitochondrial quality control: Easy come, easy go. *Biochim. Biophys. Acta* **2015**, *1853*, 2802–2811. [CrossRef]
10. Chalkiadaki, A.; Guarente, L. High-Fat Diet Triggers Inflammation-Induced Cleavage of SIRT1 in Adipose Tissue to Promote Metabolic Dysfunction. *Cell Metab.* **2012**, *16*, 180–188. [CrossRef] [PubMed]

11. Peng, J.; Wu, Y.; Deng, Z.; Zhou, Y.; Song, T.; Yang, Y.; Zhang, X.; Xu, T.; Xiaming, Z.; Cai, A.; et al. MiR-377 promotes white adipose tissue inflammation and decreases insulin sensitivity in obesity via suppression of sirtuin-1 (SIRT1). *Oncotarget* 2017, *8*, 70550–70563. [CrossRef]
12. Wu, Z.; Puigserver, P.; Andersson, U.; Zhang, C.; Adelmant, G.; Mootha, V.; Troy, A.; Cinti, S.; Lowell, B.; Scarpulla, R.C.; et al. Mechanisms Controlling Mitochondrial Biogenesis and Respiration through the Thermogenic Coactivator PGC-1. *Cell* 1999, *98*, 115–124. [CrossRef]
13. Illesca, P.; Valenzuela, R.; Espinosa, A.; Echeverría, F.; Soto-Alarcon, S.; Campos, C.; Rodriguez, A.; Vargas, R.; Magrone, T.; Videla, L.A. Protective Effects of Eicosapentaenoic Acid Plus Hydroxytyrosol Supplementation against White Adipose Tissue Abnormalities in Mice Fed a High-Fat Diet. *Molecules* 2020, *25*, 4433. [CrossRef] [PubMed]
14. DeBarmore, B.; Longchamps, R.J.; Zhang, Y.; Kalyani, R.R.; Guallar, E.; Arking, D.; Selvin, E.; Young, J.H. Mitochondrial DNA copy number and diabetes: The Atherosclerosis Risk in Communities (ARIC) study. *BMJ Open Diabetes Res. Care* 2020, *8*, e001204. [CrossRef] [PubMed]
15. Chen, K.Y.; Brychta, R.J.; Sater, Z.A.; Cassimatis, T.M.; Cero, C.; Fletcher, L.A.; Israni, N.S.; Johnson, J.W.; Lea, H.J.; Linderman, J.D.; et al. Opportunities and challenges in the therapeutic activation of human energy expenditure and thermogenesis to manage obesity. *J. Biol. Chem.* 2020, *295*, 1926–1942. [CrossRef] [PubMed]
16. Pelaz, B.; Alexiou, C.; Alvarez-Puebla, R.A.; Alves, F.; Andrews, A.M.; Ashraf, S.; Balogh, L.P.; Ballerini, L.; Bestetti, A.; Brendel, C.; et al. Diverse Applications of Nanomedicine. *ACS Nano* 2017, *11*, 2313–2381. [CrossRef] [PubMed]
17. Ruiz, A.; Ali, L.M.A.; Cáceres-Vélez, P.R.; Cornudella, R.; Gutiérrez, M.; Moreno, J.A.; Piñol, R.; Palacio, F.; Fascineli, M.L.; de Azevedo, R.B.; et al. Hematotoxicity of magnetite nanoparticles coated with polyethylene glycol: In vitro and in vivo studies. *Toxicol. Res.* 2015, *4*, 1555–1564. [CrossRef]
18. Ali, L.M.; Gutiérrez, M.; Cornudella, R.; Moreno, J.A.; Piñol, R.; Gabilondo, L.; Millán, A.; Palacio, F. Hemostasis Disorders Caused by Polymer Coated Iron Oxide Nanoparticles. *J. Biomed. Nanotechnol.* 2013, *9*, 1272–1285. [CrossRef]
19. Ali, L.M.; Marzola, P.; Nicolato, E.; Fiorini, S.; Guillamón, M.D.L.H.; Piñol, R.; Gabilondo, L.; Millán, A.; Palacio, F. Polymer-coated superparamagnetic iron oxide nanoparticles as T2 contrast agent for MRI and their uptake in liver. *Futur. Sci. OA* 2019, *5*, FSO235. [CrossRef]
20. Ali, L.M.; Shaker, S.A.; Pinol, R.; Millan, A.; Hanafy, M.Y.; Helmy, M.H.; Kamel, M.A.; Mahmoud, S.A. Effect of superparamagnetic iron oxide nanoparticles on glucose homeostasis on type 2 diabetes experimental model. *Life Sci.* 2020, *245*, 117361. [CrossRef]
21. Sharifi, S.; Daghighi, S.; Motazacker, M.M.; Badlou, B.A.; Sanjabi, B.; Akbarkhanzadeh, A.; Rowshani, A.T.; Laurent, S.; Peppelenbosch, M.P.; Rezaee, F. Superparamagnetic iron oxide nanoparticles alter expression of obesity and T2D-associated risk genes in human adipocytes. *Sci. Rep.* 2013, *3*, srep02173. [CrossRef]
22. Kamel, M.A.; Helmy, M.H.; Hanafi, M.Y.; Mahmoud, S.A.; Elfetooh, H.A.; Badr, M.S. Maternal Obesity and Malnutrition in Rats Differentially Affect Glucose Sensing in the Muscles and Adipose Tissues in the Offspring. *Int. J. Biochem. Res. Rev.* 2014, *4*, 440–469. [CrossRef]
23. Gomaa, A.A.; El-Sers, D.A.; Al-Zokeim, N.I.; Gomaa, M.A. Amelioration of experimental metabolic syndrome induced in rats by orlistat and *Corchorus olitorius* leaf extract; role of adipo/cytokines. *J. Pharm. Pharmacol.* 2018, *71*, 281–291. [CrossRef]
24. Caumo, A.; Perseghin, G.; Brunani, A.; Luzi, L. New Insights on the Simultaneous Assessment of Insulin Sensitivity and β-Cell Function with the HOMA2 Method. *Diabetes Care* 2006, *29*, 2733–2734. [CrossRef]
25. Tietz, N.W.; Burtis, C.A.; Ashwood, E.R.; Bruns, D.E. *Tietz Textbook of Clinical Chemistry and Molecular Diagnostics*; Elsevier Saunders: St. Louis, MO, USA, 2006.
26. Gowayed, M.A.; Mahmoud, S.A.; El-Sayed, Y.; Abu-Samra, N.; Kamel, M.A. Enhanced mitochondrial biogenesis is associated with the ameliorative action of creatine supplementation in rat soleus and cardiac muscles. *Exp. Ther. Med.* 2019, *19*, 384–392. [CrossRef]
27. Livak, K.J.; Schmittgen, T.D. Analysis of relative gene expression data using real-time quantitative PCR and the $2^{-\Delta\Delta CT}$ method. *Methods* 2001, *25*, 402–408. [CrossRef]
28. Björntorp, P.; Bergman, H.; Varnauskas, E. PLASMA FREE FATTY ACID TURNOVER RATE IN OBESITY. *Acta Med. Scand.* 2009, *185*, 351–356. [CrossRef]
29. Jensen, M.D.; Haymond, M.W.; Rizza, R.A.; Cryer, P.E.; Miles, J.M. Influence of body fat distribution on free fatty acid metabolism in obesity. *J. Clin. Investig.* 1989, *83*, 1168–1173. [CrossRef]
30. Itani, S.I.; Ruderman, N.B.; Schmieder, F.; Boden, G. Lipid-Induced Insulin Resistance in Human Muscle Is Associated with Changes in Diacylglycerol, Protein Kinase C, and IκB-α. *Diabetes* 2002, *51*, 2005–2011. [CrossRef]
31. Boden, G.; She, P.; Mozzoli, M.; Cheung, P.; Gumireddy, K.; Reddy, P.; Xiang, X.; Luo, Z.; Ruderman, N. Free fatty acids produce insulin resistance and activate the proinflammatory nuclear factor-κB pathway in rat liver. *Diabetes* 2005, *54*, 3458–3465. [CrossRef]
32. Boden, G. Obesity and Free Fatty Acids. *Endocrinol. Metab. Clin. N. Am.* 2008, *37*, 635–646. [CrossRef] [PubMed]
33. Santos-Alvarez, J.; Goberna, R.; Sánchez-Margalet, V. Human Leptin Stimulates Proliferation and Activation of Human Circulating Monocytes. *Cell. Immunol.* 1999, *194*, 6–11. [CrossRef]
34. Finck, B.N.; Kelley, K.W.; Dantzer, R.; Johnson, R.W. In Vivo and in Vitro Evidence for the Involvement of Tumor Necrosis Factor-α in the Induction of Leptin by Lipopolysaccharide. *Endocrinology* 1998, *139*, 2278–2283. [CrossRef] [PubMed]
35. Elmquist, J.K.; Ahima, R.S.; Maratos-Flier, E.; Flier, J.S.; Saper, C.B. Leptin activates neurons in ventrobasal hypothalamus and brainstem. *Endocrinology* 1997, *138*, 839–842. [CrossRef] [PubMed]

36. Paracchini, V.; Pedotti, P.; Taioli, E. Genetics of Leptin and Obesity: A HuGE Review. *Am. J. Epidemiol.* **2005**, *162*, 101–114. [CrossRef]
37. Boudina, S.; Graham, T.E. Mitochondrial function/dysfunction in white adipose tissue. *Exp. Physiol.* **2014**, *99*, 1168–1178. [CrossRef] [PubMed]
38. Gregoire, F.M.; Smas, C.M.; Sul, H.S. Understanding Adipocyte Differentiation. *Physiol. Rev.* **1998**, *78*, 783–809. [CrossRef]
39. Keuper, M.; Jastroch, M.; Yi, C.X.; Fischer-Posovszky, P.; Wabitsch, M.; Tschöp, M.H.; Hofmann, S.M. Spare mitochondrial respiratory capacity permits human adipocytes to maintain ATP homeostasis under hypoglycemic conditions. *FASEB J.* **2014**, *28*, 761–770. [CrossRef] [PubMed]
40. Vernochet, C.; Damilano, F.; Mourier, A.; Bezy, O.; Mori, M.A.; Smyth, G.; Rosenzweig, A.; Larsson, N.; Kahn, C.R. Adipose tissue mitochondrial dysfunction triggers a lipodystrophic syndrome with insulin resistance, hepatosteatosis, and cardiovascular complications. *FASEB J.* **2014**, *28*, 4408–4419. [CrossRef] [PubMed]
41. Virbasius, J.V.; Scarpulla, R.C. Activation of the human mitochondrial transcription factor A gene by nuclear respiratory factors: A potential regulatory link between nuclear and mitochondrial gene expression in organelle biogenesis. *Proc. Natl. Acad. Sci. USA* **1994**, *91*, 1309–1313. [CrossRef]
42. Wu, Z.; Puigserver, P.; Spiegelman, B.M. Transcriptional activation of adipogenesis. *Curr. Opin. Cell Biol.* **1999**, *11*, 689–694. [CrossRef]
43. Barroso, E.; Rodríguez-Calvo, R.; Serrano-Marco, L.; Astudillo, A.M.; Balsinde, J.; Palomer, X.; Vázquez-Carrera, M. The PPARβ/δ Activator GW501516 Prevents the Down-Regulation of AMPK Caused by a High-Fat Diet in Liver and Amplifies the PGC-1α-Lipin 1-PPARα Pathway Leading to Increased Fatty Acid Oxidation. *Endocrinology* **2011**, *152*, 1848–1859. [CrossRef]
44. Tiraby, C.; Tavernier, G.; Lefort, C.; Larrouy, D.; Bouillaud, F.; Ricquier, D.; Langin, D. Acquirement of Brown Fat Cell Features by Human White Adipocytes. *J. Biol. Chem.* **2003**, *278*, 33370–33376. [CrossRef]
45. Nicholls, D.G. Stoicheiometries of Proton Translocation by Mitochondria. *Biochem. Soc. Trans.* **1977**, *5*, 200–203. [CrossRef]
46. Stanford, K.I.; Middelbeek, R.J.; Townsend, K.L.; An, D.; Nygaard, E.B.; Hitchcox, K.M.; Markan, K.R.; Nakano, K.; Hirshman, M.F.; Tseng, Y.-H.; et al. Brown adipose tissue regulates glucose homeostasis and insulin sensitivity. *J. Clin. Investig.* **2013**, *123*, 215–223. [CrossRef]
47. Cypess, A.M.; Kahn, C.R. Brown fat as a therapy for obesity and diabetes. *Curr. Opin. Endocrinol. Diabetes Obes.* **2010**, *17*, 143–149. [CrossRef]
48. Madsen, L.; Pedersen, L.M.; Lillefosse, H.H.; Fjære, E.; Bronstad, I.; Hao, Q.; Petersen, R.K.; Hallenborg, P.; Ma, T.; De Matteis, R.; et al. UCP1 Induction during Recruitment of Brown Adipocytes in White Adipose Tissue Is Dependent on Cyclooxygenase Activity. *PLoS ONE* **2010**, *5*, e11391. [CrossRef] [PubMed]
49. Vegiopoulos, A.; Müller-Decker, K.; Strzoda, D.; Schmitt, I.; Chichelnitskiy, E.; Ostertag, A.; Diaz, M.B.; Rozman, J.; de Angelis, M.H.; Nüsing, R.M.; et al. Cyclooxygenase-2 Controls Energy Homeostasis in Mice by de Novo Recruitment of Brown Adipocytes. *Science* **2010**, *328*, 1158–1161. [CrossRef]
50. Qiang, L.; Wang, L.; Kon, N.; Zhao, W.; Lee, S.; Zhang, Y.; Rosenbaum, M.; Zhao, Y.; Gu, W.; Farmer, S.R.; et al. Brown Remodeling of White Adipose Tissue by SirT1-Dependent Deacetylation of Pparγ. *Cell* **2012**, *150*, 620–632. [CrossRef]
51. Chen, W.; Yang, Q.; Roeder, R.G. Dynamic Interactions and Cooperative Functions of PGC-1α and MED1 in TRα-Mediated Activation of the Brown-Fat-Specific UCP-1 Gene. *Mol. Cell* **2009**, *35*, 755–768. [CrossRef]
52. Lee, J.-Y.; Takahashi, N.; Yasubuchi, M.; Kim, Y.-I.; Hashizaki, H.; Kim, M.-J.; Sakamoto, T.; Goto, T.; Kawada, T. Triiodothyronine induces UCP-1 expression and mitochondrial biogenesis in human adipocytes. *Am. J. Physiol. Cell Physiol.* **2012**, *302*, C463–C472. [CrossRef]
53. Lee, P.; Greenfield, J.R.; Ho, K.K.Y.; Fulham, M. A critical appraisal of the prevalence and metabolic significance of brown adipose tissue in adult humans. *Am. J. Physiol. Metab.* **2010**, *299*, E601–E606. [CrossRef]
54. Ouellet, V.; Routhier-Labadie, A.; Bellemare, W.; Lakhal-Chaieb, L.; Turcotte, E.; Carpentier, A.C.; Richard, D. Outdoor Temperature, Age, Sex, Body Mass Index, and Diabetic Status Determine the Prevalence, Mass, and Glucose-Uptake Activity of 18F-FDG-Detected BAT in Humans. *J. Clin. Endocrinol. Metab.* **2011**, *96*, 192–199. [CrossRef] [PubMed]
55. Pettinelli, P.; del Pozo, T.; Araya, J.; Rodrigo, R.; Araya, A.V.; Smok, G.; Csendes, A.; Gutierrez, L.; Rojas, J.; Korn, O.; et al. Enhancement in liver SREBP-1c/PPAR-α ratio and steatosis in obese patients: Correlations with insulin resistance and n-3 long-chain polyunsaturated fatty acid depletion. *Biochim. Biophys. Acta (BBA) Mol. Basis Dis.* **2009**, *1792*, 1080–1086. [CrossRef]
56. O'Mara, A.E.; Johnson, J.W.; Linderman, J.D.; Brychta, R.J.; McGehee, S.; Fletcher, L.A.; Fink, Y.A.; Kapuria, D.; Cassimatis, T.M.; Kelsey, N.; et al. Chronic mirabegron treatment increases human brown fat, HDL cholesterol, and insulin sensitivity. *J. Clin. Investig.* **2020**, *130*, 2209–2219. [CrossRef]
57. Thyagarajan, B.; Foster, M.T. Beiging of white adipose tissue as a therapeutic strategy for weight loss in humans. *Horm. Mol. Biol. Clin. Investig.* **2017**, *31*. [CrossRef] [PubMed]
58. Wang, S.; Pan, M.-H.; Hung, W.-L.; Tung, Y.-C.; Ho, C.-T. From white to beige adipocytes: Therapeutic potential of dietary molecules against obesity and their molecular mechanisms. *Food Funct.* **2019**, *10*, 1263–1279. [CrossRef]
59. Baskaran, P.; Krishnan, V.; Ren, J.; Thyagarajan, B. Capsaicin induces browning of white adipose tissue and counters obesity by activating TRPV1 channel-dependent mechanisms. *J. Cereb. Blood Flow Metab.* **2016**, *173*, 2369–2389. [CrossRef] [PubMed]
60. Supinski, G.S.; Callahan, L.A. Polyethylene Glycol–Superoxide Dismutase Prevents Endotoxin-induced Cardiac Dysfunction. *Am. J. Respir. Crit. Care Med.* **2006**, *173*, 1240–1247. [CrossRef]

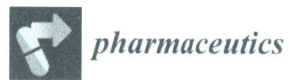

Review

Recent Advances in the Development of Drug Delivery Applications of Magnetic Nanomaterials

Alexandra Pusta [1,2], Mihaela Tertis [1], Izabell Crăciunescu [3], Rodica Turcu [3], Simona Mirel [2] and Cecilia Cristea [1,*]

[1] Department of Analytical Chemistry and Instrumental Analysis, Iuliu Hațieganu University of Medicine and Pharmacy, 4 Louis Pasteur Street, 400349 Cluj-Napoca, Romania; alexandra.pusta@umfcluj.ro (A.P.); mihaela.tertis@umfcluj.ro (M.T.)
[2] Department of Medical Devices, Iuliu Hațieganu University of Medicine and Pharmacy, 4 Pasteur Street, 400349 Cluj-Napoca, Romania; smirel@umfcluj.ro
[3] National Institute for Research and Development of Isotopic and Molecular Technologies, 400293 Cluj-Napoca, Romania; izabell.craciunescu@itim-cj.ro (I.C.); rodica.turcu@itim-cj.ro (R.T.)
* Correspondence: ccristea@umfcluj.ro; Tel.: +40-721-375-789

Abstract: With the predicted rise in the incidence of cancer, there is an ever-growing need for new cancer treatment strategies. Recently, magnetic nanoparticles have stood out as promising nanostructures for imaging and drug delivery systems as they possess unique properties. Moreover, magnetic nanomaterials functionalized with other compounds can lead to multicomponent nanoparticles with innovative structures and synergetic performance. The incorporation of chemotherapeutic drugs or RNA in magnetic drug delivery systems represents a promising alternative that can increase efficiency and reduce the side effects of anticancer therapy. This review presents a critical overview of the recent literature concerning the advancements in the field of magnetic nanoparticles used in drug delivery, with a focus on their classification, characteristics, synthesis and functionalization methods, limitations, and examples of magnetic drug delivery systems incorporating chemotherapeutics or RNA.

Keywords: magnetic nanomaterials; cancer; drug delivery systems; targeted therapy; personalized treatment

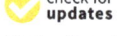

Citation: Pusta, A.; Tertis, M.; Crăciunescu, I.; Turcu, R.; Mirel, S.; Cristea, C. Recent Advances in the Development of Drug Delivery Applications of Magnetic Nanomaterials. *Pharmaceutics* 2023, 15, 1872. https://doi.org/10.3390/pharmaceutics15071872

Academic Editor: Natalia L. Klyachko

Received: 26 May 2023
Revised: 21 June 2023
Accepted: 25 June 2023
Published: 3 July 2023

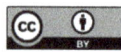

Copyright: © 2023 by the authors. Licensee MDPI, Basel, Switzerland. This article is an open access article distributed under the terms and conditions of the Creative Commons Attribution (CC BY) license (https://creativecommons.org/licenses/by/4.0/).

1. Introduction

Cancer represents a major public health problem worldwide, being the first leading cause of death in people below the age of 70 in North America, Canada, Australia, China, and numerous European countries [1]. With the increase in population and life expectancy, it is predicted that the incidence of cancer will rise in the following years, reaching 28.4 million cases annually worldwide by 2040 [2]. In this context, finding effective therapies for cancer is crucial for reducing the medical and economic burden of this disease.

Conventional cancer therapies include surgery, radiotherapy, and/or chemotherapy. Among these, chemotherapy is widely used but presents various side effects that can limit patient compliance and adherence [3]. Moreover, cancer cells can develop chemotherapy resistance through many mechanisms, rendering it ineffective [4]. Recently, non-coding RNAs such as micro RNAs (miRNA) and small interfering RNAs (siRNA) have been studied for their potential as novel cancer treatments due to their capacity to regulate gene transcription [5]. However, their applicability is limited too by their low stability, high costs, and immunological adverse reactions [6].

In recent years, nanotechnology has emerged as a tool for cancer treatment, promising improved therapeutic outcomes for both chemotherapy and RNA-based therapy, by delivering therapeutic agents in close proximity to the tumor using nano drug delivery systems (DDSs). Nano DDSs generally range in size between 10 and 100 nm, which allows sufficient circulation time and accumulation in the tumor tissue due to the enhanced permeability and retention (EPR) effect [7,8]. Numerous types of DDSs have been employed, such as polymers [9,10], lipid nanoparticles (NPs) [11], and metallic NPs [12] (silver, gold, or magnetic NPs). Among these, magnetic NPs represent a promising alternative, due to their properties such as high stability, high saturation magnetization/large magnetic moment of particles, good response to moderate magnetic fields, inherent ability to cross biological barriers, protection of the drug from rapid degradation in biological systems, provision of a large surface area for conjugating targeting ligands [7,8,13–19], low production costs [20], and superparamagnetism, which allows their guidance in the organism using an external magnetic field [7,21]. Scientific interest in NPs in general and in magnetic nanoparticles (MNPs) in particular has grown exponentially in the last decade, due to recent high-interest research on their properties and the fact that in a relatively short time, these materials have become particularly important tools in high-interest biomedical areas such as biomaterial science, biochemistry, diagnostics, magnetic drug and gene delivery, hyperthermia, magnetic resonance imaging (MRI), and theragnostics [22–31]. The increased interest in the field of MNPs is demonstrated by the number of scientific articles provided by a simple "magnetic nanoparticles" keyword search in the Scopus database. Before 1995, fewer than 100 articles were published, but after 1996, when the first successful clinical trials took place, there was an exponential increase with 3000 articles in 2010, 6500 in 2015, and up to 8700 in 2020 [32]. As a general structure, NPs are considered inorganic or organic particles of submicron size with enhanced properties relative to a similar bulk form. The specific physical and chemical properties given by nanostructuring, such as optical, electrical, and magnetic properties or increased reactivity, made these special types of NPs attractive to nanotechnology. Following the development of biotechnological applications, the term "bio-magnetic nanoparticles" (BMNPs) was introduced, describing a unique combination of physio-chemical properties of magnetic nanoparticles with their entirely biocompatible nature, which makes them particularly effective in various biomedical applications [33]. Starting from the particular requirements of each biomedical application, BMNPs are considered to have a huge potential in drug delivery applications, because their surface can be specifically functionalized with various molecular layers [7,14,24,34]. Apart from drug delivery, magnetic NPs can be used for hyperthermia applications, MRI contrast imaging, and diagnosis procedures. Recently, magneto-mechanical actuation of MNPs has also been used as an anti-cancer strategy. In this technique, the application of a magnetic field does not lead to heating (such as in hyperthermia), but to vibrations of the MNPs in the proximity of cells, leading to mechanical alterations and cell death [35,36]. Moreover, complex strategies combining more of these approaches can also be employed. The combination of hyperthermia and drug delivery in the same carrier can enhance anti-cancer efficiency destroying cancer cells through multiple mechanisms. Theragnostic approaches also represent a promising direction, combining simultaneous treatment and diagnosis for improved cancer management. These applications have been extensively covered elsewhere [7,13,20,37,38] and do not represent the scope of this review.

In this work, we will present the main types of magnetic nanomaterials and their characteristics, classification, and common synthesis procedures. A few limitations of MNPs and some considerations on the development of DDSs will be presented. In the next section, we will present and comparatively discuss examples of applications of magnetic nanomaterials used for the targeted delivery of common chemotherapeutics such as doxorubicin (DOX), platinum compounds cisplatin (CIS) and oxaliplatin (OXA), methrotrexate (MTX), sorafenib (SOR), and curcumin (Cur), with a focus on their advantages compared to chemotherapeutics alone. Targeted delivery of miRNA and siRNA will also be covered in a dedicated section. Theragnostic approaches for the simultaneous imaging and diagnosis of cancer will also be presented in a separate section, due to their promising perspectives in the field of cancer management.

2. Classification of BMNPs

In order to properly choose the most appropriate MNPs for specific biomedical applications, a very clear classification of them according to their nature, composition, and size is required, taking into account the synthesis methods used to prepare them and the specific functionalization of the surface.

Over time, several types of MNPs have been developed and researched. Generally, these MNPs can be grouped into three main categories as (i) magnetic pure metals (Fe, Co, Ni), (ii) magnetic metal oxides (Fe_2O_3, Fe_3O_4) or ferrites ($MeFe_2O_4$, Me = Fe, Co, Zn), and (iii) multicomponent magnetic nanoparticles as core/shell MNPs or magnetic nanoclusters (Figure 1). Each of these mentioned categories has both advantages and disadvantages, but their properties can be adapted to fit a particular type of application. In the following, each category will be discussed and exemplified.

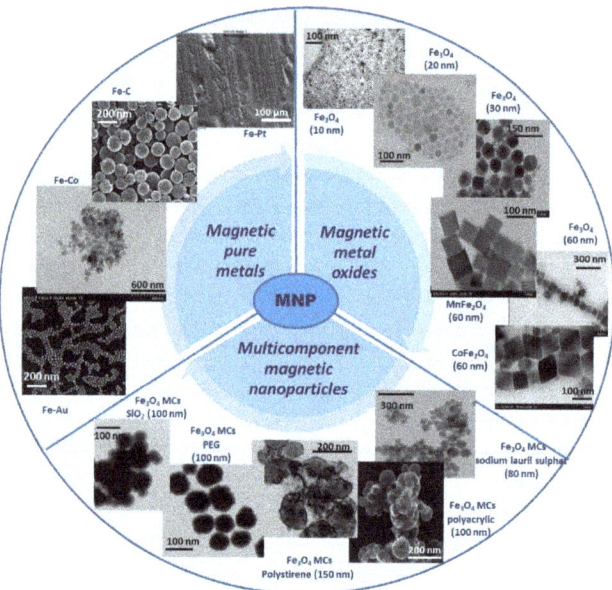

Figure 1. General classification and exemplification of magnetic nanoparticles (all images are original and belong to the authors).

2.1. Magnetic Pure Metals

Pure metal type materials exhibit some unique properties, with some of them directly dependent on the distribution of electrons in the external orbitals, and magnetic behavior is one of these properties. Transition metals, such as Fe, Ni, Co, and Mn, are the most commonly used in this class because they show good magnetic performance in several biomedical fields [39].

Iron (Fe) nanoparticles are one of the most common ferromagnetic materials used for biomedical applications. The main advantage of using this material is related to its excellent magnetic properties, which can be exploited in a wide range of biomedical applications.

In terms of synthesis methods, Fe nanoparticles can be obtained by relatively simple methods such as the reduction of iron salts in aqueous solutions in the presence of reducing agents such as sodium borohydride [40], or by thermal decomposition of $Fe(CO)_5$ on a polymer matrix [41]. Even if the synthesis methods are facile and accessible, one of the major weaknesses of these NPs is that synthesis requires rigorous control of the surface-covering shell since direct contact between the Fe surface and air leads to their combustion. Therefore, the necessity to find homogeneous and uniform coatings for this kind of nanoparticle is critical. There are studies in which tailoring the reaction parameters and changing the Fe precursor to Fe[N(SiMe$_3$)$_2$]$_2$ can result in major improvements in the reaction yield, better control of the size distribution, and a reduction in by-product formation [42].

In addition to Fe NPs, cobalt (Co) is another magnetic material commonly used in biomedical applications. Although its toxicity is higher than that of Fe NPs, beneficial effects of its use have been observed in specific MRI imaging applications and local hyperthermia of malignant tumors [43,44].

2.2. Magnetic Metal Oxides

From the general class of metal oxides, iron oxide distinguishes itself as a material with excellent magnetic properties and low toxicity compared to pure metallic forms, which, due to its unique physio-chemical properties, has potential applications in nanotechnology [39]. Over time, metal oxides have gained popularity in biomedical applications due to their physicochemical and mechanical stability, low toxicity, and biocompatibility but also for their efficiency in some special areas of biomedical science such as magnetic bio-separation of some species of interest, magnetic hyperthermia, drug carriers at target sites, and bio sensing [45,46].

There are three types of iron oxides: Iron (III) oxide, with two subspecies: Hematite (α-Fe$_2$O$_3$) and maghemite (γ-Fe$_2$O$_3$); a rare type of iron (II) oxide (FeO) called wüstite; and iron (II, III) oxide named magnetite (Fe$_3$O$_4$). This different stoichiometry due to the flexibility of the Fe oxidation state (Fe^{2+}/Fe^{3+}) is supported by the formation of different single-crystal phases with different chemical and physical properties.

Of all iron oxide structures, Fe$_3$O$_4$ has the most closely packed cubic inverted spinel structure and semi metallic properties, demonstrating great potential in biomedical fields [47]. One of the biggest advantages of these NPs is the ease of their synthesis at relatively high reaction yields by simple and conventional methods. In the beginning, conventional preparation methods such as the co-precipitation or solvothermal method [48–53] did not offer rigorous control over the size and size distribution of MNPs, so aggregation and poly dispersibility appeared, which hindered their use in biomedical applications. Over time, however, new synthesis methods were explored to obtain size-controlled NPs with a uniform size distribution. For example, by using organic iron precursors, Fe$_3$O$_4$ NPs with a narrow size distribution were obtained. By adjusting the molar ratio between metal precursors and different surfactant molecules, different particles can be obtained ranging in shape from cubic to polyhedral [54]. It can be concluded that the physicochemical properties of NPs, in particular the magnetic properties, can be adjusted according to the intended application with minimal changes in the composition and synthesis parameters.

Although iron oxides have the advantage of easy preparation, they present certain limitations related to chemical stability under biological environmental conditions, often resulting in aggregation phenomena that decrease their potential use in biomedical applications. Coating the surface of iron oxide NPs with biocompatible molecular layers increases chemical and mechanical stability, reduces surface oxidation, and decreases toxicity in biological entities. Thus, iron oxide NPs, generically called superparamagnetic iron oxide nanoparticles (SPIONs), have been developed. These particles represent small synthetic iron oxide particles with a core ranging between 10 nm and 30 nm in diameter, coated with certain biocompatible molecules, which provide chemical handles for the conjugation of therapeutic agents and improve their blood distribution profile [55]. These particles exhibit superparamagnetic properties, meaning that under an external magnetic field, they magnetize to saturation magnetization, and when the magnetic field is removed, they exhibit no residual magnetic interaction. This property is dependent on the size of the NPs and generally occurs when their size is only 10–20 nm. At such a small size, these NPs do not exhibit multiple magnetic domains, as found in larger NPs, acting as a "single super spin" that exhibits high magnetic susceptibility. Thus, upon application of a magnetic field, these NPs provide a stronger and faster magnetic response compared to bulk magnets with negligible residual magnetization and coercivity (the field required to bring the magnetism to zero) [56]. This unique property of SPIONs represents a great advantage for their use in specific biomedical applications such as controlled drug delivery where these NPs function as drug delivery vehicles because they can drag specific drug molecules to the target site, under the influence of an external magnetic field. Furthermore, once the applied magnetic field is removed, the magnetic particles do not retain any residual magnetism and aggregation phenomena are avoided, thus evading absorption by phagocytes and increasing half-life in circulation. In addition, due to their negligible tendency to agglomerate, SPIONs pose no danger of thrombosis or blockage of blood capillaries [55].

A sub-division of metal oxides, emerging from the necessity of adjusting the properties of this type of material for specific biomedical applications, is spinel ferrites ($MeFe_2O_4$), a very important magnetic material due to their combined electrical and magnetic properties, which make them useful in many technological applications [57]. The main component of these materials is iron oxide doped with a variety of bivalent transition metals such as zinc (Zn), manganese (Mn), cobalt (Co), nickel (Ni), iron (Fe), platinum (Pt), and palladium (Pd). It has been demonstrated that due to the doping of the Fe_3O_4 structure with bivalent cations, ferrites show improved electrical and magnetic properties for hyperthermia applications, for example, but also present the disadvantage of higher toxicity compared to magnetite [58]. The use of some stabilizing molecules, which also confer biocompatibility on the ferrite NPs surfaces, is essential for biomedical practical applications. In the synthesis of Co ferrite NPs, a $CoFe_2(CO)_9$ precursor and two stabilizing agents, hexadecylamine and oleic acid, were used to obtain small, relatively polydisperse MNPs. When a third stabilizing agent, lauric acid, was introduced, bigger monodispersed crystalline structures with a narrower size distribution were obtained. A decrease in the toxicity of the system was also demonstrated, with the developed system showing promising applications against tumor cells [59]. Another particularly efficient approach to using ferrite NPs in biomedical applications is their coating with biocompatible polymer layers, such as polyhydroxy and polyamine-type polymers and polyethylene glycol (PEG). It has been proven that the use of these systems in controlled drug release applications is particularly effective, with researchers also performing biocompatibility tests, which demonstrated that these materials can be successfully applied without adverse effects regarding toxicity [60]. Other ferrite-type magnetic structures have been reported in the literature, which, in addition to excellent magnetic properties, also show lower toxicity, such as Zn-, Mn-, and Ni-based ferrites [61]. There are also ferrite-type systems, with two transition metal components, Co-Zn and Mn-Zn type, in which it was highlighted that the concentration of Zn ions has an effect on the size of the final particles, i.e., increasing the concentration of Zn cations decreases the size of the particles [62].

2.3. Multicomponent Magnetic Nanoparticles

Multicomponent MNPs have been developed as a normal evolution of the technology because these systems can present multiple functionalities at the same time, by simply combining two or more components and thus offering new features that are not available in single-component materials or structures. In addition, in these multicomponent systems, improved specific properties can be obtained that may overcome the natural limitations of single-component materials. There are several types of multicomponent magnetic structures, but the most often studied and with real possibilities of application in biomedicine are the two main categories: (i) Core/shell type multicomponent MNPs and (ii) magnetic clusters (MCs).

(i) Core/shell-type multicomponent magnetic nanoparticles

Core/shell-type MNPs are the most common type of multicomponent NPs and have been widely studied. Core/shell structures were first prepared in semiconductor NPs [63] with the specific aim to modify their electrical and optical properties. The extension of this idea to magnetic systems initially emerged as an idea to protect and enhance the properties of metallic MNPs by coating them with protective layers, especially Fe NPs, which have extremely high reactivity in metallic form.

Core/shell composite structures of Fe/Fe$_3$O$_4$ type with a magnetic core consisting of iron NPs (Fe) and a thin protective coating of iron oxide (Fe$_3$O$_4$) were prepared [64]. Following the same idea of covering magnetic cores of other metals, various multicomponent magnetic systems have been developed, in which the metallic magnetic core was synthesized by the so-called seed-mediated process followed by coating with oxide layers of the same metal and/or various metallic combinations, such as Ni/NiO [65], Co/CoSe [66], Co/Co$_2$P [67], and Pt/Fe$_2$O$_3$ [68]. Another successful possibility consisted of covering metallic Fe NPs with a ferrite shell (Fe@MFe$_2$O$_4$, M = Fe, Mn, Co) [69]. The core/shell composite system kept high-level magnetic properties, presented high relaxivity, and remained mono-dispersed throughout the experiments without showing aggregation processes under the action of the biological environment.

There are also core/shell type multicomponent magnetic systems in which the magnetic core is bimagnetic, obtained by an interesting combination of two magnetic metallic species, covered as a whole with an oxide coating. A successful example of such synthesized systems is the FePt/Fe$_3$O$_4$ core/shell system where MNPs from the core were obtained by sequential decomposition of some organic precursors Fe(acac)$_3$ and Pt(acac)$_2$ and the thickness of the external shell was tailored from 0.5 nm to 5 nm by controlling the synthesis parameters [70]. The seed-mediated growth method was extended to prepare other types of core/shell binary systems such as FePt/ZnO [71], Fe$_3$O$_4$/ZnO [72], Co/CdSe [73], FePt/PbS [74], and Fe$_3$O$_4$/Cu$_{2-x}$S [75].

Another model of multicomponent core/shell systems, in which the magnetic core was made of iron oxide NPs (Fe$_3$O$_4$) covered with a noble metal coating, was also obtained. The as-prepared systems Fe$_3$O$_4$/Au [76] and Fe$_3$O$_4$/Au/Ag [77] were later functionalized appropriately for the intended biomedical application. This system not only benefits from the excellent magnetic properties of the SPION core but also from the plasmon resonance properties of the noble metals in the combination of the multicomponent magnetic system [78].

(ii) Magnetic clusters

In recent years, MC systems obtained by controlled self-assembly of superparamagnetic nanoparticles into three-dimensional clusters have gained popularity in biomedical applications, based on the new, innovative, collective properties that hold great promise for the development of advanced bio nanomaterials with novel integrated functions [79]. Depending on the preparation method and the nature of the functionalizing polymers, MNPs can be assembled with different spatial orientations resulting in clusters with different shapes and sizes (spheres, rod-like, nanoring, etc.) [80–82], which influence their properties. MCs with a polymer coating are very promising for theragnostic applications since they ensure an increase in the performance of MRI and hyperthermia and allow encapsulation of the drug that can be released at the target [80,81,83].

MCs are defined as systems consisting of a finite number of interacting spins ranging from a few hundred to several thousand, with well-controlled sizes, shapes, and compositions, which are magnetically isolated from the environment [84]. From the general definition of MCs, an important subclass of MCs is distinguished, consisting of several hundred MNPs with superparamagnetic properties [85,86], self-assembled as up to 100 nm MCs. In these systems, the spin dynamics exhibit many features similar to those of the molecular nanomagnets, such as superparamagnetic relaxation and quantized spin-wave states [87].

Since some of the properties of MCs depend on both the sizes of the MCs and the component NPs, considerable effort is required to control these two structural parameters in order to establish the optimal structure–property relationship and to obtain multicomponent magnetic systems with specific properties for biomedical applications. The development of robust synthesis protocols that allow rigorous control over the composition, size, and shape, as well as cluster surface properties and uniformity of colloidal NPs, requires a very good understanding of the mechanisms that induce aggregation phenomena. The forces involved in the controlled aggregation process of MNPs are both covalent and non-covalent such as hydrogen bonding, electrostatics, and van der Waals interactions, forces that can be controlled by the modification of synthesis parameters, such as the nature and concentration of solvents, the surfactants involved, the reaction temperatures, and reaction times [79].

The literature presents a wide variety of preparation methods for MCs, including options that involve several simple procedures integrated into a single reaction step or more complex versions that produce MC in a single reaction step. A classification of MC preparation methods can therefore be made as follows: (a) Single-step MC procedures, which integrate the synthesis of MNPs and their controlled aggregation into clusters in a single step, and (b) multi-step MC procedures, which first produce MNPs of a specific size, shape, and surface functionality and then self-assemble into clusters of required geometrical configurations in subsequent separate steps. Each of the synthesis methods has both advantages and disadvantages. While single-step processes are easier in terms of methods and more efficient in terms of producing MCs, the control of the synthesis parameters is less rigorous because the NPs' synthesis and the clustering steps take place at the same time. Multi-step processes have the advantage of being more flexible in terms of primary materials, being able to produce a wide variety of materials in cluster form with well-organized structures, but they also bring a higher complexity, as well as some disadvantages in terms of magnetic properties, which may decrease due to the functionalization of the surface with relatively thick layers of non-magnetic materials.

(a) Single step-magnetic cluster procedures

From the most popular preparation techniques for the synthesis of MCs in a single reaction step, we can list the thermolysis method and the solvothermal method. In the following, some literature references of each of these methods will be exemplified, although it should be noted that there is no generally accepted method, and each synthesis of MCs with different shapes, sizes, structures, and surface functionality will involve specific synthesis parameters that cannot be reproduced for other versions.

The thermolysis method involves the reaction of metal precursors in the presence of the capping ligand in an organic solvent at a high temperature. Due to the high temperature, the metal precursor decomposes, and the nanoparticle seed and growing reaction is initiated. At this point, the capping ligands bind to the surface of the NPs, limit their growth, and prevent the formation of interparticle bonds, also leading to the clusterization of the NPs in controlled shape and size clusters through steric interactions between ligand molecules. The nature and concentration of the capping ligands play an essential role in obtaining structurally homogeneous clusters with a uniform size distribution. Using the thermolysis method, oxide clusters of transition metals such as In_2O_3, CoO, MnO, and ZnO were prepared by reducing the concentration of stabilizing organic ligands to the point where insufficiently stabilized primary NPs agglomerated in a controlled three-dimensional form [88]. The thermolysis method has also been successfully implemented to produce MCs with Fe_3O_4 as primary MNPs in a single reaction step at a high temperature to obtain polyelectrolyte-coated MCs [89]. In this process, basic hydrolysis of the iron precursor ($FeCl_3$) using diethylene glycol as a solvent and polyacrylic acid as a surfactant took place at 220°C. The size of the MCs could be controlled by modifying the synthesis parameters, such as varying the pH and controlling the molar ratio between the metal precursor and surfactant, resulting in homogeneous geometry and narrow size distributions of MCs with sizes between 30 and 180 nm.

The solvothermal method consists of chemical reactions of metal precursors in a closed environment called and autoclave at high temperatures, higher than the boiling point of the solvent. This method has very quickly become a commonly used method due to its versatility and simplicity of application in terms of materials, methods, and cost. There are, however, several disadvantages of this method, namely the relatively high energy requirements, the reactions taking place at high temperatures for long reaction times, the limited scalability, and the lack of direct monitoring of the reaction process. In the literature, there are many studies that describe the preparation of MCs obtained by the solvothermal method [48–53].

(b) Multi-step magnetic cluster procedures

Multi-step MCs procedures involve the preliminary preparation of MNPs, using traditional methods that are subsequently assembled in one or more reaction steps in clusters with controlled shapes and sizes. This method offers the opportunity to combine the inherent properties of MNPs with innovative properties resulting from the collective interaction of NPs within the clusters. A large number of new composite materials commonly produced in the form of NPs with excellent control over size, shape, and surface properties can be developed easily and with remarkable properties, which can later be modularly assembled in the form of super-structured nanomaterials with various configurations and programmable properties.

One of the simplest methods to obtain MCs in two reaction steps was the encapsulation of the MNPs in different encapsulating agents with a specific function for controlled aggregation, protection, and surface functionalization. For the embedding process, different types of molecules were used as encapsulating agents, including polymers and/or block copolymers [90–92], micelles [93], polysaccharides [94], or hydrogels [95].

Another efficient clustering method is the emulsion method, slightly modified as the mini-emulsion method, if MCs of hundreds of nanometers in size are obtained. The mini-emulsion method can have two alternatives, direct emulsion, generically called "oil-in-water emulsion" in which oil (nonpolar solvent) droplets form micelles in an aqueous medium containing a water-soluble surfactant, or inverse emulsion, generically called "water-in-oil emulsion" in which water droplets form micelles in an organic medium with a non-polar dissolved surfactant. For the preparation of MCs, the mini-emulsion oil-in-water method is most commonly used because the pre-prepared magnetic particles can be easily dispersed in an organic solvent and used as the organic oil phase. In this process, MNPs prepared in a previous reaction step are homogeneously dispersed as a colloidal solution in a non-polar organic solvent, such as cyclohexane, dodecane, or toluene, to form an organic phase, generically called the "oil" phase. At the same time, a surfactant aqueous solution is prepared having dissolved a surfactant agent such as sodium dodecyl sulphate or cetyltrimethylammonium bromide, which has an amphiphilic structure. Using an ultrasonic finger, the two non-miscible phases are mixed to form a mini-emulsion. The mini-emulsion represents droplets of the organic phase, oil, containing the MNPs dispersed in water, where the surfactant is oriented with the hydrophobic end to the oil droplets and the hydrophilic end to the aqueous medium, creating stable oil in water micelles. The oil-in-water mini-emulsion is heated and the organic solvent from the micelles is evaporated, forming hydrophilic MCs. The size of these clusters can be adjusted by changing the concentration of NPs in the medium and the surfactant in the oil phase [96]. Using this method, composite clusters have been obtained by encapsulating various types of nanoparticles in different micelles, and/or molecular layers, polymers, and organic or inorganic layers such as γ-Fe_2O_3/TiO_2 [97], $NaYF_4$-Yb,Er/$NaYF_4$:Eu [98], CeO_2/Pd [99], polystyrene [100], and Fe_3O_4/OA-FeCo/Al_2O_3 MCs [101].

3. Limitations and Solutions to Overcome These Limitations in the Use of MNPs in Bio-Nano Medical Applications

Over time, based on a deeper understanding of the action mechanism of bio-MNPs in biomedical applications, some ideal properties, considered minimum requirements for the functionalization of MNPs, were proposed for higher performance of these materials in practical nano-bio applications (Figure 2).

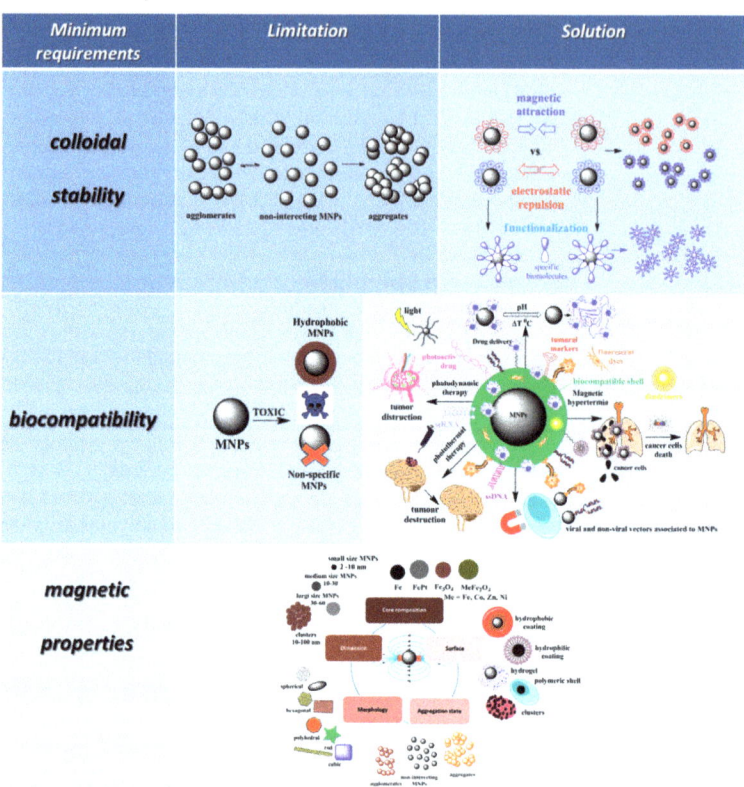

Figure 2. Strategies to bridge the gap between magnetic nanoparticles (MNPs) and bio-magnetic nanoparticles (BMNPs).

These minimum requirements have been established based on some limitations relative to the direct applications of these materials in bio-nano medicine. One of the most important is related to the colloidal stability of MNPs in the aqueous medium, when agglomeration and/or aggregation phenomena occur. Another limitation is the potential negative effects on the human body and the environment [18]. Proper surface functionalization increases the compatibility of MNPs with the biological environments, making them biocompatible and biospecific. Significant research efforts are dedicated to suitable surface modifications of magnetic nanoparticles to improve colloidal stability, prevent aggregation of nanoparticles, ensure a non-toxic state in physiological conditions, and introduce functional groups for binding of application-specific target molecules [7,14,15,18,19], thus the appropriate coating of NPs is very important to ensure their stability in physiological and biological fluids [18,19,102].

The first minimum requirement for the use of these NPs in biomedical applications is their surface functionalization to prevent MNPs from aggregation and lead to improved colloidal stability [103]. The colloidal stability of the MNPs can be improved by balancing the attractive and repulsive forces between these materials and their environment. Stabilization of MNPs can be performed by controlling the intensity of one or both repulsive forces, which are electrostatic repulsion and steric repulsion. Steric stabilization is based on coating MNPs with various molecules or a ligand shell or embedding them in an inorganic or polymeric matrix with steric properties. In these cases, the repulsive potential is given by the molecular weight and/or density of the surface coating material and its chemical and mechanical stability but also by the quality of the dispersion medium in which the functionalized magnetic material is used. The mechanism behind steric stabilization refers to the fact that if two sterically stabilized MNPs approach each other and exhibit steric properties, a connection is created between them that has the effect of reducing the entropy of the material, increasing the osmotic pressure between the functionalized MNPs, and leading to increased colloidal stability [104].

Another very important property necessary for the application of MNPs in biological environments is the compatibility of these NPs with the aqueous medium. An appropriate strategy to overcome the limitations imposed by the use of uncoated, hydrophobic, or weakly hydrophilic MNPs is crucial for the stability of MNPs in a biological environment and depends on the nature of the MNP surface. If MNPs are uncovered, the direct attachment of hydrophilic agents to the surface of uncoated MNPs in the final stage of MNP synthesis can be chosen as a compatibility strategy. If MNPs are already coated with a hydrophobic layer, the addition of amphiphilic molecules containing both a hydrophobic segment and a hydrophilic component can be used for water compatibility. In this case, the hydrophobic part forms a double-layer structure with the initial hydrophobic surface of the MNPs, while the hydrophilic groups are exposed on the outside of the NPs, which makes them water soluble. Another compatibility strategy when the surface of MNPs is hydrophobic or weakly hydrophilic is the ligand exchange method, with the direct replacement of the original surfactant with a new one, which can improve the hydrophilic properties of MNPs [105].

Another particularly important requirement when it comes to the use MNPs in biomedical applications is the magnetic properties of these materials, which depend on their nature and size. In applications where these NPs involve exposure to an external magnetic field, their shape and size, as well as magnetic properties such as their superparamagnetism and saturated magnetization value, are essential criteria for material selection. Very small-sized particles, below 10 nm, despite presenting colloidal and magnetic stability, are very difficult to process and have relatively low magnetization values. Therefore, slightly larger NPs are preferred because they are easier to manipulate magnetically, have higher magnetization values, and at the same time, have lower colloidal stability. A new and original alternative that overcomes the limitations of colloidal and magnetic instability while having superparamagnetic properties and high saturation magnetization values is represented by MCs, which are self-assembled, controlled aggregations of hundreds of single-core MNPs in the form of spherical clusters of approximately 100 nm in size.

One of the particularly important requirements for using MNPs in biomedical applications is low toxicity to the biological environment and biocompatibility of the material. It is known that, due to their large surface area and chemical reactivity, MNPs can generate reactive oxygen species that can penetrate tissues down to the cellular level, thus being extremely toxic [106,107]. MNPs can exert their toxic activity at multiple levels, leading to potential mitochondrial destruction, DNA damage, temporary or permanent cell cycle cessation, or cell membrane disruption [108]. It is known that the shape and size of MNPs, the hydrophilicity of the surface, the mass/thickness of the surface covering material, as well as the surface charge are key factors governing the biocompatibility of the material. An important strategy for improving biocompatibility and reducing toxicity is represented by the functionalization of MNPs with different agents, such as polymers, proteins, or inorganic compounds. Proteins that are abundant in human serum, such as albumin, can create a protective barrier on the surface of MNPs, increasing biocompatibility [109]. Coatings with silica, which is abundant in hydroxyl groups, also generate less-toxic MNPs [110]. Some studies suggest that coating with noble metals such as gold can also increase biocompatibility [111]. Biocompatible molecular layers covering MNPs with negative charges show better biocompatibility, while a positively charged shell on the surface shows better cooperation with bio systems but can often interact electrostatically with differently charged particles of a biological medium. Biocompatible polymeric coatings represent a useful alternative because they can decrease the density of the material, making them more stable from colloidal and magnetic points of view and, at the same time, offer advantages on further surface functionalization with different biologically active substances for specific applications. From the synthesis method point of view, MNP surface functionalization with positively or negatively charged molecular layers is easier and much more controllable, while surface coatings with polymeric layers offer much less control over the morphology of the final material, resulting in relatively thick polymeric layers and therefore slightly lower magnetic properties.

4. Considerations about the Development of Magnetic Drug Delivery Systems

The main goal of DDSs is to ensure that the chemotherapeutic drug reaches its intended site of action in the body, that is, the tumor and cancer cells, while minimizing its distribution to healthy cells, reducing side effects and increasing therapeutic efficacy.

There are several types of DSSs [112–114]:

(i) Oral drug delivery—the most common form of drug delivery, where the drug is taken orally in the form of pills, capsules, or liquids. In this case, the drug is absorbed into the bloodstream through the digestive system.

(ii) Injectable drug delivery—a method that involves injecting the drug directly into the bloodstream, intramuscularly or subcutaneously. This type of delivery is used for drugs that cannot be taken orally or that need to be delivered quickly.

(iii) Topical drug delivery—a method of delivery that involves applying the drug directly to the skin, mucous membranes, or other external surfaces of the body. Pharmaceutical formulations such as creams or ointments are commonly used in this case.

(iv) Inhalatory drug delivery—a method that involves delivering drugs through inhalation into the lungs. This type of delivery is commonly used for the treatment of respiratory diseases.

(v) Implantable drug delivery—a method of delivery that involves implanting a device or a drug-eluting implant that slowly releases the drug over a period of time. This method is commonly used for long-term treatments.

In addition to these traditional DDSs, there are also newer technologies such as targeted drug delivery, where drugs are delivered specifically to cancer cells, and nanotechnology-based drug delivery, where drugs are delivered using NPs, technologies that are still in development but hold promise for the future of drug delivery [115,116].

MNPs have drawn considerable attention in recent years due to properties that make them promising candidates for drug delivery, with numerous studies published in this field. In the successful development of magnetic DDSs, some considerations about their physical properties, targeting abilities, cargo release, and cytotoxic properties need to be taken into account.

In general, iron oxide NPs, especially magnetite, are used for the development of magnetic DDSs. The most important properties of these carriers are their size and superparamagnetism. In order to be used for in vivo applications, the size of DDSs needs to be between 10 and 100 nm in diameter [7,8]. Particles that are smaller in size are quickly eliminated by the kidneys and cannot perform their biological role in vivo, while bigger particles are recognized by the immune system and are trapped in the reticuloendothelial system [117,118]. The size of dehydrated magnetic NPs is determined experimentally using electron microscopy techniques such as transmission electron microscopy (TEM) or scanning electron microscopy. Another characteristic is the hydrodynamic size, which is the size of the hydrated NPs in an aqueous solution and is generally determined by dynamic light scattering [119].

Biomedical applications generally focus not on simple MNPs but on magnetic nanocomposites that combine the properties of MNPs with those of other components, leading to complex properties such as increased biocompatibility and stability, low toxicity, and high drug-binding capacity. The shell of these magnetic nanocomposites can be represented by polymers (PEG, chitosan, carboxymethyl chitosan, poly(methacrylic acid), polydopamine, poly(lactide-co-glycolide), polyvinyl alcohol, polyethyleneimine), mesoporous silica, layered double hydroxides, liposomes, sugars, proteins, inorganic compounds, or lipids. The successful functionalization can be confirmed by Fourier Transform Infrared Spectroscopy or Energy Dispersive Spectroscopy.

Drugs are incorporated into magnetic DDSs by interacting with the shell, either by covalent binding or electrostatic interactions. The loaded DDSs can be characterized by two parameters, namely drug-loading capacity (LC) and drug encapsulation efficiency (EE). The LC represents the amount of drug that is loaded in 100 g of DDS and helps determine the amount of drug that could be delivered by the DDS to its target. EE represents the percentage of drug that was loaded into the DDS from the feeding solution [120].

Once the DDS is obtained and loaded with the desired drug, it needs to be delivered to the target organ. In the treatment of cancer, targeting can be performed in either a passive or an active manner. Passive targeting relies on the EPR effect, which allows preferential accumulation of nano-DDSs in the tumor tissue due to increased permeability of blood vessels and retention at the tumor level due to low lymphatic drainage. However, EPR offers only a modest increase in accumulation at the tumor level compared to healthy organs, so active targeting was developed as an alternative [117,121]. Active targeting can be achieved by the functionalization of the magnetic DDSs with ligands that can specifically bind to structures present on the surface of cancer cells. Examples of such ligands are antibodies, peptides, proteins, aptamers, folic acid (FA), or hyaluronic acid (HA) [121]. In the case of magnetic DDSs, targeting can be aided by the application of an external magnetic field that guides the DDS to the desired location.

Once at the delivery site, the DDS needs to be able to release the loaded cargo. In the treatment of cancer, the special properties of the tumor microenvironment are used to preferentially deliver the drugs to the tumor. Most DDSs investigated in this review present a pH-dependent release behavior, which relies on the lower pH of the tumor microenvironment compared to that of healthy cells or blood [122]. Other examples of preferential release include the use of substrates that are degraded by enzymes overexpressed at the tumor site [123–127], redox-dependent release based on the higher concentration of glutathione (GSH) in tumor cells compared to healthy ones [128,129], or magnetic-field-mediated release [128,130–137].

Ideally, drugs encapsulated in DDSs should present higher toxicity towards tumors and lower toxicity towards healthy organs compared to the free drug. Toxicity assessments were generally carried out on cell cultures, while few studies also focused on the in vivo effects of the DDSs using animal models.

5. Chemotherapy Delivery Using Magnetic Nanoparticles

Chemotherapy represents one of the mainstays of cancer treatment. Its primary goal is to stop cancer cell proliferation and the formation of metastases [3]. There are different classes of chemotherapeutic drugs, based on their primary mechanism of action: Alkylating agents, antimetabolites, antimicrotubule agents, topoisomerase inhibitors, antibiotics, and others [138]. Despite having different mechanisms, all chemotherapeutics present toxicity towards malignant cells but also towards healthy cells, producing side effects such as myelosuppression, hair loss, nausea, and vomiting. In recent years, efforts have been made to improve the selectivity of chemotherapeutics for cancer cells and tumors by using different strategies. One such strategy is the incorporation of chemotherapeutic drugs into DDSs. DDSs offer several advantages over classical chemotherapy treatment [115,116,139,140]:

- One of the main advantages of DDSs is the ability to target specific cells or tissues, minimizing damage to healthy cells.
- DSS use reduces side effects associated with chemotherapy, because DDSs deliver drugs directly to the site of action.
- DDSs can improve the efficacy of drugs by ensuring that they are delivered to the intended site of action and in the correct dosage.
- Some DDS technologies, such as implantable drug delivery devices, can release drugs slowly over an extended period, ensuring sustained and controlled release of the drug.

- DDSs can be personalized to the individual patient, taking into account factors such as age, weight, and the specific characteristics of their cancer. This can help to ensure that the patient receives the optimal treatment for their individual case.
- DDSs can help reduce the development of drug resistance.

Overall, DDSs have the potential to provide more effective, targeted, and personalized treatments for cancer patients, while reducing the side effects and toxicity associated with classical chemotherapy.

In this section, examples of magnetic DDSs will be discussed and presented comparatively. The examples are classified based on the drug they incorporate. An overview of the main characteristics of the incorporated drugs is presented in Table 1, while examples of DDSs for each drug are presented comparatively in Table 2.

Table 1. Drugs commonly prescribed in the treatment of cancers [141–144].

Drug	Indications	Class	Mechanism of Action	Specific Side Effects
DOX	Acute lymphoblastic leukemia Hodgkin's lymphoma Breast cancer Ovarian cancer Bladder cancer Bone tumors	Anthracyclines	Intercalation into DNA double-helix Topoisomerase II inhibition Formation of oxygen reactive species	Cardiotoxicity
CIS, OXA	Ovarian cancer Breast cancer Colorectal carcinoma	Alkylating agents	Intercalation into DNA double-helix	Neurotoxicity Nephrotoxicity Ototoxicity
MTX	Non-Hodgkin's lymphoma Breast cancer Bladder cancer Osteosarcoma	Antimetabolite	Inhibition of folic acid metabolism	Immunosuppression Hepatotoxicity Respiratory failure
SOR	Hepatocellular carcinoma Renal cell carcinoma Thyroid cancer	Multi kinase inhibitor	Inhibition of cell signaling pathways Inhibition of angiogenesis	Rash Arterial hypertension

5.1. Doxorubicin

Doxorubicin (DOX) is one of the most commonly used drugs in the treatment of a variety of cancers. Many attempts have been made to reduce DOX toxicity, with its incorporation into numerous DDSs. Indeed, DOX has become a "model" molecule for the development of magnetic DDSs, with many proof-of-concept formulations using this molecule.

MNPs functionalized with different composites have been intensively used for the development of nanocarriers for DOX. Numerous recent studies present different approaches regarding the synthesis, functionalization, drug loading, delivery method, and release of DOX. In order for DDSs to be effective in targeted therapy, it is crucial to improve their biocompatibility and targeting ability. To improve biocompatibility, various materials such as biodegradable polymers [130,145,146], sugars [129,130,147], lipids [133], and proteins [148,149] have been used. These materials can be used for coating purposes to reduce the toxicity and immunogenicity of the resulting DDS.

Regarding their indication, DOX-containing DDSs were developed for a wide variety of cancers, including breast cancer [123,147,150], liver cancer [131,133,145], lung cancer [151], and colorectal carcinoma [129,132,152].

A polymer coating often used in the development of DDSs is PEG, which has proven to be suitable both for the efficient loading of different drugs and with good properties in terms of biocompatibility. Thus, MNPs and boron nanosheets coated with a pH-responsive PEG polymer were used for the fabrication of a new DDS for which highly controlled loading and release processes were optimized for DOX. Both in vitro and in vivo experiments have demonstrated that the DDS can inhibit tumor growth, induce cancer cell apoptosis, and reduce the toxic effects of DOX, a potential alternative for liver cancer therapy [145]. Polysaccharides such as chitosan or its modified forms can also be employed for the functionalization of MNPs for DOX delivery. A study reported a nanocomposite material that combines two different components, GSH and magnetic-sensitive iron oxide NPs, which provide redox-responsiveness and magnetic sensitivity, respectively. The MePEG-grafted water-soluble chitosan backbone helps achieve biocompatibility and stability of the nanocomposites. The conjugation of DOX with chitosan via a disulfide linkage ensures controlled drug release in the presence of GSH, which is often found in higher concentrations in cancer cells. In vitro experiments showed that an external magnetic stimulus helps concentrate the nanocomposites and provides efficient internalization of the nanocomposites into cancer cells [129]. The use of aminated lignosulfonate and carboxymethyl chitosan as biopolymers for DDS fabrication also offers several advantages, such as biocompatibility and pH responsiveness. The optimized NPs allowed for the encapsulation, targeted delivery, and controlled release of DOX to cancer cells. The drug-loaded particles were tested on cancer cells using MTT assay and live/dead staining experiments, and both methods showed that the drug-loaded particles had a significant inhibitory effect on the growth of cancer cells [147]. Chitosan-functionalized ferrogels were fabricated, and the resulting nanostructure possesses unique characteristics such as high porosity, ultra-low density, and superparamagnetism with high DOX loading efficiency. The ferrogels also exhibit tumor-specific pH-responsive swelling, excellent biodegradation, remotely switchable drug release, high magnetic hyperthermia potential, excellent biocompatibility, and promising cell–material interactions as substantiated by MTT assay, cytoskeleton staining, and confocal imaging [130].

An innovative DDS based on dumbbell-shaped NPs of $CoFe_2O_4/MoO_2$ was developed for liver cancer treatment using external magnetic and photothermal effects. These NPs were modified with poly(methacrylic acid), loaded with DOX, and sealed with phase-change material to prevent premature drug release. The cytotoxicity of the composite was evaluated on human liver tumor cells and the results showed that the combined procedure led to the highest killing rate of tumor cells, indicating the potential of the developed system for liver cancer treatment [131]. Magnetic nanocomposites coated with nylon-6 were also reported for the delivery of DOX. The composites were synthesized by the co-precipitation method and coated with biodegradable nylon-6 to increase biocompatibility. The magnetic composites demonstrated good loading capacity and pH-dependent release behavior. Cytotoxicity studies were performed on lung cancer cell lines and showed increased toxicity of the DDS compared to free DOX [153].

A drug-loaded magnetic microrobot that can polarize macrophages into the antitumor phenotype to target and inhibit cancer cells was developed. The in vitro tests demonstrated that the microrobots have good biocompatibility with normal cells and immune cells. DOX was loaded onto the surface of microrobots through electrostatic interactions and exhibited pH-responsive release behavior. The microrobots were able to target and kill cancer cells in a 3D tumor spheroid culture assay through dual targeting from magnetic guidance and M1 macrophages. The findings suggest that the combined use of magnetic control, macrophages, and pH-responsive drug release can improve the tumor-targeting and antitumor abilities of microrobots [151]. However, the size of the microrobots exceeds the nanometer range, indicating the possible uptake by the immune system in the case of in vivo administration. A pH-responsive mesoporous Fe_2O_3-Au-based DDS with magnetic targeting was also designed. The Fe_2O_3 particles were constructed with external mesopores and internal hollow structures, while Au NPs were connected on the surface of Fe_2O_3 through pH-responsive bonds for drug encapsulation [146]. Magnetic mesoporous silica NPs were developed as a multipurpose nanoplatform for delivering DOX and providing magnetothermal therapy to cancer cells. The core-shell-type particles were characterized for their magnetic and thermal properties, drug loading and release kinetics, and cytotoxicity against cancer cells. The results revealed high magnetic saturation and heating efficiency, efficient DOX loading and release, and significant cytotoxicity against cancer cells both in vitro and in vivo [128]. Another approach for the delivery of DOX consisted of obtaining mesoporous silica nanoparticles, which were then modified by growing magnetic NPs on their exterior. This nanocomposite was loaded with DOX and release studies were performed in different pH and temperature conditions. The results indicated that the release is both pH and temperature dependent [154]. Amino acids were also employed for MNP functionalization in the delivery of DOX. Cysteine-modified magnetite NPs loaded with DOX were extensively characterized. The release behavior proved to be pH dependent, with twice as much DOX released at acidic pH compared to neutral pH. However, the acidic pH value tested, pH 3, is lower compared to that of the tumor microenvironment (5–6). The NPs' toxicity towards melanoma cells was investigated using cytotoxicity and apoptosis assays [155]. Another nanocomposite for DOX delivery was developed from magnetite NPs covered with calcium carbonate by ion co-precipitation. The nanocomposite demonstrated a high DOX loading capacity and pH-dependent release. Cytotoxicity studies carried out on cervical and breast cancer cells proved the high anti-cancer efficiency of the synthesized composites [156].

The development and characterization of an active targeting DDS were presented. Iron oxide NPs were functionalized with FA and loaded with DOX. The results indicated the successful loading and release of DOX combined with the efficiency of the nanosystems as selective contrast agents in MRI, with the data representing an initial stage in the validation of the nanotheranostic system before in vivo evaluation [157]. FA functionalization of magnetic NPs was also reported by Gentili et al. who developed a system for DOX delivery (MNP@FA.DOX). The administration of DOX using this system resulted in an enhancement of cell death compared to the free drug, confirmed by apoptosis assay. The images observed in Figure 3A correspond to Prussian blue staining of HCT116 cells treated with MNPs (up) and free DOX (down). The images show, as expected, the absence of precipitated iron in the cells that were not treated with MNPs@FA.DOX. In the case of delivering the drug by MNPs (up), it can be seen that the amount of intracellular iron rises and HCT116 cell size increased after 8 h of NP treatment. Figure 3B (down) shows the increase in the total size of the HCT116 cells and a marked increase in the dimensions of the cell nuclei, but no atypical morphological changes were observed for DOX treatment [132].

The interaction of magnetic DDS with cellular receptors is important and has been exploited in numerous studies. A magnetic liposomal carrier was used and showed targeted delivery of DOX to cancer cells via the $\alpha v \beta 3$-integrin receptor, higher cytotoxicity in various cancer cell lines, and minimal toxicity to the heart tissue. This lipidic formulation was also found to have higher tumor accumulation and therapeutic efficacy compared to the clinical liposomal formulation of DOX (Lippod™), especially in combination with gamma radiation or magnetic hyperthermia therapy. The mechanism of chemo-radio-sensitization involved the activation of JNK-mediated pro-apoptotic signaling axis and delayed repair of DNA double-strand breaks [133]. Tannic acid-modified magnetic hydrotalcite-based MgAl NPs were synthesized for the targeted delivery of DOX to estrogen-receptor-expressing colorectal cancer cells. The in vitro release showed a pH-dependent biphasic and sustained release of DOX, while the safety and biocompatibility of the DDS were confirmed using hemolysis and MTT assays. Furthermore, higher cellular uptake in ER-positive HCT116 and LoVo cells was observed [152]. The development of a magnetic dual-responsive nanocarrier for targeted drug delivery to cancer cells overexpressing the DNA repair enzyme APE1 was described (Figure 3B).

The carrier consists of Fe_3O_4@SiO_2 NPs and a specially designed AP-DNA strand that can be hydrolyzed by APE1. DOX was loaded onto the AP-DNA to form the theragnostic nanosystem (FS@DNA-DOX). The distribution of FS@DNA-DOX NPs was evaluated by in vivo fluorescence imaging and it was observed that after magnetic attraction near the tumor, the fluorescence intensity in the tumor location was significantly higher than that in other tissues, but without magnetic attraction, a strong distribution in the other organs was observed (Figure 3C). The fluorescence intensity per unit area in the tumor area was significantly higher than that in other organs after treatment with NPs with magnetism (Figure 3D) [123]. Some cancer treatment regimens involve drug combinations in order to enhance the treatment's effectiveness. Thus, the encapsulation of different drugs in DDS is of interest for clinical practice. A novel approach, based on a core/double shells magnetic-luminescent nanomaterial was reported as nanocarrier for both MTX and DOX for simultaneous administration in breast cancer therapy. The encapsulation of the two drugs has been demonstrated with good efficiency, and a controlled pH-dependent drug release was observed. The encapsulation system has proven effective in cell line tests, being able to distinguish between normal and cancer tissues and cytotoxicity studies against MCF-7 cells demonstrated superior tumor inhibition compared to the free drugs [150].

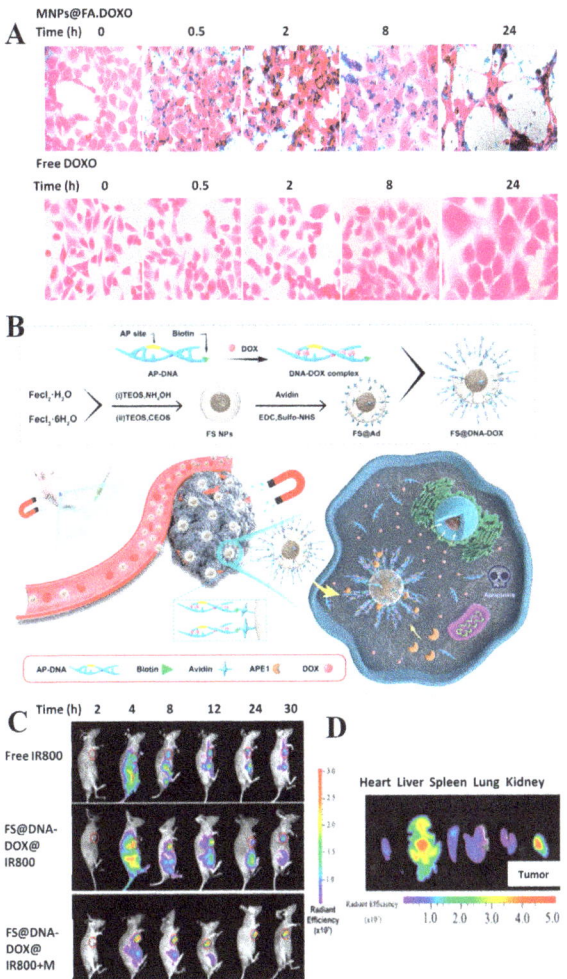

Figure 3. Analysis of (**A**) MNPs uptake and (**B**) cell morphology. (**A**) HCT116 cells treated with 1 µM MNPs@FA.DOXO. The intracellular iron from MNPs was evidenced by the Prussian blue assay. (**B**) HCT116 cells treated with free drug. The images are representative of three independent experiments. Cell staining: H&E. Magnification 400×. Reprinted with permission from Ref. [132] Copyright 2023 Elsevier; (**B**) The therapeutic mechanism of FS@DNA-DOX NPs as a magnetic-targeted and APE1-triggered drug delivery nanosystem. (**C**) Fluorescence images of mice after injection with IR800 and FS@IR800 NPs with or without magnetism. The red circles in the image represent the injection site. (**D**) The representative fluorescence images of major organs at 30 h postinjection of FS@DNA-DOX@IR800 with magnetism. Reprinted with permission from Ref. [123] Copyright 2023 Elsevier.

5.2. Platinum Compounds

Magnetic DDSs were developed for the passive or active delivery of CIS and OXA. In most cases, magnetite was used as a core, and polymers or mesoporous silica were used to cover the magnetic cores. The release mechanism was generally pH-dependent.

Magnetic NPs were functionalized with PEG and an ionic liquid for the delivery of CIS. The DDS demonstrated high platinum loading and stability in diluted human serum. The release was performed in simulated cytosolic media, which contains additives that make it more similar to real-life release conditions. However, no cytotoxicity tests were performed for the DDS [158]. Maghemite NPs were functionalized with nano graphene oxide (NGO) and the synthesis process is represented schematically in Figure 4A. The strong interactions between NGO and the CIS led to a slow-release profile, which followed reversible second-order kinetics. However, the release behavior was only tested at pH 7.4, with no tests carried out at the lower pH of the tumor microenvironment. The DDS exhibited in vitro toxicity towards U87 glioblastoma cells and the application of a magnetic field led to selective cell death in the area of magnet application [159]. Magnetite NPs covered in a silica layer and modified with dicarboxylic acid groups were developed as a potential treatment for pancreatic cancer. The DDS exhibited prolonged release at pH 7.4, with approximately 80% of loaded CIS released after 250 h. Cytotoxicity studies carried out on healthy cells and two pancreatic cell lines demonstrated selective toxicity towards cancer cells, with increased toxicity towards the highly metastatic line AspC-1 [160]. Rinaldi et al. reported polydopamine-modified MCs for the delivery of CIS. The clusters present better magnetic properties compared to magnetic NPs and can be guided more easily to the tumor tissue. The synthesis procedure was carefully optimized with respect to the surfactant, the solvent used, and the concentration of the nanoclusters, and the particles were characterized by TEM (results presented in Figure 4B–I). The resulting DDS showed pH-dependent release. The cytotoxicity of the DSS was tested on MCF-7 breast cancer cells and HeLa cervical cancer cells and demonstrated superior toxicity towards HeLa cells. The use of a magnet for the guidance of the clusters in cell cultures led to superior cytotoxic properties compared to the "no-magnet" approach, indicating the advantages of magnetic guidance [161].

Silica-coated magnetic NPs were also used for the active targeting of CIS, using HA as the targeting ligand. The developed system exhibited pH-dependent release, which followed Higuchi model kinetics. The DDS proved to be selectively toxic towards CT26 colorectal cancer cells compared to embryonic kidney cells and its cytotoxicity was higher compared to that of free CIS in cancer cells. In vivo experiments demonstrated that both the half-life and the area under the curve for CIS were increased when it was incorporated into the DDS, compared to CIS alone. Moreover, histological analyses revealed no toxic effects of the DDS on the kidneys, hearts, and lungs of tested rats [162]. Xie's group also developed active targeting methods for the delivery of CIS, using either peptides [118] or FA [163]. In both cases, the toxicity of the constructed DDSs was higher compared to that of CIS alone in HNE-1 nasopharyngeal carcinoma cells, due to increased cellular uptake.

A passive OXA delivery approach was proposed by Darroudi et al. who developed chitosan functionalized magnetite NPs that displayed toxicity towards CT-26 colon cancer cells. However, more studies need to be performed, since the release behavior was not studied and the toxicity was not compared to that of free OXA [164]. Another passive approach involved the use of biomimetic magnetite NPs loaded with OXA. The release of OXA from these carriers followed a pH-dependent model. Moreover, upon application of a magnetic field, the release improved due to the hyperthermia effect, leading to a total release of 80% after 2.5 h. The DDS exhibited higher cytotoxicity compared to free OXA in T-84, HT-29, SW480, HCT-15, and MC-38 colon cancer cell lines [165].

Antibodies were used for the active targeting of OXA towards colorectal [119] and gastric cancer cells, respectively [166]. Magnetite particles were coated with poly(lactide-co-glycolide) and an anti-CD33 antibody was conjugated to the DDS. The DDS achieved a slow-release profile of OXA at pH 7.4, and its successful internalization in CaCo-2 cells via receptor-mediated endocytosis was demonstrated by fluorescence, indicating the successful co-localization of NPs and OXA in cancer cells (Figure 4J) [119]. Another antibody, Herceptin, was conjugated to iron-gold NPs for the targeted delivery of OXA. The DDS exhibited pH-dependent drug release and successful cell internalization. Moreover, animal studies demonstrated the specific accumulation of the DDS in tumor masses, indicating the selectivity of the DDS and its capacity to be used as a targeted delivery device.

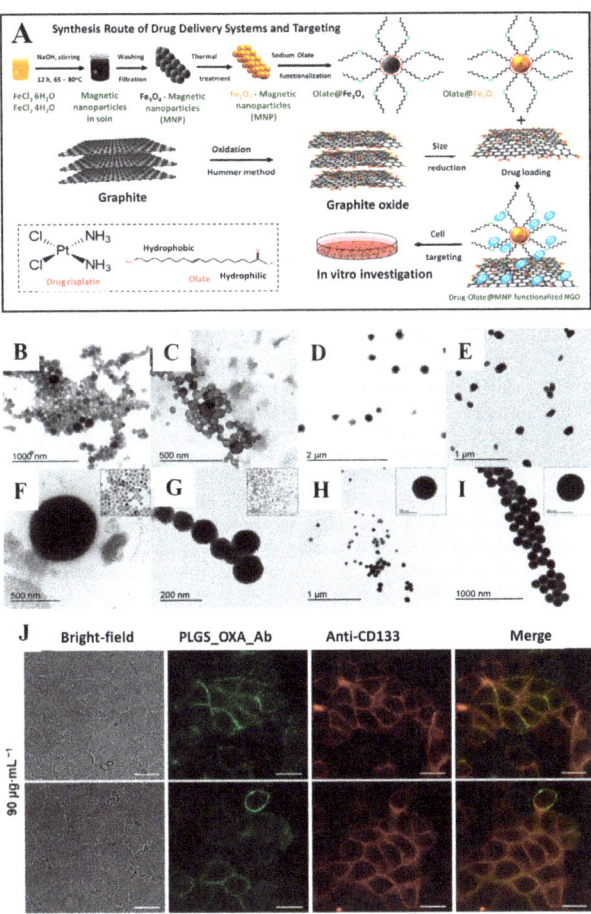

Figure 4. (**A**) Schematic representation of the synthesis process of maghemite NPs functionalized with nano graphene oxide for CIS-targeted delivery. Reprinted from Ref. [159]. (Open access); TEM images of Magnetic Nanoclusters synthesized using (**B**) low concentration of SDS surfactant; (**C**) low concentration of SPIONs; (**D**) SPIONs dispersed in THF; (**E**) SPIONs dispersed in hexane; (**F**) SPIONs with size of 12 nm; (**G**) SPIONs with size of 7 nm; (**H**) scaled up one-fold; (**I**) scaled up five-fold. Insets show SPIONs with size of (**F**) 7 nm and (**G**) 12 nm, low-magnification (**H**) MNCs scaled up one-fold and (**I**) MNCs scaled up five-fold. Reprinted with permission from Ref. [161]. Copyright 2023 American Chemical Society. (**J**) Fluorescence microscopy images of human cells derived from colorectal carcinoma (CaCo-2) treated with oxaliplatin-containing PLGA nanoparticles coated with anti-CD133 antibody conjugated to Alexa Fluor 488 (PLGA_OXA_Ab) and co-stained with antiCD133 Atto 565. The CaCo-2 cells were treated with 90 μg·mL^{-1} concentration of the PLGA_OXA_Ab for 30 min. From left: Bright-field images of the cells; fluorescence emission of cells treated with PLGA_OXA_Ab; cells stained with anti-CD133-Atto 565; merge of the fluorescence images. The scale bars correspond to 20 μm. Reprinted from Ref. [119] (Open access).

5.3. Methotrexate

Several attempts have been made at encapsulating MTX into magnetic DDSs. Some of these used magnetite NPs functionalized with amino acids such as L-lysine (Fe-Lys) [124], arginine (Fe-Arg) [125], glycine (Fe-Gly) [126], or proteins such as bovine serum albumin (Fe-BSA) [127] in order to covalently bind MTX. The amino groups of the amino acids/proteins were covalently bound to the carboxyl groups of MTX to form an amide bond. Among these DDSs, Fe-Arg presented the smallest diameter, while Fe-BSA was the largest in size. The highest MTX loading efficiency was observed in the case of Fe-Lys. In all cases, the release of MTX from the carriers was dependent on the presence of proteinases, due to their capacity to cleave the amide bond in lysosomal conditions (acid pH). For the amino-acid-modified DDSs, the release of MTX took place in less than 12 h, while for the BSA-modified DDS, the release was slower. In the case of Fe-Gly, the release behavior was also pH-dependent and followed a Michaelis–Menten model, fitting an enzyme-dependent kinetics profile. Fe-Arg, Fe-Gly, and Fe-BSA demonstrated hemocompatibility in the hemolysis assay, while Fe-Arg and Fe-Gly also demonstrated biocompatibility towards fibroblasts. Fe-Gly and Fe-Arg demonstrated higher cytotoxicity towards breast cancer MCF-7 cells compared to MTX alone, while Fe-Lys and Fe-BSA demonstrated similar cytotoxicity compared to MTX alone.

Polymers and cyclodextrins have also been used to develop magnetic DDSs for the delivery of MTX. Magnetite superparamagnetic particles were covered with poly 3-hydroxybutyrate-co-3-hydroxyvalerate using a method optimized by the Box–Behnken design. The average size of the DDS was around 90 nm; however, large variations were noticed, with some particles exceeding 200 nm in diameter, which could be too large for EPR entrapment. The release of MTX at pH 6.8 from the carriers was slower compared to the release of free MTX in the same conditions, indicating a slow-release behavior. The toxicity of the DDS was higher compared to free MTX on SW-480 colorectal cancer cells [167]. Cationic polymers and cyclodextrins were also used as functionalizing agents for magnetite-based DDSs. MTX was loaded due to the electrostatic interactions between the cationic polymer and the negative charges of MTX at neutral pH. At the acidic pH of the tumor environment, the MTX was protonated, and the interactions were lost, leading to the pH-dependent release of MTX. The MTX was quickly released from the DDS and was successfully internalized in the cytoplasm of Saos-2 osteosarcoma cells. The cytotoxicity of the DDS was marginally higher than that of free MTX [168].

Active targeting was also employed for MTX delivery, using HA [169] or FA antibodies [170] as targeting agents. The HA-modified DDS displayed high drug encapsulation efficiency and the drug release was pH-dependent, with a higher than 10-fold increase in released MTX at pH 5.5 compared to pH 7.4. The DDS proved to be cytotoxic towards A549 lung cancer cells, with IC_{50} values much lower compared to those of MTX alone. Moreover, the DDS caused an increase in the expression of pro-apoptotic genes in cancer cells and a decrease in the expression of the gene encoding the pro-inflammatory cytokine tumor necrosis factor α (TNF-α). This demonstrates that the DDS has potential anticancer activity in A549 lung cancer cells, a type of cell that has high resistance to MTX [169]. Antibodies against folate receptors were synthesized and conjugated to MTX-modified magnetic NPs. The resulting DDS had high encapsulation efficiency for MTX and high binding efficiency for the antibody. The release of MTX was pH dependent and the DDS exhibited higher toxicity towards HeLa cervical cancer cells compared to MTX alone. Immunohistochemistry demonstrated the attachment of the DDS to FA receptors in mouse tumor tissue, and fluorescence analysis revealed the internalization of the DDS in cancer cells by endocytosis [170].

5.4. Curcumin

Curcumin (Cur) is a natural compound extracted from *Curcuma longa* and has attracted attention as a possible anticancer agent. Some studies have suggested that curcumin can help reduce the side effects of chemotherapy when used in association with it and can also improve patient survival due to its anti-oxidant and anti-angiogenic effects [171,172]. Despite its good safety profile and promising preliminary results, Cur has very poor bioavailability and water solubility, making it difficult to formulate and administer [172]. Different liposomal formulations have been fabricated to increase their bioavailability [172], and many proof-of-concept studies have associated Cur with magnetic NPs for both passive and active targeted delivery.

A passive targeted delivery approach used magnetite NPs covered with a layered double hydroxide (LDH), loaded with Cur, and finally covered with polydopamine [173]. The DDS demonstrated pH-dependent release in vitro and the polydopamine coating degraded progressively, allowing a controlled release of 63% of the drug after a period of 28 h. The DDS had lower cytotoxicity towards HepG2 liver cancer cells compared to Cur alone at the same concentration due to the time it took for the uptake, cleavage, and release of the drug from the DDS. However, cellular uptake studies demonstrated that Cur from the DDS could be efficiently internalized into HepG2 cells by endocytosis [173]. The same group also proposed an active targeting strategy for Cur, using polymer-modified magnetite NPs. The two monomers used were PEG methyl ether methacrylate and 4-vinylphenylboronic acid (VB), with the latter acting as both a site for the covalent binding of Cur and a ligand for the overexpressed sialic acid residues on the surface of cancer cells. The DDS showed a lower drug-loading capacity compared to the previous approach and pH-dependent release. Due to the stability of the boronate ester bond between Cur and VB at neutral pH, the DDS exhibited remarkable pH-dependent release, with only 2.5% of Cur released at pH 7.2 and 78% at pH 5.4, demonstrating good selectivity for cancer cells. Moreover, selectivity was also confirmed by cellular uptake studies that showed that the particles can be successfully internalized into HepG2 cells, while no internalization occurs in normal L02 hepatocytes [174]. Other active targeting techniques used FA as the cancer-cell-targeting agent. Danafar's group reported magnetite NPs coated with BSA and FA for Cur delivery [175]. Although the drug-loading capacity of the proposed DDS was small, it demonstrated good selectivity towards HepG2 cancer cells. Cellular uptake studies showed that the FA-modified DDS could be more efficiently internalized into HepG2 cells compared to their FA-free analogs. Apoptosis assay also indicated a higher rate of cell death in the case of FA-modified DDS. The release of Cur from the DDS was pH dependent, with 70% of Cur released at pH 4.5 after 30 h compared to 55% at pH 7.4 [175]. Another FA-modified DDS comprised of superparamagnetic magnetite NPs and quantum dots was developed. The release of Cur followed a pseudo-second-order kinetics model and was pH-dependent, with approximately twice as much Cur released at pH 5.5 compared to pH 7.4.

Cytotoxicity studies were performed on a breast cancer line and an osteosarcoma cell line and revealed that, at low concentrations, the DDS exhibited better cytotoxicity compared to Cur alone. Moreover, the selectivity of the FA-modified DDS was demonstrated by cytotoxicity tests, because the toxicity of the FA-modified system was greater than that of the unmodified carrier [176].

Table 2. Magnetic nanoparticles for the targeted delivery of chemotherapeutic drugs.

Carrier, Drug	Cancer	Targeting	Size (nm)	LC	LE	Release Mechanism	Ref.
Fe_3O_4/BNN/PEG, DOX	Liver	Magnetic	151–216	$19 \pm 0.54\%$	$83 \pm 0.33\%$	pH dependent	[145]
Achiral nanorobot, DOX	Breast, liver	Magnetic, macrophages	40000	-	45%	pH dependent	[151]
Mesoporous Fe_2O_3–Au, DOX	Lung	Magnetic	100	-	-	pH dependent	[146]
Fe_3O_4/chitosan aerogel, DOX	Osteosarcoma	Magnetic	-	40%	-	pH swelling, AMF	[130]
Fe_3O_4/CMCS/ALS, DOX	Breast	Magnetic	90–170	48.68%	86.23%	pH dependent	[147]
Fe_3O_4/Nylon/DOX	Lung	Magnetic	28 ± 4	73.2%	-	pH dependent	[153]
Fe_3O_4/SiO_2-AP-DNA, DOX	Breast	Magnetic, enzymatic	70	-	-	Enzymatic	[123]
Fe_3O_4/SiO_2-CS-FA, DOX	Cervical	Magnetic, Active, FA	100	-	15%	Redox, pH dependent AMF	[128]
Fe_3O_4/SiO_2/DOX	Breast	Magnetic	5–10	62%	-	pH, temperature dependent	[154]
Fe_3O_4/L-cys/DOX	Melanoma	Magnetic	3–34	-	-	pH dependent	[155]
Fe_3O_4/$CaCO_3$/DOX	Breast, cervical	Magnetic	135	1900 μg/mg	-	pH dependent	[156]
$CoFe_2O_4$/MoO_2/PMMA/DOX/TD, DOX	Liver	Magnetic	20	20%	51%	AMF, photothermal	[131]
Fe_3O_4/HT/TA, DOX	Colorectal	Magnetic	70	8.17%	95%	pH dependent	[152]
Fe_3O_4/FA, DOX	Colorectal	Magnetic, Active, FA	10	7.15%	-	Magnetic, pH dependent	[132,157]
Fe_2O_3/ChitoPEG, DOX	Colorectal	Magnetic	148.9	-	-	Redox responsive	[129]
Lipo/SPION/ICG/cRGD, DOX	Fibrosarcoma	Magnetic, Active, cRGD	166 ± 42	-	47.5%	AMF	[133]
MNC/PDO, CIS	Cervical, breast	Magnetic	90–100	0.067%	-	pH dependent	[161]
MNP/PEG/IL,CIS	-	Passive	15.1 ± 1.7	36 g Pt/ g Fe	-	Cytosolic media	[158]
Fe_2O_3/NGO, CIS	Glioblastoma	Magnetic	10	37%	-	-	[159]
Fe_3O_4/SiO_2/ dicarboxylic acid groups CIS	Pancreatic	Passive	54 ± 9	11%	23%	pH dependent	[160]
Fe_3O_4/SiO_2/EDTA/HA, CIS	Colorectal	Magnetic, Active, HA	70–100	34.11%	82.85	pH dependent	[162]
Fe_3O_4/ASA/PEG/TAT, CIS	Nasopharyngeal	Magnetic, Active, TAT	49.42 ± 9.5	-	-	-	[118]
Fe_3O_4/FA/CBD, CIS	Nasopharyngeal	Magnetic, Active, FA, CBD	20 ± 1	6.32%	61.35%	-	[163]
Fe_3O_4/CS, OXA, IRI	Colon	Passive	36.77	-	-	-	[164]
Fe_3O_4/Ma/C, OXA	Colon	Magnetic	34 ± 10	40%	-	pH dependent	[165]
Fe_3O_4/Au/Herceptin, OXA	Gastric	Magnetic, Active, Ab	8–20	-	-	pH dependent	[166]
Fe_3O_4/PLGA/anti-CD133 Ab, OXA	Colorectal carcinoma	Active, Ab	166 ± 25	22%	44%	-	[119]
Fe_3O_4/l-lysine, MTX	Breast	Passive	43.72 ± 4.73	8.9%	-	Enzymatic	[164]
Fe_3O_4/Arg, MTX	Breast	Passive	26.99 ± 7.31	$8.25 \pm 0.29\%$	-	Enzymatic	[125]
Fe_3O_4/Gly, MTX	Breast	Passive	46.82 ± 5.03	4.2%	-	pH dependent, enzymatic	[126]
Fe_3O_4/BSA, MTX	Breast	Passive	105.7 ± 3.81	3.5%	-	Enzymatic	[127]
Fe_3O_4/PHBV, MTX	Colorectal	Passive	90	$6.79 \pm 0.01\%$	84%	-	[167]

Table 2. Cont.

Carrier, Drug	Cancer	Targeting	Size (nm)	LC	LE	Release Mechanism	Ref.
Fe_3O_4/Cat/Ciclo, MTX	Osteosarcoma	Passive	20–80	8.92%	89.27%	pH dependent	[168]
Fe_3O_4/DPA/PEG/HA, MTX	Lung	Active, HA	103	42.94%	88.11%	pH dependent	[169]
Fe_3O_4/FRab, MTX	Cervical	Active, FR ab	50–100	-	90.62%	pH dependent	[170]
Fe_3O_4/Cur-LDH/PDO, Cur	Liver	Passive	179.4 ± 29.8	38%	-	pH dependent	[173]
Fe_3O_4/C-VB-PEGMA, Cur	Liver	Active, VB	10.3 ± 1.3	25%	67.7%	pH dependent	[174]
Fe_3O_4/BSA, Cur	Liver	Active, FA	60.21 ± 12.32	5%	-	pH dependent	[175]
Fe_3O_4/GQD, Cur	Breast, osteosarcoma	Active, FA	34.3	-	-	pH dependent	[176]
Fe_3O_4/PVA/LDH, SOR	Liver	Passive	19	54%	-	pH dependent	[177]
Fe_3O_4/PEG/LDH, SOR	Liver	Passive	17	69%	-		
Fe_3O_4/PVA/LDH, SOR	Liver	Passive	19	87%	-	pH dependent	[178]
Fe_3O_4/Alg, SOR	Liver	Passive	10–15	-	58.8%	Biphasic release	[179]

67 µg of Pt per 100 mg of MNC@PDO, mg Pt/mg DDS, mg OXA/mg magnetite. BNN—boron nitride nanosheets; CMCS—carboxymethyl chitosan; ALS—aminated lignosulfonate; CS—chitosan; FA—folic acid; AMF—alternating magnetic field; PMMA—poly(methacrylic acid); TD—1-tetradecanol; ChitoPEG—methoxy polyethylene glycol grafted to chitosan; Lipo—lipsome; SPION—superparamagnetic iron oxide nanoparticle; ICG—indocyaninde green; CIS—cisplatin; MNC—magnetic nanoclusters; PDO—polydopamine; IL—ionic liquid; NGO—nanographene oxide; ASA—aldehyde sodium alginate; TAT—transcription activator peptide; CBD—intracellular aggregation ability peptide; OXA—oxaliplatin; IRI—irinotecan; Ab—antibody; PLGA—poly(lactide-co-glycolide); DPA—dopamine; MTX—methotrexate; Gly—glycine; FR—folate receptor; Cat—cationic polymer; cyclo—cyclodextrin; Arg—arginine; BSA—bovine serum albumin; Cur—curcumin; LDH—layered double hydroxide; VB—4-vinylphenylboronic acid; PEGMA—polyethylene glycol methyl ether methacrylate; GQD—graphene quantum dots; SOR—sorafenib; PVA—polyvinyl alcohol; LDH—layered double hydroxide; Alg—alginate; L-cys—cysteine.

5.5. Sorafenib

Sorafenib (SOR) presents systemic side effects, low bioavailability, and water solubility [144], which can be limited by encapsulating it in DDSs.

Several attempts have been made to use magnetite NPs for the delivery of SOR in the treatment of hepatocellular carcinoma. Anionic compounds, such as LDH or alginate, were used to functionalize the core particles and allow SOR binding. Pastorin's group developed superparamagnetic iron oxide NPs modified with polyvinyl alcohol (PVA) or PEG and double-layered magnesium-aluminum hydroxide for the delivery of SOR [177]. PEG-coated NPs demonstrated a higher drug-loading capacity, smaller hydrodynamic diameter, and narrower size distribution. Both carriers exhibited a sustained, pseudo-second-order kinetics, pH-dependent release behavior, in vitro. Due to PEG's higher solubility in water compared to PVA, the release from the PEG-modified particles was faster than from the PVA-modified ones. The same group reported magnetite NPs modified with PVA and zinc-aluminum LDH [178]. Compared to the previous approach, the drug-loading capacity was significantly increased. The release of SOR from the SOR-functionalized carriers was higher than from a simple physical mixture of SOR and carriers demonstrating the advantage of the nanoformulation. The release was pH-dependent and followed pseudo-second-order kinetics [178]. Cytotoxicity studies were carried out on fibroblasts and HepG2 hepatocellular carcinoma cells and demonstrated that all nanoformulations had superior cytotoxicity compared to SOR alone on cancer cells, while displaying good biocompatibility with fibroblasts [177,178]. Another approach consisted of the encapsulation of SPIONs into alginate microspheres containing SOR. The system demonstrated acceptable drug-loading efficiency and a biphasic release profile, with 54% of the total SOR released in the first hour. Since the release profile was studied at pH 7.4, which is the normal pH of serum, not of the tumor environment, this could raise the question of the safety of the system, since SOR could be released in serum before reaching the tumor. The formulation exhibited cytotoxicity towards HepG2 cells; however, no comparison to SOR alone was performed [179].

6. RNA Delivery Using Magnetic Nanoparticles

Non-coding RNAs, such as miRNA and siRNAs, have recently emerged as promising therapeutic tools for cancer management. The main limitations of RNA use in therapy are related to its limited ability to pass through cellular membranes, due to its hydrophilic nature, negative charge, and instability in the presence of serum enzymes [180]. For these reasons, numerous attempts have been made at encapsulating RNA in DDSs that could enhance its pharmacokinetics and stability.

In the development of magnetic DDSs for RNA delivery, magnetite has been the most commonly used magnetic core. Cationic polymers, especially polyethyleneimine (PEI), were generally used for the functionalization of the cores, due to their ability to interact electrostatically with the negatively charged RNA cargo. MicroRNAs and siRNAs were loaded into the magnetic carriers. Some studies also included chemotherapy drugs, such as DOX (Figure 5A–F) together with siRNA for enhanced in vivo efficiency. The release of the RNA was mostly achieved by alternating magnetic field (AMF) triggering, but also by pH-dependent mechanisms. Targeting was generally passive, with some examples of magnetic or active targeting also present.

Controlled delivery of miR-1484 mimic was achieved by magnetite NPs covered with a thermo-liable Diels-Alder cycloadduct that released the RNA in A549 lung cancer cells in the presence of an AMF that led to heating and subsequent cleavage of the Diels-Alder bond. The cytotoxicity of the DDS was higher towards A549 in the presence of AMF than in its absence, indicating its importance in the release of the RNA cargo. A high concentration of NPs was used to compensate for the relatively low RNA loading efficiency, which could pose safety concerns [134]. Two similar approaches for the delivery of miR-34 for the treatment of neuroblastoma were developed using PEI [135] and PEI and tripolyphosphate (TPP) [136], respectively. The carriers were similar in size and demonstrated AMF-triggered release of the RNA due to an increase in temperature and shell softening. TPP conjugation decreased the inherent toxicity associated with PEI. Genetic analyses demonstrated that both approaches led to the inhibition of the MYCN oncogene.

Magnetic guidance was used in several examples for the delivery of siRNA to tumor cells. Iron oxide NPs were functionalized with caffeic acid, calcium phosphate, PEG, and siRNA and their cytotoxic potential was evaluated in an HER2-positive breast cancer cell line. HER2 expression levels were decreased after incubation with the DDS and expression levels decreased further when a magnetic field was applied. Cell internalization was also increased in the presence of a magnetic field [181]. In order to reduce the toxicity of PEI, while also maintaining the DDS' (FFP@MNP) capacity to escape endosomal entrapment, Zhang et al., developed magnetite NPs functionalized with PEI and fluorinated PEG. Figure 5G shows the effect of FPP@MNPs on cell viability, which was characterized by the CCK8 kit. Different concentrations of FPP@MNP were added to HeLa cells and then cultured for 24 h or 48 h. It was observed that the viability of HeLa decreased with the incubation time and FPP@MNPs were toxic for concentrations ≥ 8 µg/mL. The results of FPP@MNPs-induced HeLa cell apoptosis are shown in Figure 5G(a–e), and the analysis of cell viability is shown in Figure 5G(ii). The cells were scanned layer by layer and three-dimensionally reconstructed by laser confocal microscopy (Figure 5H). HeLa, A549, and 4 T1 cells were transfected with FPP@MNPs under external magnetic field enhancement (MagTrans). The commercial nucleic acid vector Invitrogen Lipofectamine 3000 (Lipo3000) was used as the control. For each group of cells, it is evident that the amount of siRNA inside MagTrans-treated cells is significantly higher than Lipo3000 transfected cells. For Lipo3000-transfected cells, the distribution of siRNA can be observed in almost every cell, but the amount of siRNA contained in a single cell is far less than that of cells treated by MagTrans. Transfection methods used were magnetic field-enhanced F7-PEG-PEI@MNP transfection (MagTrans) or Lipo3000 transfection (Lipo 3000) [182]. Iron oxide NPs were integrated into non-ionic surfactant vesicles (niosomes) and used for the combined delivery of siRNA and transtuzumab/erlotinib to breast cancer cells. The schematic representation of the experimental protocol for DDS fabrication is represented in Figure 5I. High siRNA encapsulation was obtained, and in the case of both drugs, siRNA significantly increased the activation of apoptotic pathways, especially after the application of a magnetic field. The representative fluorescent images showing the occurrence of apoptosis of BT-474 cells after administration of siRNA/FexOy/NIO with erlotinib, free siRNA with erlotinib, erlotinib, and control cells are presented in Figure 5J [183].

PEI was also used as a shell for magnetite NPs used in the delivery of siRNA. Zhang et al., reported a DDS for the combined delivery of two siRNAs for applications in oral cancer treatment. The NPs demonstrated a high affinity for RNA and gene silencing potential comparable to that of lipofectamine, which was used as a positive control. Moreover, cancer cell migration was also impaired by the DDS [137]. Another approach using PEI as a modifier for the delivery of siRNA in the treatment of glioblastoma was also reported. Magnetic nanoparticles modified with PEI and ATN-RNA were synthesized, and the schematic diagram of preparation and its application in RNAi therapy of glioblastoma cells is presented in Figure 5K. The optimized complexes of Mag@PEI/ATN-RNA were submitted to an agarose gel electrophoresis assay to visualize the linking of ATN-RNA to Mag@PEI NPs (Figure 5L). Analysis revealed that two weight equivalents were sufficient to bind almost all of the ATN-RNA used in the experiment. However, to gain a deeper insight into this process, ATN-RNA concentration in the supernatant was investigated by UV-Vis spectroscopy (Figure 5M). A colocalization analysis was also performed to further demonstrate the transfer of Mag@PEI/ATN-RNA complexes into glioblastoma cells, demonstrated via a colocalization analysis (Figure 5N). A visible colocalization between the ATTO 550-labeled Mag@PEI nanoparticles (red color) and the FITC-labeled ATN-RNA (green color) in the cytoplasm was obtained, suggesting high transfection efficiency of the synthesized nanoparticles [184]. Another study reported gelatin-covered magnetite NPs loaded with siRNA, which demonstrated cytotoxicity towards Caco-2 colorectal cancer cells [185]. Their toxicity was higher or similar to that of HiPerFect®, a commercial RNA transfection agent. However, no gene expression or cell migration assays were reported.

Active targeting of siRNA and chemotherapeutic drugs such as paclitaxel and DOX was achieved by coupling functionalized magnetic NPs with folate and T7 peptide [186] and epidermal growth factor receptor (EGFR) ligand, respectively [187]. The complex approach to paclitaxel and siRNA delivery involved the combination of magnetic NPs with polylactic acid-PEG and FA, peptide T7, and chitosan-spermine. The DDS exhibited higher encapsulation efficiency for siRNA than for the drug, and the release behavior was pH-dependent. Transfection efficiency was similar to that of lipofectamine in MCF-7 breast cancer cells. Active delivery of survivin siRNA and DOX was achieved by using a DDS comprised of maghemite NPs functionalized with carboxymethyl chitosan (CMCS), PEI, heparin, and EGF, labeled as eMNNS. The preparation of eMNNS was performed in three main steps: (1) Synthesis of the core followed by TPP-mediated encapsulation of CMCS; (2) PEI coating via EDC/NHS crosslinking; and (3) conjugation of Heparin and EGF with MNNS to form eMMNS (Figure 5A), while the targeted co-delivery of therapeutic siRNAs and DOX for GSC treatments is presented in Figure 5B. In vitro analyses were conducted to evaluate the tumor-suppressing effect of the DDS to inhibit the growth of glioblastoma stem cells (GSCs). In vivo experiments were conducted on BALB/c nude mice bearing glioblastoma U251 cell-induced tumors (Figure 5C,D). The mice were divided into three groups and administered different formulations to assess the safety and efficacy of eMNNS for cancer therapy. The first group was treated with Sur siRNA-MNNS (Figure 5C(a)), the second group with DOX/Sur siRNA-eMNNS (Figure 5C(b)), and the third group served as a control group (Figure 5C(c)). The results showed that the tumor size of the mice treated with Sur siRNA-MNNS decreased compared to the control group, while the mice treated with DOX/Sur siRNA-eMNNS exhibited the smallest tumor size and the best anti-tumor capacity. Moreover, histological analysis revealed extensive necrosis areas within the tumor mass treated with DOX/Sur siRNA-eMNNS. It was observed that the tumor size of the mice treated with Sur siRNA-MNNS decreased compared to the control group, and the mice treated with DOX/Sur siRNA-eMNNS exhibited the smallest tumor size and the best anti-tumor capacity (Figure 5C–E). Moreover, the histological analyses revealed extensive necrosis areas within the tumor mass treated with DOX/Sur siRNA-eMNNS (Figure 5F) [187].

Some examples of magnetic nanoparticles applied for RNA delivery are presented in Table 3.

Table 3. Magnetic nanoparticles for the targeted delivery of RNA.

Carrier, RNA	Cancer	Targeting	Size (nm)	LC	EE	Release Mechanism	Ref.
Fe_3O_4/DAC, miR-1484 mimic	Lung	Passive	10.1 ± 0.5	2.5×10^{-10} moles/mg NPs	8.4%	AMF	[134]
Fe_3O_4/PEI/TPP, miR-34a	Neuroblastoma	Passive	20	-	-	AMF	[136]
Fe_3O_4/PEI, miR-34a	Neuroblastoma	Passive	10–20	-	-	AMF	[135]
Fe_3O_4/PEI, siRNA	Glioblastoma	Passive	8–12	-	90%		[184]
Fe_3O_4/PEI, siRNA	Oral	Passive	7.95	-	100%	AMF	[137]
Fe_3O_4/Gel, siRNA	Colorectal	Passive	60	-	41.5%		[185]
Fe_2O_3-Fe_3O_4/Caf/CaP/PEG-Pa siRNA	Breast	Magnetic	14	1.5 ± 0.1 μM			[181]
Fe_3O_4/FPP/PEI, siRNA	Cervical	Magnetic	12	-	-		[182]
FexOy/noisome siRNA + erlotinib siRNA + transtuzumab	Breast	Magnetic	100	-	99%	-	[183]
Fe_3O_4/PCS/PPF/PPT siRNA/PTX	Breast	Active, FA, T7 peptide	197 ± 16	-	68.52% (siRNA) 41.31 ± 3.6% (PTX)	pH dependent	[186]
Fe_3O_4/CMCS/PEI/Hep siRNA/DOX	Glioblastoma	Active, EGF	40–50	3.86% (DOX)	-	-	[187]

Gel—gelatin; DAC—Diels-Alder cycloadduct; PEI—polyethyleneimine; TPP—tripolyphosphate; PCS—Polylactic acid-Chitosan-Spermine; PPF—poly-lactic acid polyethylene glycol-folate; PPT—Poly-lactic acid-PEG-T7 peptide; CMCS—carboxymethylchitosan; Hep –heparin; EGF—epidermal growth factor; Caf—caffeic acid; CaP—calcium phosphate; PEG-Pa—polyethylene glycol anionic polymer; FPP—Heptafluorobutyryl-polyethylene glycol-polyethyleneimine.

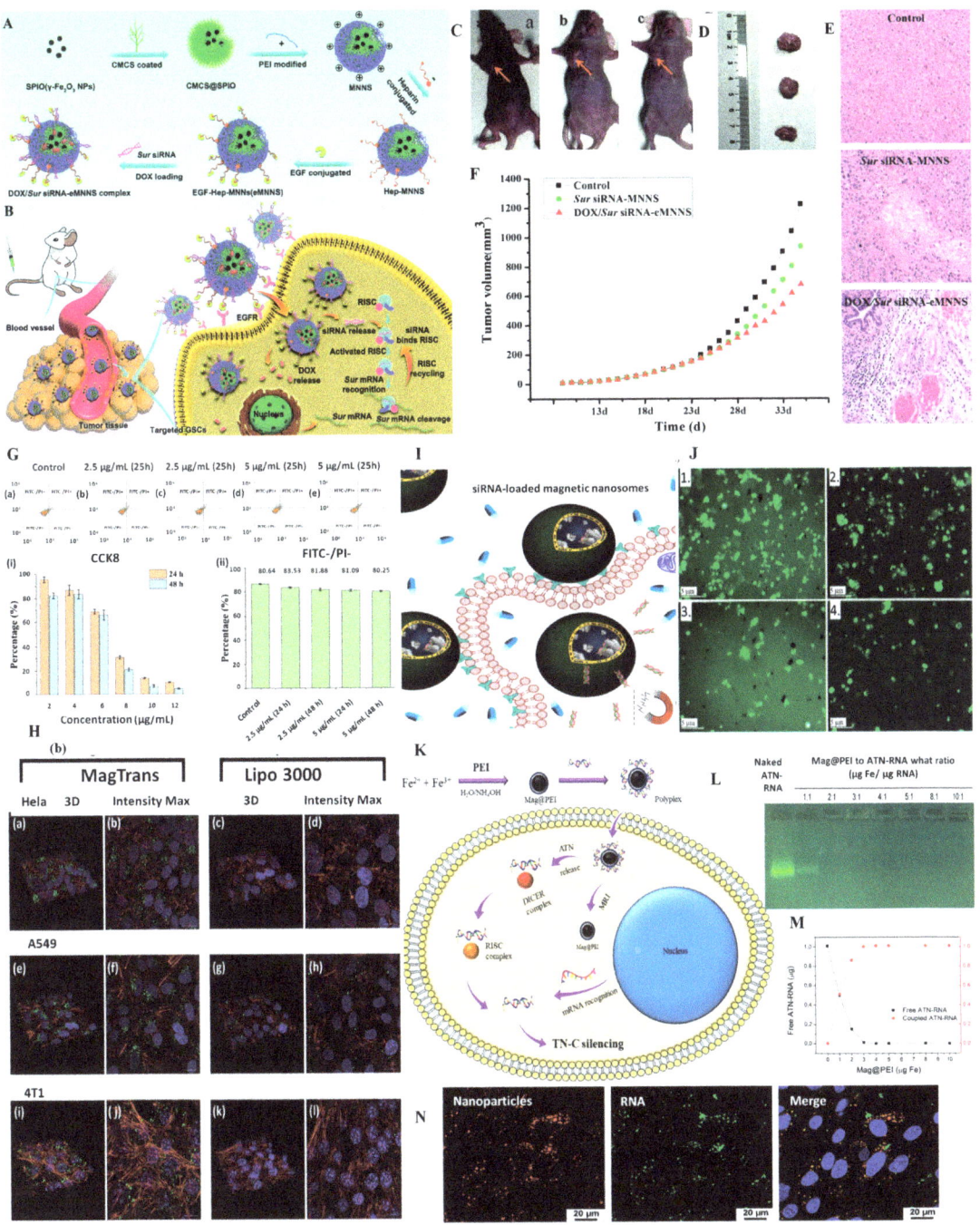

Figure 5. (**A**) Schematic illustration of the fabrication of the EGFR-targeted theragnostic nanoplatform, and (**B**) targeted co-delivery of therapeutic siRNAs and DOX for GSC treatments. (**C**) Typical photographs showing the size of tumors (indicated by arrows) in mice on day 2 weeks with three different treatments. Photo-images of excised tumors from mice bearing glioblastoma U251-induced

tumors 2 weeks after different treatments. a: Control; b: Sur siRNA MNNS; c: DOX/Sur siRNA-eMNNS. (**D**) Tumor growth inhibition for the mice bearing glioblastoma U251-induced tumors after treatment with various formulations (n = 3). (**E**) Representative histology (H&E) images of the tumor tissue in the control, Sur siRNA-MNNS, and DOX/Sur siRNA-eMNNS groups. (**F**) Active targeting co-delivery of therapeutic Sur siRNA and an antineoplastic drug via epidermal growth factor receptor-mediated magnetic nanoparticles for synergistic programmed cell death in glioblastoma stem cells. Adapted with permission from Ref. [187] Copyright 2023 Royal Society of Chemistry. (**G**) Fluorinated PEG-PEI Coated Magnetic Nanoparticles for siRNA Delivery and CXCR4 Knockdown (a–e) Scatter diagram of HeLa cells apoptosis stained by Annexin V-FITC/PI measured by flow cytometry. (i) Relative cell viability measured by CCK8 kit. (ii) Analysis of cell viability measured by flow cytometry (a–e). (**H**) Results of FAM-siRNA transfection captured by confocal microscopy. Blue is Hoechst33342-stained nuclei, Green is FAM-labeled siRNA NC, and Red is Rhodamine-Phalloidin-stained F-actin (a–d) HeLa, (e–h) A549, (i–l) 4 T1.) Reprinted from Ref. [182] (Open access). In vitro Application of Magnetic Hybrid Niosomes: (**I**) Targeted siRNA-Delivery for Enhanced Breast Cancer Therapy—schematic representation of the experimental protocol. (**J**) Representative fluorescent images (using the Calbryte-520 Assay Kit) showing occurring apoptosis (light green) of BT-474 cells after administration of (1) siRNA/FexOy/NIO with erlotinib, (2) free siRNA with erlotinib, (3) erlotinib and (4) control cells and subsequent magnetic treatment. Reprinted from Ref. [183] (Open access). Nano-mediated delivery of double-stranded RNA for gene therapy of glioblastoma multiforme. (**K**) Schematic diagram of preparation of Mag@PEI/ATN-RNA complexes and its application in RNAi therapy of GBM cells. Binding of ATN-RNA to Mag@PEI NPs. (**L**) Agarose gel electrophoresis of Mag@PEI/ATN-RNA complexes at the different mass ratio. (**M**) Binding capability of Mag@PEI NPs towards ATN-RNA recorded using Nanodrop. (**N**) Colocalization of Mag@PEI NPs and ATN-RNA in U-118 cells. The representatives of the colors are blue (Hoechst 33342) for nuclei, green (FITC) for ATN-RNA, and red (ATTO550) for Mag@PEI nanoparticles. Reprinted from Ref. [184] (Open access).

7. Theragnostic Agents

Theragnostic approaches are emerging as innovative techniques in cancer management. Nanotechnology offers a vast array of nanosized devices known as nanotheragnostics, which combine diagnostic and therapeutic capabilities for real-time disease monitoring and treatment at the cellular and molecular levels. To effectively diagnose and treat diseases using nanotheragnostics, it is crucial for these nanomedicines to circulate throughout the body without being eliminated by the immune system.

One important aspect of nanotheranostics is their ability to target specific organs or tissues by attaching biological ligands to their surface. This targeting mechanism improves the efficiency and specificity of drug delivery, ensuring that the therapeutic agents reach the intended site of action [188]. Combining drug delivery and imaging can achieve early detection and enhanced treatment [189].

In the field of diagnostics, non-invasive techniques have gained significant attention. MNPs are being used as novel diagnostic agents, particularly in MRI for imaging various diseases, providing detailed anatomical and functional information. However, recent advancements have enabled the utilization of MNPs not only for imaging but also for drug targeting to the cellular membrane and for multi-modal imaging. By incorporating therapeutic agents and imaging capabilities into a single nanotheragnostic system, it becomes possible to simultaneously monitor the disease progression and deliver treatment directly to the affected cells or tissues. This approach holds promise for more effective and personalized medicine, as it allows for real-time monitoring of treatment response and adjustment of therapeutic strategies as needed in personalized medicine [190].

In recent years, MNPs and nanocomposites have been employed for the development of theragnostic agents. In Table 4, some examples of theragnostic approaches using MNPs are summarized.

Table 4. Theragnostic agents for the simultaneous treatment and diagnosis of cancer.

Agent	Cancer	Type of action	Ref.
Fe_3O_4/Chi/GO	Breast	DOX delivery + MRI	[191]
Fe_3O_4/PEG-b-PLA	Breast	DOX delivery + MPI	[192]
SPION/Lipo/Pept	Breast	PTX delivery + MRI	[193]
SPION/Lipo	CNS lymphoma	RTX delivery + MRI	[194]
Zn-doped SPION/Den/Apt/Fluo	Breast	DOX delivery + gene silencing + hyperthermia + NIR/MR imaging	[195]

Chi—chitosan; MRI—magnetic resonance imaging; PEG-b-PLA—polyethylene glycol-block-poly lactic acid copolymer; MPI—magnetic particle imaging; Lipo—liposome; Pept—pH responsive peptide; PTX—paclitaxel; CNS—central nervous system; RTX—rituximab; Den—dendrimer; Apt—aptamer; Fluo—fluorescent dye; NIR—near infra-red.

8. Perspectives and Conclusions

Chemotherapy is currently one of the primary methods for treating cancer, but its effectiveness can be limited by inefficient drug delivery and damage to normal tissues caused by uncontrolled drug release. The use of RNA-mediated cancer therapy is a novel therapeutic strategy that still faces some limitations. Nanomedicine delivery systems have been developed to address these challenges by improving the specificity and efficiency of drug delivery to cancer cells while minimizing harm to healthy tissues. Magnetic nanoparticles have been extensively studied in recent years for their potential applications as DDSs, diagnosis, or theragnostic tools. Different types of magnetic nanomaterials can be used, such as magnetic pure metals, magnetic oxides, multicomponent MNPs (MCs), or magnetic nanocomposites, each exhibiting unique properties. To be used in medical applications, these NPs need to meet minimal requirements such as biocompatibility, improved stability in biological fluids, adequate size, and superparamagnetism.

Moreover, adequate drug loading and controlled release need to be achieved for the successful use of magnetic DDSs in drug delivery applications. Uncontrolled drug release can lead to toxicity and damage to healthy tissues. Thus, researchers are exploring various strategies for achieving controlled drug release, such as pH-responsive or stimuli-responsive DDS. DDSs have been developed for the targeted delivery of chemotherapeutics such as doxorubicin, platinum compounds, methotrexate, sorafenib, and curcumin, as well as for RNA-mediated therapeutics. Their effects were mostly tested in vitro, with a few examples of strategies also tested in vivo. The magnetic properties of MNPs represent an advantage due to the possibility of applying a magnetic field to guide them. Moreover, the application of magnetic fields can also improve the anti-cancer efficiency, by using hyperthermia or magneto-mechanical actuation of MNPs. Magnetic hyperthermia is a well-known technique that can be combined with drug delivery to enhance tumor-killing properties by increasing temperature at the tumor site. Apart from this, magneto-mechanical actuation of MNPs has recently emerged as a tool in cancer treatment. In this technique, an alternating magnetic field is applied to MNPs, causing them to vibrate and produce mechanical alterations the cells. In the future, this technique could be combined with drug delivery to enhance cancer cell destruction.

Theragnostic approaches have also been developed for combined drug delivery and imaging. This technique offers perspectives for personalized medicine using MNPs. Simultaneous imaging and treatment could potentially lead to better delivery of the drug in the proximity of the tumor, real-life treatment monitoring, and improved outcomes for the patient.

There are several ways to incorporate MNPs into clinical practice. By leveraging nanotechnology, interdisciplinary collaboration, and standardization, MNPs can offer early disease detection, targeted delivery of treatments to diseased areas, and non-invasive monitoring of novel therapies. The review briefly discusses the importance of MNPs (including SPIONs) and their synthesis, stability through surface modification, and applications for

DDSs and medical treatment. The size, shape, and surface chemistry of MNPs impact their pharmacokinetics and toxicity. By fine-tuning these properties, improved passive, active, and magnetic targeting approaches can be achieved. Attention must be given to the choice of targeting agent and the attachment method for MNPs to maximize sensitivity in active targeting approaches.

In the future, more research needs to be carried out in the field of MNPs to fully assess their toxicity, drug-loading potential, and in vivo properties. However, the existing results show the promising impact of MNP-based DDSs for the treatment of cancer. Polymer-functionalized MNPs show perspective for future studies due to their increased biocompatibility, drug-loading capacity, and improved stability. The preliminary results obtained in this field show promise for improved drug delivery and personalized medicine; however, many challenges still remain until the advent of the use of magnetic DDSs in a clinical setting. With recent advances in the synthesis and modification of MNPs, as well as increased awareness of the potential immunomodulatory effects of nanoscale heat, MNPs continue to hold promise as a valuable tool for both physicians and patients.

Author Contributions: Conceptualization, A.P., M.T. and C.C.; resources, C.C. and R.T.; writing—original draft preparation, A.P., M.T., I.C. and S.M.; writing—review and editing C.C., R.T., A.P., M.T. and I.C. All authors have read and agreed to the published version of the manuscript.

Funding: M.T. acknowledges project no TE 125/2022, PN-III-P1-1.1-TE-2021-1543. For I.C. and R.T. this work was supported by the projects funded by the Ministry of Research, Innovation, and Digitalisation through Programme 1—Development of the National Research and Development System, Subprogramme 1.2—Institutional Performance—Funding Projects for Excellence in RDI, Contract No. 37PFE/30.12.2021 and by CNCS/CCCDI—UEFISCDI, project number PN-III-P2-2.1-PED-2021-2049, within PNCDI III.

Institutional Review Board Statement: Not applicable.

Informed Consent Statement: Not applicable.

Data Availability Statement: Not applicable.

Acknowledgments: A.P. acknowledges UMF internal grant no. 773/9/11.01.2023.

Conflicts of Interest: The authors declare no conflict of interest.

References

1. World Health Organization. Global Health Estimates (2020). Available online: who.int/data/gho/data/themes/mortality-and-global-health-estimates/ghe-leading-causes-of-death (accessed on 3 March 2023).
2. Sung, H.; Ferlay, J.; Siegel, R.L.; Laversanne, M.; Soerjomataram, I.; Jemal, A.; Bray, F. Global Cancer Statistics 2020: GLOBOCAN Estimates of Incidence and Mortality Worldwide for 36 Cancers in 185 Countries. *CA Cancer J. Clin.* **2021**, *71*, 209–249. [CrossRef] [PubMed]
3. Cancer Chemotherapy-StatPearls-NCBI Bookshelf. Available online: https://www.ncbi.nlm.nih.gov/books/NBK564367/ (accessed on 15 February 2023).
4. Bukowski, K.; Kciuk, M.; Kontek, R. Mechanisms of multidrug resistance in cancer chemotherapy. *Int. J. Mol. Sci.* **2020**, *21*, 3233. [CrossRef] [PubMed]
5. Cuciniello, R.; Filosa, S.; Crispi, S. Novel approaches in cancer treatment: Preclinical and clinical development of small non-coding RNA therapeutics. *J. Exp. Clin. Cancer Res.* **2021**, *40*, 383. [CrossRef] [PubMed]
6. Zare, M.; Pemmada, R.; Madhavan, M.; Shailaja, A.; Ramakrishna, S.; Kandiyil, S.P.; Donahue, J.M.; Thomas, V. Encapsulation of miRNA and siRNA into Nanomaterials for Cancer Therapeutics. *Pharmaceutics* **2022**, *14*, 1620. [CrossRef]
7. Vangijzegem, T.; Lecomte, V.; Ternad, I.; Van Leuven, L.; Muller, R.N.; Stanicki, D.; Laurent, S. Superparamagnetic Iron Oxide Nanoparticles (SPION): From Fundamentals to State-of-the-Art Innovative Applications for Cancer Therapy. *Pharmaceutics* **2023**, *15*, 236. [CrossRef]
8. Chavan, N.; Dharmaraj, D.; Sarap, S.; Surve, C. Magnetic nanoparticles–A new era in nanotechnology. *J. Drug Deliv. Sci. Technol.* **2022**, *77*, 103899. [CrossRef]
9. Calzoni, E.; Cesaretti, A.; Polchi, A.; Di Michele, A.; Tancini, B.; Emiliani, C. Biocompatible Polymer Nanoparticles for Drug Delivery Applications in Cancer and Neurodegenerative Disorder Therapies. *J. Funct. Biomater.* **2019**, *10*, 4. [CrossRef]
10. Begines, B.; Ortiz, T.; Pérez-Aranda, M.; Martínez, G.; Merinero, M.; Argüelles-Arias, F.; Alcudia, A. Polymeric nanoparticles for drug delivery: Recent developments and future prospects. *Nanomaterials* **2020**, *10*, 1403. [CrossRef]

11. Xu, L.; Wang, X.; Liu, Y.; Yang, G.; Falconer, R.J.; Zhao, C.-X. Lipid Nanoparticles for Drug Delivery. *Adv. NanoBiomed Res.* **2022**, *2*, 2100109. [CrossRef]
12. Chandrakala, V.; Aruna, V.; Angajala, G. Review on metal nanoparticles as nanocarriers: Current challenges and perspectives in drug delivery systems. *Emergent Mater.* **2022**, *5*, 1593–1615. [CrossRef]
13. Sankaranarayanan, S.A.; Thomas, A.; Revi, N.; Ramakrishna, B.; Rengan, A.K. Iron oxide nanoparticles for theranostic applications- Recent advances. *J. Drug Deliv. Sci. Technol.* **2022**, *70*, 103196. [CrossRef]
14. Mai, B.T.; Conteh, J.S.; Gavilán, H.; Di Girolamo, A.; Pellegrino, T. Clickable Polymer Ligand-Functionalized Iron Oxide Nanocubes: A Promising Nanoplatform for "Local Hot Spots" Magnetically Triggered Drug Release. *ACS Appl. Mater. Interfaces* **2022**, *14*, 48476–48488. [CrossRef] [PubMed]
15. Mekseriwattana, W.; Guardia, P.; Herrero, B.T.; de la Fuente, J.M.; Kuhakarn, C.; Roig, A.; Katewongsa, K.P. Riboflavin-citrate conjugate multicore SPIONs with enhanced magnetic responses and cellular uptake in breast cancer cells. *Nanoscale Adv.* **2022**, *4*, 1988–1998. [CrossRef] [PubMed]
16. Mishra, S.K.; Herman, P.; Crair, M.; Constable, R.T.; Walsh, J.J.; Akif, A.; Verhagen, J.V.; Hyder, F. Fluorescently-tagged magnetic protein nanoparticles for high-resolution optical and ultra-high field magnetic resonance dual-modal cerebral angiography. *Nanoscale* **2022**, *14*, 17770–17788. [CrossRef] [PubMed]
17. Aires, A.; Fernández-Afonso, Y.; Guedes, G.; Guisasola, E.; Gutiérrez, L.; Cortajarena, A.L. Engineered Protein-Driven Synthesis of Tunable Iron Oxide Nanoparticles as T1 and T2 Magnetic Resonance Imaging Contrast Agents. *Chem. Mater.* **2022**, *34*, 10832–10841. [CrossRef] [PubMed]
18. Portilla, Y.; Fernández-Afonso, Y.; Pérez-Yagüe, S.; Mulens-Arias, V.; Morales, M.P.; Gutiérrez, L.; Barber, D.F. Different coatings on magnetic nanoparticles dictate their degradation kinetics in vivo for 15 months after intravenous administration in mice. *J. Nanobiotechnol.* **2022**, *20*, 543. [CrossRef]
19. Yan, B.; Wang, S.; Liu, C.; Wen, N.; Li, H.; Zhang, Y.; Wang, H.; Xi, Z.; Lv, Y.; Fan, H.; et al. Engineering magnetic nano-manipulators for boosting cancer immunotherapy. *J. Nanobiotechnol.* **2022**, *20*, 547. [CrossRef]
20. Li, X.; Li, W.; Wang, M.; Liao, Z. Magnetic nanoparticles for cancer theranostics: Advances and prospects. *J. Control. Release* **2021**, *335*, 437–448. [CrossRef]
21. kianfar, E. Magnetic Nanoparticles in Targeted Drug Delivery: A Review. *J. Supercond. Nov. Magn.* **2021**, *34*, 1709–1735. [CrossRef]
22. Anik, M.I.; Hossain, M.K.; Hossain, I.; Mahfuz, A.M.U.B.; Rahman, M.T.; Ahmed, I. Recent progress of magnetic nanoparticles in biomedical applications: A review. *Nano Sel.* **2021**, *2*, 1146–1186. [CrossRef]
23. Shabatina, T.I.; Vernaya, O.I.; Shabatin, V.P.; Melnikov, M.Y. Magnetic nanoparticles for biomedical purposes: Modern trends and prospects. *Magnetochemistry* **2020**, *6*, 30. [CrossRef]
24. Socoliuc, V.; Peddis, D.; Petrenko, V.I.; Avdeev, M.V.; Susan-Resiga, D.; Szabó, T.; Turcu, R.; Tombácz, E.; Vékás, L. Magnetic nanoparticle systems for nanomedicine—A materials science perspective. *Magnetochemistry* **2020**, *6*, 2. [CrossRef]
25. Hepel, M. Magnetic nanoparticles for nanomedicine. *Magnetochemistry* **2020**, *6*, 3. [CrossRef]
26. Wu, K.; Su, D.; Liu, J.; Saha, R.; Wang, J.P. Magnetic nanoparticles in nanomedicine: A review of recent advances. *Nanotechnology* **2019**, *30*, 502003. [CrossRef]
27. Mittal, A.; Roy, I.; Gandhi, S. Magnetic Nanoparticles: An Overview for Biomedical Applications. *Magnetochemistry* **2022**, *8*, 107. [CrossRef]
28. Kudr, J.; Haddad, Y.; Richtera, L.; Heger, Z.; Cernak, M.; Adam, V.; Zitka, O. Magnetic nanoparticles: From design and synthesis to real world applications. *Nanomaterials* **2017**, *7*, 243. [CrossRef]
29. Anderson, S.D.; Gwenin, V.V.; Gwenin, C.D. Magnetic Functionalized Nanoparticles for Biomedical, Drug Delivery and Imaging Applications. *Nanoscale Res. Lett.* **2019**, *14*, 188. [CrossRef]
30. Chouhan, R.S.; Horvat, M.; Ahmed, J.; Alhokbany, N.; Alshehri, S.M.; Gandhi, S. Magnetic nanoparticles—A multifunctional potential agent for diagnosis and therapy. *Cancers* **2021**, *13*, 2213. [CrossRef]
31. Bruschi, M.L.; de Alcântara Sica de Toledo, L. Pharmaceutical Applications of Iron-Oxide. *Magnetichemistry* **2019**, *5*, 50. [CrossRef]
32. Petrov, K.; Chubarov, A. Magnetite Nanoparticles for Biomedical Applications. *Encyclopedia* **2022**, *2*, 1811–1828. [CrossRef]
33. Cardoso, V.F.; Francesko, A.; Ribeiro, C.; Bañobre-López, M.; Martins, P.; Lanceros-Mendez, S. Advances in Magnetic Nanoparticles for Biomedical Applications. *Adv. Healthc. Mater.* **2018**, *7*, 1700845. [CrossRef]
34. Stanicki, D.; Vangijzegem, T.; Ternad, I.; Laurent, S. An update on the applications and characteristics of magnetic iron oxide nanoparticles for drug delivery. *Expert Opin. Drug Deliv.* **2022**, *19*, 321–335. [CrossRef] [PubMed]
35. Nikitin, A.A.; Ivanova, A.V.; Semkina, A.S.; Lazareva, P.A.; Abakumov, M.A. Magneto-Mechanical Approach in Biomedicine: Benefits, Challenges, and Future Perspectives. *Int. J. Mol. Sci.* **2022**, *23*, 11134. [CrossRef] [PubMed]
36. Naud, C.; Thébault, C.; Carrière, M.; Hou, Y.; Morel, R.; Berger, F.; Diény, B.; Joisten, H. Cancer treatment by magneto-mechanical effect of particles, a review. *Nanoscale Adv.* **2020**, *2*, 3632–3655. [CrossRef] [PubMed]
37. Zhou, J.; Chen, L.; Chen, L.; Zhang, Y.; Yuan, Y. Emerging role of nanoparticles in the diagnostic imaging of gastrointestinal cancer. *Semin. Cancer Biol.* **2022**, *86*, 580–594. [CrossRef]
38. Dadfar, S.M.; Roemhild, K.; Drude, N.I.; von Stillfried, S.; Knüchel, R.; Kiessling, F.; Lammers, T. Iron oxide nanoparticles: Diagnostic, therapeutic and theranostic applications. *Adv. Drug Deliv. Rev.* **2019**, *138*, 302–325. [CrossRef]
39. Nosheen, S.; Irfan, M.; Abidi, S.H.; Syed, Q.; Habib, F.; Asghar, A.; Waseem, B.; Soomro, B.; Butt, H. Mubashar Akram a review: Development of magnetic nano vectors for biomedical applications. *GSC Adv. Res. Rev.* **2021**, *8*, 85–110. [CrossRef]

40. Yoon, T.J.; Shao, H.; Weissleder, R.; Lee, H. Oxidation kinetics and magnetic properties of elemental iron nanoparticles. *Part. Part. Syst. Charact.* **2013**, *30*, 667–671. [CrossRef]
41. Farrell, D.; Majetich, S.A.; Wilcoxon, J.P. Preparation and Characterization of Monodisperse Fe Nanoparticles. *J. Phys. Chem. B* **2003**, *107*, 11022–11030. [CrossRef]
42. Dumestre, F.; Chaudret, B.; Amiens, C.; Renaud, P.; Fejes, P. Superlattices of iron nanocubes synthesized from Fe[N(SiMe$_3$)$_2$]$_2$. *Science* **2004**, *303*, 821–823. [CrossRef]
43. Petit, C.; Taleb, A.; Pileni, M.P. Cobalt nanosized particles organized in a 2D superlattice: Synthesis, characterization, and magnetic properties. *J. Phys. Chem. B* **1999**, *103*, 1805–1810. [CrossRef]
44. Murray, C.B.; Sun, S.; Doyle, H.; Betley, T. Monodisperse 3d Transition-Metal (Co, Ni, Fe) Nanoparticles and Their Assembly intoNanoparticle Superlattices. *MRS Bull.* **2001**, *26*, 985–991. [CrossRef]
45. Wu, W.; He, Q.; Jiang, C. Magnetic iron oxide nanoparticles: Synthesis and surface functionalization strategies. *Nanoscale Res. Lett.* **2008**, *3*, 397–415. [CrossRef] [PubMed]
46. Sun, C.; Lee, J.S.H.; Zhang, M. Magnetic nanoparticles in MR imaging and drug delivery. *Adv. Drug Deliv. Rev.* **2008**, *60*, 1252–1265. [CrossRef] [PubMed]
47. Quinto, C.A.; Mohindra, P.; Tong, S.; Bao, G. Multifunctional superparamagnetic iron oxide nanoparticles for combined chemotherapy and hyperthermia cancer treatment. *Nanoscale* **2015**, *7*, 12728–12736. [CrossRef]
48. Zhu, Y.; Zhao, W.; Chen, H.; Shi, J. A simple one-pot self-assembly route to nanoporous and monodispersed Fe$_3$O$_4$ particles with oriented attachment structure and magnetic property. *J. Phys. Chem. C* **2007**, *111*, 5281–5285. [CrossRef]
49. Xuan, S.; Wang, F.; Wang, Y.X.J.; Yu, J.C.; Leung, K.C.F. Facile synthesis of size-controllable monodispersed ferrite nanospheres. *J. Mater. Chem.* **2010**, *20*, 5086–5094. [CrossRef]
50. Xuan, S.; Wang, Y.X.J.; Yu, J.C.; Leung, K.C.F. Tuning the grain size and particle size of superparamagnetic Fe$_3$O$_4$ microparticles. *Chem. Mater.* **2009**, *21*, 5079–5087. [CrossRef]
51. Liu, J.; Sun, Z.; Deng, Y.; Zou, Y.; Li, C.; Guo, X.; Xiong, L.; Gao, Y.; Li, F.; Zhao, D. Highly water-dispersible biocompatible magnetite particles with low cytotoxicity stabilized by citrate groups. *Angew. Chemie-Int. Ed.* **2009**, *48*, 5875–5879. [CrossRef]
52. Fang, X.L.; Chen, C.; Jin, M.S.; Kuang, Q.; Xie, Z.X.; Xie, S.Y.; Huang, R.B.; Zheng, L.S. Single-crystal-like hematite colloidal nanocrystal clusters: Synthesis and applications in gas sensors, photocatalysis and water treatment. *J. Mater. Chem.* **2009**, *19*, 6154–6160. [CrossRef]
53. Deng, H.; Li, X.; Peng, Q.; Wang, X.; Chen, J.; Li, Y. Monodisperse magnetic single-crystal ferrite microspheres. *Angew. Chemie-Int. Ed.* **2005**, *44*, 2782–2785. [CrossRef]
54. Zeng, H.; Rice, P.M.; Wang, S.X.; Sun, S. Shape-Controlled Synthesis and Shape-Induced Texture of MnFe2O4 Nanoparticles. *J. Am. Chem. Soc.* **2004**, *126*, 11458–11459. [CrossRef]
55. Wahajuddin; Arora, S. Superparamagnetic iron oxide nanoparticles: Magnetic nanoplatforms as drug carriers. *Int. J. Nanomedicine* **2012**, *7*, 3445–3471. [CrossRef]
56. Dave, S.R.; Gao, X. Monodisperse magnetic nanoparticles for biodetection, imaging, and drug delivery: A versatile and evolving technology. *Wiley Interdiscip. Rev. Nanomed. Nanobiotechnol.* **2009**, *1*, 583–609. [CrossRef]
57. Hossain, A.; Sarker, M.S.I.; Khan, M.K.R.; Khan, F.A.; Kamruzzaman, M.; Rahman, M.M. Structural, magnetic, and electrical properties of sol–gel derived cobalt ferrite nanoparticles. *Appl. Phys. A* **2018**, *124*, 608. [CrossRef]
58. Veiseh, O.; Sun, C.; Fang, C.; Bhattarai, N.; Gunn, J.; Kievit, F.; Du, K.; Pullar, B.; Lee, D.; Ellenbogen, R.G.; et al. Specific targeting of brain tumors with an optical/magnetic resonance imaging nanoprobe across the blood-brain barrier. *Cancer Res.* **2009**, *69*, 6200–6207. [CrossRef] [PubMed]
59. Lee, J.H.; Huh, Y.M.; Jun, Y.W.; Seo, J.W.; Jang, J.T.; Song, H.T.; Kim, S.; Cho, E.J.; Yoon, H.G.; Suh, J.S.; et al. Artificially engineered magnetic nanoparticles for ultra-sensitive molecular imaging. *Nat. Med.* **2007**, *13*, 95–99. [CrossRef] [PubMed]
60. Osorio-Cantillo, C.; Santiago-Miranda, A.N.; Perales-Perez, O.; Xin, Y. Size- and phase-controlled synthesis of cobalt nanoparticles for potential biomedical applications. *J. Appl. Phys.* **2012**, *111*, 07B324. [CrossRef]
61. Sharifi, I.; Shokrollahi, H.; Amiri, S. Ferrite-based magnetic nanofluids used in hyperthermia applications. *J. Magn. Magn. Mater.* **2012**, *324*, 903–915. [CrossRef]
62. Ben Ali, M.; El Maalam, K.; El Moussaoui, H.; Mounkachi, O.; Hamedoun, M.; Masrour, R.; Hlil, E.K.; Benyoussef, A. Effect of zinc concentration on the structural and magnetic properties of mixed Co-Zn ferrites nanoparticles synthesized by sol/gel method. *J. Magn. Magn. Mater.* **2016**, *398*, 20–25. [CrossRef]
63. Kortan, A.R.; Hull, R.; Opila, R.L.; Bawendi, M.G.; Steigerwald, M.L.; Carroll, P.J.; Brus, L.E. Nucleation and Growth of CdSe on ZnS Quantum Crystallite Seeds, and Vice Versa, in Inverse Micelle Media. *J. Am. Chem. Soc.* **1990**, *112*, 1327–1332. [CrossRef]
64. Lee, H.; Yoon, T.J.; Weissleder, R. Ultrasensitive Detection of Bacteria Using Core Shell Nanoparticles and an NMR-Filter. *Angew. Chem. Int. Ed. Engl.* **2009**, *48*, 5657–5660. [CrossRef]
65. Lee, I.S.; Lee, N.; Park, J.; Kim, B.H.; Yi, Y.-W.; Kim, T.; Kim, T.K.; Lee, I.H.; Paik, S.R.; Hyeon, T. Ni/NiO Core/Shell Nanoparticles for Selective Binding and Magnetic Separation of Histidine-Tagged Proteins. *J. Am. Chem. Soc.* **2006**, *128*, 10658–10659. [CrossRef] [PubMed]
66. Yin, Y.; Rioux, R.M.; Erdonmez, C.K.; Hughes, S.; Somorjal, G.A.; Alivisatos, A.P. Formation of Hollow Nanocrystals Through the Nanoscale Kirkendall Effect. *Science* **2004**, *304*, 711–714. [CrossRef] [PubMed]

67. Ha, D.-H.; Moreau, L.M.; Bealing, C.R.; Zhang, H.; Hennig, R.G.; Robinson, R.D. The structural evolution and diffusion during the chemical transformation from cobalt to cobalt phosphide nanoparticles. *J. Mater. Chem.* **2011**, *21*, 11498–11510. [CrossRef]
68. Teng, X.; Black, D.; Watkins, N.J.; Gao, Y.; Yang, H. Platinum-Maghemite Core−Shell Nanoparticles Using a Sequential Synthesis. *Nano Lett.* **2003**, *3*, 261–264. [CrossRef]
69. Yoon, T.J.; Lee, H.; Shao, H.; Weissleder, R. Highly magnetic core-shell nanoparticles with a unique magnetization mechanism. *Angew. Chemie-Int. Ed.* **2011**, *50*, 4663–4666. [CrossRef] [PubMed]
70. Zeng, H.; Li, J.; Wang, Z.L.; Liu, J.P.; Sun, S. Bimagnetic Core/Shell FePt/Fe_3O_4. *Nanoparticles* **2004**, *4*, 187–190.
71. Zhou, T.; Lu, M.; Zhang, Z.; Gong, H.; Chin, W.S.; Liu, B. Synthesis and characterization of multifunctional FePt/ ZnO core/Shell nanoparticles. *Adv. Mater.* **2010**, *22*, 403–406. [CrossRef]
72. Cho, N.H.; Cheong, T.C.; Min, J.H.; Wu, J.H.; Lee, S.J.; Kim, D.; Yang, J.S.; Kim, S.; Kim, Y.K.; Seong, S.Y. A multifunctional core-shell nanoparticle for dendritic cell-based cancer immunotherapy. *Nat. Nanotechnol.* **2011**, *6*, 675–682. [CrossRef]
73. Kim, H.; Achermann, M.; Balet, L.P.; Hollingsworth, J.A.; Klimov, V.I. Synthesis and characterization of Co/CdSe core/shell nanocomposites: Bifunctional magnetic-optical nanocrystals. *J. Am. Chem. Soc.* **2005**, *127*, 544–546. [CrossRef] [PubMed]
74. Lee, J.-S.; Bodnarchuk, M.I.; Shevchenko, E.V.; Talapin, D.V. "Magnet-in-the-Semiconductor" FePt−PbS and FePt−PbSe Nanostructures: Magnetic Properties, Charge Transport, and Magnetoresistance. *J. Am. Chem. Soc.* **2010**, *132*, 6382–6391. [CrossRef]
75. Tian, Q.; Hu, J.; Zhu, Y.; Zou, R.; Chen, Z.; Yang, S.; Li, R.; Su, Q.; Han, Y.; Liu, X. Sub-10 nm Fe_3O_4@$Cu_{2-x}S$ Core−Shell Nanoparticles for Dual-Modal.pdf. *J. Am. Chem. Soc.* **2013**, *135*, 8571–8577. [CrossRef] [PubMed]
76. Xu, Z.; Hou, Y.; Sun, S. Magnetic core/shell Fe3O4/Au and Fe3O 4/Au/Ag nanoparticles with tunable plasmonic properties. *J. Am. Chem. Soc.* **2007**, *129*, 8698–8699. [CrossRef] [PubMed]
77. Wang, L.; Luo, J.; Fan, Q.; Suzuki, M.; Suzuki, I.S.; Engelhard, M.H.; Lin, Y.; Kim, N.; Wang, J.Q.; Zhong, C.J. Monodispersed core-shell Fe 3O 4@Au nanoparticles. *J. Phys. Chem. B* **2005**, *109*, 21593–21601. [CrossRef]
78. Shi, W.; Zeng, H.; Sahoo, Y.; Ohulchanskyy, T.Y.; Ding, Y.; Wang, Z.L.; Swihart, M.; Prasad, P.N. A General Approach to Binary and Ternary Hybrid Nanocrystals. *Nano Lett.* **2006**, *6*, 875–881. [CrossRef] [PubMed]
79. Lu, Z.; Yin, Y. Colloidal nanoparticle clusters: Functional materials by design. *Chem. Soc. Rev.* **2012**, *41*, 6874–6887. [CrossRef]
80. Guimarães, T.R.; Lansalot, M.; Bourgeat-Lami, E. Polymer-encapsulation of iron oxide clusters using macroRAFT block copolymers as stabilizers: Tuning of the particle morphology and surface functionalization. *J. Mater. Chem. B* **2020**, *8*, 4917–4929. [CrossRef]
81. Li, Y.; Wang, N.; Huang, X.; Li, F.; Davis, T.P.; Qiao, R.; Ling, D. Polymer-Assisted Magnetic Nanoparticle Assemblies for Biomedical Applications. *ACS Appl. Bio Mater.* **2020**, *3*, 121–142. [CrossRef]
82. Tadic, M.; Kralj, S.; Kopanja, L. Synthesis, particle shape characterization, magnetic properties and surface modification of superparamagnetic iron oxide nanochains. *Mater. Charact.* **2019**, *148*, 123–133. [CrossRef]
83. Storozhuk, L.; Besenhard, M.O.; Mourdikoudis, S.; LaGrow, A.P.; Lees, M.R.; Tung, L.D.; Gavriilidis, A.; Thanh, N.T.K. Stable Iron Oxide Nanoflowers with Exceptional Magnetic Heating Efficiency: Simple and Fast Polyol Synthesis. *ACS Appl. Mater. Interfaces* **2021**, *13*, 45870–45880. [CrossRef]
84. Furrer, A. Magnetic cluster excitations. *J. Phys. Conf. Ser.* **2011**, *325*, 012001. [CrossRef]
85. Kratz, H.; Taupitz, M.; De Schellenberger, A.A.; Kosch, O.; Eberbeck, D.; Wagner, S.; Trahms, L.; Hamm, B.; Schnorr, J. Novel magnetic multicore nanoparticles designed for MPI and other biomedical applications: From synthesis to first in vivo studies. *PLoS ONE* **2018**, *13*, e0190214. [CrossRef] [PubMed]
86. Hobson, N.J.; Weng, X.; Siow, B.; Veiga, C.; Ashford, M.; Thanh, N.T.K.; Schätzlein, A.G.; Uchegbu, I.F. Clustering superparamagnetic iron oxide nanoparticles produces organ-Targeted high-contrast magnetic resonance images. *Nanomedicine* **2019**, *14*, 135–1152. [CrossRef] [PubMed]
87. Hennion, M.; Pardi, L. Neutron study of mesoscopic magnetic clusters. *Phys. Rev. B-Condens. Matter Mater. Phys.* **1997**, *56*, 8819–8827. [CrossRef]
88. Narayanaswamy, A.; Xu, H.; Pradhan, N.; Peng, X. Crystalline nanoflowers with different chemical compositions and physical properties grown by limited ligand protection. *Angew. Chemie-Int. Ed.* **2006**, *45*, 5361–5364. [CrossRef] [PubMed]
89. Ge, J.; Hu, Y.; Biasini, M.; Beyermann, W.P.; Yin, Y. Superparamagnetic magnetite colloidal nanocrystal clusters. *Angew. Chemie-Int. Ed.* **2007**, *46*, 4342–4345. [CrossRef]
90. Dan, M.; Scott, D.F.; Hardy, P.A.; Wydra, R.J.; Hilt, J.Z.; Yokel, R.A.; Bae, Y. Block copolymer cross-linked nanoassemblies improve particle stability and biocompatibility of superparamagnetic iron oxide nanoparticles. *Pharm. Res.* **2013**, *30*, 552–561. [CrossRef]
91. Bernad, S.I.; Craciunescu, I.; Sandhu, G.S.; Dragomir-Daescu, D.; Tombacz, E.; Vekas, L.; Turcu, R. Fluid targeted delivery of functionalized magnetoresponsive nanocomposite particles to a ferromagnetic stent. *J. Magn. Magn. Mater.* **2021**, *519*, 167489. [CrossRef]
92. Turcu, R.; Craciunescu, I.; Garamus, V.M.; Janko, C.; Lyer, S.; Tietze, R.; Alexiou, C.; Vekas, L. Magnetic microgels for drug targeting applications: Physical-chemical properties and cytotoxicity evaluation. *J. Magn. Magn. Mater.* **2015**, *380*, 307–314. [CrossRef]
93. Larsen, B.A.; Haag, M.A.; Serkova, N.J.; Shroyer, K.R.; Stoldt, C.R. Controlled aggregation of superparamagnetic iron oxide nanoparticles for the development of molecular magnetic resonance imaging probes. *Nanotechnology* **2008**, *19*, 265102. [CrossRef]

94. Lim, E.K.; Jang, E.; Kim, B.; Choi, J.; Lee, K.; Suh, J.S.; Huh, Y.M.; Haam, S. Dextran-coated magnetic nanoclusters as highly sensitive contrast agents for magnetic resonance imaging of inflammatory macrophages. *J. Mater. Chem.* **2011**, *21*, 12473–12478. [CrossRef]
95. Craciunescu, I.; Petran, A.; Daia, C.; Marinica, O.; Vekas, L.; Turcu, R. Stimuli responsive magnetic nanogels for biomedical application. *AIP Conf. Proc.* **2013**, *1565*, 203–207. [CrossRef]
96. Kostopoulou, A.; Lappas, A. Colloidal magnetic nanocrystal clusters: Variable length-scale interaction mechanisms, synergetic functionalities and technological advantages. *Nanotechnol. Rev.* **2015**, *4*, 595–624. [CrossRef]
97. Lu, Z.; Duan, J.; He, L.; Hu, Y.; Yin, Y. Mesoporous TiO2 nanocrystal clusters for selective enrichment of phosphopeptides. *Anal. Chem.* **2010**, *82*, 7249–7258. [CrossRef]
98. Li, P.; Peng, Q.; Li, Y. Dual-Mode luminescent colloidal spheres from monodisperse rare-earth fluoride nanocrystals. *Adv. Mater.* **2009**, *21*, 1945–1948. [CrossRef]
99. Chen, C.; Nan, C.; Wang, D.; Su, Q.; Duan, H.; Liu, X.; Zhang, L.; Chu, D.; Song, W.; Peng, Q.; et al. Mesoporous multicomponent nanocomposite colloidal spheres: Ideal high-temperature stable model catalysts. *Angew. Chemie-Int. Ed.* **2011**, *50*, 3725–3729. [CrossRef] [PubMed]
100. Xu, F.; Cheng, C.; Xu, F.; Zhang, C.; Xu, H.; Xie, X.; Yin, D.; Gu, H. Superparamagnetic magnetite nanocrystal clusters: A sensitive tool for MR cellular imaging. *Nanotechnology* **2009**, *20*, 405102. [CrossRef] [PubMed]
101. Craciunescu, I.; Chițanu, E.; Codescu, M.M.; Iacob, N.; Kuncser, A.; Kuncser, V.; Socoliuc, V.; Susan-Resiga, D.; Bălănean, F.; Ispas, G.; et al. High performance magnetorheological fluids: Very high magnetization FeCo–Fe$_3$O$_4$ nanoclusters in a ferrofluid carrier. *Soft Matter* **2022**, *18*, 626–639. [CrossRef] [PubMed]
102. Castellanos-Rubio, I.; Barón, A.; Luis-Lizarraga, O.; Rodrigo, I.; de Muro, I.G.; Orue, I.; Martínez-Martínez, V.; Castellanos-Rubio, A.; López-Arbeloa, F.; Insausti, M. Efficient Magneto-Luminescent Nanosystems based on Rhodamine-Loaded Magnetite Nanoparticles with Optimized Heating Power and Ideal Thermosensitive Fluorescence. *ACS Appl. Mater. Interfaces* **2022**, *14*, 50033–50044. [CrossRef]
103. Bohara, R.A.; Thorat, N.D.; Pawar, S.H. Role of functionalization: Strategies to explore potential nano-bio applications of magnetic nanoparticles. *RSC Adv.* **2016**, *6*, 43989–44012. [CrossRef]
104. Einarson, M.B.; Berg, J.C. Electrosteric stabilization of colloidal latex dispersions. *J. Colloid Interface Sci.* **1993**, *155*, 165–172. [CrossRef]
105. Rui, H.; Xing, R.; Xu, Z.; Hou, Y.; Goo, S.; Sun, S. Synthesis, functionalization, and biomedical applications of multifunctional magnetic nanoparticles. *Adv. Mater.* **2010**, *22*, 2729–2742. [CrossRef]
106. Wu, L.; Wen, W.; Wang, X.; Huang, D.; Cao, J.; Qi, X.; Shen, S. Ultrasmall iron oxide nanoparticles cause significant toxicity by specifically inducing acute oxidative stress to multiple organs. *Part. Fibre Toxicol.* **2022**, *19*, 24. [CrossRef] [PubMed]
107. Jiang, Z.; Shan, K.; Song, J.; Liu, J.; Rajendran, S.; Pugazhendi, A.; Jacob, J.A.; Chen, B. Toxic effects of magnetic nanoparticles on normal cells and organs. *Life Sci.* **2019**, *220*, 156–161. [CrossRef]
108. Malhotra, N.; Lee, J.S.; Liman, R.A.D.; Ruallo, J.M.S.; Villaflore, O.B.; Ger, T.R.; Hsiao, C. Der Potential toxicity of iron oxide magnetic nanoparticles: A review. *Molecules* **2020**, *25*, 3159. [CrossRef]
109. Chubarov, A.S. Serum Albumin for Magnetic Nanoparticles Coating. *Magnetochemistry* **2022**, *8*, 13. [CrossRef]
110. Sadjadi, S.; Sadjadi, S. 4-Covalent Functionalized Silica-Coated Magnetic Nanoparticles: Classification, Synthetic Methods and Their Applications. In *Woodhead Publishing Series in Electronic and Optical Materials*; Hussain, C.M., Patankar, K.K., Eds.; Woodhead Publishing: Cambridge, UK, 2022; pp. 117–152. [CrossRef]
111. Moraes Silva, S.; Tavallaie, R.; Sandiford, L.; Tilley, R.D.; Gooding, J.J. Gold coated magnetic nanoparticles: From preparation to surface modification for analytical and biomedical applications. *Chem. Commun.* **2016**, *52*, 7528–7540. [CrossRef] [PubMed]
112. Raghav, N.; Sharma, M.R.; Kennedy, J.F. Nanocellulose: A mini-review on types and use in drug delivery systems. *Carbohydr. Polym. Technol. Appl.* **2021**, *2*, 100031. [CrossRef]
113. Utomo, E.; Stewart, S.A.; Picco, C.J.; Domínguez-Robles, J.; Larrañeta, E. Classification, Material Types, and Design Approaches of Long-Acting and Implantable Drug Delivery Systems. In *Long-Acting Drug Delivery Systems: Pharmaceutical, Clinical, and Regulatory Aspects*; Woodhead Publishing: Cambridge, UK, 2022; pp. 17–59. [CrossRef]
114. Zhang, H.; Fan, T.; Chen, W.; Li, Y.; Wang, B. Recent advances of two-dimensional materials in smart drug delivery nano-systems. *Bioact. Mater.* **2020**, *5*, 1071–1086. [CrossRef]
115. Zhang, W.; Zhang, Z.; Fu, S.; Ma, Q.; Liu, Y.; Zhang, N. Micro/nanomotor: A promising drug delivery system for cancer therapy. *ChemPhysMater* **2022**, *2*, 114–125. [CrossRef]
116. Brindhadevi, K.; Garalleh, H.; Alalawi, A.; Al-Sarayreh, E.; Pugazhendi, A. Carbon nanomaterials: Types, synthesis strategies and their application as drug delivery system for Cancer therapy. *Biochem. Eng. J.* **2023**, *192*, 108828. [CrossRef]
117. Nakamura, Y.; Mochida, A.; Choyke, P.L.; Kobayashi, H. Nano-drug delivery: Is the enhanced permeability and retention (EPR) effect sufficient for curing cancer? *Bioconjucation Chem.* **2016**, *27*, 2225–2238. [CrossRef] [PubMed]
118. Weng, H.; Bejjanki, N.K.; Zhang, J.; Miao, X.; Zhong, Y.; Li, H.; Xie, H.; Wang, S.; Li, Q.; Xie, M. TAT peptide-modified cisplatin-loaded iron oxide nanoparticles for reversing cisplatin-resistant nasopharyngeal carcinoma. *Biochem. Biophys. Res. Commun.* **2019**, *511*, 597–603. [CrossRef]

119. Zumaya, A.L.V.; Rimpelová, S.; Štějdířová, M.; Ulbrich, P.; Vilčáková, J.; Hassouna, F. Antibody Conjugated PLGA Nanocarriers and Superparmagnetic Nanoparticles for Targeted Delivery of Oxaliplatin to Cells from Colorectal Carcinoma. *Int. J. Mol. Sci.* **2022**, *23*, 1200. [CrossRef] [PubMed]
120. Rus, I.; Tertis, M.; Cristea, C.; Sandulescu, R. Modern Analytical Techniques for Drug Delivery Systems Characterization. *Curr. Anal. Chem.* **2020**, *16*, 1–10. [CrossRef]
121. Attia, M.F.; Anton, N.; Wallyn, J.; Omran, Z.; Vandamme, T.F. An overview of active and passive targeting strategies to improve the nanocarriers efficiency to tumour sites. *J. Pharm. Pharmacol.* **2019**, *71*, 1185–1198. [CrossRef] [PubMed]
122. Jin, M.Z.; Jin, W.L. The updated landscape of tumor microenvironment and drug repurposing. *Signal Transduct. Target. Ther.* **2020**, *5*, 166. [CrossRef]
123. Peng, Z.; Ning, K.; Tang, X.; He, R.; Zhang, D.Y.; Ma, Y.; Guan, S.; Zhai, J. A multifunctional DNA repair enzyme and magnetic dual-triggered theranostic nanosystem for intelligent drug delivery. *Mater. Des.* **2023**, *226*, 111611. [CrossRef]
124. Nosrati, H.; Salehiabar, M.; Davaran, S.; Danafar, H.; Manjili, H.K. Methotrexate-conjugated L-lysine coated iron oxide magnetic nanoparticles for inhibition of MCF-7 breast cancer cells. *Drug Dev. Ind. Pharm.* **2018**, *44*, 886–894. [CrossRef]
125. Attari, E.; Nosrati, H.; Danafar, H.; Kheiri Manjili, H. Methotrexate anticancer drug delivery to breast cancer cell lines by iron oxide magnetic based nanocarrier. *J. Biomed. Mater. Res.-Part A* **2019**, *107*, 2492–2500. [CrossRef] [PubMed]
126. Nosrati, H.; Mojtahedi, A.; Danafar, H.; Kheiri Manjili, H. Enzymatic Stimuli-Responsive Methotrexate-Conjugated Magnetic Nanoparticles for Target Delivery to Breast Cancer Cells and Release Study in Lysosomal Condition. *J. Bimedical Res. Part A* **2018**, *106*, 1646–1654. [CrossRef] [PubMed]
127. Azizi, S.; Nosrati, H.; Danafar, H. Simple surface functionalization of magnetic nanoparticles with methotrexate-conjugated bovine serum albumin as a biocompatible drug delivery vehicle. *Appl. Organomet. Chem.* **2020**, *34*, e5479. [CrossRef]
128. Zhao, Q.; Xie, P.; Li, X.; Wang, Y.; Zhang, Y.; Wang, S. Magnetic mesoporous silica nanoparticles mediated redox and pH dual-responsive target drug delivery for combined magnetothermal therapy and chemotherapy. *Colloids Surfaces A Physicochem. Eng. Asp.* **2022**, *648*, 129359. [CrossRef]
129. Yoon, H.M.; Kang, M.S.; Choi, G.E.; Kim, Y.J.; Bae, C.H.; Yu, Y.B.; Jeong, Y. Il Stimuli-responsive drug delivery of doxorubicin using magnetic nanoparticle conjugated poly(Ethylene glycol)-g-chitosan copolymer. *Int. J. Mol. Sci.* **2021**, *22*, 13169. [CrossRef] [PubMed]
130. Sumitha, N.S.; Krishna, N.G.; Sailaja, G.S. Multifunctional chitosan ferrogels for targeted cancer therapy by on-demand magnetically triggered drug delivery and hyperthermia. *Biomater. Adv.* **2022**, *142*, 213137. [CrossRef]
131. Mao, H.; Chang, Q.; Zhang, Z.; Feng, J.; Zhou, X.; Hu, Z. Synthesis of CoFe2O4/MoO2 dumbbell-shaped nanoparticles with enhanced AMF/NIR induced drug delivery for liver cancer treatment. *Ceram. Int.* **2022**, *48*, 28640–28648. [CrossRef]
132. Martín, M.J.; Azcona, P.; Lassalle, V.; Gentili, C. Doxorubicin delivery by magnetic nanotheranostics enhances the cell death in chemoresistant colorectal cancer-derived cells. *Eur. J. Pharm. Sci.* **2021**, *158*, 105681. [CrossRef]
133. Shetake, N.G.; Ali, M.; Kumar, A.; Bellare, J.; Pandey, B.N. Theranostic magnetic nanoparticles enhance DNA damage and mitigate doxorubicin-induced cardio-toxicity for effective multi-modal tumor therapy. *Biomater. Adv.* **2022**, *142*, 213147. [CrossRef]
134. Arrizabalaga, J.H.; Casey, J.S.; Becca, J.C.; Liu, Y.; Jensen, L.; Hayes, D.J. Development of magnetic nanoparticles for the intracellular delivery of miR-148b in non-small cell lung cancer. *Biomed. Eng. Adv.* **2022**, *3*, 100031. [CrossRef]
135. Mdlovu, N.V.; Lin, K.S.; Chen, Y.; Wu, C.M. Formulation of magnetic nanocomposites for intracellular delivery of micro-RNA for MYCN inhibition in neuroblastoma. *Colloids Surfaces A Physicochem. Eng. Asp.* **2021**, *615*, 126264. [CrossRef]
136. Mdlovu, N.V.; Chen, Y.; Lin, K.S.; Hsu, M.W.; Wang, S.S.S.; Wu, C.M.; Lin, Y.S.; Ohishi, K. Multifunctional nanocarrier as a potential micro-RNA delivery vehicle for neuroblastoma treatment. *J. Taiwan Inst. Chem. Eng.* **2019**, *96*, 526–537. [CrossRef]
137. Jin, L.; Wang, Q.; Chen, J.; Wang, Z.; Xin, H.; Zhang, D. Efficient delivery of therapeutic siRNA by Fe3O4 magnetic nanoparticles into oral cancer cells. *Pharmaceutics* **2019**, *11*, 615. [CrossRef] [PubMed]
138. Tilsed, C.M.; Fisher, S.A.; Nowak, A.K.; Lake, R.A.; Lesterhuis, W.J. Cancer chemotherapy: Insights into cellular and tumor microenvironmental mechanisms of action. *Front. Oncol.* **2022**, *12*, 960317. [CrossRef]
139. Cernat, A.; Florea, A.; Rus, I.; Truta, F.; Dragan, A.-M.; Cristea, C.; Tertis, M. Applications of magnetic hybrid nanomaterials in Biomedicine. *Biopolym. Nanomater.* **2021**, 639–675. [CrossRef]
140. Fatima, H.; Shukrullah, S.; Hussain, H.; Aslam, H.; Naz, M.Y. Utility of Various Drug Delivery Systems and Their Advantages and Disadvantages. In *Nanotechnology for Drug Delivery and Pharmaceuticals*; Academic Press: Cambridge, MA, USA, 2023; pp. 235–258. [CrossRef]
141. Sritharan, S.; Sivalingam, N. A comprehensive review on time-tested anticancer drug doxorubicin. *Life Sci.* **2021**, *278*, 119527. [CrossRef] [PubMed]
142. Zhang, C.; Xu, C.; Gao, X.; Yao, Q. Platinum-based drugs for cancer therapy and anti-tumor strategies. *Theranostics* **2022**, *12*, 2115–2132. [CrossRef]
143. Koźmiński, P.; Halik, P.K.; Chesori, R.; Gniazdowska, E. Overview of dual-acting drug methotrexate in different neurological diseases, autoimmune pathologies and cancers. *Int. J. Mol. Sci.* **2020**, *21*, 3483. [CrossRef]
144. Kong, F.H.; Ye, Q.F.; Miao, X.Y.; Liu, X.; Huang, S.Q.; Xiong, L.; Wen, Y.; Zhang, Z.J. Current status of sorafenib nanoparticle delivery systems in the treatment of hepatocellular carcinoma. *Theranostics* **2021**, *11*, 5464–5490. [CrossRef]

145. Carrera Espinoza, M.J.; Lin, K.S.; Weng, M.T.; Kunene, S.C.; Lin, Y.S.; Liu, S.Y. Magnetic boron nitride nanosheets-based on pH-responsive smart nanocarriers for the delivery of doxorubicin for liver cancer treatment. *Colloids Surfaces B Biointerfaces* **2023**, *222*, 113129. [CrossRef]
146. Wang, J.; Zhu, F.; Li, K.; Xu, J.; Li, P.; Fan, Y. pH-responsive mesoporous Fe2O3–Au nanomedicine delivery system with magnetic targeting for cancer therapy. *Med. Nov. Technol. Devices* **2022**, *15*, 100127. [CrossRef]
147. Liu, Q.; Tan, Z.; Zheng, D.; Qiu, X. pH-responsive magnetic Fe3O4/carboxymethyl chitosan/aminated lignosulfonate nanoparticles with uniform size for targeted drug loading. *Int. J. Biol. Macromol.* **2022**, *225*, 1182–1192. [CrossRef]
148. Zhang, J.; Su, X.; Weng, L.; Tang, K.; Miao, Y.; Teng, Z.; Wang, L. Gadolinium-hybridized mesoporous organosilica nanoparticles with high magnetic resonance imaging performance for targeted drug delivery. *J. Colloid Interface Sci.* **2023**, *633*, 102–112. [CrossRef] [PubMed]
149. Demina, P.A.; Saveleva, M.S.; Anisimov, R.A.; Prikhozhdenko, E.S.; Voronin, D.V.; Abalymov, A.A.; Cherednichenko, K.A.; Timaeva, O.I.; Lomova, M.V. Degradation of Hybrid Drug Delivery Carriers with a Mineral Core and a Protein– Tannin Shell under Proteolytic Hydrolases. *Biomimetics* **2022**, *7*, 61. [CrossRef] [PubMed]
150. Ghazimoradi, M.; Tarlani, A.; Alemi, A.; Hamishehkar, H.; Ghorbani, M. pH-responsive, magnetic-luminescent core/shell carriers for co-delivery of anticancer drugs (MTX & DOX) for breast cancer treatment. *J. Alloys Compd.* **2023**, *936*, 168257. [CrossRef]
151. Song, X.; Fu, W.; Cheang, U.K. Immunomodulation and delivery of macrophages using nano-smooth drug-loaded magnetic microrobots for dual targeting cancer therapy. *iScience* **2022**, *25*, 104507. [CrossRef]
152. Gonbadi, P.; Jalal, R.; Akhlaghinia, B.; Ghasemzadeh, M.S. Tannic acid-modified magnetic hydrotalcite-based MgAl nanoparticles for the in vitro targeted delivery of doxorubicin to the estrogen receptor-overexpressing colorectal cancer cells. *J. Drug Deliv. Sci. Technol.* **2022**, *68*, 103026. [CrossRef]
153. Kovrigina, E.; Poletaeva, Y.; Zheng, Y.; Chubarov, A. Nylon-6-Coated Doxorubicin-Loaded Magnetic Nanoparticles and Nanocapsules for Cancer Treatment. *Magnetochemistry* **2023**, *9*, 106. [CrossRef]
154. Santhamoorthy, M.; Thirupathi, K.; Krishnan, S.; Guganathan, L.; Dave, S.; Phan, T.T.V.; Kim, S.-C. Preparation of Magnetic Iron Oxide Incorporated Mesoporous Silica Hybrid Composites for pH and Temperature-Sensitive Drug Delivery. *Magnetochemistry* **2023**, *9*, 81. [CrossRef]
155. Toderascu, L.I.; Sima, L.E.; Orobeti, S.; Florian, P.E.; Icriverzi, M.; Maraloiu, V.A.; Comanescu, C.; Iacob, N.; Kuncser, V.; Antohe, I.; et al. Synthesis and Anti-Melanoma Activity of L-Cysteine-Coated Iron Oxide Nanoparticles Loaded with Doxorubicin. *Nanomaterials* **2023**, *13*, 621. [CrossRef]
156. Popova, V.; Poletaeva, Y.; Chubarov, A. pH-Responsible Doxorubicin-Loaded Fe_3O_4@$CaCO_3$ Nanocomposites for Cancer Treatment. *Pharmaceutics* **2023**, *15*, 771. [CrossRef]
157. Azcona, P.L.; Montiel Schneider, M.G.; Grünhut, M.; Lassalle, V.L. Stimuli-responsive nanotheranostics intended for oncological diseases:: In vitro evaluation of their target, diagnostic and drug release capabilities. *New J. Chem.* **2019**, *43*, 2126–2133. [CrossRef]
158. Kuznetsova, O.V.; Timerbaev, A.R. Magnetic nanoparticles for highly robust, facile and efficient loading of metal-based drugs. *J. Inorg. Biochem.* **2022**, *227*, 111685. [CrossRef]
159. Makharza, S.A.; Cirillo, G.; Vittorio, O.; Valli, E.; Voli, F.; Farfalla, A.; Curcio, M.; Iemma, F.; Nicoletta, F.P.; El-Gendy, A.A.; et al. Magnetic graphene oxide nanocarrier for targeted delivery of cisplatin: A perspective for glioblastoma treatment. *Pharmaceuticals* **2019**, *12*, 76. [CrossRef] [PubMed]
160. Ferreira, B.J.M.L.; Martel, F.; Silva, C.; Santos, T.M.; Daniel-da-Silva, A.L. Nanostructured functionalized magnetic platforms for the sustained delivery of cisplatin: Synthesis, characterization and in vitro cytotoxicity evaluation. *J. Inorg. Biochem.* **2020**, *213*, 111258. [CrossRef] [PubMed]
161. Mandriota, G.; Di Corato, R.; Benedetti, M.; De Castro, F.; Fanizzi, F.P.; Rinaldi, R. Design and Application of Cisplatin-Loaded Magnetic Nanoparticle Clusters for Smart Chemotherapy. *ACS Appl. Mater. Interfaces* **2019**, *11*, 1864–1875. [CrossRef]
162. Zarkesh, K.; Heidari, R.; Iranpour, P.; Azarpira, N.; Ahmadi, F.; Mohammadi-Samani, S.; Farjadian, F. Theranostic Hyaluronan Coated EDTA Modified Magnetic Mesoporous Silica Nanoparticles for Targeted Delivery of Cisplatin. *J. Drug Deliv. Sci. Technol.* **2022**, *77*, 103903. [CrossRef]
163. Bejjanki, N.K.; Xu, H.; Xie, M. GSH triggered intracellular aggregated-cisplatin-loaded iron oxide nanoparticles for overcoming cisplatin resistance in nasopharyngeal carcinoma. *J. Biomater. Appl.* **2021**, *36*, 45–54. [CrossRef]
164. Farmanbar, N.; Mohseni, S.; Darroudi, M. Green synthesis of chitosan-coated magnetic nanoparticles for drug delivery of oxaliplatin and irinotecan against colorectal cancer cells. *Polym. Bull.* **2022**, *79*, 10595–10613. [CrossRef]
165. Jabalera, Y.; Garcia-Pinel, B.; Ortiz, R.; Iglesias, G.; Cabeza, L.; Prados, J.; Jimenez-Lopez, C.; Melguizo, C. Oxaliplatin–biomimetic magnetic nanoparticle assemblies for colon cancer-targeted chemotherapy: An in vitro study. *Pharmaceutics* **2019**, *11*, 395. [CrossRef]
166. Liu, D.; Li, X.; Chen, C.; Li, C.; Zhou, C.; Zhang, W.; Zhao, J.; Fan, J.; Cheng, K.; Chen, L. Target-specific delivery of oxaliplatin to HER2-positive gastric cancer cells in vivo using oxaliplatin-au-fe3o4-herceptin nanoparticles. *Oncol. Lett.* **2018**, *15*, 8079–8087. [CrossRef] [PubMed]
167. Baqeri, N.; Shahsavari, S.; Dahouee, I.A.; Shirmard, L.R. Design of slow-release methotrexate drug delivery system using PHBV magnetic nanoparticles and evaluation of its cytotoxicity. *J. Drug Deliv. Sci. Technol.* **2022**, *77*, 103854. [CrossRef]

168. Ahmadi, D.; Zarei, M.; Rahimi, M.; Khazaie, M.; Asemi, Z.; Mir, S.M.; Sadeghpour, A.; Karimian, A.; Alemi, F.; Rahmati-Yamchi, M.; et al. Preparation and in-vitro evaluation of pH-responsive cationic cyclodextrin coated magnetic nanoparticles for delivery of methotrexate to the Saos-2 bone cancer cells. *J. Drug Deliv. Sci. Technol.* **2020**, *57*, 101584. [CrossRef]
169. Dou, J.; Mi, Y.; Daneshmand, S.; Heidari Majd, M. The effect of magnetic nanoparticles containing hyaluronic acid and methotrexate on the expression of genes involved in apoptosis and metastasis in A549 lung cancer cell lines. *Arab. J. Chem.* **2022**, *15*, 104307. [CrossRef]
170. Lodhi, M.S.; Khalid, F.; Khan, M.T.; Samra, Z.Q.; Muhammad, S.; Zhang, Y.J.; Mou, K. A Novel Method of Magnetic Nanoparticles Functionalized with Anti-Folate Receptor Antibody and Methotrexate for Antibody Mediated Targeted Drug Delivery. *Molecules* **2022**, *27*, 261. [CrossRef]
171. Mansouri, K.; Rasoulpoor, S.; Daneshkhah, A.; Abolfathi, S.; Salari, N.; Mohammadi, M.; Rasoulpoor, S.; Shabani, S. Clinical effects of curcumin in enhancing cancer therapy: A systematic review. *BMC Cancer* **2020**, *20*, 791. [CrossRef] [PubMed]
172. Giordano, A.; Tommonaro, G. Curcumin and cancer. *Nutrients* **2019**, *11*, 2376. [CrossRef]
173. Liu, Z.; Wang, X.; Chen, X.; Cui, L.; Li, Z.; Bai, Z.; Lin, K.; Yang, J.; Tian, F. Construction of pH-Responsive Polydopamine Coated Magnetic Layered Hydroxide for Intracellular Drug Delivery. *SSRN Electron. J.* **2022**, *182*, 12–20. [CrossRef]
174. Li, Z.; Wan, W.; Bai, Z.; Peng, B.; Wang, X.; Cui, L.; Liu, Z.; Lin, K.; Yang, J.; Hao, J.; et al. Construction of pH-responsive nanoplatform from stable magnetic nanoparticles for targeted drug delivery and intracellular imaging. *Sensors Actuators B Chem.* **2023**, *375*, 132869. [CrossRef]
175. Felenji, H.; Johari, B.; Moradi, M.; Gharbavi, M.; Danafar, H. Folic Acid-Conjugated Iron Oxide Magnetic Nanoparticles Based on Bovine Serum Albumin (BSA) for Targeted Delivery of Curcumin to Suppress Liver Cancer Cells. *Chem. Africa* **2022**, *5*, 1627–1939. [CrossRef]
176. Seyyedi Zadeh, E.; Ghanbari, N.; Salehi, Z.; Derakhti, S.; Amoabediny, G.; Akbari, M.; Asadi Tokmedash, M. Smart pH-responsive magnetic graphene quantum dots nanocarriers for anticancer drug delivery of curcumin. *Mater. Chem. Phys.* **2023**, *297*, 127336. [CrossRef]
177. Ebadi, M.; Bullo, S.; Buskara, K.; Hussein, M.Z.; Fakurazi, S.; Pastorin, G. Release of a liver anticancer drug, sorafenib from its PVA/LDH- and PEG/LDH-coated iron oxide nanoparticles for drug delivery applications. *Sci. Rep.* **2020**, *10*, 21521. [CrossRef] [PubMed]
178. Ebadi, M.; Buskaran, K.; Bullo, S.; Hussein, M.Z.; Fakurazi, S.; Pastorin, G. Drug delivery system based on magnetic iron oxide nanoparticles coated with (polyvinyl alcohol-zinc/aluminium-layered double hydroxide-sorafenib). *Alexandria Eng. J.* **2021**, *60*, 733–747. [CrossRef]
179. Alpdemir, Ş.; Vural, T.; Kara, G.; Bayram, C.; Haberal, E.; Denkbaş, E.B. Magnetically responsive, sorafenib loaded alginate microspheres for hepatocellular carcinoma treatment. *IET Nanobiotechnol.* **2020**, *14*, 623–627. [CrossRef]
180. Winkle, M.; El-Daly, S.M.; Fabbri, M.; Calin, G.A. Noncoding RNA therapeutics—Challenges and potential solutions. *Nat. Rev. Drug Discov.* **2021**, *20*, 629–651. [CrossRef] [PubMed]
181. Cristofolini, T.; Dalmina, M.; Sierra, J.A.; Silva, A.H.; Pasa, A.A.; Pittella, F.; Creczynski-Pasa, T.B. Multifunctional hybrid nanoparticles as magnetic delivery systems for siRNA targeting the HER2 gene in breast cancer cells. *Mater. Sci. Eng. C* **2020**, *109*, 110555. [CrossRef]
182. Cao, Y.; Zhang, S.; Ma, M.; Zhang, Y. Fluorinated PEG-PEI Coated Magnetic Nanoparticles for siRNA Delivery and CXCR4 Knockdown. *Nanomaterials* **2022**, *12*, 1692. [CrossRef]
183. Maurer, V.; Altin, S.; Seleci, D.A.; Zarinwall, A.; Temel, B.; Vogt, P.M.; Strauß, S.; Stahl, F.; Scheper, T.; Bucan, V.; et al. In-vitro application of magnetic hybrid niosomes: Targeted sirna-delivery for enhanced breast cancer therapy. *Pharmaceutics* **2021**, *13*, 394. [CrossRef]
184. Grabowska, M.; Grześkowiak, B.F.; Szutkowski, K.; Wawrzyniak, D.; Głodowicz, P.; Barciszewski, J.; Jurga, S.; Rolle, K.; Mrówczyński, R. Nano-mediated delivery of double-stranded RNA for gene therapy of glioblastoma multiforme. *PLoS ONE* **2019**, *14*, e0213852. [CrossRef]
185. Selimovic, A.; Kara, G.; Denkbas, E.B. Magnetic gelatin nanoparticles as a biocompatible carrier system for small interfering RNA in human colorectal cancer: Synthesis, optimization, characterization, and cell viability studies. *Mater. Today Commun.* **2022**, *33*, 104616. [CrossRef]
186. Amani, A.; Dustparast, M.; Noruzpour, M.; Zakaria, R.A.; Ebrahimi, H.A. Design and Invitro Characterization of Green Synthesized Magnetic Nanoparticles Conjugated with Multitargeted Poly Lactic Acid Copolymers for Co-delivery of siRNA and Paclitaxel. *Eur. J. Pharm. Sci.* **2021**, *167*, 106007. [CrossRef] [PubMed]
187. Wang, X.; Li, R.; Zhu, Y.; Wang, Z.; Zhang, H.; Cui, L.; Duan, S.; Guo, Y. Active targeting co-delivery of therapeutic: Sur siRNA and an antineoplastic drug via epidermal growth factor receptor-mediated magnetic nanoparticles for synergistic programmed cell death in glioblastoma stem cells. *Mater. Chem. Front.* **2020**, *4*, 574–588. [CrossRef]
188. Setia, A.; Mehata, A.K.; Vikas; Malik, A.K.; Viswanadh, M.K.; Muthu, M.S. Theranostic magnetic nanoparticles: Synthesis, properties, toxicity, and emerging trends for biomedical applications. *J. Drug Deliv. Sci. Technol.* **2023**, *81*, 104295. [CrossRef]
189. Ferreira, M.; Sousa, J.; Pais, A.; Vitorino, C. The Role of Magnetic Nanoparticles in Cancer Nanotheranostics. *Materials* **2020**, *13*, 266. [CrossRef] [PubMed]

190. Mirković, M.; Milanović, Z.; Perić, M.; Vranješ-Đurić, S.; Ognjanović, M.; Antić, B.; Kuraica, M.; Krstić, I.; Kubovcikova, M.; Antal, I.; et al. Design and preparation of proline, tryptophan and poly-l-lysine functionalized magnetic nanoparticles and their radiolabeling with 131I and 177Lu for potential theranostic use. *Int. J. Pharm.* **2022**, *628*, 122288. [CrossRef] [PubMed]
191. Baktash, M.S.; Zarrabi, A.; Avazverdi, E.; Reis, N.M. Development and optimization of a new hybrid chitosan-grafted graphene oxide/magnetic nanoparticle system for theranostic applications. *J. Mol. Liq.* **2021**, *322*, 114515. [CrossRef]
192. Fuller, E.G.; Scheutz, G.M.; Jimenez, A.; Lewis, P.; Savliwala, S.; Liu, S.; Sumerlin, B.S.; Rinaldi, C. Theranostic nanocarriers combining high drug loading and magnetic particle imaging. *Int. J. Pharm.* **2019**, *572*, 118796. [CrossRef]
193. Zheng, X.C.; Ren, W.; Zhang, S.; Zhong, T.; Duan, X.C.; Yin, Y.F.; Xu, M.Q.; Hao, Y.L.; Li, Z.T.; Li, H.; et al. The theranostic efficiency of tumor-specific, pH-responsive, peptide-modified, liposome-containing paclitaxel and superparamagnetic iron oxide nanoparticles. *Int. J. Nanomed.* **2018**, *13*, 1495–1504. [CrossRef]
194. Saesoo, S.; Sathornsumetee, S.; Anekwiang, P.; Treetidnipa, C.; Thuwajit, P.; Bunthot, S.; Maneeprakorn, W.; Maurizi, L.; Hofmann, H.; Rungsardthong, R.U.; et al. Characterization of liposome-containing SPIONs conjugated with anti-CD20 developed as a novel theranostic agent for central nervous system lymphoma. *Colloids Surf. B Biointerfaces* **2018**, *161*, 497–507. [CrossRef]
195. Chen, Z.; Peng, Y.; Li, Y.; Xie, X.; Wei, X.; Yang, G.; Zhang, H.; Li, N.; Li, T.; Qin, X.; et al. Aptamer-Dendrimer Functionalized Magnetic Nano-Octahedrons: Theranostic Drug/Gene Delivery Platform for Near-Infrared/Magnetic Resonance Imaging-Guided Magnetochemotherapy. *ACS Nano* **2021**, *15*, 16683–16696. [CrossRef]

Disclaimer/Publisher's Note: The statements, opinions and data contained in all publications are solely those of the individual author(s) and contributor(s) and not of MDPI and/or the editor(s). MDPI and/or the editor(s) disclaim responsibility for any injury to people or property resulting from any ideas, methods, instructions or products referred to in the content.

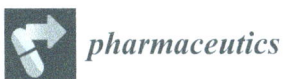

Review

Bioimaging Probes Based on Magneto-Fluorescent Nanoparticles

Sayan Ganguly * and Shlomo Margel *

Department of Chemistry, Institute of Nanotechnology and Advanced Materials (BINA), Bar-Ilan University, Ramat-Gan 5290002, Israel
* Correspondence: sayanganguly2206@gmail.com (S.G.); shlomo.margel@biu.ac.il (S.M.)

Abstract: Novel nanomaterials are of interest in biology, medicine, and imaging applications. Multimodal fluorescent-magnetic nanoparticles demand special attention because they have the potential to be employed as diagnostic and medication-delivery tools, which, in turn, might make it easier to diagnose and treat cancer, as well as a wide variety of other disorders. The most recent advancements in the development of magneto-fluorescent nanocomposites and their applications in the biomedical field are the primary focus of this review. We describe the most current developments in synthetic methodologies and methods for the fabrication of magneto-fluorescent nanocomposites. The primary applications of multimodal magneto-fluorescent nanoparticles in biomedicine, including biological imaging, cancer treatment, and drug administration, are covered in this article, and an overview of the future possibilities for these technologies is provided.

Keywords: nanoparticles; biomedical; magneto-fluorescent; multimodal imaging

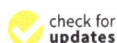

Citation: Ganguly, S.; Margel, S. Bioimaging Probes Based on Magneto-Fluorescent Nanoparticles. *Pharmaceutics* 2023, 15, 686. https://doi.org/10.3390/pharmaceutics15020686

Academic Editor: Constantin Mihai Lucaciu

Received: 3 February 2023
Revised: 14 February 2023
Accepted: 16 February 2023
Published: 17 February 2023

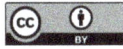

Copyright: © 2023 by the authors. Licensee MDPI, Basel, Switzerland. This article is an open access article distributed under the terms and conditions of the Creative Commons Attribution (CC BY) license (https://creativecommons.org/licenses/by/4.0/).

1. Introduction

There are several definitions of "imaging". Most people consider imaging to be a subset of photography. These limitations are by no means present in scientific imaging [1]. Nuclear magnetic resonance (also known as magnetic resonance imaging; MRI) [2,3]; radioimaging with respective nuclides [4,5]; computed tomography (CT) [6,7]; positron emission tomography (PET) [8]; electrochemical imaging with rastering electrodes; mechanical methods, such as atomic force microscopy (AFM) [9]; and even more sophisticated scanning methods, such as laser ablation (ICP-MS) [10], mass spectrometry (MALDI) [11], and the like, can all be used to produce images. While many of these techniques are inapplicable to living systems or intact tissues due to their destructive nature or the substantial sample preparation they require, some are. Over the previous decade, several fluorescent microscopic instruments have been created [12,13], allowing for the visualization of biological functions at sizes ranging from the molecular to the cellular to the organ to the complete organism [14]. For instance, because of advances in super-resolution microscopy, scientists are now able to pinpoint the locations of individual molecules within cells with an accuracy greater than 10 nm [15]. This study aims to familiarize the reader with the wide variety of nanomaterials now available for fluorescence imaging and to help in choosing the best one for a given application.

A significant reduction in phototoxicity may be achieved with the utilization of light-sheet illumination, which also enables the rapid collection of sufficient data in a condensed amount of time to enable volumetric imaging [16]. The ability to see biological mechanisms has been revolutionized as a whole as a result of the combination of sensitive high-speed detectors, strong lasers, and speedy computers [17]. However, in order to provide an accurate representation of biological processes, these more sophisticated instruments require stronger reporting systems. Molecular imaging allows us to see and learn about individual molecules and tissues in living organisms [18,19]. Tracking cells after transplantation into a patient and subsequently detecting illnesses at an early stage before biochemical problems cause changes in anatomical structure is a rapidly growing field of study. Position emission tomography (PET), single photon emission computed tomography (SPECT), magnetic resonance imaging (MRI), optical imaging (OI), and ultrasonography (USG) are all examples of molecular imaging modalities that have recently become more useful in the diagnosis of a wide range of disorders [20–22]. Figure 1 details the capabilities of several of the most widely used medical imaging techniques. There is no perfect imaging modality that can offer all the necessary data because each modality has its own set of benefits and drawbacks [23]. As a result, it makes sense to mix imaging modalities in a way that maximizes the benefits of one while mitigating the drawbacks of the others. Nanoparticles (NPs) that are 100–10,000 orders of magnitude smaller than cells can be manipulated to cross cell membranes and aggregate in specific places. Owing to their distinct chemical and physical features, they can transport medications and imaging agents more effectively [24,25]. The use of NP-based multimodal imaging probes, which can be identified by multiple imaging modalities, has grown in importance because it paves the way for simultaneous multitargeting and monitoring, increasing diagnostic and therapeutic effects [26].

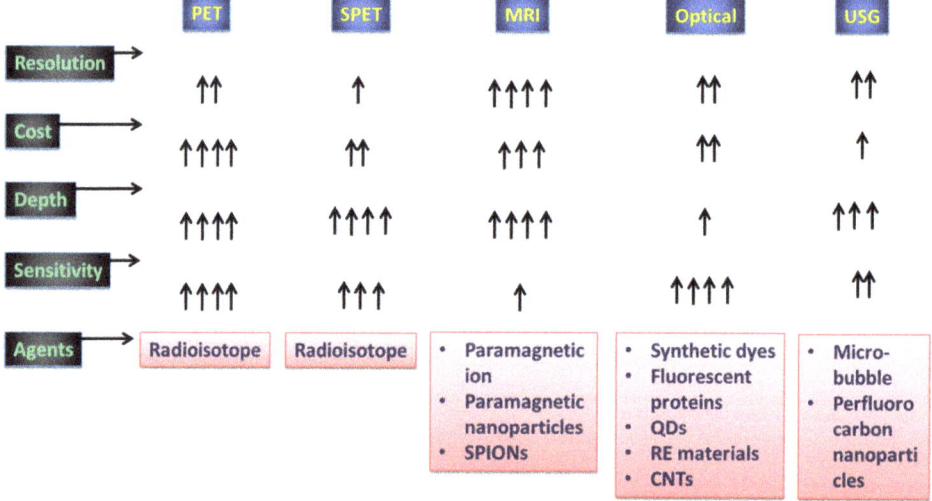

Figure 1. Aspects of diagnostic imaging systems employed in practice. The conventional diagnostic tools and their viabilities with respect to signal capturing are shown. A single arrow represents the minimum viability, and four arrows represents high viability.

Many biological applications might benefit from the use of magnetic NPs, which possess a wide variety of desirable features. After the advent of X-ray technology, research into imaging agents took off, eventually expanding to encompass the radiolabeling of cells and tissues to better aid in the diagnosis and tracking of disease. Each product's generic and commercial names were recorded, as was the company that received the first FDA approval (at a minimum, the year, and ideally the month and day). The FDA's records often revealed the current distributors of products approved before or around the mid-1990s (and not necessarily the innovator organization if the product had changed hands as a result of licensing or acquisitive activities). Although much work went into reducing the toxicity of Collargol and other pioneering compounds, newer and safer contrast agents eventually supplanted colloidal silver [27]. Similarly, J. Edwards Burns introduced thallium nitrate as a contrast agent in 1915 [28]. Moses Swick made an important contribution to the development of urographic imaging [29]. The imaging method for breast cancer, especially melanoma staging, makes use of sulfur colloids [30]. The iron oxide nanoparticle Ferumoxytol (Feraheme™, AMAG Pharmaceuticals) is coated with polyglucose sorbitol carboxymethylether and displays superparamagnetic characteristics [31]. Iron deficiency anemia (IDA) may be effectively and rapidly treated with ferumoxytol when it is injected intravenously (i.v.) at a dose of 510 mg. Gadolinium chelates are widely used because they are the safest MR contrast media. They are regarded as being less dangerous than nonionic iodinated contrast agents [32]. First-generation commercialized, FDA-approved ultrasound contrast agents (UCAs) were either nitrogen-based gases encased in peptide capsules (Albunex; Molecular Biosystems, Inc., San Diego, CA, USA) or powdered, hydrophilic particulate matter (Levovist; Bayer AG, Leverkusen, Germany) [33]. In order to aid doctors in ruling out Alzheimer's disease as the only cause of cognitive decline, the Food and Drug Administration (FDA) has just green-lit a novel radiopharmaceutical agent. Individuals with cognitive impairment who are being tested for Alzheimer's disease or other causes of cognitive decline may benefit from a positron-emission tomographic (PET) scan of the brain with an injection of florbetapir F18 (Amyvid, Eli Lilly, Indianapolis, IN, USA) [34]. When an external magnetic field is applied, magnetic NPs, for instance, can be directed to a single cell or organ of interest. Cancer hyperthermia treatment relies on the fact that an alternating magnetic field may be utilized to selectively heat the region in which magnetic particles are concentrated [35]. It is also possible to employ aqueous dispersions of superparamagnetic NPs as contrast agents for MRI (MRI) [36]. Combining magnetic and other features into a single nanocomposite structure paves the way for novel nanomaterials with interesting multimodal capabilities. Examples of potential biological applications include multimodal biological imaging, medical diagnostics, and drug-delivery systems, all of which might benefit from the creation of fluorescent-magnetic nanocomposites [37]. These nanocomposites have the potential to be used in multimodal tests for both in vitro and in vivo bioimaging techniques, including MRI and fluorescence microscopy [38]. They have both photodynamic and hyperthermic capabilities, making them potential bimodal medicines for cancer treatment [39]. The ability to readily regulate and monitor these nanocomposites using fluorescent or confocal microscopy and MRI makes cell tracking, cytometry, and magnetic separation fascinating new applications. Our analysis will be limited to the most up-to-date findings concerning magneto-fluorescent nanomaterials and a few of their therapeutic systems.

2. Types of Magnetic and Fluorescent Nanoparticles

2.1. Superparamagnetic Nanoparticles

Unlike their bulk counterparts, magnetic NPs have completely distinct magnetic properties. A huge number of magnetic domains make up the majority of ferromagnetic materials, and each domain has parallel magnetic moments that are isolated by domain walls [40]. Domain walls arise when magnetostatic energy and domain-wall energy are in equilibrium [41,42]. The domain-wall energy is responsible for the larger interfacial area between domains, and the magnetostatic energy grows proportionately with the volume of the material [43]. The energy required to create domain barriers is substantially more than the magnetostatic energy required to maintain a single-domain NP; hence, there is a critical value below which a stable single-domain NP can be established when the size of ferromagnetic materials is lowered to the nanoscale level [44]. As illustrated in Figure 2, the critical size (r_c) of an NP may be stated according to Equation (1) when the magnetostatic energy is equal to the domain-wall energy and the NP is transitioning from the multidomain state to the single-domain state [45].

$$r_c = 18 \frac{\sqrt{AK_{eff}}}{\mu_0 M^2} \quad (1)$$

where A represents the exchange constant, K_{eff} is the anisotropy constant, 0 is the vacuum permeability, and M is the saturation magnetization. The critical diameter of magnetic NPs is generally between 10 and 100 nm.

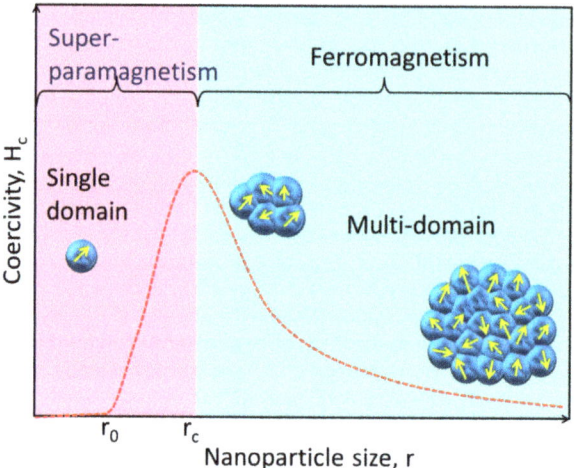

Figure 2. This simplified diagram shows how the magnetic coercivity (H_c, the magnetic field needed to decrease the magnetization to zero) of a magnetic NP varies with its physical dimensions. As an NP is shrunk to the critical size (r_c), the domain wall vanishes and the H_c rises. The NP reaches the superparamagnetic domain and exhibits zero coercivity if its size is further reduced to r_0, where the thermal agitation energy is greater than the magnetic anisotropy energy and the magnetic moment of the NP varies freely.

The magnetic spins of ferromagnetic NPs are linked and parallel-aligned inside a single domain, as was indicated before. When the magnetic moments are kept in a single domain of ferromagnetic NPs, the magnetic anisotropy energy [46] (ΔE) is calculated as follows:

$$\Delta E = K_{eff} V \qquad (2)$$

Figure 3 shows how to calculate the volume of an NP using Equation (2).

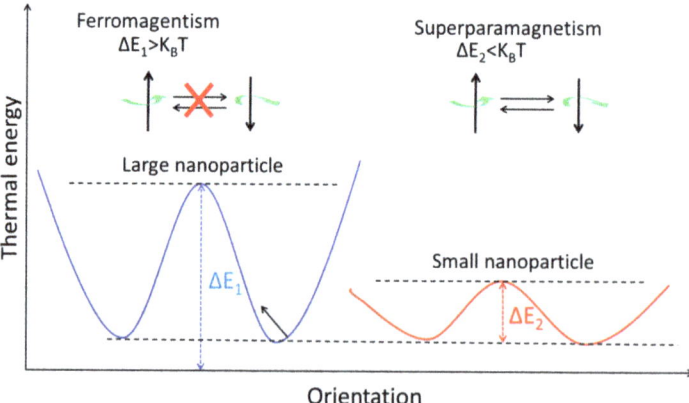

Figure 3. The energy levels of magnetic NPs with varying magnetic spin orientations. When it comes to stopping the magnetization from rotating, thermal energy ($K_B T$) is the limiting factor. Both ferromagnetism and superparamagnetism may be seen in the large and small NPs, respectively.

2.2. Fluorescent Nanoparticles

Over the course of the last ten years, research and development efforts have been heavily concentrated on fluorescent NPs [37,47–51]. These NPs include semiconductor

NPs (quantum dots), metal NPs, silica NPs, polymer NPs, and many more [52–54]. In comparison to traditional fluorescent organic dyes, fluorescent NPs exhibit a more brilliant fluorescence, increased photostability, and enhanced biocompatibility. In addition, the NPs have a distinct set of chemical and optical characteristics [55,56]. Several different kinds of fluorescent NPs have emerged for bioimaging over the past few decades. These include organic-dye-doped silica NPs, organic polymer NPs, metallic NPs, carbon-based NPs (nanotubes and nanodots) [57], quantum dots (QDs) [58–60], and lanthanide-doped upconverting nanoparticles (UCNPs) [61–63]. In terms of their composition, fluorescent NPs employed in bioimaging may be roughly divided into two categories: organic and inorganic NPs. In order to be considered among the best fluorescent probes for imaging, fluorescent NPs should generally meet the following characteristics: high signal-to-background ratio, big strokes to prevent self-quenching, excellent stability under physiological settings, little cytotoxicity, and minimum disruption of biological activities, to name only a few. They also have limited fluorescence durations, typically around 10^{-9} s, which is insufficient for efficiently separating short-lived fluorescence interference from dispersed excitation light.

Optical biosensors based on fluorescence may be divided into two categories: those that use downconversion fluorescence and those that use upconversion fluorescence. Downconversion fluorescence, the foundation of most existing optical biosensors, works by transforming the energy of light, often in the ultraviolet to visible light range, into a more usable form. These probes excel in chemical, photochemical, and thermal stability, and their long fluorescence lifetimes make them ideal for biosensing applications. They are vulnerable to photobleaching and blinking, and their overlapping excitation and emission spectra are a challenge for multiplexing applications [64]. In addition, biological samples include endogenous fluorophores, such as hemoglobin, which strongly absorb and scatter light below 700 nm, resulting in a high background fluorescence that can only penetrate biological media superficially. These limitations of downconversion-based biosensors have severely stymied their use in biosensing and bioimaging. Nanoparticles based on upconversion fluorescence (UCNPs) have significant potential for use in biomedical settings due to their ability to convert near-infrared (NIR) light into visible light [65]. Due to its providing an optically clear window onto biological tissues, NIR light has attracted a lot of attention as an excitation source for biosensing and bioimaging in recent years [66].

2.3. Types of Noninvasive Imaging

Recently, a variety of noninvasive optical imaging techniques, including computed tomography (CT), magnetic resonance (MR), positron emission tomography (PET), single-photon emission CT (SPECT), ultrasound (US), and optical imaging (OI), as well as their variants and subcategories, have been described [67,68]. Each one is distinct from the others in respect of resolution and sensitivity complexity, the length of time required to obtain data, and cost. The selection of an imaging modality is largely determined by the precise question that needs answering, and various imaging modalities are often complimentary rather than in competition. Medical imaging with magnetic resonance (MRI) is another technique that has expanded greatly in recent years. MRI is particularly useful for diagnosing conditions affecting soft tissues [69]. Furthermore, the drawbacks of each approach, such as MRI's low sensitivity and OI's lack of anatomical background information, cancel each other out.

2.4. Magnetic Resonance Imaging (MRI)

The MRI method was developed from the foundations of nuclear magnetic resonance. NMR signals obtained from hydrogen nuclei placed in various physiological contexts throughout an organism are used to create tissue contrasts, which are then used for diagnostic purposes. The frequencies at which nuclear spins resonate when a specimen is immersed in a homogeneous, static magnetic field are proportional to the strength of the magnetic field. Specimens are activated by a radiofrequency pulse at their resonance frequency in order to alter their net magnetization once they have established an equilibrium magnetization. Three-dimensional pictures of the body are constructed by measuring the variations in generated electromagnetic signals in the presence of linear field gradients. MRI is a powerful diagnostic tool for detecting lesions in the brain and spinal cord due to its high tissue specificity. Figure 4 shows the main contributors to the overall signal and contrast levels obtained from a sample.

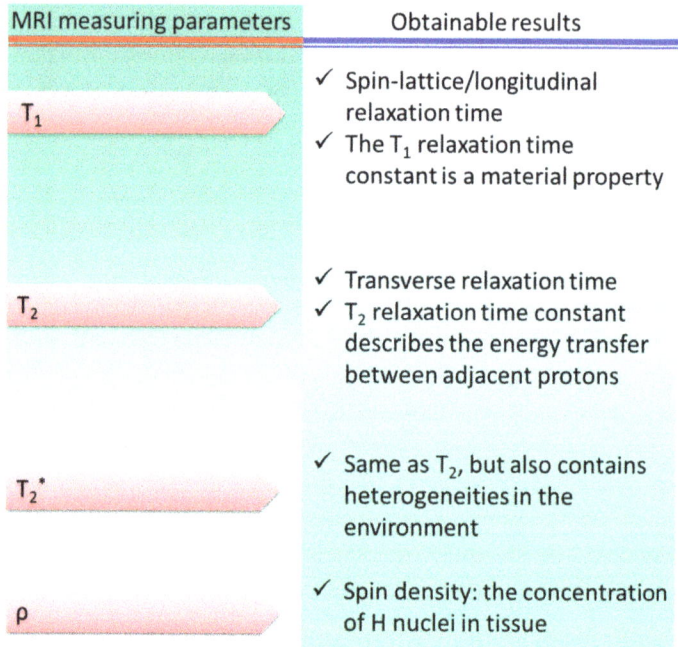

Figure 4. Parameters of magnetic resonance imaging: sources of signal variation. * represents a separate variable.

2.5. Computed Tomography (CT)

Over the past decade, there has been a meteoric surge in the number of papers published on the use of microcomputed tomography (CT) imaging in preclinical in vivo research [70,71]. Better spatial and temporal resolution has enabled researchers to acquire more precise anatomical pictures of small animals and track the development of illnesses in small-animal models. Although organs and tumors are not easily visible on CT images without the use of iodinated contrast agents, CT has poor soft-tissue contrast for malignancies and surrounding tissues [72–74]. At first, CT had great spatial resolution but low contrast in soft tissues. The noninvasive examination of high-contrast structures, such as bones and implants, was hence the primary emphasis of the earliest publications on the utilization of CT. There have been significant increases in the temporal and geometrical resolutions, as well as the readout speeds, of X-ray detectors as technology has developed. A μCT method with a spatial resolution of 1–100 μm is denoted as μCT [75]. μCT has the potential to supplant the laborious serial staining procedures needed for the histomorphometric examination of thin slices, and it might also be used to conduct longitudinal in vivo investigations in tiny animals. Given CT's short imaging duration and great spatial resolution, it can be utilized to examine lung cancers and bone metastases. μCT has been employed in high-throughput phenotyping methods for a large number of transgenic mice, allowing for the detection of gross defects. To examine cell trafficking, tumor development, and response to treatment in vivo, μCT images showing tumor structural features were coregistered with bioluminescence pictures. This approach to image processing has the potential to be employed in evaluating hematological reconstitution after bone-marrow transplantation. CT is useful because of the high spatial resolution (12–50 µm) that is required to observe minute anatomical features. Functional imaging methods can be used with CT to reveal metabolic and dynamic details. Comparisons of in vivo trabecular structures and mineralization densities between mice strains were made in osseous disease investigations to account for any variations in experimental design and data collection [76]. Similar to CT angiography (CTA) in humans, contrast-agent injection is required for in vivo examination of vascular systems using CT in small animals. Vessel analysis in rats after sacrifice [13] was possible with the older, somewhat slow CT scanners, with scanning periods extending up to hours, employing perfusion with radiopaque polymerizing chemicals [77] or shock freezing of the contrast-agent-perfused material [78].

3. Synthesis and Fabrication of Magneto-Fluorescent Nanoparticles

Nanotechnology has grown rapidly over the past few decades as a new discipline that bridges previously separate scientific disciplines, such as biology, medicine, chemistry, materials engineering, quantum mechanics, and electronics. The benefits of nanomaterials, such as their high surface-to-volume ratios, unique optical characteristics, and nanoscale physical phenomena, have led to their widespread usage in scientific study and medical practice. Superparamagnetism at room temperature is a defining characteristic of MNPs (e.g., Fe_3O_4, γ-Fe_2O_3, or a combination of the two) when their size is small enough [79]. Molecular nanoparticles (MNPs) have the potential to be used in ferrofluid technology [80] and heterogeneous catalysis due to their extremely high surface-to-volume ratios and in the cleanup of polluted or contaminated environmental media [81]. Furthermore, it has recently been considered that MNPs might be used for a variety of biological applications (magnetic contrast agents, hyperthermia agents, magnetic vectors for drug administration, etc.). While MNPs have great potential for biomedical applications, they must first meet a number of requirements that are often contradictory. These include: (a) extremely low toxicity to the human body; (b) outstanding magnetic properties; (c) a relatively narrow size distribution; and (d) the ability to have their surfaces easily modified (through coating) in order to allow their functionalization for particular bioagents. Since magnetite (Fe_3O_4) and maghemite (γ-Fe_2O_3) NPs have been shown to be biocompatible, they are good choices to meet the first two requirements [79]. Additionally, MNPs with high stability, biocompatibility, and low toxicity may be created and employed in a wide range of biomedical applications after being modified by functional components [82].

The creation of specific magneto-fluorescent NPs has attracted a lot of attention in recent years. Although these nanocomposites have a wide range of compositions and morphologies, we have categorized the preparation techniques into two types of synthetic strategy: the coupling approach and the encapsulation method, based on reports from a variety of sources. Table 1 lists several common methods for synthesizing composite NPs and the various ways they might be employed.

Table 1. Synthetic tailored magneto-fluorescent multimodal nanoparticles (NPs) and potential uses.

Nanoparticles	Method	Targeting Ligand	Application	Ref.
Fe_3O_4/anti-IgG/GQD/BSA	Coupling	Human IgG	Urine renal disease	[83]
Ab (anti-aflatoxin B1)–CdS–Fe_3O_4 bioconjugates	Coupling	Aflatoxin B1	Detection of aflatoxin B_1 B_1 in corn samples	[84]
Dox-loaded carbon dot (CD)–4-carboxyphenylboronic acid (CBBA)–$MnFe_2O_4$ NPs [DCCM]	Coupling	Sialic acid	HeLa cells	[85]
Iron oxide superparamagnetic NPs-PEG-Cypher5E/folic acid	Coupling	Folic acid	MR imaging and fluorescence imaging	[86]
Fe_3O_4(MNP)-Cds(QDs)-folic acid	Coupling	Folic acid	As a delivery agent and an in vitro imaging diagnostic agent	[87]

Table 1. Cont.

Nanoparticles	Method	Targeting Ligand	Application	Ref.
MTX-PEG-CS-IONPs-Cy5.5	Coupling	Folic acid	Dual-model imaging and synergistically self-targeted cancer therapy	[88]
Fe_3O_4-dopamine hydrobromide (DPA)-PEG-FA/FITC NPs	Coupling	Folic acid	Targeted imaging of various tumors	[89]
Fe_3O_4-CdTe-humanized monoclonal antibody CC49 (hCC49 antibody)	Coupling	Tumor-associated glycoprotein-72 (TAG-72)	Cancer cell imaging	[90]
Fe_3O_4@$mSiO_2$–triphenylphospine (TPP)/CD	Coupling	Mitochondria	Mitochondrial diseases	[91]
BRCAA1 antibody-FMNPs (Fe_3O_4-CdTe)	Encapsulation	BRCAA1 protein	In vivo dual-model imaging of gastric cancer	[92]
FMN (flavin mononucleotide)-coated ultrasmall superparamagnetic iron oxide (FLUSPIO)	Encapsulation	Riboflavin (Rf)	Prostate cancer xenografts	[93]
MNPs@OPE[oligo(p-phenylene ethynylene)]-PEG-FA		Folate receptor	Targeted magnetic resonance and two-photon optical imaging in vitro and in vivo	[94]
Fe_3O_4@SiO_2/RhBITC-anti-HER2 antibody NPs	Encapsulation	Human epidermal growth factor receptor 2 (HER2)	Discrimination of HER2-positive breast cancer cells	[95]
Fe_3O_4@SiO_2(FITC)-FA/AICAR(5-aminoimidazole-4-carboxamide-1-β-D-ribofuranoside)/DOX	Encapsulation	Folate receptor	Inhibition of cancer cell growth	[96]
PTX/Fe_3O_4 NPs/$CuInS_2$/ZnS QDs@biotin–PEG–PCD [abiotin–poly(ethylene glycol)–poly(curcumin-dithiodipropionic acid) copolymer]	Encapsulation	Biotin receptor	Treatment of multidrug-resistant breast cancer at the cellular level	[97]
Trastuzumab-conjugated Lipo[MNP@m-SiO_2(FITC)]	Encapsulation	Her2/neu	In vitro fluorescence and MR imaging of Her2/neu-positive breast cancer	[98]
Fe_3O_4/$CuInS_2$(CIS)@SiO_2(Gd–DTPA)–RGD (arginine-glycine-aspartic acid)	Encapsulation	$\alpha V \beta 3$ integrin	MR and fluorescence imaging of pancreatic cancer	[99]

There have been few attempts made to construct hybrid systems, despite the rising interest in and the relevance of SPIONs and SiQDs to the fabrication of biodegradable and biocompatible nanoprobes for biomedical use. Conjugation of the two systems and studies of their conjugated characteristics are scarce, and obstacles such as charge or energy transfer processes and iron oxide's high absorption in the visible spectrum make even their simple fabrication by quenching QD/SiQDs PL difficult [100]. Long interparticular spacers are usually employed to avoid such disadvantages and ensure the flourishing of both luminous and magnetic characteristics [101]. Covalent binding and electrostatic absorption are used to couple the magnetic and fluorescent species shown in Figure 5 after they have been synthesized and functionalized independently. In this procedure, the coupling strategy for magnetic and fluorescent NPs is determined by the modifications made to their surfaces. Thiol, carboxyl, and amino groups are all examples of functional moieties that may be found in the coupling agents [102]. The formation of core–shell structures on the surfaces of magnetic materials often involves loading fluorescent elements onto the top of a magnetic material by either bond formation or charge attraction. After that, conjugation of specific ligands onto the surfaces of the magneto-fluorescent NPs is often performed. In another method, which is illustrated in Figure 5, the cores of new composite micro- or nanospheres are formed by encasing prefabricated fluorescent NPs and magnetic NPs in various materials, such as silica or polymer beads, protein, chitosan, and liposomes. This results in the formation of new NPs. In order to create these composite nanospheres, two different approaches have been utilized. These materials give the NPs favorable features, such as strong biocompatibility and stability and facile functionalization, to enable the inclusion of ligands so that the NPs may be selectively targeted physiologically. These materials also make the incorporation of ligands easier [103]. Since the existing coupling techniques are straightforward and provide a number of important benefits, a wide variety of magneto-fluorescent NPs have been fabricated and put to use in a variety of subfields of biomedicine. However, the stability of NPs generated in this manner frequently shifts in response to varied settings; as a result, their applications in biomedicine are restricted. When compared to magneto-fluorescent NPs created using the coupling approach, those prepared using the encapsulation method provide a number of benefits, including the ones listed below:

(a) NPs can be covalently modified with diverse targeted ligands using the surface functionalities of silica or polymer nanospheres without a stable structure.
(b) However, controlling the proportion of MNPs to luminescent NPs is difficult, making the production of well-dispersed, homogeneous, multimodal NPs complicated.
(c) Additionally, the outer layer of silica or polymer, which may serve as a screen, may play a role in preventing unwanted particles from entering.

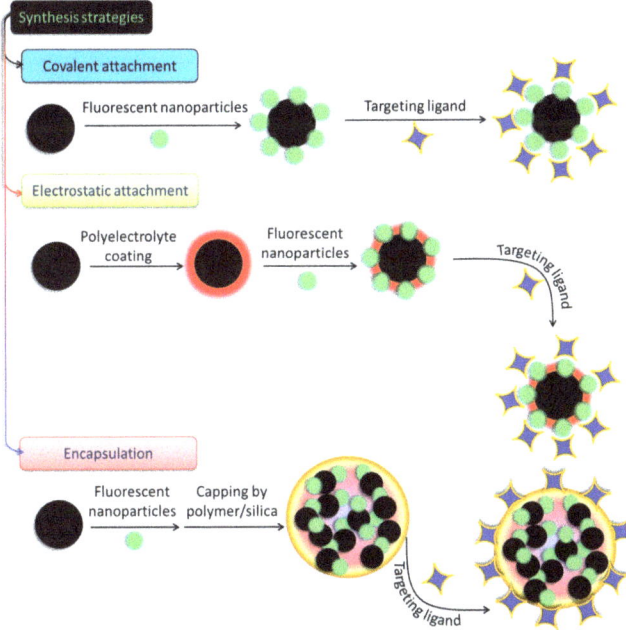

Figure 5. Different approaches to prepare fluorescent-nanoparticle-decorated magnetic nanostructures.

4. Magento-Fluorescent Nanobioprobe for Cancer Targeting

The health sector can benefit greatly from fluorescent and magnetic materials. Due to their unique optical and magnetic capabilities, typical materials such as quantum dots (QDs) and iron-oxide NPs have attracted the attention of scientists for decades. Nanomaterials such as quantum dots (QDs) have the potential to revolutionize in vitro biolabeling, in vivo targeting, and imaging thanks to their unique combination of broad and continuous absorption, narrow and symmetric fluorescence emission, and intense and steady fluorescence. Bioseparation, immobilization of cells and enzymes, medication administration, magnetic resonance imaging, and thermotherapy are just a few of the many applications of magnetic nanoparticles. QDs and magnetic nanoparticles have been found to coexist in nanocomposites in recent years. Macrophages and related immune cells have been intensively explored for insights into the internalization pathways of synthetic NPs, such as superparamagnetic iron oxide nanoparticles (SPIONs) and gold NPs. Upon internalization of SPIONs, multivesicular bodies are formed in the cytoplasm via a time-dependent vesicle-bound route. It is generally agreed that some internalized SPIONs are degraded in lysosomes, while others are released into the cytoplasmic compartments for continued metabolism [104]. Previous research has shown that NPs such as gold NPs are subject to varying degrees of absorption by HeLa cells depending on various factors, including particle size and shape [105]. A simplified graphical illustration has been given in Figure 6 for easy visualization.

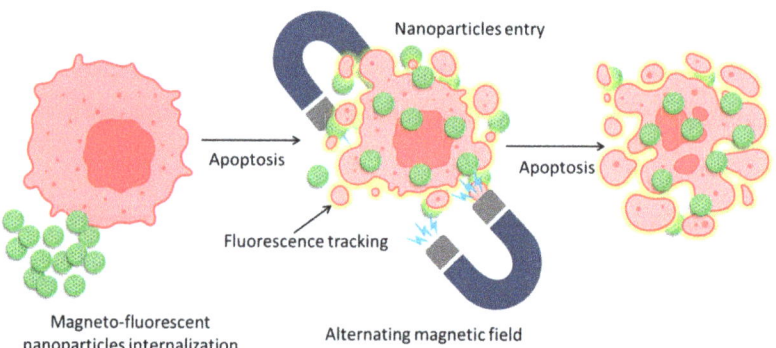

Figure 6. Mechanism of magnetic nanoparticle internalization into cancer cells and their tracking and apoptotic behavior against an alternating magnetic field.

Quantum dots (QDs) were immobilized on the surface of superparamagnetic polystyrene nanospheres, and the novel combination of fluorescence emission and hyperthermia engineered in these nanocomposites is expected to be used in therapeutic trials for concurrent in vivo imaging and local therapy via hyperthermia [106]. Similarly, in another study, CdTe/CdS quantum dots (QDs) and Fe_3O_4 NPs were encapsulated in silica-coated magnetic polystyrene nanospheres (MPNs) [107]. Although the bioconjugates were useful in identifying and sorting cancer cells, they were unable to perform these functions in the case of K562 cells because they lacked surface expression of human epidermal growth factor receptor (EGFR). By using a direct amide coupling procedure, iron oxide nanoparticles and CdS quantum dots were successfully synthesized to form a multifunctional hybrid nanocomposite material [108]. These NPs were further coupled with folic acid to test their potential as a molecular imaging probe. Cell uptake and cytotoxicity experiments were performed on normal mouse splenocytes, C6 rat glioma cells, and A549 human lung adenocarcinoma epithelial cells. C6 cell green fluorescence emission demonstrated uptake of nanoparticles. Research using Prussian blue staining has hinted at the existence of iron oxide within cells. To add to this, it was shown that folic acid-conjugated nanocomposites were considerably hazardous to C6 cells only after 48 h, but not to A549 cells or splenocytes.

Chitosan-encapsulated NPs of iron oxide (for use as MRI contrast agents), cadmium sulfide (for use as a fluorescence probe), and podophyllotoxin (for use as an anticancer medication) were produced and described as multifunctional hybrid nanocomposite materials [109]. KB, C6, and A549 cancer cell lines were used to test the efficacy of these nanocomposites in combating various forms of the disease. The existence of these nanocomposites in KB and C6 cells, but not A549 cells, was verified by fluorescence imaging and Perl's Prussian blue staining. Experiments on cytotoxicity demonstrated that the nanocomposites covered with biopolymers were only slightly harmful to cancer cells. For targeted tumor imaging, NPs with strong near-infrared (NIR) fluorescence were produced for use in T_1- and T_2-weighted MR imaging. Wang et al. combined T_1- and T_2-weighted magnetic resonance imaging (MRI) with fluorescence imaging of malignancies by incorporating ultrasmall Fe_3O_4 NPs (2–3 nm) with an NIR-emitting semiconducting polymer [110]. Multimodal fluorescent magnetic nanoparticles (FMNPs) with folic acid functionalization glow brightly under fluorescent light and relax slowly. In a different study, the thiol-induced assembly of magneto-fluorescent nanoparticles mimicking hydrangea flowers was described [111]. Thiol-metal bonding and surface functionalization allow for a straightforward strategy for creating magneto-fluorescent Fe_3O_4-SH@QD NPs which have the form of flowers like hydrangeas. MRI and biolabels, targeting and photodynamic treatment, cell tracking and separation, amongst other technologies, might all benefit from magneto-fluorescent Fe_3O_4-SH@QD NPs' efficient fluorescence, superparamagnetism at room temperature, and fast reaction to an external field. For fluorescence and magnetic resonance imaging of cancer cells, setua et al. developed a nanobioprobe based on doped Y_2O_3 nanocrystals [112]. Up to this point, the vast majority of research efforts have been focused on creating C-dots doped with nonmetals. Furthermore, there have been very few reports of investigations concerning the production and usage of heavy-metal-doped C-dots. Gadolinium-doped C-dots, also known as Gd-CQDs, are dual-fluorescence and MRI probes that were recently synthesized by Yang Xu et al. [113]. Both in vitro and in vivo testing demonstrated that they have low toxicity levels and are highly biocompatible. Due to the large amount of Gd present in Gd–CQDs and their hydrophilicity, it was shown that these particles had a greater MR response than gadopentetic acid dimeglumine (Gd–DTPA) (Figure 7). The authors discovered that Gd–CQDs dispersed themselves in tissues in a heterogeneous manner: some of them penetrated the tissue cells, while others were identified less often in the extracellular matrix. In order to detect Fe^{3+} ions, Quan Xu and colleagues created Cu-doped C-dots to use as fluorescent-sensing probes [114]. Recent research carried out by our team has resulted in the successful development of Ag/C-dot and Au/C-dot nanohybrids derived from lemon extract for the purpose of cancer cellular imaging [115]. To begin with, metal-oxide NPs, such as iron-oxide (Fe_2O_3/Fe_3O_4), manganese dioxide (MnO), yttrium dioxide (Gd_2O_3), and dysprosium dioxide (Dy_2O_3), were used [116–118]. Pakkath et al. used lemon extract and an efficient, one-pot, microwave-assisted pyrolysis process (Figure 8) to produce transition-metal-ion-doped C-dots (TMCDs) containing Mn^{2+}, Fe^{2+}, Co^{2+}, and Ni^{2+} within 6 min [119].

The success of these magneto-fluorescent NPs will depend heavily on their sizes, which must be programmable, the magnetic and optical signals, their long-term stability, and the variety of surface functionalities. The MRI contrast agent is encapsulated in a fluorescent quantum dot (QD) core that is enclosed inside a hollow magnetic shell, as shown by pahari et al. [120]. As can be observed in Figure 9A–D, a fluorescence quantum efficiency of roughly 16% (measured in buffered aqueous media) is adequate for optical microscopy imaging of 3D cell growth. Images taken with a wide-field optical microscope revealed a single drop of 3D cell culture on a Matrigel scaffold, originating from mouse cerebral tissue, on a 32 mm cell-culture dish. CdSe@CdS@Fe_2O_3 nanoparticle markers were added to the Sprague–Dawley rat embryonic cells 6 days before harvesting the cells at day 13 in vitro. Red fluorescent NPs (620 nm peak) were likely to be localized inside the cells, as they were found in close proximity to the nuclei.

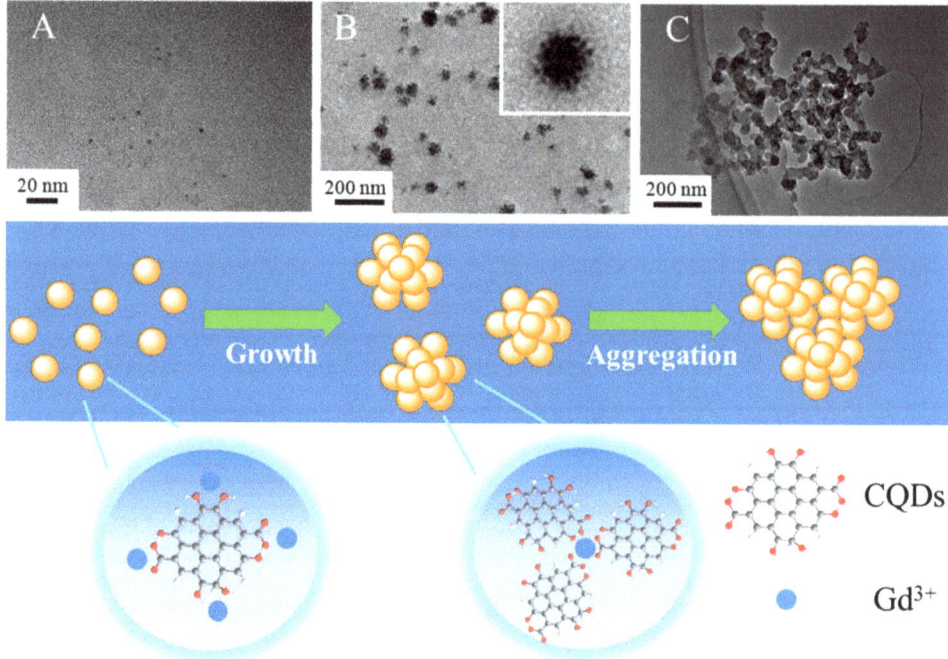

Figure 7. (**A**) TEM photos of the hydrothermal products after varied incubation durations, including (**A**) 1 h, (**B**) 3 h, and (**C**) 5 h, as well as a schematic illustration of the process of Gd–CQD synthesis [113].

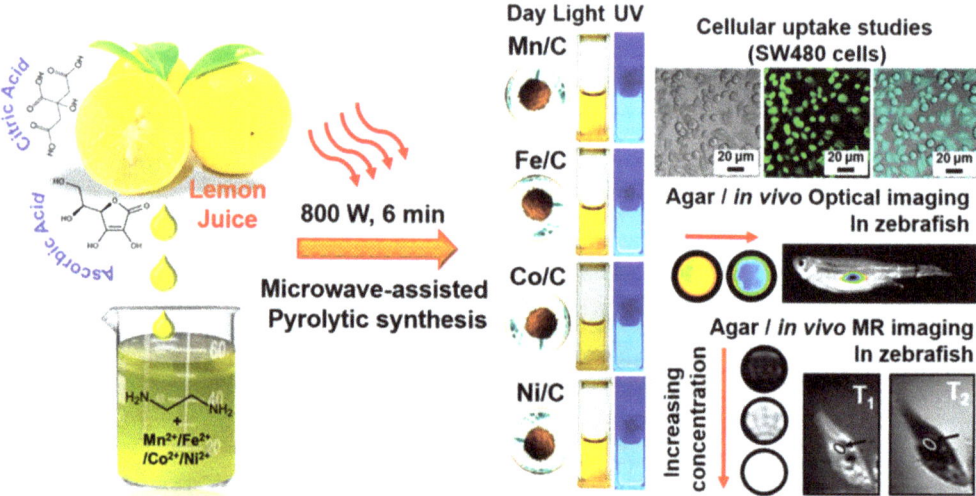

Figure 8. Microwave-assisted pyrolytic synthesis of EDA-functionalized TMCDs as possible nanoprobes for magneto-fluorescent bioimaging depicted schematically [119].

High-efficiency cellular imaging was achieved by preparing and using new fluorescent/magnetic NPs [121]. The nanoparticles covered in modified chitosan had a magnetic oxide core and a fluorescent dye linked to it through covalent bonds. We tested how well the NPs worked at marking cancer cells. Flow cytometry and magnetic resonance imaging both showed that the nanoparticles had a strong affinity for cells. The findings demonstrated that the nanoparticles' efficacy in labeling cells was sensitive to both the length of incubation and the concentration of the nanoparticles used.

It is becoming increasingly obvious that techniques for identifying multiple key targets in size-limited clinical specimens will be essential in order to assess the temporal and spatial conditions of signal transduction networks and to realize the goal of personalized medicine. The molecular diversity of human cells, especially cancer cells, is quite high. Western blotting, flow cytometry, immunofluorescence imaging, and immunohistochemistry require extraordinarily high cell densities, cannot be multiplexed, and have low throughputs. As a result, these approaches are restricted in terms of the quantity of information that can be retrieved from clinical specimens. Improved intracellular biomarker sensing using nanoparticles was reported by Haun et al.; the method used is based on bio-orthogonal chemistry [122]. They also demonstrated that this method could detect protein biomarkers and phosphoprotein signal mediators in the cytosol and nucleus, respectively, using either magnetic or fluorescence modalities. In order to enclose highly ferrimagnetic nanoparticles and ZnS/InP quantum dots, Song et al. described the use of an amphiphilic block copolymer containing a flowable hydrophobic chain [123]. The uniform diameter of the resulting ferrimagnetic fluorescent micelle (FMFM) was around 180 nm. Common poly(D,L-lactide) (PLA)-based amphiphilic block copolymer with a stiff hydrophobic chain unavoidably led to greater aggregation (400 nm in diameter), which was easily removed by the reticuloendothelial system (RES). Long-term colloidal stability in the flowable FMFM was seen within one month, and the necessary fluorescent stability was achieved within 84 h. Iron-based nanoparticles (IBNs) are ideal because they are biocompatible and may be directed at a tumor by a variety of methods (passive targeting, active targeting, or magnetic targeting). When necessary, IBNs can also be combined with other well-known fluorescent substances, such as dyes, ICG that has been authorized for therapeutic use, fluorescent proteins, and quantum dots. Depending on whether or not IBNs are paired with a fluorescent substance, they may also be stimulated and identified by means of existing optical techniques that rely on scattering or fluorescence processes. Systems that combine IBNs with optical techniques are versatile, allowing for several approaches to tumor detection. Such methods can also identify solitary tumor cells by combining IBNs with near-field scanning optical, dark-field, confocal, and super-resolution microscopy and recognize interactive manifestations, such as the permeation of a chromophore substance in an organism by utilizing photoluminescence lifetime imaging and fluorescence correlation spectroscopy. There is significant promise in the biological sciences for site-specific multimodal nanoplatforms with fluorescent-magnetic characteristics. By linking the human holo-transferrin to an optically and magnetically active bimodal nanosystem composed of quantum dots and iron oxide nanoparticles, Filho et al. created a multimodal nanoprobe (BNP-Tf) (Tf) [124]. There are several types of magneto-fluorescence for multimodal imaging and drug-delivery purposes, as shown in Table 2. The new BNP-Tf nanoplatform was effective in labeling the TfR at doses that did not produce any substantial toxic impact in HeLa cells for at least 24 h and remained active for at least two months. Using MRI, flow cytometry, and fluorescence microscopy, we showed that HeLa cells tagged specifically with BNP-Tf not only generated a strong fluorescence but also displayed a high r_2/r_1 relaxivity ratio, making it potentially an appealing probe for obtaining fluorescence and T_2-weighted MR images. Enumerating and analyzing CTCs in circulation has become a powerful tool in cancer diagnosis and prognosis. However, for accurate and sensitive CTC detection, it is a major difficulty to successfully harvest lowly abundant CTCs with high purity from blood samples in a quick and high-throughput way. To rapidly magnetically isolate CTCs from human blood with high capture efficiency and purity approaching 80%, a novel class of DNA-templated magnetic nanoparticle-quantum dot (QD)-aptamer copolymers (MQAPs) were designed. QD photoluminescence (PL) is used to concurrently profile the phenotypes of CTCs at the single-cell level. These MQAPs are built via a hybridization chain process to boost the magnetic response, increase the binding selectivity for target cells over background cells, and make the QD PL in the ensemble extremely bright, allowing for single-cell identification. Nonspecific binding does not occur on MQAPs, ensuring that captured cells are as pure as possible. For the purpose of magnetically isolating rare cancer cells, li et al. produced a new class of MNP-QD-aptamer copolymers with high CE and CP that are advantageous for practical applications. These MQAPs are ideal for isolating and identifying CTCs in challenging environments thanks to their linear compact construction, strong magnetic sensitivity, excellent selectivity, and high PL intensity [125]. This method not only has excellent capture purity, but also identifies CTC phenotypes without the need for any further fixation or permeabilization processes. It was possible to successfully release the MQAPs from the cells while the cells themselves remained alive upon isolation. This provides new opportunities for the bioinspired design of tunable inorganic magneto-fluorescent materials for use in healthcare. Cancer molecular imaging (MI) is an emerging area of diagnostic imaging that offers new ways to study cancer biology in living organisms. In an effort to improve signal and/or contrast, binding avidity, and targeting specificity in the early detection of cancer, a wide range of targeted nanoprobes (NPs) have been created. Cancer cells differ from normal cells in their overexpression patterns of folate receptors (FRs) on the cell surface. Therefore, there has been a lot of interest in using folic acid (FA) or folate-conjugated NPs as diagnostic agents and treatments and even their combination usage as theranostics to target FR-overexpressing tumor cells. Owing to the strong binding between the ligand and its receptor, FR-specific MI methods have a number of advantages. Magnetic resonance imaging (MRI), computed tomography (CT), optical and nuclear imaging (ONI), and ultrasonography (US) are just a few of the clinical imaging modalities that may be tailored for use with NPs.

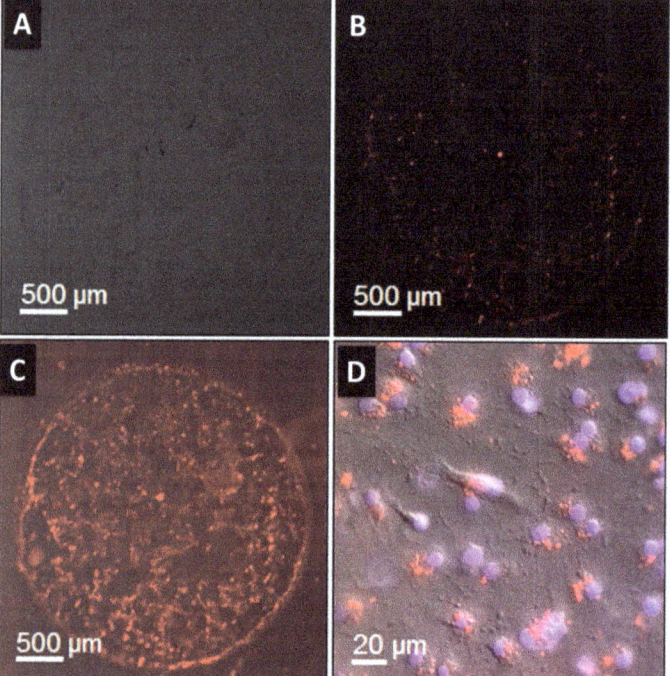

Figure 9. (**A**) Bright-field picture showing all cells; (**B**) red fluorescence image revealing QD in nanoparticles, which are specifically localized using a Rhodamine filter; (**C**) merged image; (**D**) magnification of (**C**) showing few individual cells. Hoechst staining marks cell nuclei blue. Nanoparticles (red dots) near nuclei indicate cell localization [120].

Table 2. Different types of magneto-fluorescent nanoparticles, their magnetic characters, and specific applications.

Magnetic Part	Fluorescent Part	Size (nm)	Magnetization (emu/g)	Application	Ref.
Fe_3O_4	FITC	125	-	Cell imaging	[126]
Fe_3O_4	RhB	30	8	Cell membrane imaging	[127]
$CoFe_2O_4$–Cr_2O_3	-	30	5	Cell imaging	[128]
γ-Fe_2O_3	FITC	9	-	MRI and fluorescence imaging	[129]
Fe_3O_4	Poly(methacrylic acid)	280	30–60	Cell labeling and drug delivery	[130]
Fe_3O_4	CdSe/CdS QDs	9	15	Mouse brain imaging	[131]
Fe_3O_4	RITC/SiO_2	60	-	MRI and fluorescence imaging (tumor)	[132]
Fe_3O_4	QDs/PEG	150	-	Circulatory fluorescence imaging	[133]
Fe_3O_4	CdSe/ZnS	35–45	-	Cell imaging	[134]
Fe_3O_4	CdTe/ZnS	185	37	Anticancer drug release and imaging	[135]
Fe_3O_4	FITC	11	-	Fluorescence imaging	[136]
Fe_3O_4/Fe_2O_3	Cy5.5	97	-	Neovasculature	[137]
Fe_3O_4	Yb^{3+}/Er^{3+}/Tm^{3+}/$NaYF_4$	80	38	Cell imaging	[138]
Fe_3O_4	CdSe	-	-	Cell imaging	[139]
Fe_3O_4	RhB	-	-	Cell imaging	[140]
Fe_3O_4	CdTe	70–80	6	Cell imaging and drug delivery	[141]
Fe_3O_4	CdTe	50–1000	-	Field-assisted cell alignment	[142]
Fe_3O_4	CdTe	34	60	Cell imaging	[143]
Fe_3O_4	FITC	14	55	MRI contrast agent	[121]
Fe_3O_4	Atto 390/fluorescein/Rh6G	100–400	-	Magneto-sensitive fluorescence imaging	[144]
Fe_3O_4	Ce6	20–30	50	Tumor cell imaging	[145]
$CoFe_2O_4$	RhB/RITC	60	-	Cell imaging	[146]
FePt	CdS	10	5	Cell imaging	[147]
Fe_3O_4	FITC	600–700	17	Cell imaging	[148]
Fe_3O_4	ZnS	100	30	Cell imaging	[149]
Fe_3O_4	CdTe/CdS	8	-	Cell imaging	[150]
$Zn_{0.4}Fe_{2.6}O_4$	Drug	160	-	Drug release and imaging	[151]
FePt	Atto 590	5	-	Cell imaging	[152]
Iron oxide	Cy7	21	-	MRI	[153]
Fe_3O_4	PDI-PAA	60	7	Cell imaging	[154]
Fe_3O_4	FITC	36	23	Cell imaging	[155]
Fe_3O_4	Squarylium indocyanine	51	8	Cell imaging	[24]

5. Magento-Fluorescent Nanobioprobe for MRI

Magneto-fluorescent particles are known to be promising new materials for cutting-edge uses. However, it has been difficult to synthesize magneto-fluorescent nanomaterials with desirable characteristics, such as uniform and adjustable size, high-magnetic-content loading, maximum fluorophore coverage at the surface, and flexible surface functioning. An easy method was revealed by chem et al. for combining magnetic nanoparticles with fluorescent quantum dots to create colloidal magneto-fluorescent supernanoparticles [131]. The core of these supernanoparticles is made up of tightly packed magnetic nanoparticles, while the shell is made up entirely of fluorescent quantum dots. High colloidal stability and biocompatibility, as well as adaptable surface functionality, are all provided by a thin layer of silica coating. Following surface pegylation, we showed that these silica-coated magneto-fluorescent supernanoparticles may be magnetically controlled inside live cells while being optically monitored. Quantum dots (QDs) doped with gadolinium paramagnetic ions have been identified as promising materials for fluorescence and magnetic-field-driven aquatic applications. Some intensely fluorescent Gd-doped AgInS2 QDs were supposedly synthesized at Gd molar ratios of 18–20 [156]. The new materials showed improved PL characteristics at greater Gd loadings than state-of-the-art materials, which showed poor PL features at higher Gd loadings. Aging, and the subsequent formation of a smaller particle size distribution, was linked to an improvement in PL characteristics. Increased medication delivery, water purification, and pollution monitoring are only some of the potential uses of this material, as demonstrated by the increased and sustained fluorescence at increasing magnetic Gd loadings. In order to meet the demand for magneto-fluorescent properties in a single unit, core–shell multifunctional nanostructures were produced [157]. High stability and integrity of the core and shell were achieved in the development of CdS quantum dots (QDs) on the surface of SrFe 12O19 nanoparticle cores, as evidenced by UV-visible spectroscopy, photoluminescence spectroscopy, VSM, and FTIR. Optical investigations can rule out the presence of flaws or core–shell structures and reveal comprehensive data on the emergence of any new phase at the interface. For nanostructures with core–shell geometries, the single magnetic domain structure is evinced by a small Stoner–Wohlfarth value. The goal of achieving anisotropy in only one direction, or "uniaxiality", was successfully met. The use of water in the synthesis broadens the potential range of uses for these nanostructures, especially in biology. Chitosan-encapsulated NPs of iron oxide (as MRI contrast agents), cadmium sulfide (as a fluorescent probe), and podophyllotoxin (as an anticancer medicine) were produced and described to create a multifunctional hybrid nanocomposite material [109]. Human oral cancer (KB) cells, rat glioma (C6) cells, and human lung adenocarcinoma (A549) cells were used for the in vitro research. Both fluorescence imaging and Perl's Prussian blue staining revealed the intracellular localization of these nanocomposites. The feasibility of these nanocomposites as dual-mode imaging probes was demonstrated by in vivo fluorescence imaging and Prussian blue staining investigations. Deposition of these nanocomposites in lung cells was seen in Wistar rat model biodistribution and toxicity tests, with no obvious ill effects on other essential organs. Cd-free Ag-In-S ternary quantum dots (t-QDs) with fluorescence lifetimes (LTs) of several hundred nanoseconds (ns) were paired with superparamagnetic Fe_3O_4 nanoparticles (SPIONs) and mesoporous $CaCO_3$ microbeads (Figure 10) to create a magneto-fluorescent bead platform, as described by Martynenko et al. [158], who also evaluated the feasibility of using these magneto-fluorescent microbeads as magneto-fluorescent carriers with distinct LT signatures for time-resolved flow cytometry in the biological sciences and biotechnology (LT-FCM). For a recently designed flow cytometer using photon counting detection and polymeric carrier beads doped with various organic dyes, we recently proved this encoding technique.

Carbon-coated core–shell multifunctional SPION (MFCSNP)-based drug delivery nanocarriers (MFCSNPs-FA-CHI-5FU nanocarriers) targeting folic acid and chitosan (FA-CHI) have been produced [159]. In addition to serving as a site-specific drug carrier, the pH-responsive release of 5-FU from MFCSNPs-FA-CHI-5FU nanocarriers demonstrates the utility of folic acid in this context. It was also discovered that MFCSNPs-FA-CHI-5FU nanocarriers show potential as T2-weighted MR contrast agents, and their contrast augmentation (signal darkening) in MR imaging is promising. Results from in vitro cytotoxicity tests as well as confocal microscopy imaging showed that MFCSNPs-FA-CHI-5FU nanocarriers are selective for folate-receptor-positive cancer cells and may be internalized via accumulation in the cell cytoplasm. Preliminary biological examination further supports the hemocompatibility and biocompatibility of the nanocarriers, allowing these multifunctional magnetic fluorescent NPs to be used as novel targeted theranostic devices. The effectiveness of MFCSNPs-FA-CHI-5FU nanocarriers as contrast agents was investigated using magnetic resonance imaging. By decreasing the magnitude of the transverse relaxation time, it has been proven that magnetic NPs can attenuate MR signal strength. Figure 11 shows a T2-weighted magnetic resonance image.

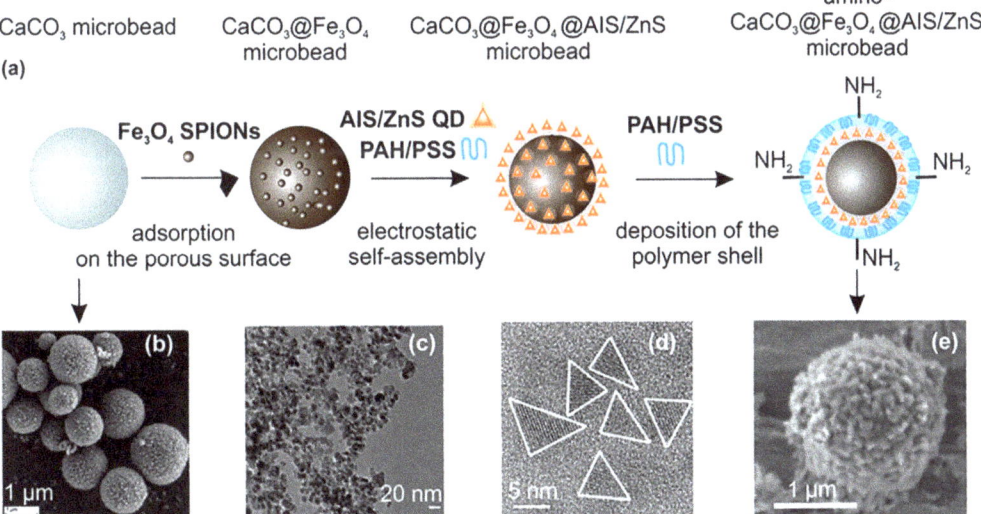

Figure 10. (**a**) Illustration of multistep synthesis of aminated magneto-fluorescent $CaCO_3$ microbeads and (**b–e**) SEM and TEM pictures of building blocks: (**b**) $CaCO_3$ spherical microparticles, (**c**) Fe_3O_4 SPIONs capped with PSS, (**d**) AIS/ZnS QDs stabilized with MPA, and (**e**) $CaCO_3@Fe_3O_4@AIS/ZnS$ microbeads containing amino surface groups for further bioconjugation [158].

In order to be useful in diagnostic imaging, bimodal magneto-fluorescent materials require surface-engineered nanoparticles with excellent biosafety, pronounced colloidal stability, large magnetic moments, and robust photoluminescence (PL) emission. For in vivo magneto-resonance and fluorescence dual-mode imaging of malignant tumors, Mohandes et al. proposed polymer-coated nanoparticles (PCNPs) based on manganese ferrites covered with a thin shell of nitrogen-doped carbon dots. Hybrid magneto-fluorescent nanoparticles may be easily synthesized by in situ thermolysis of metal oxalates and phenylenediamine in diphenyl ether [160]. After 60 min, the tumor may be seen clearly since the fluorescence intensity in the area containing the tumor tissue appears to rise with time. The remarkable efficacy of PCNPs as T2 contrast agents in clinical diagnosis has also been demonstrated by magnetic resonance imaging (MRI) of phantoms and animal instances. High-resolution MRI imaging of cardiomyocyte death in vivo has the potential to advance the discovery of effective new cardioprotective treatments. Thus, in vitro comparisons were made between the new nanoparticle AnxCLIO-Cy5.5 and annexin V-FITC for detecting apoptosis in cardiomyocytes, and both demonstrated a significant degree of colocalization [161]. Five mice were administered AnxCLIO-Cy5.5 and four were given CLIO-Cy5.5, both at a dosage of 2 mg Fe/kg, followed by temporary blockage of the left anterior descending

(LAD) artery, and MRI was performed. In vivo measurements of MR signal strength and myocardial T2* were taken in hypokinetic areas of the LAD distribution. To back up the in vivo results, fluorescence imaging was performed outside of living organisms. Mice treated with AnxCLIO-Cy5.5 had substantially shorter myocardial T2*s (8.1 vs. 13.2 ms, P 0.01) and a greater fluorescent target-to-background ratio (2.1 vs. 1.1, P 0.01). One more study described the use of a magneto-fluorescent theranostic nanocomplex targeted to neutrophil gelatinase-associated lipocalin (NGAL) for imaging and treatment of pancreatic cancer [162]. The agent was made up of a nanoshell with a silica core and a gold shell. An outer layer of silica encased approved NIR (ICG) and MR (iron oxide) contrast agents. Antibodies attached to the outsides of the complexes helped direct the agents to cells that made too much NGAL. Nanocomplex sizes were changed to give a plasmon resonance at about 808 nm.

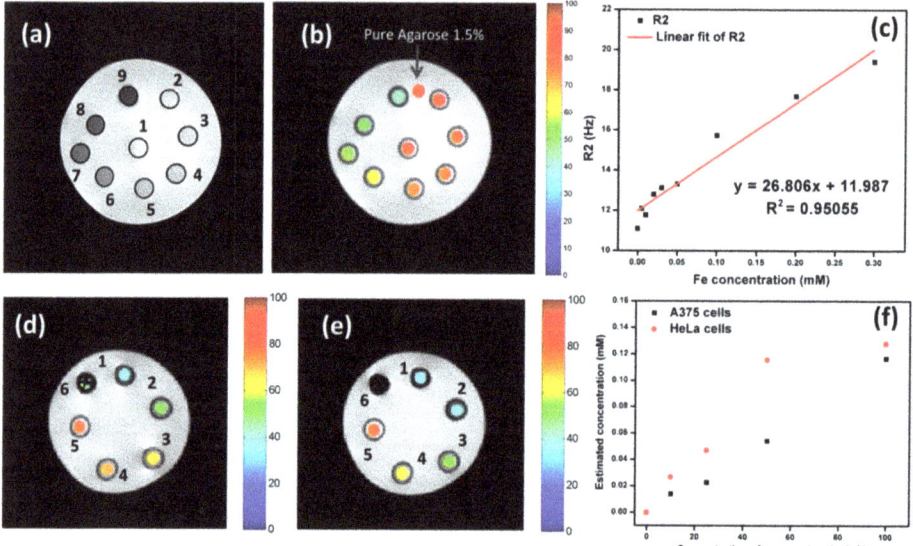

Figure 11. MRI (**a**) with a T2 weighting and (**b**) with a T2 map (ms) superimposed in color. MFCSNPs-FA-CHI-5FU nanocarrier concentrations are shown in part as numbers (1–9) that correspond to areas representing miniature phantom tubes. (**c**) Different concentrations of MFCSNPs in agarose (1.5%) were used to create phantoms, as detailed in the Experimental section. Fe concentration against R2 plot for MFCSNPs-FA-CHI-5FU nanocarriers (red line represents a linear fitting). MRI scans with color overlays of (**d**) A375 and (**e**) HeLa cells. Small phantom tubes containing A375 and HeLa cells were treated with varying quantities of MFCSNPs-FA-CHI-5FU nanocarriers (0–200 g/mL), as shown by the numbers (0 refers to cells only and 2–6 correspond to various concentrations of nanocarriers (0–200 g/mL)). (**f**) A concentration vs. relaxivity plot of nanocarriers incubated with cancer cells, with the y-axis representing the estimated concentration of internalized nanocarriers.

6. Magneto-Fluorescent Nanobioprobe for Positron Emission Tomography (PET) Imaging

It has gradually become apparent that the behavior of cells in vivo is significantly different from that observed in vitro, due to factors such as the presence of many cell types, complicated anatomical characteristics, fluid flow forces, and combinations of cytokines and chemokines. Hence, there is a pressing need to create and verify imaging methods permitting the study of cells in their natural environments. With the advent of new cell-tracking imaging techniques, cells delivered in animal models may be observed with an unparalleled level of detail and specificity. Nuclear-medicine imaging techniques, such as PET scans, are available. Radiotracers are radioactive substances used in nuclear medicine that are administered intravenously and at extremely low doses. In contrast to other types of imaging, PET scans may detect changes in metabolic processes and cellular activity. They may now be able to detect illness in its infancy. Radiotracers are taken up at a higher rate by diseased cells than by healthy ones. The term for these areas of high uptake is "hot spots". A PET scanner is able to detect this radiation and provide pictures of the afflicted tissue. PET scan pictures are combined with CT-scan X-rays to create a PET/CT scan. PET imaging's distinctive characteristics of very high sensitivity and precise determination of in vivo concentrations of radiotracers stem from the physics of the emission and the detection of the coinciding photons. In oncology, cardiology, and neurology, PET imaging has become an integral part of clinical practice. Preclinical research has also benefited greatly from PET imaging, especially when it comes to studying mouse models of illness and other small-animal models. However, PET imaging systems encounter a number of obstacles. Issues including integration with X-ray computed tomography and magnetic resonance imaging, as well as the basic trade-offs between resolution and noise, need to be addressed.

PET imaging can detect high-energy photons from decaying radioactive isotopes at low levels with far greater sensitivity than MRI. Nanoparticle labeling with PET isotopes such as ^{18}F has effectively lowered the detection threshold and increased sensitivity [163]. At a clinically relevant dosage, a fluorescently derivatized CLIO was coupled with ^{18}F by copper-catalyzed azide-alkyne cycloaddition, yielding a trimodal nanoparticle detectable through positron emission tomography (PET), fluorescence molecular tomography (FMT), and magnetic resonance imaging (MRI) (Figure 12). To put this another way, PET was 200 times more sensitive than MRI (16 times) and 50 times more sensitive than FMT (5 times) when it came to detecting 18F-magnetic nanoparticles. A strong positive correlation ($r^2 > 0.99$) exists between PET and FMT signals in agar-based phantoms when CLIO-based particles are used that contain 18F and the fluorescent dye VT680.

Imaging using 18F-CLIO PET-CT revealed considerably increased PET signals in murine aortic aneurysms compared to normal aortas, likely because 18F-CLIO targeted monocytes and macrophages within the aneurysm [164]. Radionuclide, fluorescent, histologic, and flow cytometric tests all corroborated the cellular probe distribution. Presently, risk indicators, such as aneurysm diameter, gathered from the community are used to determine whether or not the surgical excision of an aneurysm is warranted. Therapeutic choices might be made on an individual basis using nanoparticle-PET agent conjugates in response to molecular illness indicators, such as cellular inflammatory activity in the aneurysm. Using PET for in vivo imaging of leukocytes enables researchers in the field of immunology to monitor the selective recruitment of particular immune cells at various points in the pathogenesis of an illness, locate infectious or inflammatory hotspots, and create evidence-based therapy plans [165]. The use of CNs for ^{89}Zr leukocyte labeling for PET imaging of inflammation was described by Fairclough et al. [166]. The purpose of this research was to perfect the process of labeling leukocytes by enhancing the CN preparation for maximum ^{89}Zr-loading and cell uptake. The effectiveness of cell uptake has been studied with respect to the nanoparticles' size and surface charge. The absorption and retention of ^{89}Zr-loaded CNs in mixed human leukocyte cells, as well as CNs' affinity for ^{89}Zr, have been studied. A novel technique for radiolabeling white blood cells with zirconium-89 (^{89}Zr) or copper-64 (^{64}Cu) for PET imaging was assessed. Ionotropic gelation was employed to create chitosan nanoparticles (CNs) that were then used to transport radiometals into white blood cells. Using the same ^{89}Zr-labeled DNPs described previously, Keliher et al. performed PET-CT imaging in a mouse model of cancer. On account of its popularity for studying tumor infiltrating host cells, a syngeneic colon cancer (CT26) mouse model was employed [167]. Images from a variety of xenografted animals are shown in Figure 13. In certain animals, the concentration of RES in tumors was higher than in any other organ of the reticuloendothelial system, which was an unexpected finding. Through thorough correlative histology and flow cytometry experiments, we were able to ascertain whether tumoral accumulation was the result of cellular uptake or extraversion and interstitial accumulation. After removing tumors, we cut them into thin slices (1 mm) and used autoradiography to image them next to slides stained with Mac-3 (a stain that identifies macrophages). All in all, the "hot areas" and the Mac3 optimism across the chapters were in accord (Figure 13). Histological examination revealed selective uptake of fluorescent DNPs by Mac3+ cells and a general lack of absorption by Mac3 cells (Figure 14).

Mammary carcinoma is the second most frequent malignant tumor (after lung cancer) in adult women and the fifth leading cause of cancer-related mortality worldwide [168]. While existing clinical techniques may not be perfect, there is room for improvement in the diagnosis and monitoring of lymphatic involvement and recurrence. For the time being, the sentinel-lymph-node technique is the most reliable method for identifying nodal invasion in the lymphatic axillary chain. This method, however, is fairly intrusive, since it relies on a surgical biopsy of the first lymph node of the axillary chain detected using lymph scintigraphy with ^{99m}Tc [169]. After designing and testing a wide variety of bifunctional magneto-fluorescent nanoparticle systems (MFNs), Corsi et al. narrowed down to one MFN type that met the aforementioned requirements with respect to sensitivity, in vitro safety, and physiological behavior. Accordingly, the MFN-based multifunctional contrast agent we disclose here appears to possess all the necessary features for its future development for the in vitro and in vivo imaging of early mammary cancer. Size, shape, zeta potential, fluorescence intensity, T_2 relaxivity enhancement in water protons, and stability are all factors in determining the quality of these nanoparticles. Therefore, two were created, and their internalization processes, intracellular destinies, and toxicities in MCF-7 cancer cells were investigated.

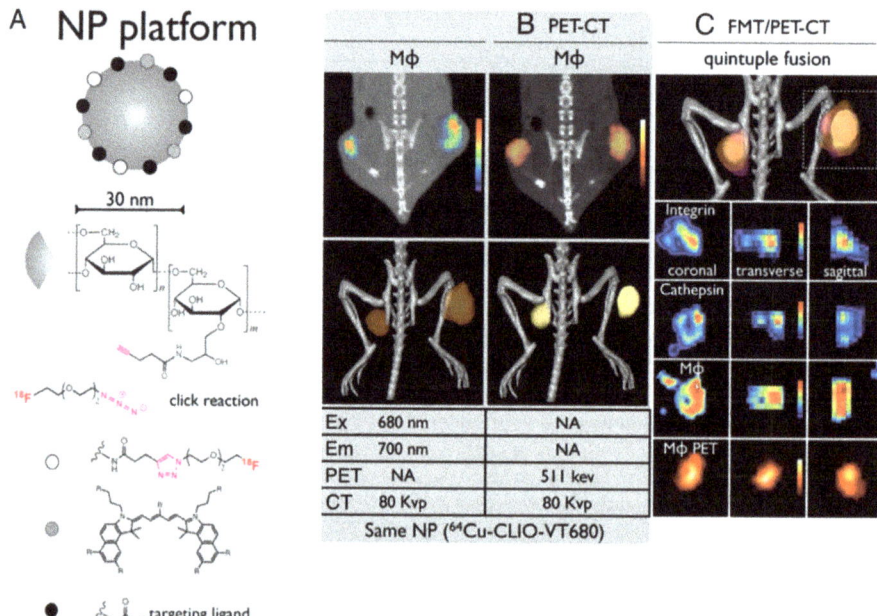

Figure 12. Nanoparticle-based multimodality PET imaging. (**A**) The broad range of targeted ligands that may be conjugated to CLIO, including, but not limited, to 18F through click chemistry and peptides. Tumor-bearing mice were coinjected with a fluorescent peptide against integrins, a fluorescent cathepsin sensor, and ^{64}Cu-CLIO-VT680, and then subjected to in vivo multichannel PET-CT (**B**) and FMT/PET-CT (**C**) [163].

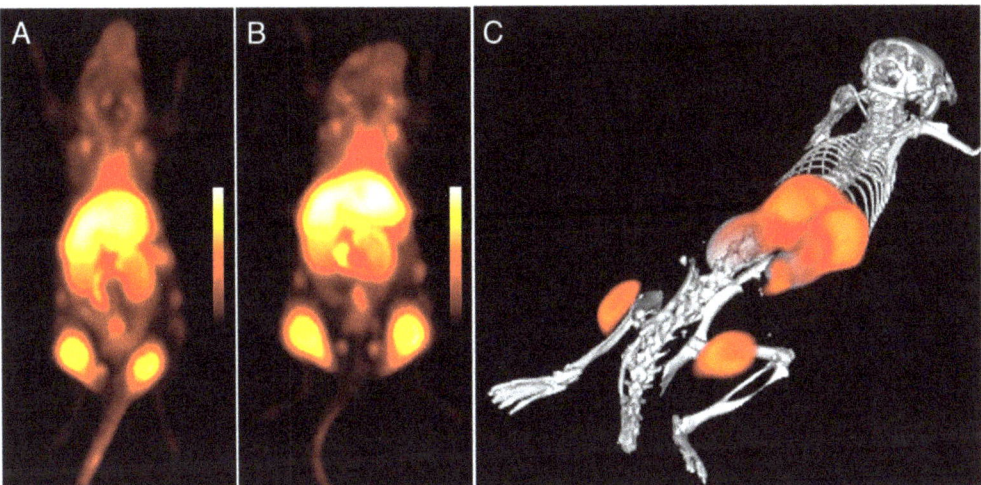

Figure 13. Imaging using 89Zr-labeled DNPs using PET in mice with bilateral flank tumors (24 h after administration). (**A**,**B**) Two distinct animals with almost identical tumor distributions (coronal stacks). Panel A depicts an animal; panel (**C**) depicts a three-dimensional model of the animal [167].

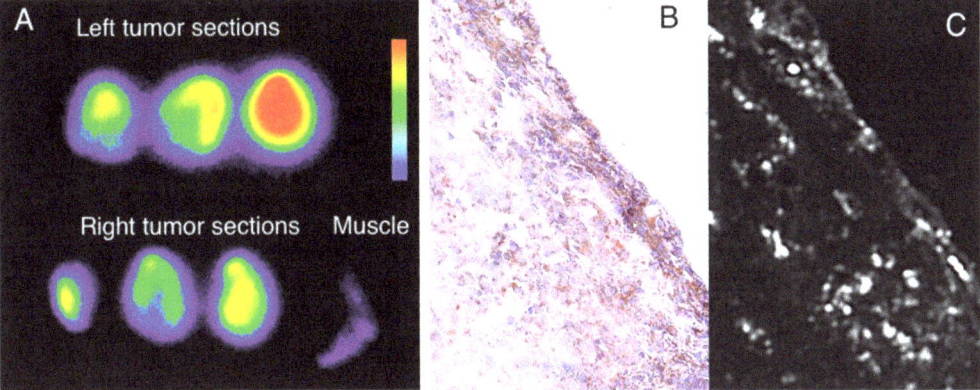

Figure 14. The study of DNP distribution using autoradiography and histopathology. Sections of tumor and adjacent normal tissue (**A**) autoradiographed to highlight predominant accumulations in malignancies. In (**B**), a typical Mac3 immunohistology specimen can be seen. The sections next to B show the distribution of fluorescent DNPs in Mac3-positive cells (**C**) [167].

7. Quantum Dot-Magnetic Nanoparticle Assembly as a Site-Specific Imaging Probe

Since their beginnings, nanoscience and nanotechnology have revolved around the concept of fluorescent quantum dots (QDs), which are typically described as having a diameter size of 10 nm. Several distinct structural, electrochemical, and photochemical features of QDs make them potentially useful platforms for sensing applications. Nanocrystals of semiconductor elements from groups II–VI, III–V, and IV are commonly referred to as quantum dots because of their luminous properties [170]. Their sub-10 nanometer dimensions provide them with unique optical and electrical characteristics compared to those of bulk materials. These 1D nanomaterials are amenable to surface changes for added functionality. Some QDs have reactive functional groups, such as amines, carboxylic acids, alcohols, and thiols, in their coats because they are stabilized in aqueous solutions. A simple method was provided for producing quantum dots (QDs) magnetically doped with Fe with a size range of 3–6 nm that are water-dispersible and emit in the near-infrared (NIR). In situ hydrothermal doping of alloyed CdTeS nanocrystals with Fe was used to achieve this [171]. Using N-acetyl-cysteine (NAC) ligands, which have both thiol and carboxylic acid functional groups, anchored magnetic quantum dots (MQDs) showed high saturation magnetization (85 emu g^{-1}). These NPs could also emit fluorescence in the NIR range and had a proton transverse relaxivity of 3.6 mM^{-1} s^{-1}. Phantom and in vitro investigations have shown that NIR MQD functionality may be evaluated. These unaggregated Fe-doped CdTeS MQDs have the potential to operate as multimodal contrast agents for tracking living cells due to their water-dispersibility, NIR emission, and MR contrast. Using the free-radical polymerization approach, nanocomposites consisting of ZnS:Mn2+ quantum dots (QDs) and Fe$_3$O$_4$ QDs/SiO$_2$/P(NIPAAm-co-AAm) core–shell-shell structures have been effectively synthesized [172]. HeLa cell cytoplasm fluoresces red, demonstrating its usefulness for biolabeling. Citric acid and manganese tetraphenyl porphyrin were used as carbon sources in an aqueous medium to create manganese-doped carbon quantum dots (MnCQDs) in a single hydrothermal process [173]. X-ray photoelectron spectroscopy, transmission electron microscopy, and diffraction confirmed the MnCQD structures. Under UV irradiation (365 nm), MnCQDs emit strong green luminescence with a peak at 482 nm and a fluorescence quantum yield of 13%. At a detection limit of 220 nM, ferric ion in aqueous solution may be detected with the use of MnCQDs as a fluorescent probe. MnCQDs were shown to have little cytotoxicity in an MTT experiment using HeLa cells. In MnC-QDs, the presence of paramagnetic ions results in an improved magnetic resonance (MR) signal. Therefore, MnCQDs can function as good MRI contrast agents. A nanoprobe for fluorescence and magnetic resonance (MR) imaging synthesized with ease was described by shi et al. via a method in which Gd3+ ions are chelated onto the surface of cDTPAA-functionalized carbon quantum dots. This allows the nanoprobe to have bright fluorescence and significantly improved relaxivity (CQDs) [174]. The CQD–DTPA–Gd nanoprobe that was created as a consequence has exceptional water solubility, great fluorescence efficiency, exceptionally high relaxivity, and almost no cytotoxicity. Superparamagnetic nitrogen-doped carbon-iron oxide hybrid quantum dots (C-Fe$_3$O$_4$ QDs) might also be employed for FL/MR/CT bioimaging [175]. For example, C-Fe$_3$O$_4$ QDs are produced by a green and straightforward one-pot hydrothermal technique that employs poly(-glutamic acid) as a precursor and stabilizer. As-prepared C-Fe$_3$O$_4$ QDs have high water miscibility, spectral FL properties with high quantum yields of 21.6%, exceptional photostability, robust superparamagnetic characteristics, and cytocompatibility. Additional proof that as-prepared C-Fe$_3$O$_4$ QDs are ready for use in FL/MR/CT triple-modal tumor imaging came from in vivo bioimaging of tumor-bearing nude mice, which combined FL, MR, and CT images. Mn-doped quantum dots (QDs), and in particular Mn-doped ZnS (ZnSe) QDs, are appealing for fluorescence/magnetic resonance imaging (MRI) dual-mode imaging because of their distinctive fluorescent and magnetic characteristics [176]. However, for MRI imaging, a minimal concentration of dopant (Mn^{2+}) is sufficient to maximize fluorescence in QDs. Here, an enrichment technique with mesoporous silica (MSN) loading (Figure 15) was investigated for the purpose of producing a highly luminescent/paramagnetic Mn-doped ZnSe QD assembly (MSN@QD) for enhanced MRI/optical dual-model imaging. The QD loading density in MSNs was calculated to be 152 ± 12. The MSN@QD assembly fluorescence was enriched with QDs (enrichment factor = 143) upon loading. No significant concentration quenching was seen, despite the huge Stokes shift (200 nm). Enhanced local Mn^{2+} concentration also led to a boost in T_1 MR contrast (Figure 16), allowing for signal enrichment to be achieved in magnetic resonance imaging (MRI).

A carbon quantum dot (CQD)-stabilized gadolinium hybrid nanoprobe (Gd-CQD) was described by Xu et al., which was made by hydrothermally treating citrate acid, ethanediamine, and GdCl$_3$ in one pot at 200 °C for 4 h [113]. High biocompatibility and minimal toxicity were proven by in vitro and in vivo testing. Due to their high Gd contents and hydrophilicity, the Gd-CQDs were shown to have a greater MR response than gadopentetic acid dimeglumine (Gd-DTPA). Finally, Gd-CQDs retained their CQD-derived fluorescence. Zebrafish embryos and mice were used to verify that Gd-CQDs may be imaged in vivo using both magnetic resonance (MR) and fluorescence. High affinity for U87 cancer cells was achieved by targeted imaging using Gd-CQDs modified with arginine-glycine-aspartic acid (RGD) tripeptide. In order to create multimodal nanoprobes that make use of both optical and magnetic imaging, gadolinium (Gd) complexes containing CDs were generated by a one-step microwave technique [177]. The generated Gd-CDs showed strong fluorescence and had great water solubility and biocompatibility. It was shown that apoferritin (AFn) nanocages labelled with Gd-CD compounds might serve as good T_1 contrast agents for magnetic resonance imaging because Gd-doped CDs dramatically improved the circulation duration and lowered the toxicity of Gd^{3+} in vitro and in vivo magnetic resonance imaging. Cancer theranostics is a promising area for the application of self-assembling multifunctional Gd-CDs/AFn (DOX)/FA nanoparticles. When designing multifunctional nanostructures for use in biological imaging, it is preferable to include luminescent imaging agents and MRI contrast agents. Fluorescence microscopy and magnetic resonance imaging (MRI) may both make use of luminescent biocompatible silicon quantum dots (SiQDs). This is the first report of the production of a nanocomplex including SiQDs and gadolinium ions (Gd^{3+}) for use in biology [178]. The optical characteristics of the probes were confirmed to be unaltered after they were taken up by cells and transported into the intracellular space. It was found that the nanostructures had a magnetic resonance relaxivity of 2.4 $mM^{-1} s^{-1}$ (in terms of Gd^{3+} concentration), which works out at around 6000 $mM^{-1} s^{-1}$ per nanoconstruct. The newly developed probe's appealing optical and relaxivity characteristics pave the way for SiQDs to be used in future multimodal applications, such as cancer imaging. The virtues of nanoscale ternary chalcogenides, including their adaptability and wide range of energy and biomedical uses, have resulted in a surge in their study. Aqueous synthesis of silver indium sulfide quantum dots with dual ligands of glutathione and polyethyleneimine has been reported [179]. The resulting silver indium sulfide quantum dots have a long lifespan of 3.69 s, great fluorescence stability, and minimal cytotoxicity, making them a promising tool for live-cell imaging. Since it offers a practical and novel technique to control the inherent characteristics of carbon quantum dots (CQDs) and graphene quantum dots (GQDs), doping fluorescent carbon dots (DFCDs) with heteroatoms has lately gained a lot of interest in comparison to conventional fluorescent materials.

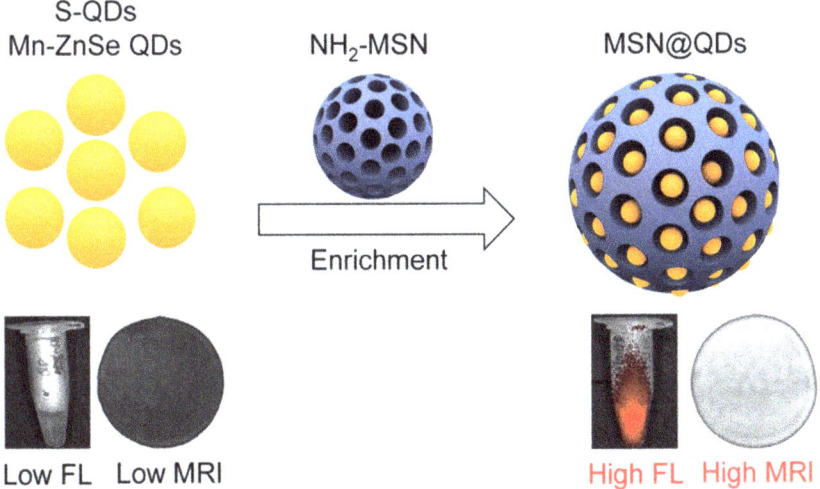

Figure 15. Improved Dual-Modal Imaging Through Enrichment Process Schematic [176].

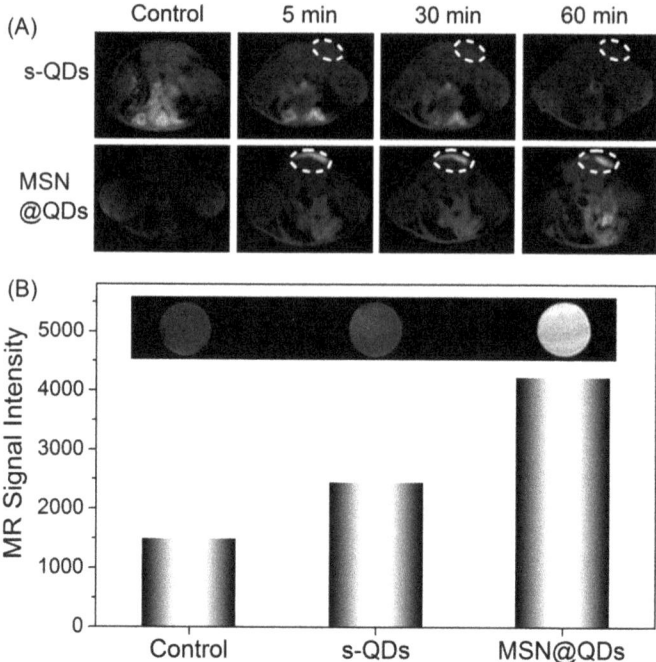

Figure 16. Comparison of pre- and post-injection MR images of a Balb/c mouse injected with s-QDs and MSN@QDs: MR coronal pictures at T1 weighting (**A**) and the associated MR signal intensity (**B**) as measured in vitro [176].

The photostability and luminosity of QDs can be greatly improved by including them in nano- or micromatrix composites [180]. Putting quantum dots and other functional nanoparticles in the same matrix is predicted to provide imaging probes that can detect many modalities. Making nanoprobes out of common nanomaterials (such as quantum dots, gold nanoparticles, and iron oxide nanoparticles) is a crucial step towards improving in vivo multimodality imaging. Strong processes and low-toxicity synthetic techniques for multimodality nanoprobes are urgently needed in nanomedicine domains [181]. Using magnetic nanoparticles (high T2 relaxivity), visible-light-emitting CdSe/ZnS quantum dots (QDs; Em = 600 nm), and near-infrared (NIR)-emitting CdSeTe/CdS QDs, MA et al. developed a simple and robust technique for developing multilayered nanoparticles (MQQ-probe) (Em 780 nm) [182]. A variety of nanoparticles were coated in layers of silica. Core–shell nanoprobes have many layers, each of which can give a unique set of features depending on the nanoparticles they contain. In order to facilitate easy, quick, and selective cell extraction, fluorescent labeling, and counting, Tran et al. demonstrated a prototype smartphone-based imaging platform (SIP) coupled with magneto-luminescent suprananoparticle assemblies [183]. As shown in Figure 17, the author provided several instances of high-magnification photographs of the separated cells that were taken with a microscope designed for scientific study. For the four colors of the MNP@QDs, the signal-to-noise ratios (SNRs) on the SIP were 7 3 (SD), 8 3, 14 5, and 9 3 for cells labelled with MNP@QD485, MNP@QD575, MNP@QD605, and MNP@QD635, respectively. The production of these suprananoparticle assemblies and their immunoconjugates by self-assembly is extremely beneficial, and the ultrabright PL of these assemblies makes it possible to image single cells while maintaining a high signal-to-noise ratio. Proof of concept was achieved by isolating and counting HER2-positive SK-BR3 breast cancer cells against a background of HER2-negative MBA-MD-231 breast cancer cells. This allowed for comparison of the two populations. The extraordinary physical and chemical capabilities of inorganic nanoparticles have led to their introduction into biological systems as effective probes for in vitro diagnostics and in vivo imaging. To combine the strengths of MR and fluorescence imaging, a novel class of color-tunable quantum dots (QDs) called Gd-Zn-Cu-In-S/ZnSs (GZCIS/ZnSs) have been synthesized and put to use [184]. By integrating Gd into ZCIS/ZnS QDs, we were able to successfully fabricate GZCIS/ZnS QDs with significant MR enhancement and without sacrificing the fluorescence characteristics of the original ZCIS/ZnS QDs. High PL quantum yield and "color-tunable" PL emission from 550 to 725 nm may be achieved by varying the Zn/Cu feeding ratio in the as-prepared GZCIS/ZnS QDs (QY). A bovine serum albumin (BSA) coating was used to introduce the GZCIS/ZnS QDs into water.

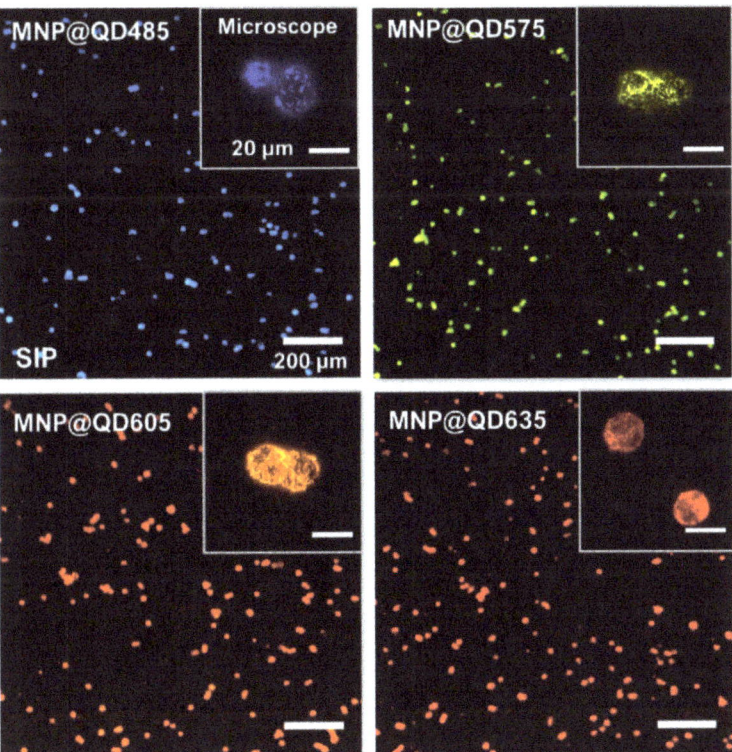

Figure 17. Smartphone (main images, scale bar = 200 m) and microscope (insets, scale bar = 20 m) images of fixed SK-BR3 cells isolated with MNP@QDs of different colors: QD485, QD575, QD605, and QD635. The notation for the QDs indicates the QDs' peak PL emission wavelengths. The smartphone pictures were taken in RGB color format. The microscope images were given "false colors" based on the monochrome intensity values [183].

8. Conclusions and Perspectives

This review was motivated by the plethora of ground-breaking studies conducted all across the world. Insight into the manufacturing of fluorescent NPs and the methods for imbuing them with magnetic properties may be gained from this debate. There are extremely high requirements for and interest in these resources. Based on what has been said, it is evident that magneto-fluorescent nanocomposites provide novel avenues for research in chemistry, biology, and medicine. Despite recent advancements, the field of fluorescent-magnetic nanocomposite materials is still in its infancy, and much work needs to be done to further improve these materials and their applications. Magneto-fluorescent hybrids of varying sizes, architectures, dispersions, and surface modifications have been synthesized using the various approaches discussed here. In point of fact, surface modifications of these nanoparticles with other compounds, polymers, and silica lead to the stabilization of the nanosystems as well as decrease in toxicity, which allows for biological applications. In spite of the fact that toxicological studies have been conducted on some of these NPs, the precise mechanism by which nanoparticles cause toxicity is still unknown. As a result, a more in-depth investigation into the toxicity and biocompatibility of fluorescent-magneto hybrid NPs and the constituents that make them up is required. Significant progress has been achieved in the synthesis of nanoparticles with adaptable designs, paving the way for both intelligent delivery and individualized therapy. Nanoparticles with many functions, such as magneto-fluorescent nanoparticles, are without a doubt the most helpful instruments now available. Although there is an immediate need for various modifications and new insights into the manufacturing of magneto-fluorescent nanoparticles and their toxicities, these particles show significant promise for use in medical diagnosis and other applications. Recently, several kinds of luminous materials, including semiconductor quantum dots (QDs) and organic urophores, have been linked with magnetic units to produce MFNPs. These MFNPs may operate both as optical and magnetic probes due to the coupling of the two types of materials. The fact that these QDs often include heavy metals, such as cadmium, lead, and other substances, which have the potential to be poisonous, have lower water solubility, and pose environmental risks limits the range of uses for these materials.

9. Present Market and Future Development

Magnetic particle imaging (MPI) is a novel imaging technique that, like MRI and positron emission tomography, has the potential for high-resolution imaging without requiring any intrusive procedures (PET). It is anticipated that MPI will be able to follow cells for cancer-therapy monitoring. A possibility exists that CAR T cells will take up SPIONs. SPIONs may be taken up by macrophages in active phagocytic sites or by atherosclerotic plaques if they are delivered systemically [185]. In a magnetic particle imager, the signals produced by SPIONs of different sorts and with varied features, such as core size, or by the same SPIONs in different settings can be easily distinguished. Both bound and unbound SPIONs provide distinguishable signals which can prove useful in preclinical research. The variations in the produced signals may be used to create multicolored pictures, with each hue representing a unique SPION or a SPION in a distinct environment [186]. The amplifier noise level can be lowered to the same level as the patient noise contribution via processes such as cryogenic cooling of the amplifiers and adjusted tuning. Industrial efforts to create an MPI/MRI scanner which combines the benefits of these two imaging modalities are quite promising [187]. One of the pillars of future technologies that will allow for the development of superior systems with high spatial and temporal resolution is the creation of multimodal imaging systems that use fluorescence imaging. Ongoing research and development of new algorithms is also contributing to overcoming the shortcomings of present imaging systems, particularly with respect to depth of penetration. Fluorescence imaging has become a widely utilized and increasingly popular tool in preclinical biomedical research as a result of its sensitivity, cost-effectiveness, and safety, as well as the availability of a wide range of functionalized fluorophores. Possible future applications of fluorescence imaging in clinical medicine may be seen in its current applications, such as cancer detection and therapy and surgical planning. Fluorescence imaging is projected to play a larger role in the clinical care of patients as technology improves, opening the door to imaging-driven tailored therapy. Cost estimates were derived from an analysis of publicly accessible financial data from the annual reports of major firms producing and selling imaging agents. We compared these figures with the extensive data and analysis we have on the price of creating medicinal medications. When compared to the current revenues of blockbuster imaging medicines, which are between USD 200 and 400 million, it is clear that the development and commercialization of a drug for diagnostic imaging is rather expensive. All of the top-selling radiological agents have been available for quite some time. The market size for imaging agents is substantially smaller than that for therapeutic medications. In 2004, sales in the United States, which account for over half of global sales, amounted to USD 2.8 billion [188]. From a commercial perspective, there are five primary manufacturers of imaging agents. Among them are GE, BMS, Bracco, Schering, and Tyco, which were formerly a part of Amersham. While researchers try to perfect magnetic scanning devices, others refine nanoparticles for injection into patients or for the delivery of medications. The ultimate goal is to create universally effective nanoparticles that can cross biological barriers that are not homogeneous [189]. The use of artificial intelligence (AI) in radiography is a hotly debated issue at the moment. Machine learning, representation learning, and deep learning are the three primary subfields in artificial intelligence [190]. The fields of deep learning and machine learning are the most applicable to radiology. Inevitably, as time goes on, many of the existing technological flaws will be fixed, allowing for the creation of a highly sensitive and secure imaging system for medical diagnosis, which is desperately needed to satisfy societal expectations.

Author Contributions: Conceptualization, S.G. and S.M.; resources, S.G.; writing—original draft preparation, S.G.; writing—review and editing, S.G. and S.M.; visualization, S.G.; supervision, S.M.; project administration, S.M. All authors have read and agreed to the published version of the manuscript.

Funding: This research received no external funding.

Institutional Review Board Statement: Not applicable.

Informed Consent Statement: Not applicable.

Data Availability Statement: Not applicable.

Conflicts of Interest: The authors declare no conflict of interest.

References

1. De la Encarnación, C.; de Aberasturi, D.J.; Liz-Marzán, L.M. Multifunctional plasmonic-magnetic nanoparticles for bioimaging and hyperthermia. *Adv. Drug Deliv. Rev.* **2022**, *189*, 114484. [CrossRef] [PubMed]
2. Wang, Y.; Gu, H. Core–shell-type magnetic mesoporous silica nanocomposites for bioimaging and therapeutic agent delivery. *Adv. Mater.* **2015**, *27*, 576–585. [CrossRef]
3. Mirza, S.; Ahmad, M.S.; Shah, M.I.A.; Ateeq, M. Magnetic nanoparticles: Drug delivery and bioimaging applications. In *Metal Nanoparticles for Drug Delivery and Diagnostic Applications*; Elsevier: Amsterdam, The Netherlands, 2020; pp. 189–213.
4. Deller, A.; Moldon, J.; Miller-Jones, J.; Patruno, A.; Hessels, J.; Archibald, A.; Paragi, Z.; Heald, G.; Vilchez, N. Radio imaging observations of PSR J1023+ 0038 in an LMXB state. *Astrophys. J.* **2015**, *809*, 13. [CrossRef]
5. Galperin, A.; Margel, D.; Baniel, J.; Dank, G.; Biton, H.; Margel, S. Radiopaque iodinated polymeric nanoparticles for X-ray imaging applications. *Biomaterials* **2007**, *28*, 4461–4468. [CrossRef]
6. Ganguly, S.; Grinberg, I.; Margel, S. Layer by layer controlled synthesis at room temperature of tri-modal (MRI, fluorescence and CT) core/shell superparamagnetic IO/human serum albumin nanoparticles for diagnostic applications. *Polym. Adv. Technol.* **2021**, *32*, 3909–3921. [CrossRef]
7. Pelc, N.J. Recent and future directions in CT imaging. *Ann. Biomed. Eng.* **2014**, *42*, 260–268. [CrossRef] [PubMed]
8. Kreisl, W.C.; Kim, M.-J.; Coughlin, J.M.; Henter, I.D.; Owen, D.R.; Innis, R.B. PET imaging of neuroinflammation in neurological disorders. *Lancet Neurol.* **2020**, *19*, 940–950. [CrossRef] [PubMed]
9. Ando, T. High-speed atomic force microscopy. *Curr. Opin. Chem. Biol.* **2019**, *51*, 105–112. [CrossRef]
10. Van Malderen, S.J.; Van Acker, T.; Vanhaecke, F. Sub-micrometer nanosecond LA-ICP-MS imaging at pixel acquisition rates above 250 Hz via a low-dispersion setup. *Anal. Chem.* **2020**, *92*, 5756–5764. [CrossRef]
11. Ryan, D.J.; Spraggins, J.M.; Caprioli, R.M. Protein identification strategies in MALDI imaging mass spectrometry: A brief review. *Curr. Opin. Chem. Biol.* **2019**, *48*, 64–72. [CrossRef]
12. Ganguly, S.; Margel, S. 3D printed magnetic polymer composite hydrogels for hyperthermia and magnetic field driven structural manipulation. *Prog. Polym. Sci.* **2022**, *131*, 101574. [CrossRef]
13. Ganguly, S.; Margel, S. Design of magnetic hydrogels for hyperthermia and drug delivery. *Polymers* **2021**, *13*, 4259. [CrossRef] [PubMed]
14. Kasouni, A.; Chatzimitakos, T.; Stalikas, C. Bioimaging applications of carbon nanodots: A review. *C* **2019**, *5*, 19. [CrossRef]

15. Bon, P.; Cognet, L. On Some Current Challenges in High-Resolution Optical Bioimaging. *ACS Photonics* **2022**, *9*, 2538–2546. [CrossRef] [PubMed]
16. Gibbs, J.H.; Zhou, Z.; Kessel, D.; Fronczek, F.R.; Pakhomova, S.; Vicente, M.G.H. Synthesis, spectroscopic, and in vitro investigations of 2, 6-diiodo-BODIPYs with PDT and bioimaging applications. *J. Photochem. Photobiol. B Biol.* **2015**, *145*, 35–47. [CrossRef]
17. Saikia, M.J.; Kanhirodan, R.; Mohan Vasu, R. High-speed GPU-based fully three-dimensional diffuse optical tomographic system. *Int. J. Biomed. Imaging* **2014**, *2014*, 3. [CrossRef]
18. Gahlmann, A.; Moerner, W. Exploring bacterial cell biology with single-molecule tracking and super-resolution imaging. *Nat. Rev. Microbiol.* **2014**, *12*, 9–22. [CrossRef]
19. Braeken, Y.; Cheruku, S.; Ethirajan, A.; Maes, W. Conjugated polymer nanoparticles for bioimaging. *Materials* **2017**, *10*, 1420. [CrossRef]
20. Han, X.; Xu, K.; Taratula, O.; Farsad, K. Applications of nanoparticles in biomedical imaging. *Nanoscale* **2019**, *11*, 799–819. [CrossRef]
21. Reisch, A.; Klymchenko, A.S. Fluorescent polymer nanoparticles based on dyes: Seeking brighter tools for bioimaging. *Small* **2016**, *12*, 1968–1992. [CrossRef]
22. Yao, S.; Belfield, K.D. Two-photon fluorescent probes for bioimaging. *Eur. J. Org. Chem.* **2012**, *2012*, 3199–3217. [CrossRef]
23. Sharma, P.; Brown, S.; Walter, G.; Santra, S.; Moudgil, B. Nanoparticles for bioimaging. *Adv. Colloid Interface Sci.* **2006**, *123*, 471–485. [CrossRef] [PubMed]
24. Lu, Y.; He, B.; Shen, J.; Li, J.; Yang, W.; Yin, M. Multifunctional magnetic and fluorescent core–shell nanoparticles for bioimaging. *Nanoscale* **2015**, *7*, 1606–1609. [CrossRef] [PubMed]
25. Erathodiyil, N.; Ying, J.Y. Functionalization of Inorganic Nanoparticles for Bioimaging Applications. *Acc. Chem. Res.* **2011**, *44*, 925–935. [CrossRef] [PubMed]
26. Xu, L.; Jiang, X.; Liang, K.; Gao, M.; Kong, B. Frontier luminous strategy of functional silica nanohybrids in sensing and bioimaging: From ACQ to AIE. *Aggregate* **2022**, *3*, e121. [CrossRef]
27. Muller, G.L. Experimental Bone Marrow Reactions: I. Anemia Produced by Collargol. *J. Exp. Med.* **1926**, *43*, 533. [CrossRef]
28. Burns, J.E. Thorium—A New Agent for Pyelography: Preliminary report. *J. Am. Med. Assoc.* **1915**, *64*, 2126–2127. [CrossRef]
29. Swick, M. Intravenous urography by means of the sodium salt of 5-iodo2-pyridon-N-acetic acid. *J. Am. Med. Assoc.* **1930**, *95*, 1403–1409. [CrossRef]
30. Newman, E.A.; Newman, L.A. Lymphatic mapping techniques and sentinel lymph node biopsy in breast cancer. *Surg. Clin. N. Am.* **2007**, *87*, 353–364. [CrossRef]
31. Coyne, D.W. Ferumoxytol for treatment of iron deficiency anemia in patients with chronic kidney disease. *Expert Opin. Pharmacother.* **2009**, *10*, 2563–2568. [CrossRef]
32. Runge, V.M. Safety of approved MR contrast media for intravenous injection. *J. Magn. Reson. Imaging Off. J. Int. Soc. Magn. Reson. Med.* **2000**, *12*, 205–213. [CrossRef]
33. Feinstein, S.B.; Cheirif, J.; Ten Cate, F.J.; Silverman, P.R.; Heidenreich, P.A.; Dick, C.; Desir, R.M.; Armstrong, W.F.; Quinones, M.A.; Shah, P.M. Safety and efficacy of a new transpulmonary ultrasound contrast agent: Initial multicenter clinical results. *J. Am. Coll. Cardiol.* **1990**, *16*, 316–324. [CrossRef] [PubMed]
34. Lilly, E. Highlights of prescribing information Amyvid (florbetapir F 18 injection). *Revis. Dec.* **2019**.
35. Kumar, P.; Fabre, F.; Durand, A.; Clua-Provost, T.; Li, J.; Edgar, J.H.; Rougemaille, N.; Coraux, J.; Marie, X.; Renucci, P.; et al. Magnetic Imaging with Spin Defects in Hexagonal Boron Nitride. *Phys. Rev. Appl.* **2022**, *18*, L061002. [CrossRef]
36. de Gille, R.W.; McCoey, J.M.; Hall, L.T.; Tetienne, J.-P.; Malkemper, E.P.; Keays, D.A.; Hollenberg, L.C.L.; Simpson, D.A. Quantum magnetic imaging of iron organelles within the pigeon cochlea. *Proc. Natl. Acad. Sci. USA* **2021**, *118*, e2112749118. [CrossRef] [PubMed]
37. Das, P.; Ganguly, S.; Margel, S.; Gedanken, A. Tailor made magnetic nanolights: Fabrication to cancer theranostics applications. *Nanoscale Adv.* **2021**, *3*, 6762–6796. [CrossRef]
38. Ganguly, S. Preparation/processing of polymer-graphene composites by different techniques. In *Polymer Nanocomposites Containing Graphene*; Woodhead Publishing, Elsevier: Amsterdam, The Netherlands, 2022; pp. 45–74. [CrossRef]
39. Ganguly, S.; Margel, S. Review: Remotely controlled magneto-regulation of therapeutics from magnetoelastic gel matrices. *Biotechnol. Adv.* **2020**, *44*, 107611. [CrossRef]
40. Chen, D.-X.; Sanchez, A.; Taboada, E.; Roig, A.; Sun, N.; Gu, H.-C. Size determination of superparamagnetic nanoparticles from magnetization curve. *J. Appl. Phys.* **2009**, *105*, 083924. [CrossRef]
41. Manukyan, K.V.; Chen, Y.-S.; Rouvimov, S.; Li, P.; Li, X.; Dong, S.; Liu, X.; Furdyna, J.K.; Orlov, A.; Bernstein, G.H. Ultrasmall α-Fe^{2}O^3 superparamagnetic nanoparticles with high magnetization prepared by template-assisted combustion process. *J. Phys. Chem. C* **2014**, *118*, 16264–16271. [CrossRef]
42. Marcus, M.; Smith, A.; Maswadeh, A.; Shemesh, Z.; Zak, I.; Motiei, M.; Schori, H.; Margel, S.; Sharoni, A.; Shefi, O. Magnetic targeting of growth factors using iron oxide nanoparticles. *Nanomaterials* **2018**, *8*, 707. [CrossRef]
43. Lukawska, A.; Jagoo, Z.; Kozlowski, G.; Turgut, Z.; Kosai, H.; Sheets, A.; Bixel, T.; Wheatley, A.; Abdulkin, P.; Knappett, B. Ac magnetic heating of superparamagnetic Fe and Co nanoparticles. In *Defect and Diffusion Forum*; Trans Tech Publications Ltd.: Zurich, Switzerland, 2013; pp. 159–167.

44. Chalise, D.; Cahill, D.G. Highly Sensitive and High-Throughput Magnetic Resonance Thermometry of Fluids Using Superparamagnetic Nanoparticles. *Phys. Rev. Appl.* **2023**, *19*, 014055. [CrossRef]
45. Melo, L.G.; Soares, T.R.; Neto, O.P.V. Analysis of the magnetostatic energy of chains of single-domain nanomagnets for logic gates. *IEEE Trans. Magn.* **2017**, *53*, 1–10. [CrossRef]
46. Nozaki, T.; Yamamoto, T.; Miwa, S.; Tsujikawa, M.; Shirai, M.; Yuasa, S.; Suzuki, Y. Recent progress in the voltage-controlled magnetic anisotropy effect and the challenges faced in developing voltage-torque MRAM. *Micromachines* **2019**, *10*, 327. [CrossRef] [PubMed]
47. Parameswaranpillai, J.; Das, P.; Ganguly, S. Introduction to Quantum Dots and Their Polymer Composites. In *Quantum Dots and Polymer Nanocomposites*; CRC Press: Boca Raton, FL, USA, 2023; pp. 1–19.
48. Parameswaranpillai, J.; Das, P.; Ganguly, S. *Quantum Dots and Polymer Nanocomposites: Synthesis, Chemistry, and Applications*; CRC Press: Boca Raton, FL, USA, 2022.
49. Saravanan, A.; Maruthapandi, M.; Das, P.; Ganguly, S.; Margel, S.; Luong, J.H.; Gedanken, A. Applications of N-doped carbon dots as antimicrobial agents, antibiotic carriers, and selective fluorescent probes for nitro explosives. *ACS Appl. Bio Mater.* **2020**, *3*, 8023–8031. [CrossRef] [PubMed]
50. Das, P.; Ganguly, S.; Maity, P.P.; Srivastava, H.K.; Bose, M.; Dhara, S.; Bandyopadhyay, S.; Das, A.K.; Banerjee, S.; Das, N.C. Converting waste Allium sativum peel to nitrogen and sulphur co-doped photoluminescence carbon dots for solar conversion, cell labeling, and photobleaching diligences: A path from discarded waste to value-added products. *J. Photochem. Photobiol. B Biol.* **2019**, *197*, 111545. [CrossRef]
51. Das, P.; Bose, M.; Das, A.K.; Banerjee, S.; Das, N.C. One-step synthesis of fluorescent carbon dots for bio-labeling assay. *Macromol. Symp.* **2018**, *382*, 1800077. [CrossRef]
52. Das, P.; Ganguly, S.; Saravanan, A.; Margel, S.; Gedanken, A.; Srinivasan, S.; Rajabzadeh, A.R. Naturally Derived Carbon Dots In Situ Confined Self-Healing and Breathable Hydrogel Monolith for Anomalous Diffusion-Driven Phytomedicine Release. *ACS Appl. Bio Mater.* **2022**, *5*, 5617–5633. [CrossRef]
53. Das, P.; Ganguly, S.; Margel, S.; Gedanken, A. Immobilization of heteroatom-doped carbon dots onto nonpolar plastics for antifogging, antioxidant, and food monitoring applications. *Langmuir* **2021**, *37*, 3508–3520. [CrossRef]
54. Das, P.; Maruthapandi, M.; Saravanan, A.; Natan, M.; Jacobi, G.; Banin, E.; Gedanken, A. Carbon dots for heavy-metal sensing, pH-sensitive cargo delivery, and antibacterial applications. *ACS Appl. Nano Mater.* **2020**, *3*, 11777–11790. [CrossRef]
55. Das, P.; Ganguly, S.; Saha, A.; Noked, M.; Margel, S.; Gedanken, A. Carbon-dots-initiated photopolymerization: An in situ synthetic approach for MXene/poly (norepinephrine)/copper hybrid and its application for mitigating water pollution. *ACS Appl. Mater. Interfaces* **2021**, *13*, 31038–31050. [CrossRef]
56. Das, P.; Ganguly, S.; Mondal, S.; Ghorai, U.K.; Maity, P.P.; Choudhary, S.; Gangopadhyay, S.; Dhara, S.; Banerjee, S.; Das, N.C. Dual doped biocompatible multicolor luminescent carbon dots for bio labeling, UV-active marker and fluorescent polymer composite. *Luminescence* **2018**, *33*, 1136–1145. [CrossRef]
57. Ahmed, S.R.; Sherazee, M.; Srinivasan, S.; Rajabzadeh, A.R. Nanozymatic detection of thiocyanate through accelerating the growth of ultra-small gold nanoparticles/graphene quantum dots hybrids. *Food Chem.* **2022**, *379*, 132152. [CrossRef]
58. Das, P.; Ganguly, S.; Banerjee, S.; Das, N.C. Graphene based emergent nanolights: A short review on the synthesis, properties and application. *Res. Chem. Intermed.* **2019**, *45*, 3823–3853. [CrossRef]
59. Das, P.; Ganguly, S.; Maity, P.P.; Bose, M.; Mondal, S.; Dhara, S.; Das, A.K.; Banerjee, S.; Das, N.C. Waste chimney oil to nanolights: A low cost chemosensor for tracer metal detection in practical field and its polymer composite for multidimensional activity. *J. Photochem. Photobiol. B Biol.* **2018**, *180*, 56–67. [CrossRef] [PubMed]
60. Ganguly, S.; Das, P.; Das, T.K.; Ghosh, S.; Das, S.; Bose, M.; Mondal, M.; Das, A.K.; Das, N.C. Acoustic cavitation assisted destratified clay tactoid reinforced in situ elastomer-mimetic semi-IPN hydrogel for catalytic and bactericidal application. *Ultrason. Sonochem.* **2020**, *60*, 104797. [CrossRef]
61. Wu, F.; Su, H.; Zhu, X.; Wang, K.; Zhang, Z.; Wong, W.-K. Near-infrared emissive lanthanide hybridized carbon quantum dots for bioimaging applications. *J. Mater. Chem. B* **2016**, *4*, 6366–6372. [CrossRef]
62. Martinić, I.; Eliseeva, S.V.; Petoud, S. Near-infrared emitting probes for biological imaging: Organic fluorophores, quantum dots, fluorescent proteins, lanthanide(III) complexes and nanomaterials. *J. Lumin.* **2017**, *189*, 19–43. [CrossRef]
63. Das, P.; Ganguly, S.; Ahmed, S.R.; Sherazee, M.; Margel, S.; Gedanken, A.; Srinivasan, S.; Rajabzadeh, A.R. Carbon Dot Biopolymer-Based Flexible Functional Films for Antioxidant and Food Monitoring Applications. *ACS Appl. Polym. Mater.* **2022**, *4*, 9323–9340. [CrossRef]
64. Dempsey, G.T.; Bates, M.; Kowtoniuk, W.E.; Liu, D.R.; Tsien, R.Y.; Zhuang, X. Photoswitching mechanism of cyanine dyes. *J. Am. Chem. Soc.* **2009**, *131*, 18192–18193. [CrossRef] [PubMed]
65. Smith, A.M.; Mancini, M.C.; Nie, S. Second window for in vivo imaging. *Nat. Nanotechnol.* **2009**, *4*, 710–711. [CrossRef] [PubMed]
66. Li, C.; Liu, J.; Alonso, S.; Li, F.; Zhang, Y. Upconversion nanoparticles for sensitive and in-depth detection of Cu^{2+} ions. *Nanoscale* **2012**, *4*, 6065–6071. [CrossRef] [PubMed]
67. Mahmood, U.; Weissleder, R. Some Tools for Molecular Imaging. *Acad. Radiol.* **2002**, *9*, 629–631. [CrossRef] [PubMed]
68. Plewes, D.B.; Kucharczyk, W. Physics of MRI: A primer. *J. Magn. Reson. Imaging* **2012**, *35*, 1038–1054. [CrossRef]

69. Santra, S.; Bagwe, R.P.; Dutta, D.; Stanley, J.T.; Walter, G.A.; Tan, W.; Moudgil, B.M.; Mericle, R.A. Synthesis and Characterization of Fluorescent, Radio-Opaque, and Paramagnetic Silica Nanoparticles for Multimodal Bioimaging Applications. *Adv. Mater.* **2005**, *17*, 2165–2169. [CrossRef]
70. Sarma, A.; Heilbrun, M.E.; Conner, K.E.; Stevens, S.M.; Woller, S.C.; Elliott, C.G. Radiation and chest CT scan examinations: What do we know? *Chest* **2012**, *142*, 750–760. [CrossRef] [PubMed]
71. Ghosh, S.; Ganguly, S.; Maruthi, A.; Jana, S.; Remanan, S.; Das, P.; Das, T.K.; Ghosh, S.K.; Das, N.C. Micro-computed tomography enhanced cross-linked carboxylated acrylonitrile butadiene rubber with the decoration of new generation conductive carbon black for high strain tolerant electromagnetic wave absorber. *Mater. Today Commun.* **2020**, *24*, 100989. [CrossRef]
72. Ghosh, S.; Das, P.; Ganguly, S.; Remanan, S.; Das, T.K.; Bhattacharyya, S.K.; Baral, J.; Das, A.K.; Laha, T.; Das, N.C. 3D-enhanced, high-performing, super-hydrophobic and electromagnetic-interference shielding fabrics based on silver paint and their use in antibacterial applications. *ChemistrySelect* **2019**, *4*, 11748–11754. [CrossRef]
73. Bartling, S.H.; Budjan, J.; Aviv, H.; Haneder, S.; Kraenzlin, B.; Michaely, H.; Margel, S.; Diehl, S.; Semmler, W.; Gretz, N. First multimodal embolization particles visible on x-ray/computed tomography and magnetic resonance imaging. *Investig. Radiol.* **2011**, *46*, 178–186. [CrossRef]
74. Aviv, H.; Bartling, S.; Grinberg, I.; Margel, S. Synthesis and characterization of Bi2O3/HSA core-shell nanoparticles for X-ray imaging applications. *J. Biomed. Mater. Res. Part B Appl. Biomater.* **2013**, *101*, 131–138. [CrossRef]
75. Schladitz, K. Quantitative micro-CT. *J. Microsc.* **2011**, *243*, 111–117. [CrossRef]
76. Jiang, Y.; Zhao, J.; White, D.; Genant, H. Micro CT and Micro MR imaging of 3D architecture of animal skeleton. *J. Musculoskelet Neuron. Interact* **2000**, *1*, 45–51.
77. Abruzzo, T.; Tumialan, L.; Chaalala, C.; Kim, S.; Guldberg, R.E.; Lin, A.; Leach, J.; Khoury, J.C.; Morgan, A.E.; Cawley III, C.M. Microscopic computed tomography imaging of the cerebral circulation in mice: Feasibility and pitfalls. *Synapse* **2008**, *62*, 557–565. [CrossRef]
78. Dorr, A.; Sled, J.G.; Kabani, N. Three-dimensional cerebral vasculature of the CBA mouse brain: A magnetic resonance imaging and micro computed tomography study. *Neuroimage* **2007**, *35*, 1409–1423. [CrossRef] [PubMed]
79. Riani, P.; Napoletano, M.; Canepa, F. Synthesis, characterization and ac magnetic analysis of magnetite nanoparticles. *J. Nanoparticle Res.* **2011**, *13*, 7013–7020. [CrossRef]
80. Raj, K.; Moskowitz, B.; Casciari, R. Advances in ferrofluid technology. *J. Magn. Magn. Mater.* **1995**, *149*, 174–180. [CrossRef]
81. Bell, A.T. The impact of nanoscience on heterogeneous catalysis. *Science* **2003**, *299*, 1688–1691. [CrossRef]
82. Takahashi, M.; Mohan, P.; Nakade, A.; Higashimine, K.; Mott, D.; Hamada, T.; Matsumura, K.; Taguchi, T.; Maenosono, S. Ag/FeCo/Ag core/shell/shell magnetic nanoparticles with plasmonic imaging capability. *Langmuir* **2015**, *31*, 2228–2236. [CrossRef]
83. Jiang, D.; Ni, D.; Liu, F.; Zhang, L.; Liu, L.; Pu, X. A fluorescent imaging assay of cast in renal disease based on graphene quantum dots and Fe3O4 nanoparticles. *Clin. Chim. Acta* **2016**, *454*, 94–101. [CrossRef]
84. Liu, Y.; Zhang, X.; Fang, F.; Kuang, G.; Wang, G. Sandwich immunoassays of multicomponent subtrace pathogenic DNA based on magnetic fluorescent encoded nanoparticles. *BioMed Res. Int.* **2016**, *2016*, 7324384. [CrossRef]
85. Fahmi, M.Z.; Chen, J.-K.; Huang, C.-C.; Ling, Y.-C.; Chang, J.-Y. Phenylboronic acid-modified magnetic nanoparticles as a platform for carbon dot conjugation and doxorubicin delivery. *J. Mater. Chem. B* **2015**, *3*, 5532–5543. [CrossRef]
86. Chen, Y.-C.; Chang, W.-H.; Wang, S.-J.; Hsieh, W.-Y. Fluorescent magnetic nanoparticles with specific targeting functions for combinded targeting, optical imaging and magnetic resonance imaging. *J. Biomater. Sci. Polym. Ed.* **2012**, *23*, 1903–1922. [CrossRef] [PubMed]
87. Wen, C.-Y.; Xie, H.-Y.; Zhang, Z.-L.; Wu, L.-L.; Hu, J.; Tang, M.; Wu, M.; Pang, D.-W. Fluorescent/magnetic micro/nano-spheres based on quantum dots and/or magnetic nanoparticles: Preparation, properties, and their applications in cancer studies. *Nanoscale* **2016**, *8*, 12406–12429. [CrossRef] [PubMed]
88. Lin, J.; Li, Y.; Li, Y.; Wu, H.; Yu, F.; Zhou, S.; Xie, L.; Luo, F.; Lin, C.; Hou, Z. Drug/dye-loaded, multifunctional PEG–chitosan–iron oxide nanocomposites for methotraxate synergistically self-targeted cancer therapy and dual model imaging. *ACS Appl. Mater. Interfaces* **2015**, *7*, 11908–11920. [CrossRef] [PubMed]
89. Majd, M.H.; Barar, J.; Asgari, D.; Valizadeh, H.; Rashidi, M.R.; Kafil, V.; Shahbazi, J.; Omidi, Y. Targeted fluoromagnetic nanoparticles for imaging of breast cancer mcf-7 cells. *Adv. Pharm. Bull.* **2013**, *3*, 189.
90. Ahmed, S.R.; Dong, J.; Yui, M.; Kato, T.; Lee, J.; Park, E.Y. Quantum dots incorporated magnetic nanoparticles for imaging colon carcinoma cells. *J. Nanobiotechnol.* **2013**, *11*, 28. [CrossRef]
91. Zhang, Y.; Shen, Y.; Teng, X.; Yan, M.; Bi, H.; Morais, P.C. Mitochondria-targeting nanoplatform with fluorescent carbon dots for long time imaging and magnetic field-enhanced cellular uptake. *ACS Appl. Mater. Interfaces* **2015**, *7*, 10201–10212. [CrossRef]
92. Wang, K.; Ruan, J.; Qian, Q.; Song, H.; Bao, C.; Zhang, X.; Kong, Y.; Zhang, C.; Hu, G.; Ni, J. BRCAA1 monoclonal antibody conjugated fluorescent magnetic nanoparticles for in vivo targeted magnetofluorescent imaging of gastric cancer. *J. Nanobiotechnol.* **2011**, *9*, 23. [CrossRef]
93. Jayapaul, J.; Arns, S.; Bunker, M.; Weiler, M.; Rutherford, S.; Comba, P.; Kiessling, F. In vivo evaluation of riboflavin receptor targeted fluorescent USPIO in mice with prostate cancer xenografts. *Nano Res.* **2016**, *9*, 1319–1333. [CrossRef]

94. Yin, C.; Hong, B.; Gong, Z.; Zhao, H.; Hu, W.; Lu, X.; Li, J.; Li, X.; Yang, Z.; Fan, Q. Fluorescent oligo (p-phenyleneethynylene) contained amphiphiles-encapsulated magnetic nanoparticles for targeted magnetic resonance and two-photon optical imaging in vitro and in vivo. *Nanoscale* **2015**, *7*, 8907–8919. [CrossRef]
95. Li, J.; An, Y.-L.; Zang, F.-C.; Zong, S.-F.; Cui, Y.-P.; Teng, G.-J. A dual mode targeting probe for distinguishing HER2-positive breast cancer cells using silica-coated fluorescent magnetic nanoparticles. *J. Nanoparticle Res.* **2013**, *15*, 1980. [CrossRef]
96. Daglioglu, C.; Okutucu, B. Synthesis and characterization of AICAR and DOX conjugated multifunctional nanoparticles as a platform for synergistic inhibition of cancer cell growth. *Bioconjugate Chem.* **2016**, *27*, 1098–1111. [CrossRef] [PubMed]
97. Wang, S.; Li, W.; Yuan, D.; Song, J.; Fang, J. Quantitative detection of the tumor-associated antigen large external antigen in colorectal cancer tissues and cells using quantum dot probe. *Int. J. Nanomed.* **2016**, *11*, 235.
98. Jang, M.; Yoon, Y.I.; Kwon, Y.S.; Yoon, T.-J.; Lee, H.J.; Hwang, S.I.; La Yun, B.; Kim, S.M. Trastuzumab-conjugated liposome-coated fluorescent magnetic nanoparticles to target breast cancer. *Korean J. Radiol.* **2014**, *15*, 411–422. [CrossRef] [PubMed]
99. Shen, J.; Li, Y.; Zhu, Y.; Yang, X.; Yao, X.; Li, J.; Huang, G.; Li, C. Multifunctional gadolinium-labeled silica-coated Fe_3O_4 and $CuInS_2$ nanoparticles as a platform for in vivo tri-modality magnetic resonance and fluorescence imaging. *J. Mater. Chem. B* **2015**, *3*, 2873–2882. [CrossRef]
100. Sathe, T.R.; Agrawal, A.; Nie, S. Mesoporous Silica Beads Embedded with Semiconductor Quantum Dots and Iron Oxide Nanocrystals: Dual-Function Microcarriers for Optical Encoding and Magnetic Separation. *Anal. Chem.* **2006**, *78*, 5627–5632. [CrossRef]
101. You, X.; He, R.; Gao, F.; Shao, J.; Pan, B.; Cui, D. Hydrophilic high-luminescent magnetic nanocomposites. *Nanotechnology* **2007**, *18*, 035701. [CrossRef]
102. Shen, M.; Jia, W.; Lin, C.; Fan, G.; Jin, Y.; Chen, X.; Chen, G. Facile synthesis of folate-conjugated magnetic/fluorescent bifunctional microspheres. *Nanoscale Res. Lett.* **2014**, *9*, 1–8. [CrossRef]
103. Margulis-Goshen, K.; Netivi, H.D.; Major, D.T.; Gradzielski, M.; Raviv, U.; Magdassi, S. Formation of organic nanoparticles from volatile microemulsions. *J. Colloid Interface Sci.* **2010**, *342*, 283–292. [CrossRef]
104. Gu, J.; Xu, H.; Han, Y.; Dai, W.; Hao, W.; Wang, C.; Gu, N.; Xu, H.; Cao, J. The internalization pathway, metabolic fate and biological effect of superparamagnetic iron oxide nanoparticles in the macrophage-like RAW264. 7 cell. *Sci. China Life Sci.* **2011**, *54*, 793–805. [CrossRef]
105. Chithrani, B.D.; Ghazani, A.A.; Chan, W.C. Determining the size and shape dependence of gold nanoparticle uptake into mammalian cells. *Nano Lett.* **2006**, *6*, 662–668. [CrossRef]
106. Shi, D.; Cho, H.S.; Chen, Y.; Xu, H.; Gu, H.; Lian, J.; Wang, W.; Liu, G.; Huth, C.; Wang, L. Fluorescent polystyrene–Fe_3O_4 composite nanospheres for in vivo imaging and hyperthermia. *Adv. Mater.* **2009**, *21*, 2170–2173. [CrossRef]
107. Wu, Y.; Chu, M.; Shi, B.; Li, Z. A novel magneto-fluorescent nano-bioprobe for cancer cell targeting, imaging and collection. *Appl. Biochem. Biotechnol.* **2011**, *163*, 813–825. [CrossRef] [PubMed]
108. Acharya, A.; Rawat, K.; Bhat, K.A.; Patial, V.; Padwad, Y.S. A multifunctional magneto-fluorescent nanocomposite for visual recognition of targeted cancer cells. *Mater. Res. Express* **2015**, *2*, 115401. [CrossRef]
109. Walia, S.; Sharma, S.; Kulurkar, P.M.; Patial, V.; Acharya, A. A bimodal molecular imaging probe based on chitosan encapsulated magneto-fluorescent nanocomposite offers biocompatibility, visualization of specific cancer cells in vitro and lung tissues in vivo. *Int. J. Pharm.* **2016**, *498*, 110–118. [CrossRef] [PubMed]
110. Wang, G.; Zhang, X.; Liu, Y.; Hu, Z.; Mei, X.; Uvdal, K. Magneto-fluorescent nanoparticles with high-intensity NIR emission, T 1-and T 2-weighted MR for multimodal specific tumor imaging. *J. Mater. Chem. B* **2015**, *3*, 3072–3080. [CrossRef]
111. Chen, S.; Zhang, J.; Song, S.; Xiong, C.; Dong, L. Hydrangea-like magneto-fluorescent nanoparticles through thiol-inducing assembly. *Mater. Res. Express* **2017**, *4*, 015008. [CrossRef]
112. Setua, S.; Menon, D.; Asok, A.; Nair, S.; Koyakutty, M. Folate receptor targeted, rare-earth oxide nanocrystals for bi-modal fluorescence and magnetic imaging of cancer cells. *Biomaterials* **2010**, *31*, 714–729. [CrossRef]
113. Xu, Y.; Jia, X.-H.; Yin, X.-B.; He, X.-W.; Zhang, Y.-K. Carbon quantum dot stabilized gadolinium nanoprobe prepared via a one-pot hydrothermal approach for magnetic resonance and fluorescence dual-modality bioimaging. *Anal. Chem.* **2014**, *86*, 12122–12129. [CrossRef]
114. Xu, Q.; Wei, J.; Wang, J.; Liu, Y.; Li, N.; Chen, Y.; Gao, C.; Zhang, W.; Sreeprased, T.S. Facile synthesis of copper doped carbon dots and their application as a "turn-off" fluorescent probe in the detection of Fe^{3+} ions. *RSC Adv.* **2016**, *6*, 28745–28750. [CrossRef]
115. Sajid, P.; Chetty, S.S.; Praneetha, S.; Murugan, A.V.; Kumar, Y.; Periyasamy, L. One-pot microwave-assisted in situ reduction of Ag^+ and Au^{3+} ions by Citrus limon extract and their carbon-dots based nanohybrids: A potential nano-bioprobe for cancer cellular imaging. *RSC Adv.* **2016**, *6*, 103482–103490. [CrossRef]
116. Balasubramaniam, S.; Kayandan, S.; Lin, Y.-N.; Kelly, D.F.; House, M.J.; Woodward, R.C.; St. Pierre, T.G.; Riffle, J.S.; Davis, R.M. Toward design of magnetic nanoparticle clusters stabilized by biocompatible diblock copolymers for T 2-weighted MRI contrast. *Langmuir* **2014**, *30*, 1580–1587. [CrossRef] [PubMed]
117. Na, H.B.; Lee, J.H.; An, K.; Park, Y.I.; Park, M.; Lee, I.S.; Nam, D.H.; Kim, S.T.; Kim, S.H.; Kim, S.W. Cover Picture: Development of a T1 Contrast Agent for Magnetic Resonance Imaging Using MnO Nanoparticles (Angew. Chem. Int. Ed. 28/2007). *Angew. Chem. Int. Ed.* **2007**, *46*, 5247. [CrossRef]

118. Liu, J.; Tian, X.; Luo, N.; Yang, C.; Xiao, J.; Shao, Y.; Chen, X.; Yang, G.; Chen, D.; Li, L. Sub-10 nm monoclinic Gd_2O_3: Eu3+ nanoparticles as dual-modal nanoprobes for magnetic resonance and fluorescence imaging. *Langmuir* **2014**, *30*, 13005–13013. [CrossRef] [PubMed]
119. Rub Pakkath, S.A.; Chetty, S.S.; Selvarasu, P.; Vadivel Murugan, A.; Kumar, Y.; Periyasamy, L.; Santhakumar, M.; Sadras, S.R.; Santhakumar, K. Transition metal ion (Mn^{2+}, Fe^{2+}, Co^{2+}, and Ni^{2+})-doped carbon dots synthesized via microwave-assisted pyrolysis: A potential nanoprobe for magneto-fluorescent dual-modality bioimaging. *ACS Biomater. Sci. Eng.* **2018**, *4*, 2582–2596. [CrossRef] [PubMed]
120. Pahari, S.K.; Olszakier, S.; Kahn, I.; Amirav, L. Magneto-fluorescent yolk–shell nanoparticles. *Chem. Mater.* **2018**, *30*, 775–780. [CrossRef]
121. Ge, Y.; Zhang, Y.; He, S.; Nie, F.; Teng, G.; Gu, N. Fluorescence modified chitosan-coated magnetic nanoparticles for high-efficient cellular imaging. *Nanoscale Res. Lett.* **2009**, *4*, 287–295. [CrossRef]
122. Haun, J.B.; Devaraj, N.K.; Marinelli, B.S.; Lee, H.; Weissleder, R. Probing intracellular biomarkers and mediators of cell activation using nanosensors and bioorthogonal chemistry. *ACS Nano* **2011**, *5*, 3204–3213. [CrossRef]
123. Song, Y.; Zhu, Y.; Jiang, K.; Liu, X.; Dong, L.; Li, D.; Chen, S.; Xing, H.; Yan, X.; Lu, Y. Self-assembling ferrimagnetic fluorescent micelles for bioimaging guided efficient magnetic hyperthermia therapy. *Nanoscale* **2023**, *15*, 365–375. [CrossRef]
124. Cabral Filho, P.E.; Cabrera, M.P.; Cardoso, A.L.; Santana, O.A.; Geraldes, C.F.; Santos, B.S.; de Lima, M.C.P.; Pereira, G.A.; Fontes, A. Multimodal highly fluorescent-magnetic nanoplatform to target transferrin receptors in cancer cells. *Biochim. Biophys. Acta Gen. Subj.* **2018**, *1862*, 2788–2796. [CrossRef]
125. Li, Z.; Wang, G.; Shen, Y.; Guo, N.; Ma, N. DNA-templated magnetic nanoparticle-quantum dot polymers for ultrasensitive capture and detection of circulating tumor cells. *Adv. Funct. Mater.* **2018**, *28*, 1707152. [CrossRef]
126. Zahin, N.; Anwar, R.; Tewari, D.; Kabir, M.T.; Sajid, A.; Mathew, B.; Uddin, M.S.; Aleya, L.; Abdel-Daim, M.M. Nanoparticles and its biomedical applications in health and diseases: Special focus on drug delivery. *Environ. Sci. Pollut. Res.* **2020**, *27*, 19151–19168. [CrossRef] [PubMed]
127. Bertorelle, F.; Wilhelm, C.; Roger, J.; Gazeau, F.; Ménager, C.; Cabuil, V. Fluorescence-modified superparamagnetic nanoparticles: Intracellular uptake and use in cellular imaging. *Langmuir* **2006**, *22*, 5385–5391. [CrossRef] [PubMed]
128. Borgohain, C.; Senapati, K.K.; Mishra, D.; Sarma, K.C.; Phukan, P. A new $CoFe_2O_4$–Cr_2O_3–SiO_2 fluorescent magnetic nanocomposite. *Nanoscale* **2010**, *2*, 2250–2256. [CrossRef]
129. Chekina, N.; Horák, D.; Jendelová, P.; Trchová, M.; Beneš, M.J.; Hrubý, M.; Herynek, V.; Turnovcová, K.; Syková, E. Fluorescent magnetic nanoparticles for biomedical applications. *J. Mater. Chem.* **2011**, *21*, 7630–7639. [CrossRef]
130. Chen, D.; Jiang, M.; Li, N.; Gu, H.; Xu, Q.; Ge, J.; Xia, X.; Lu, J. Modification of magnetic silica/iron oxide nanocomposites with fluorescent polymethacrylic acid for cancer targeting and drug delivery. *J. Mater. Chem.* **2010**, *20*, 6422–6429. [CrossRef]
131. Chen, O.; Riedemann, L.; Etoc, F.; Herrmann, H.; Coppey, M.; Barch, M.; Farrar, C.T.; Zhao, J.; Bruns, O.T.; Wei, H. Magneto-fluorescent core-shell supernanoparticles. *Nat. Commun.* **2014**, *5*, 5093. [CrossRef]
132. Cho, Y.-S.; Yoon, T.-J.; Jang, E.-S.; Hong, K.S.; Lee, S.Y.; Kim, O.R.; Park, C.; Kim, Y.-J.; Yi, G.-C.; Chang, K. Cetuximab-conjugated magneto-fluorescent silica nanoparticles for in vivo colon cancer targeting and imaging. *Cancer Lett.* **2010**, *299*, 63–71. [CrossRef]
133. Cho, H.-S.; Dong, Z.; Pauletti, G.M.; Zhang, J.; Xu, H.; Gu, H.; Wang, L.; Ewing, R.C.; Huth, C.; Wang, F. Fluorescent, superparamagnetic nanospheres for drug storage, targeting, and imaging: A multifunctional nanocarrier system for cancer diagnosis and treatment. *ACS Nano* **2010**, *4*, 5398–5404. [CrossRef]
134. Cho, M.; Contreras, E.Q.; Lee, S.S.; Jones, C.J.; Jang, W.; Colvin, V.L. Characterization and optimization of the fluorescence of nanoscale iron oxide/quantum dot complexes. *J. Phys. Chem. C* **2014**, *118*, 14606–14616. [CrossRef]
135. Ding, Y.; Yin, H.; Shen, S.; Sun, K.; Liu, F. Chitosan-based magnetic/fluorescent nanocomposites for cell labelling and controlled drug release. *New J. Chem.* **2017**, *41*, 1736–1743. [CrossRef]
136. Ebrahiminezhad, A.; Ghasemi, Y.; Rasoul-Amini, S.; Barar, J.; Davaran, S. Preparation of novel magnetic fluorescent nanoparticles using amino acids. *Colloids Surf. B Biointerfaces* **2013**, *102*, 534–539. [CrossRef] [PubMed]
137. Fu, A.; Wilson, R.J.; Smith, B.R.; Mullenix, J.; Earhart, C.; Akin, D.; Guccione, S.; Wang, S.X.; Gambhir, S.S. Fluorescent magnetic nanoparticles for magnetically enhanced cancer imaging and targeting in living subjects. *ACS Nano* **2012**, *6*, 6862–6869. [CrossRef] [PubMed]
138. Gai, S.; Yang, P.; Li, C.; Wang, W.; Dai, Y.; Niu, N.; Lin, J. Synthesis of magnetic, Up-Conversion luminescent, and mesoporous core–Shell-Structured nanocomposites as drug carriers. *Adv. Funct. Mater.* **2010**, *20*, 1166–1172. [CrossRef]
139. Gao, J.; Zhang, W.; Huang, P.; Zhang, B.; Zhang, X.; Xu, B. Intracellular spatial control of fluorescent magnetic nanoparticles. *J. Am. Chem. Soc.* **2008**, *130*, 3710–3711. [CrossRef] [PubMed]
140. Gallagher, J.J.; Tekoriute, R.; O'Reilly, J.-A.; Kerskens, C.; Gun'ko, Y.K.; Lynch, M. Bimodal magnetic-fluorescent nanostructures for biomedical applications. *J. Mater. Chem.* **2009**, *19*, 4081–4084. [CrossRef]
141. Gao, Y.; Zou, X.; Zhao, J.X.; Li, Y.; Su, X. Graphene oxide-based magnetic fluorescent hybrids for drug delivery and cellular imaging. *Colloids Surf. B Biointerfaces* **2013**, *112*, 128–133. [CrossRef]
142. Gaponik, N.; Radtchenko, I.L.; Sukhorukov, G.B.; Rogach, A.L. Luminescent polymer microcapsules addressable by a magnetic field. *Langmuir* **2004**, *20*, 1449–1452. [CrossRef]
143. Hong, X.; Li, J.; Wang, M.; Xu, J.; Guo, W.; Li, J.; Bai, Y.; Li, T. Fabrication of magnetic luminescent nanocomposites by a layer-by-layer self-assembly approach. *Chem. Mater.* **2004**, *16*, 4022–4027. [CrossRef]

144. Howes, P.; Green, M.; Bowers, A.; Parker, D.; Varma, G.; Kallumadil, M.; Hughes, M.; Warley, A.; Brain, A.; Botnar, R. Magnetic conjugated polymer nanoparticles as bimodal imaging agents. *J. Am. Chem. Soc.* **2010**, *132*, 9833–9842. [CrossRef]
145. Huang, P.; Li, Z.; Lin, J.; Yang, D.; Gao, G.; Xu, C.; Bao, L.; Zhang, C.; Wang, K.; Song, H. Photosensitizer-conjugated magnetic nanoparticles for in vivo simultaneous magnetofluorescent imaging and targeting therapy. *Biomaterials* **2011**, *32*, 3447–3458. [CrossRef]
146. Hwang, D.W.; Song, I.C.; Lee, D.S.; Kim, S. Smart magnetic fluorescent nanoparticle imaging probes to monitor microRNAs. *Small* **2010**, *6*, 81–88. [CrossRef] [PubMed]
147. Jha, D.K.; Saikia, K.; Chakrabarti, S.; Bhattacharya, K.; Varadarajan, K.S.; Patel, A.B.; Goyary, D.; Chattopadhyay, P.; Deb, P. Direct one-pot synthesis of glutathione capped hydrophilic FePt-CdS nanoprobe for efficient bimodal imaging application. *Mater. Sci. Eng. C* **2017**, *72*, 415–424. [CrossRef] [PubMed]
148. Kaewsaneha, C.; Opaprakasit, P.; Polpanich, D.; Smanmoo, S.; Tangboriboonrat, P. Immobilization of fluorescein isothiocyanate on magnetic polymeric nanoparticle using chitosan as spacer. *J. Colloid Interface Sci.* **2012**, *377*, 145–152. [CrossRef] [PubMed]
149. Koc, K.; Karakus, B.; Rajar, K.; Alveroglu, E. Synthesis and characterization of ZnS@ Fe_3O_4 fluorescent-magnetic bifunctional nanospheres. *Superlattices Microstruct.* **2017**, *110*, 198–204. [CrossRef]
150. Koktysh, D.; Bright, V.; Pham, W. Fluorescent magnetic hybrid nanoprobe for multimodal bioimaging. *Nanotechnology* **2011**, *22*, 275606. [CrossRef]
151. Lee, J.H.; Chen, K.J.; Noh, S.H.; Garcia, M.A.; Wang, H.; Lin, W.Y.; Jeong, H.; Kong, B.J.; Stout, D.B.; Cheon, J. On-demand drug release system for in vivo cancer treatment through self-assembled magnetic nanoparticles. *Angew. Chem. Int. Ed.* **2013**, *52*, 4384–4388. [CrossRef]
152. Lehmann, A.D.; Parak, W.J.; Zhang, F.; Ali, Z.; Röcker, C.; Nienhaus, G.U.; Gehr, P.; Rothen-Rutishauser, B. Fluorescent–Magnetic Hybrid Nanoparticles Induce a Dose-Dependent Increase in Proinflammatory Response in Lung Cells in vitro Correlated with Intracellular Localization. *Small* **2010**, *6*, 753–762. [CrossRef]
153. Levy, I.; Sher, I.; Corem-Salkmon, E.; Ziv-Polat, O.; Meir, A.; Treves, A.J.; Nagler, A.; Kalter-Leibovici, O.; Margel, S.; Rotenstreich, Y. Bioactive magnetic near Infra-Red fluorescent core-shell iron oxide/human serum albumin nanoparticles for controlled release of growth factors for augmentation of human mesenchymal stem cell growth and differentiation. *J. Nanobiotechnol.* **2015**, *13*, 34. [CrossRef]
154. Lu, Y.; Zheng, Y.; You, S.; Wang, F.; Gao, Z.; Shen, J.; Yang, W.; Yin, M. Bifunctional magnetic-fluorescent nanoparticles: Synthesis, characterization, and cell imaging. *ACS Appl. Mater. Interfaces* **2015**, *7*, 5226–5232. [CrossRef]
155. Lu, X.; Jiang, R.; Fan, Q.; Zhang, L.; Zhang, H.; Yang, M.; Ma, Y.; Wang, L.; Huang, W. Fluorescent-magnetic poly (poly (ethyleneglycol) monomethacrylate)-grafted Fe_3O_4 nanoparticles from post-atom-transfer-radical-polymerization modification: Synthesis, characterization, cellular uptake and imaging. *J. Mater. Chem.* **2012**, *22*, 6965–6973. [CrossRef]
156. May, B.M.; Fakayode, O.J.; Bambo, M.F.; Sidwaba, U.; Nxumalo, E.N.; Mishra, A.K. Stable magneto-fluorescent gadolinium-doped AgInS2 core quantum dots (QDs) with enhanced photoluminescence properties. *Mater. Lett.* **2021**, *305*, 130776. [CrossRef]
157. Rawat, D.; Singh, R.R. Avant-grade magneto/fluorescent nanostructures for biomedical applications: Organized and comprehensive optical and magnetic evaluation. *Nano Struct. Nano Objects* **2021**, *26*, 100714. [CrossRef]
158. Martynenko, I.V.; Kusic, D.; Weigert, F.; Stafford, S.; Donnelly, F.C.; Evstigneev, R.; Gromova, Y.; Baranov, A.V.; Rühle, B.; Kunte, H.-J. Magneto-fluorescent microbeads for bacteria detection constructed from superparamagnetic Fe_3O_4 nanoparticles and AIS/ZnS quantum dots. *Anal. Chem.* **2019**, *91*, 12661–12669. [CrossRef] [PubMed]
159. Tiwari, A.; Singh, A.; Debnath, A.; Kaul, A.; Garg, N.; Mathur, R.; Singh, A.; Randhawa, J.K. Multifunctional magneto-fluorescent nanocarriers for dual mode imaging and targeted drug delivery. *ACS Appl. Nano Mater.* **2019**, *2*, 3060–3072. [CrossRef]
160. Mohandes, F.; Dehghani, H.; Angizi, S.; Ramedani, A.; Dolatyar, B.; Farani, M.R.; Müllen, K.; Simchi, A. Magneto-fluorescent contrast agents based on carbon Dots@ Ferrite nanoparticles for tumor imaging. *J. Magn. Magn. Mater.* **2022**, *561*, 169686. [CrossRef]
161. Sosnovik, D.E.; Schellenberger, E.A.; Nahrendorf, M.; Novikov, M.S.; Matsui, T.; Dai, G.; Reynolds, F.; Grazette, L.; Rosenzweig, A.; Weissleder, R. Magnetic resonance imaging of cardiomyocyte apoptosis with a novel magneto-optical nanoparticle. *Magn. Reson. Med. Off. J. Int. Soc. Magn. Reson. Med.* **2005**, *54*, 718–724. [CrossRef]
162. McCarthy, J.R.; Kelly, K.A.; Sun, E.Y.; Weissleder, R. Targeted delivery of multifunctional magnetic nanoparticles. *Future Med.* **2007**, *2*, 153–167. [CrossRef]
163. Tassa, C.; Shaw, S.Y.; Weissleder, R. Dextran-coated iron oxide nanoparticles: A versatile platform for targeted molecular imaging, molecular diagnostics, and therapy. *Acc. Chem. Res.* **2011**, *44*, 842–852. [CrossRef]
164. Nahrendorf, M.; Keliher, E.; Marinelli, B.; Leuschner, F.; Robbins, C.S.; Gerszten, R.E.; Pittet, M.J.; Swirski, F.K.; Weissleder, R. Detection of macrophages in aortic aneurysms by nanoparticle positron emission tomography–computed tomography. *Arterioscler. Thromb. Vasc. Biol.* **2011**, *31*, 750–757. [CrossRef]
165. Fairclough, M.; Ellis, B.; Boutin, H.; Jones, A.; McMahon, A.; Alzabin, S.; Gennari, A.; Prenant, C. Development of a method for the preparation of zirconium-89 radiolabelled chitosan nanoparticles as an application for leukocyte trafficking with positron emission tomography. *Appl. Radiat. Isot.* **2017**, *130*, 7–12. [CrossRef]
166. Fairclough, M.; Prenant, C.; Ellis, B.; Boutin, H.; McMahon, A.; Brown, G.; Locatelli, P.; Jones, A. A new technique for the radiolabelling of mixed leukocytes with zirconium-89 for inflammation imaging with positron emission tomography. *J. Label. Compd. Radiopharm.* **2016**, *59*, 270–276. [CrossRef] [PubMed]

167. Keliher, E.J.; Yoo, J.; Nahrendorf, M.; Lewis, J.S.; Marinelli, B.; Newton, A.; Pittet, M.J.; Weissleder, R. 89Zr-labeled dextran nanoparticles allow in vivo macrophage imaging. *Bioconjugate Chem.* **2011**, *22*, 2383–2389. [CrossRef] [PubMed]
168. Rose, P.G. Endometrial carcinoma. *N. Engl. J. Med.* **1996**, *335*, 640–649. [CrossRef]
169. Veronesi, U.; Paganelli, G.; Galimberti, V.; Viale, G.; Zurrida, S.; Bedoni, M.; Costa, A.; De Cicco, C.; Geraghty, J.G.; Luini, A. Sentinel-node biopsy to avoid axillary dissection in breast cancer with clinically negative lymph-nodes. *Lancet* **1997**, *349*, 1864–1867. [CrossRef] [PubMed]
170. Iga, A.M.; Robertson, J.H.; Winslet, M.C.; Seifalian, A.M. Clinical potential of quantum dots. *J. Biomed. Biotechnol.* **2007**, *2007*, 076087. [CrossRef]
171. Saha, A.K.; Sharma, P.; Sohn, H.-B.; Ghosh, S.; Das, R.K.; Hebard, A.F.; Zeng, H.; Baligand, C.; Walter, G.A.; Moudgil, B.M. Fe doped CdTeS magnetic quantum dots for bioimaging. *J. Mater. Chem. B* **2013**, *1*, 6312–6320. [CrossRef]
172. Cao, J.; Niu, H.; Du, J.; Yang, L.; Wei, M.; Liu, X.; Liu, Q.; Yang, J. Fabrication of P (NIPAAm-co-AAm) coated optical-magnetic quantum dots/silica core-shell nanocomposites for temperature triggered drug release, bioimaging and in vivo tumor inhibition. *J. Mater. Sci. Mater. Med.* **2018**, *29*, 169. [CrossRef]
173. Yue, L.; Li, H.; Liu, Q.; Guo, D.; Chen, J.; Sun, Q.; Xu, Y.; Wu, F. Manganese-doped carbon quantum dots for fluorometric and magnetic resonance (dual mode) bioimaging and biosensing. *Microchim. Acta* **2019**, *186*, 315. [CrossRef]
174. Shi, Y.; Pan, Y.; Zhong, J.; Yang, J.; Zheng, J.; Cheng, J.; Song, R.; Yi, C. Facile synthesis of gadolinium (III) chelates functionalized carbon quantum dots for fluorescence and magnetic resonance dual-modal bioimaging. *Carbon* **2015**, *93*, 742–750. [CrossRef]
175. Liu, X.; Jiang, H.; Ye, J.; Zhao, C.; Gao, S.; Wu, C.; Li, C.; Li, J.; Wang, X. Nitrogen-doped carbon quantum dot stabilized magnetic iron oxide nanoprobe for fluorescence, magnetic resonance, and computed tomography triple-modal in vivo bioimaging. *Adv. Funct. Mater.* **2016**, *26*, 8694–8706. [CrossRef]
176. Zhou, R.; Sun, S.; Li, C.; Wu, L.; Hou, X.; Wu, P. Enriching Mn-doped ZnSe quantum dots onto mesoporous silica nanoparticles for enhanced fluorescence/magnetic resonance imaging dual-modal bio-imaging. *ACS Appl. Mater. Interfaces* **2018**, *10*, 34060–34067. [CrossRef] [PubMed]
177. Yao, H.; Su, L.; Zeng, M.; Cao, L.; Zhao, W.; Chen, C.; Du, B.; Zhou, J. Construction of magnetic-carbon-quantum-dots-probe-labeled apoferritin nanocages for bioimaging and targeted therapy. *Int. J. Nanomed.* **2016**, *11*, 4423. [CrossRef] [PubMed]
178. Erogbogbo, F.; Chang, C.-W.; May, J.L.; Liu, L.; Kumar, R.; Law, W.-C.; Ding, H.; Yong, K.T.; Roy, I.; Sheshadri, M. Bioconjugation of luminescent silicon quantum dots to gadolinium ions for bioimaging applications. *Nanoscale* **2012**, *4*, 5483–5489. [CrossRef] [PubMed]
179. Jiao, M.; Li, Y.; Jia, Y.; Li, C.; Bian, H.; Gao, L.; Cai, P.; Luo, X. Strongly emitting and long-lived silver indium sulfide quantum dots for bioimaging: Insight into co-ligand effect on enhanced photoluminescence. *J. Colloid Interface Sci.* **2020**, *565*, 35–42. [CrossRef] [PubMed]
180. Yang, J.; Dave, S.R.; Gao, X. Quantum dot nanobarcodes: Epitaxial assembly of nanoparticle−polymer complexes in homogeneous solution. *J. Am. Chem. Soc.* **2008**, *130*, 5286–5292. [CrossRef] [PubMed]
181. Han, M.; Gao, X.; Su, J.Z.; Nie, S. Quantum-dot-tagged microbeads for multiplexed optical coding of biomolecules. *Nat. Biotechnol.* **2001**, *19*, 631–635. [CrossRef]
182. Ma, Q.; Nakane, Y.; Mori, Y.; Hasegawa, M.; Yoshioka, Y.; Watanabe, T.M.; Gonda, K.; Ohuchi, N.; Jin, T. Multilayered, core/shell nanoprobes based on magnetic ferric oxide particles and quantum dots for multimodality imaging of breast cancer tumors. *Biomaterials* **2012**, *33*, 8486–8494. [CrossRef]
183. Tran, M.V.; Susumu, K.; Medintz, I.L.; Algar, W.R. Supraparticle assemblies of magnetic nanoparticles and quantum dots for selective cell isolation and counting on a smartphone-based imaging platform. *Anal. Chem.* **2019**, *91*, 11963–11971. [CrossRef]
184. Guo, W.; Yang, W.; Wang, Y.; Sun, X.; Liu, Z.; Zhang, B.; Chang, J.; Chen, X. Color-tunable Gd-Zn-Cu-In-S/ZnS quantum dots for dual modality magnetic resonance and fluorescence imaging. *Nano Res.* **2014**, *7*, 1581–1591. [CrossRef]
185. Wáng, Y.X.J.; Idée, J.-M.; Corot, C. Scientific and industrial challenges of developing nanoparticle-based theranostics and multiple-modality contrast agents for clinical application. *Nanoscale* **2015**, *7*, 16146–16150. [CrossRef]
186. Rahmer, J.; Halkola, A.; Gleich, B.; Schmale, I.; Borgert, J. First experimental evidence of the feasibility of multi-color magnetic particle imaging. *Phys. Med. Biol.* **2015**, *60*, 1775. [CrossRef] [PubMed]
187. Franke, J.; Heinen, U.; Lehr, H.; Weber, A.; Jaspard, F.; Ruhm, W.; Heidenreich, M.; Schulz, V. System characterization of a highly integrated preclinical hybrid MPI-MRI scanner. *IEEE Trans. Med. Imaging* **2016**, *35*, 1993–2004. [CrossRef]
188. BIO-TECH Report #200, The Market for PET Radiopharmaceuticals & PET Imaging. Available online: http://biotechsystems.com/reports/200/default.asp (accessed on 6 July 2005).
189. Mitchell, M.J.; Billingsley, M.M.; Haley, R.M.; Wechsler, M.E.; Peppas, N.A.; Langer, R. Engineering precision nanoparticles for drug delivery. *Nat. Rev. Drug Discov.* **2021**, *20*, 101–124. [CrossRef] [PubMed]
190. Wang, X.; Chao, L.; Liu, X.; Xu, X.; Zhang, Q. Association between HLA genotype and cutaneous adverse reactions to antiepileptic drugs among epilepsy patients in northwest China. *Front. Neurol.* **2019**, *10*, 1. [CrossRef] [PubMed]

Disclaimer/Publisher's Note: The statements, opinions and data contained in all publications are solely those of the individual author(s) and contributor(s) and not of MDPI and/or the editor(s). MDPI and/or the editor(s) disclaim responsibility for any injury to people or property resulting from any ideas, methods, instructions or products referred to in the content.

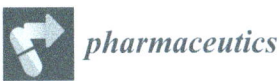

Review

Iron-Based Ceramic Composite Nanomaterials for Magnetic Fluid Hyperthermia and Drug Delivery

Ming-Hsien Chan [1,†], Chien-Hsiu Li [1,†], Yu-Chan Chang [2] and Michael Hsiao [1,3,*]

1. Genomics Research Center, Academia Sinica, Taipei 115, Taiwan
2. Department of Biomedical Imaging and Radiological Sciences, National Yang Ming Chiao Tung University, Taipei 112, Taiwan
3. Department and Graduate Institute of Veterinary Medicine, School of Veterinary Medicine, National Taiwan University, Taipei 106, Taiwan
* Correspondence: mhsiao@gate.sinica.edu.tw
† These authors contributed equally to this work.

Abstract: Because of the unique physicochemical properties of magnetic iron-based nanoparticles, such as superparamagnetism, high saturation magnetization, and high effective surface area, they have been applied in biomedical fields such as diagnostic imaging, disease treatment, and biochemical separation. Iron-based nanoparticles have been used in magnetic resonance imaging (MRI) to produce clearer and more detailed images, and they have therapeutic applications in magnetic fluid hyperthermia (MFH). In recent years, researchers have used clay minerals, such as ceramic materials with iron-based nanoparticles, to construct nanocomposite materials with enhanced saturation, magnetization, and thermal effects. Owing to their unique structure and large specific surface area, iron-based nanoparticles can be homogenized by adding different proportions of ceramic minerals before and after modification to enhance saturation magnetization. In this review, we assess the potential to improve the magnetic properties of iron-based nanoparticles and in the preparation of multifunctional composite materials through their combination with ceramic materials. We demonstrate the potential of ferromagnetic enhancement and multifunctional composite materials for MRI diagnosis, drug delivery, MFH therapy, and cellular imaging applications.

Keywords: iron-based nanoparticles; ceramic nanocomposites; magnetic resonance imaging; magnetic fluid hyperthermia; drug delivery

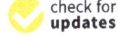

Citation: Chan, M.-H.; Li, C.-H.; Chang, Y.-C.; Hsiao, M. Iron-Based Ceramic Composite Nanomaterials for Magnetic Fluid Hyperthermia and Drug Delivery. *Pharmaceutics* 2022, 14, 2584. https://doi.org/10.3390/pharmaceutics14122584

Academic Editor: Constantin Mihai Lucaciu

Received: 7 October 2022
Accepted: 21 November 2022
Published: 24 November 2022

Publisher's Note: MDPI stays neutral with regard to jurisdictional claims in published maps and institutional affiliations.

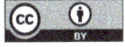

Copyright: © 2022 by the authors. Licensee MDPI, Basel, Switzerland. This article is an open access article distributed under the terms and conditions of the Creative Commons Attribution (CC BY) license (https://creativecommons.org/licenses/by/4.0/).

1. Introduction

Magnetic materials are functional materials with great potential that are widely used in biomedicine [1–3]. Their unique magnetic signals allow them to be used as sensors in imaging medicine, based on the detection of geomagnetic fields, and in noncontact magnetic-field-heating therapy [4–6]. Magnetic materials can even integrate all the conditions of nanoparticles when their particle size is limited to within a range of 1–100 nm. Nanoparticles can be used as contrast agents, target drug carriers, and multifunctional magnetic biomedical materials for controlled and focused therapy. In recent years, nanoparticles have been compounded with other materials possessing low toxicity and superparamagnetic and biocompatible properties. The resulting compounds can be applied for using in similar applications as for nanoparticles mentioned earlier [7–9]. Once nanosized, these nanomaterials exhibit many novel and excellent properties [10]. The field of nano-biomedical materials involves the integration of nanomaterials/nanotechnology with biomedical materials or drugs, and these developments have substantially contributed to the progress of human medicine.

In all mammalian cells, iron is an indispensable element for the processes of cell growth and differentiation. Because of the unique physicochemical properties of magnetic iron-based nanoparticles, such as superparamagnetism, high saturation magnetization, and high effective surface area, they have been applied in biomedical fields such as diagnostic imaging, disease treatment, and biochemical separation [11]. Iron-based nanoparticles have been used in magnetic resonance imaging (MRI) to produce clearer and more detailed images, and they have therapeutic applications in magnetic fluid hyperthermia (MFH) [12,13]. The combination of the treatment and diagnosis approach into one system for cancer treatment indicates their potential for ushering in the "iron age". In recent years, clay minerals, such as ceramic materials with iron-based nanoparticles, have been used to construct nanocomposite materials to enhance their saturation magnetization and thermal effects. Due to their unique structure and large specific surface area, iron-based nanoparticles can be homogenized by adding different proportions of ceramic minerals before and after modification to enhance saturation magnetization. In this review, we assess the potential to improve the magnetic properties of iron-based nanoparticles and in the preparation of multifunctional composite materials through their combination with ceramic materials. We demonstrate the potential of ferromagnetic enhancement and multifunctional composite materials for MRI diagnosis, drug delivery, MFH therapy, and cellular imaging applications [14].

Multifunctional nanocomposites have been a hot area of research in recent years. In this review, we hoped to identify iron-based nanocomposite materials that can enhance saturation magnetization (Ms) and be applied to optimize MRI contrast. In addition, a magnetic nanocomposite material with improved biocompatibility is needed for biomedical applications. As for the choice of the composite material, examples of low-cost, high-adsorption, and biocompatible ceramic materials, montmorillonite silicate, kaolinite minerals, or bioglass can be used to produce multifunctional nanocomposite materials with both magnetic properties and high adsorption performance.

2. Magnetic Properties of Nanoparticles

Nanotechnology has become ubiquitous in everyday life through its use in the aerospace, electronic, cosmetic, and pharmaceutical industries, among others. These developments have enabled improvement of the existing nanoparticle properties and the introduction of new optical, electrical, and mechanical functions. In addition, nano-sized materials experience small size, surface, quantum tunneling, Coulomb blocking, and quantum-limiting effects distinctly from macroscopic materials.

Hence, the optical, thermal, and electrical effects as well as magnetic, mechanical, and other properties of nanomaterials differ from those of the corresponding bulk materials (Figure 1a). Because of the unique properties of magnetic nanoparticles, such as superparamagnetism, high saturation magnetization, and high effective surface area, they are mainly used as contrast agents, to improve image contrast, and as carriers for drug delivery in disease treatment. In addition, when injected into the body, magnetic nanoparticles can generate heat energy through the use of an applied magnetic field to kill cancer cells, avoiding the damage to normal cells observed in conventional chemotherapy and inhibiting cancer cell growth by MFH. Because of their excellent magnetic properties, the application of nanomaterials is constantly being improved and refined [15–17]. All substances have a certain degree of magnetization, which is usually dependent on the material's atomic structure and surrounding temperature, and the magnetic susceptibility (χ) can be used to express the difficulty of magnetization. When a material is placed under an applied magnetic field (H), its magnetization (M) will change, and the relationship between the two is as follows (Figure 1b):

$$M = \chi H \qquad (1)$$

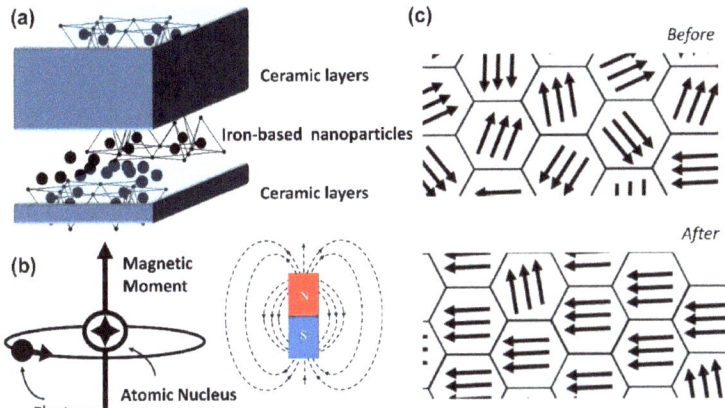

Figure 1. Magnetic variation in iron-based nanoparticles compounded with ceramic materials. Schematic diagram of (**a**) composite material composition; (**b**) magnetic dipole moment of composite material; and (**c**) nonmagnetic/magnetic zone structures.

A magnetic material has a "magnetic domain", in which the crystalline structure of the energy state itself is divided into several different regions, and these magnetic domains are all oriented in the same direction. Nevertheless, the order of each magnetic domain is not necessarily the same, and there will be mutual offset, as shown in Figure 1c. Assuming that the net magnetic moment is precisely zero, the material is not magnetic. Conversely, when the net magnetic moment is not zero, the material is magnetic [18]. Most materials have the property of being weakly magnetic, even in the absence of an applied magnetic field. The former has an approximate magnetization rate ranging from 10^{-6} to 10^{-1} in order of magnitude, while the latter only ranges from 10^{-6} to 10^{-3} in order of magnitude. In contrast, some materials can exhibit highly magnetic properties under the action of weak magnetic fields, or even without the application of magnetic fields, such as in the case of ferromagnetic, ferrimagnetic, and antiferromagnetic materials (Figure 2a). In such cases, only a minimal magnetic field is needed to saturate magnetization, and the representative materials are iron, cobalt, and nickel.

From a microscopic point of view, a large-size ferromagnetic material with multiple magnetic regions exhibits a minor hysteresis effect, as shown in Figure 2b. When the size of the material is reduced to a single domain (generally nanoscale; the critical size varies from material to fabric), the hysteresis effect is the largest (i.e., it has the most substantial coercive force). However, when the scope continues to shrink, the coercive force decreases to zero (i.e., no hysteresis occurs). With the change in the external magnetic field, the data points obtained from the magnetization process of the superparamagnetic nanoparticles can form a hysteresis curve, as shown in Figure 2d. Therefore, the superparamagnetic nanoparticles are not magnetic at room temperature without the applied magnetic field, and when the applied magnetic field is removed, the material's magnetic properties immediately disappear. For example, in iron oxide, nanoparticles usually need to reach a size of several nanometers to become superparamagnetic, as shown in Figure 2c [19].

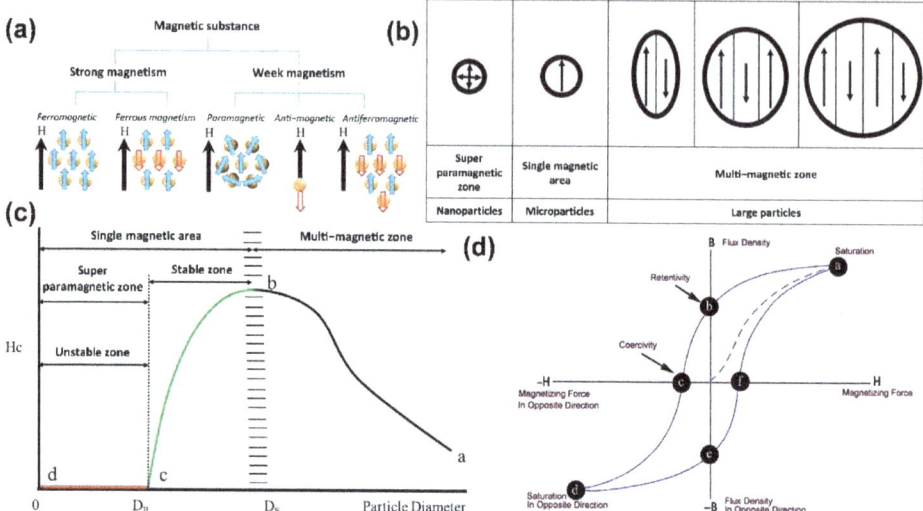

Figure 2. Theories and principles of nanometer sizing and superparamagnetism: (**a**) classification of magnetic substances; (**b**) schematic diagrams of structures of multimagnetic/single-magnetic/superparamagnetic regions; (**c**) relationship between particle size and coercivity. The multi-magnetic region is represented by the curve from a to b, where the coercivity of magnetic particles tends to increase, and the coercivity of the material shows a maximum size at Ds; between b and c is the single-magnetic region, where the particles in this size range show stability; from c to d is the superparamagnetic region, where the material shows an unstable state due to high surface activity at the nanoscale. At D_P, the material is demagnetized by external thermal effects, resulting in zero coercivity (HC = 0); the zone to the left is called superparamagnetic; and (**d**) hysteresis curves.

2.1. Properties of Iron Oxide Nanoparticles

Iron oxide nanoparticles are widely known examples of nanomaterials. Iron tetroxide (Fe_3O_4) is a biocompatible material that has been known of and used in biomedicine for almost 40 years, and it is approved for use in the human body based on its safety profile. Fe_3O_4 magnetic nanoparticles are water-soluble and can enter delicate tissues; they are commonly produced by coprecipitation (aqueous phase), thermal decomposition (organic phase), and synthetic methods (Figure 3a–c) [11]. For use in biomedical applications, nanoparticles must be: (1) non-biotoxic; (2) water-soluble; and (3) biocompatible. The biomedical applications in which nanoparticles of iron tetroxide are applied are diverse [20]. The most remarkable instances are those where their magnetic properties are exploited, for example, in thermotherapy and drug magnetic guidance therapy. For example, in the case of a rat with a tumor on its back, we can inject magnetic nanoparticles through the tail and use carefully positioned magnets around the rat to achieve guided drug treatment for the cancer [21–23].

Heat therapy aims to increase the temperature to a level that is tolerated by normal human cells but not cancer cells, at which point the cancer cells begin to die. The current research indicates that thermotherapy can effectively eliminate tumors that are smaller than 7 mm [24]. Still, in clinical trials, uniform tumor heating is impossible on animals with larger tumors (15 mm). The cancer is unevenly heated because of the uneven shape of the tumor, and it is hard to effectively destroy the entire cancer all at one time during treatment, which results in continued tumor growth [25]. Because of this, we want to develop magnetic particles that can be used to accelerate and increase the temperature of the cancerous tissue. One possibility is to dope magnetic particles into ceramic nanostructures to generate nanocomposite materials. The composite particles enable the faster elimination of cancer cells, thus achieving more effective treatment, and they are expected to more efficiently inhibit the formation of tumors. In addition, we can use the method to encapsulate magnetic nanoparticles and drugs at the same time. This problem can be resolved through ceramic-material-compounding technology, which is thermosensitive and biocompatible. Moreover, microcellular surface carriers with specific surface modifications can deliver magnetic nanoparticles and drugs to specific tumor cells. The magnetic nanoparticles are heated to 40 °C for a few seconds under an applied magnetic field, upon which the ceramic material releases the drug and magnetic nanoparticles into tumor cells [21]. Therefore, this two-pronged approach allows incorporating an additional aspect to drug therapy.

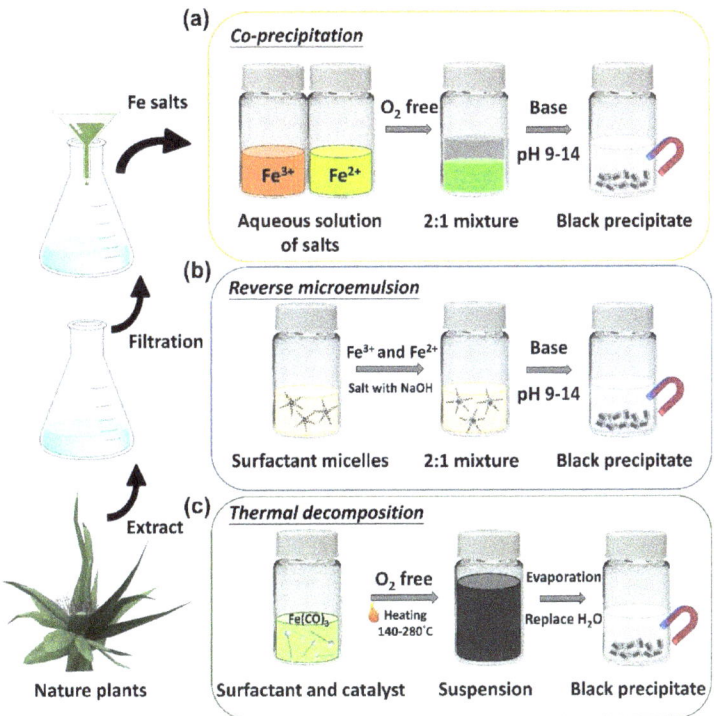

Figure 3. Synthesis of iron oxide nanoparticles by: (**a**) coprecipitation; (**b**) reverse microemulsion; (**c**) thermal decomposition under green synthesis process.

2.2. Properties of Iron–Platinum Nanoparticles

Iron–platinum nanoparticles are a magnetic material that is used in recording media with the chemical formula FePt. There are four phases of ferroplatinum: the (1) unordered γ-phase; (2) ordered paramagnetic γ1-Fe_3Pt phase (L12); (3) ferromagnetic γ2-FePt phase (L10); and (4) antiferromagnetism γ3-$FePt_3$ phase (L12). The structure of the $FePt_3$ phase (L12) depends on the FePt atomic ratio. The structure of unordered Fe platinum is chemically disordered face-centered cubic (FCC), and that of ordered Fe platinum is chemically ordered face-centered tetragonal (FCT) [26], as shown in Figure 4 [27]. In addition, the atomic lattice position of the unordered face-centered cubic is determined by the percentage of Fe and Pt atoms that form a soft magnetic structure with a small coercivity field [28]. In contrast, in the ordered face-centered cubic in iron–platinum, the iron atoms are stacked at positions (0, 1/2, 1/2) and (1/2, 0, 1/2), the platinum atoms are stacked at positions (0, 0, 0) and (1/2, 1/2, 0), and the atomic radii cause the lattice to expand in the a-axis and compress in the c-axis [29–32]. The magneto-crystal anisotropy coefficient (Ku) can reach 107 Jm^{-3} [33], which is the highest among the existing hard magnetic materials, due to spin–orbit coupling and hybridization interactions between the 3D orbital domain of

Fe and 5D orbital domain of Pt [34,35]. This alignment provides FePt with higher chemical stability than Fe, Co, or other materials (e.g., Fe_3O_4) with high coercivity fields [36]. The high Ku of FePt can allow superparamagnetic phenomena to be avoided when the particle size decreases [37]. In addition to having superior superparamagnetic properties, FePt nanoparticles also have high absorption coefficients for X-rays (Pt absorption coefficient at 50 keV: 6.95 cm^2/g). Chou et al. injected 12 nm FePt nanoparticles into mice with tumors by tail-intravenous injection, and the contrast between the MRI and computed tomography (CT) images was substantially improved, which indicates that we can use FePt to track the location of the material in two diagnostic MRI and CT imaging modalities to detect the area in which the MFH and drug release are taking place.

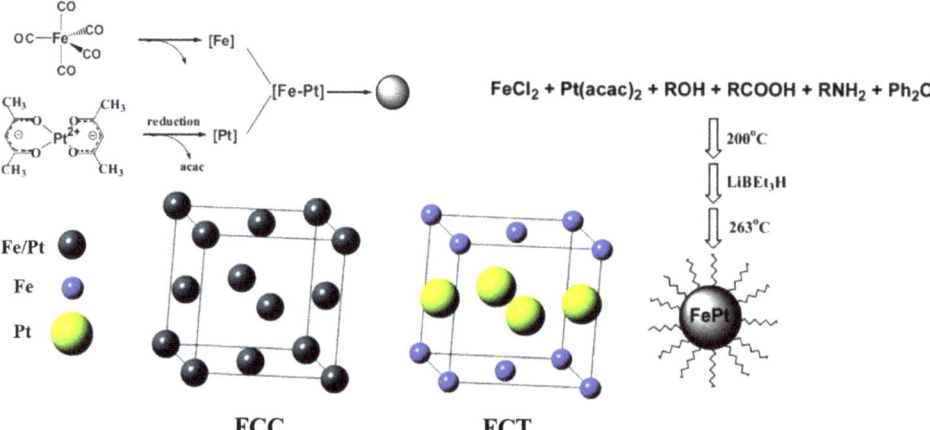

Figure 4. Schematic diagram of synthesizing disordered and ordered structures using Fe(acac)$_3$ and Pt(acac)$_2$, forming iron–platinum (FePt) nanoparticles from pyrolytic iron and reduced platinum precursors and using ferrous chloride instead of iron pentacarbonyl.

3. Surface Modification of Iron-Based Nanoparticles

The key to the technology is how to use ligands for surface modification and increase the function of magnetic nanoparticles. Generally, two methods are used: (1) Crosslinkers or spacer molecules as well as polymer ligands are used to form covalent connections [38]. The body is modified on the surface of the magnetic nanoparticles to include iron nanoparticles as the core and ligands as the shell [39]. The affinity between nanoparticles and polymer ligands depends on the type and quantity of the ligands on the surfaces of the nanoparticles; thus, how to make and select the surface ligands for linking is important [40]. Amines, carboxylates, hydroxyl groups, and thiol groups are commonly used as ligands [41]. In some cases, additional spacer molecules or crosslinking agents are required to facilitate bonding of the nanocomposites [42]. (2) In layer-by-layer coating [43], with magnetic nanoparticles as the core, other materials are coated, layer by layer, around the nanoparticles based on the electrostatic attraction between opposing charges [44]. The advantages include the ability to fabricate a single-layer structure and adjust the thickness of the functional shell [45]. According to the above two approaches, we take the carboxylation of chitosan to covalently bond to the surfaces and core–shell structures of the nanoparticles as an example, and we discuss the advantages of ceramic materials for modification of iron-based nanoparticles in the next section (Figure 5).

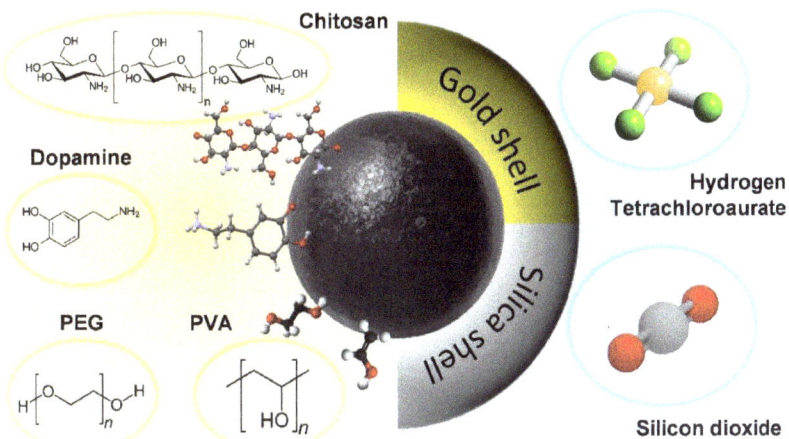

Figure 5. Schematic representation of the surface modification of iron-based nanoparticles. Iron-based nanoparticle with different crosslinker or spacer molecules and layer-by-layer coating. From left to right, the molecules are chitosan, dopamine, polyethylene glycol (PEG), polyvinyl alcohol (PVA), silicon dioxide (SiO_2), and hydrogen tetrachloroaurate ($AuCl_4$).

Chitosans are natural polysaccharides with hydrophilic, biocompatible, biodegradable, and antibacterial properties. They have a good affinity for many biomolecules, which makes them suitable for various biomedical and biotechnology applications. Degradable polymers are more commonly used for the controlled release of drugs [46]. Polysaccharides are nontoxic and biodegradable natural polymers that form particles to coat drugs in acidic environments, such as in the stomach, where they act as antacids to prevent acid damage to drugs. Therefore, they are an ideal material for drug-release-control systems. For drug-targeting applications, magnetic nanoparticles modified with chitosans can adsorb the anticancer drug epirubicin, which indicates a strong interaction between chitosans and epirubicin. In epirubicin-adsorption experiments, the equilibration time is only a few minutes, which means that there is no intrapore diffusion resistance in the adsorption process. Through regulation of the acidic environment in cancer cells at a pH of 4, chitosan is subjected to disintegration. Epirubicin adsorbed on nanomagnetic carriers is expected to be released in in vivo experiments to achieve therapeutic cancer effects [47].

The surface modification of iron-based nanoparticles with core–shell structures is close to that of iron-based nanocomposite particles combined with ceramic materials, which is the focus of this review: i.e., enhancement of the applicability of iron nanoparticles by incorporating other materials. Here, we search for an example of self-assembled nanocomposite materials for iron core–gold shells to link the advantages of ceramic materials combined with iron nanoparticles [48]. The iron core–gold shell composite nanoparticles are selectively toxic to cancer cells. Still, after being placed in water or air for a suitable period, they are no longer harmful to cancer cells [49]. Researchers found that freshly produced iron core–gold shell composite nanoparticles are not toxic to cancer cells when placed in water. Water molecules will penetrate through the grain interface of the gold shell and react with iron at the gold–iron interface to produce ferrous ions, which are gradually released to kill cancer cells. However, the dissolved oxygen in the water will also spread to the gold–iron interface through the grain interface of the gold shell, oxidizing the iron into iron oxide, which forms a protective layer to prevent the continued production and release of ferrous ions and, thus, no longer having a toxic killing function and achieving the effect of self-liquidation [50]. Likewise, protection is also provided by the ceramic material compounded with iron-based nanoparticles. In addition, due to its porous nature, the ceramic material can also offer drug loading and delivery of iron nanoparticles, similarly to chitosan mentioned above.

4. Combination of Iron-Based Nanocomposite Particles with Ceramic Materials

Clay minerals are one of the most important industrial minerals in nature. In this section, we focus on white clay ore-containing water, which is mainly made from aluminosilicate minerals, such as feldspar, and is formed by climate or water heat capacity. Because clay is easily shaped in moist conditions and can be cured after sintering, many products, such as road bricks and sewage pipes, contain clay minerals as raw material. In addition, clay minerals are white and resistant to high temperatures; thus, they are used in the porcelain, paper making, rubber, and refractory industries. As a new type of drug delivery system, ceramic nanocarriers have high mechanical strength, good body response, and low or non-existing biodegradability. Ceramic nanocarriers can protect the drug and the composite nanoparticles from pH and temperature effects. However, despite the high biocompatibility shown in current studies, there is still a lack of information on their clinical use [51]. The research journey for future applications of ceramic nanocarriers is still long; thus, this section will focus on the improvements brought by ceramic materials composites.

4.1. Bioactive Glasses

The development of suitable biomaterials for application in bone regeneration and disease treatment is a substantial challenge in current regenerative medicine. Synthetic biomaterials can be prepared using flexible synthetic methods to combine the best possible properties, such as bioactivity, degradation, and controllable drug delivery [52]. This allows various imaging, cell-specific-targeting, and controlled-drug-release functions to be incorporated into a single platform designed for simultaneous tracing and convenient therapeutic use without losing the individual properties of each component [53,54]. However, combining these different functions on the same platform is extremely difficult, which is because competition between the various functional groups could be generated when on the same material platform. As the application of a synthetic biological scaffold, bioactive glasses (BGs) are the leading group of surface-reactive glass–ceramic biomaterials. Due to the excellent biocompatibility of these glasses, they have been widely investigated by researchers for use as implant materials in the human body to fill and repair bone defects [55]. BGs were discovered in 1971 by the research group of Hench [56]. In the physiological environment of the human body, BGs can react with simulated body fluid (SBF) to form dense biologically active hydroxyapatite (HA) layers on their surface and biologically bond with damaged bone. HA is the main mineral component of bone that leads to effective physical interactions and fixes bone tissue onto the material surface [57]. Researchers have developed different families of BGs for bone tissue restoration and replacement because such materials do not cause biological toxicity, inflammation, or elicit an immune response [58]. Because of these characteristics, BGs have been extended to many different applications in the medical field, such as implants in theoretical bone repair, tissue engineering, drug delivery, and bone cancer treatment [52,53].

In 2004, Yan et al. used advanced science and proficient technology to develop a novel family of biomaterials called mesoporous bioactive glasses (MBGs). Compared with conventional BGs, MBGs have higher specific surface areas and pore volumes. MBGs exhibit improved bioactive behavior with even faster apatite phase formation than conventional BGs [55,56,59–63]. In 2006, Chang et al. produced a well-ordered MBG as a drug delivery carrier [64]. In numerous recently published studies, researchers have developed MBGs as a biomaterial extensively applied in drug delivery systems and bone tissue engineering [53,65–70]. In the latest technique, Zhang et al. fabricated a composite scaffold containing mesoporous bioactive glass to encapsulate magnetic Fe_3O_4 nanoparticles by 3D-printing technology. According to the results, the MBG scaffold structure comprises uniformly sized 400 μm macropores. The magnetic Fe_3O_4 nanoparticles can be incorporated into the scaffold without affecting its hydroxyapatite mineralization ability while endowing it with excellent magnetic heating ability. In addition, the pore structure can be loaded with doxorubicin (DOX), which is an anticancer drug, and it can thus be used for local drug delivery therapy. The 3D-printed Fe_3O_4/MBG scaffold shows potential versatility for enhanced osteogenic activity, local anticancer drug delivery, and magnetothermal therapy [71].

4.2. Biocompatible Nanolayer Ceramics

The basic structural layer of nanolayer ceramics, which is composed of silicate minerals, consists of a silicon–oxygen tetrahedron and an aluminum–oxygen octahedron, each of which has three oxygen atoms in the same plane and one oxygen atom at the top. The aluminum–oxygen octahedron consists of a stack of oxygen atoms and hydroxide ions, with the cation at the center of the octahedron and each cation bonded to six oxygen atoms (or hydroxide ions) to form an octahedron, as shown in Figure 6a [52]. According to the ratio of the tetrahedral and octahedral sheets contained in each layer of the clay minerals, they can be divided into two types: (1) the 1:1-layer type, in which the interlayer formed by stacking one tetrahedral sheet and one octahedral sheet is called the TO layer, whereas the tetrahedral plane on top and adjacent octahedral OH surface below form the coordination of OHO, which is the simplest crystalline structure of layered silicate clay minerals [72]; (2) the 2:1-layer type, in which each layer is composed of two tetrahedral sheets that are sandwiched between octahedral sheets, which forms a three-layer structure of TOT, similar to a sandwich [73].

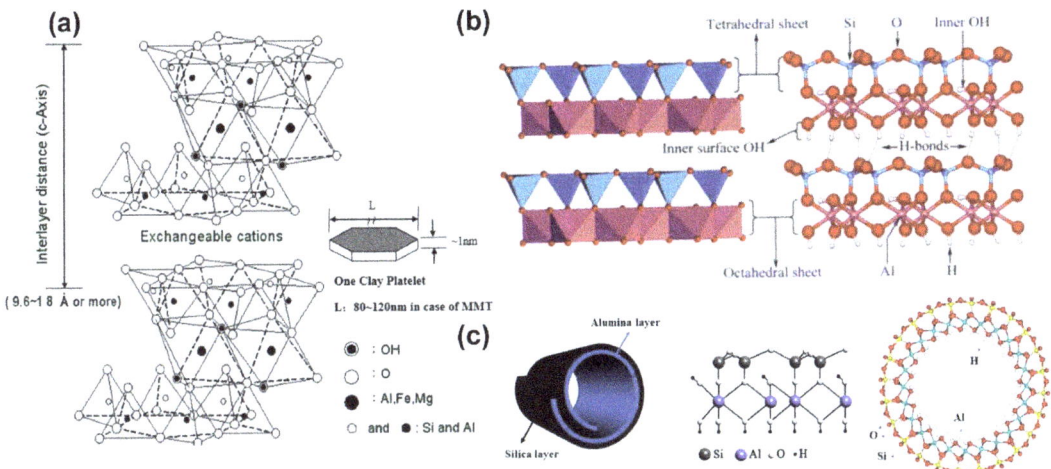

Figure 6. Suitable ceramic carriers of composite iron-based nanomaterials: (**a**) structural diagram of montmorillonite; (**b**) schematic diagram of kaolinite structure; (**c**) schematic diagram of hardystonite structure.

For example, montmorillonite is a 2:1-layer silicate, and each molecular formula has from 0.2 to 0.6 units of charge. The interlayer cations of montmorillonite, such as Na^+, Ca^{2+}, and Mg^{2+}, are exchangeable cations with high hydration. The interlayer distance is about 9.6×10^{-1} nm when there are no water or polar molecules in the interlayer, whereas the interlayer distance of montmorillonite containing divalent cations (Ca^{2+} or Mg^{2+}) increases to 14×10^{-1} nm at an average humidity of 40–60% because the interlayer contains two water molecules in the water layer. If monovalent cations (Na^+) are present in the interlayer of montmorillonite under the same humidity conditions, then the interlayer distance is 12.5×10^{-1} nm [74]. Another characteristic of montmorillonite is that it contains many exchangeable cations. Because the negative charges in the montmorillonite structure are concentrated in the central octahedral layer, the interlayer cations are weakly bound and can be easily replaced. The typical chemical formula of montmorillonite is

$(1/2Ca,Na)_{0.7}(Al,Mg,Fe)_4(Si,Al)_8O_{20}(OH)_4 \cdot nH_2O$, in which Ca^{2+} and Na^+ are exchangeable cations. The theoretical chemical composition is 49.0% SiO_2, 23% Al_2O_3, and 0.3% Fe_2O_3.

For ceramic kaolinite, the basic structural layer is composed of silicate minerals, each of which has three oxygen atoms in the same plane and one oxygen atom at the top. The aluminum–oxygen octahedron consists of a stack of oxygen atoms and hydroxide ions, with the cation at the center of the octahedron and each cation bonded to six oxygen atoms (or hydroxide ions) to form an octahedron [29]. We present the structure of kaolinite in Figure 6b, which consists of a layer of silica–oxygen tetrahedra and a layer of alumina–oxygen octahedra that are connected by a standard oxygen linkage to form a bilayer structure. In contrast, the layers are covalently bonded by providing oxygen atoms on the silica–oxygen side and hydroxide ions on the alumina–oxygen side to form hydrogen bonds. As previously mentioned, kaolinite has a stable chemical structure, uniformly distributed pore structure, and high adsorption capacity, and it can adsorb different substances in its layered structure, such as FePt nanoparticles or chemotherapeutic drugs. With the adsorption effect provided by kaolinite, FePt nanoparticles can be highly concentrated in a specific space. The nanoparticles can effectively accumulate in a magnetic-field environment according to the influence of the magnetic force to achieve a magnetically controlled MRI effect. If magnetic control is used to guide the accumulation of drugs into tumor tissue, then the side effects caused by chemotherapeutic drugs can be substantially reduced. Currently, a single treatment is not enough to achieve the substantial inhibition of tumor tissue. Cocktail-style therapies have become standard in current cancer treatments. FePt nanoparticles have excellent magnetocaloric effects, and when combined with kaolinite, their heating capacity can be substantially increased. The temperature can be increased to nearly 50 °C; thus, hepatocellular cancer cells can be killed using MFH. At the same time, if kaolinite is loaded with chemotherapeutic drugs, such as Dox, then the system can further inhibit cell growth at the tumor center.

4.3. Biocompatible Nanotube Ceramics

Hardystonite or akermanite nanotubes belong to the kaolinite group of aluminosilicate clay minerals and were discovered by the Belgian geologist d'Omalius d'Halloy and named by Pierre Berthier in 1826. Depending on the mining site and geological conditions, they can be tubular, spherical, or plate-like particles. Among these forms, the most representative is the tubular form with cavities, which has received substantial attention in various research fields due to its particular morphology, ease of mixing with multiple polymers, and good biocompatibility. The basic structure of the silicate mineral composition consists of a silicon–oxygen tetrahedron and an aluminum–oxygen octahedron, each of which has three oxygen atoms in the same plane and one oxygen atom at the top.

The cation is located at the center of the octahedron, and each cation forms a bond with six oxygen atoms (or hydroxide ions) to form the octahedron, as shown in Figure 6c [27]. Hardystonite is similar to kaolinite, but the layers in hardystonite are separated by a single layer of water molecules and are classified according to their hydrated state. Akermanite is a hydrate elite (10×10^{-1} nm), and when dried, it irreversibly loses the interlayered water to form a dehydrated elite (7×10^{-1} nm), which is more stable than the hydrated akermanite. The structure is caused by the mismatch between the silica–oxygen tetrahedra and aluminum–oxygen octahedral sheets in the layers. The tetrahedra and octahedra are connected through sharing of the top oxygen of the tetrahedra. This stress is transferred to the Si plane and the base oxygen plane through the Si–O bond, but it is also reduced by the angular elasticity of the Si–O bond. In most of the current tubular materials that are compounded with iron-based nanoparticles, carbon nanotubes are used as the carrier, and the hardystonite or akermanite structure is coated with a layer to multiply the nanoparticles. Alternatively, the iron-based nanoparticles can be doped with alpha-Al_2O_3 crystal to affect carbon nanotube growth in polycrystalline ceramics. Celik et al. prepared Fe-doped Al_2O_3 ceramics of different textures through templated grain growth and synthesized them into carbon nanotubes via catalytic chemical vapor deposition [75]. According to the experimental results, this novel nanocomposite material has the potential to be used for future biomedical diagnostic and drug delivery applications.

5. Magnetic Resonance Imaging (MRI) with Ceramic Material Composite Iron Nanoparticles

Among the many screening and diagnostic methods, magnetic resonance imaging (MRI) can provide high-resolution images of the liver without the need for ionizing radiation. Consequently, MRI is the best choice for initial tumor diagnosis. For this reason, iron-based nanomaterials have become candidates for MRI imaging because of their excellent T2 contrast ability [76]. However, most of the commonly used magnetic vibrating carriers currently available in the market are iron oxide particles or strontium ion complexes, which may cause side effects, such as nausea, allergic reactions, and kidney injury [77]. To address this, the goal of current research is to improve the performance of magnetic carriers through the development of a multifunctional composite nanocarrier that can be used for high-resolution MRI with low toxicity and a therapeutic effect [78].

Positively charged atomic nuclei spin in random environments. In this case, the nuclear spin axes are arranged in a random pattern, and when placed in a static magnetic field, the nucleus spins in the direction of the applied magnetic field. The spin frequency is called the Larmor frequency, and it is related to the properties of the nucleus itself and is proportional to the strength of the applied magnetic field. The effect is that the iron-based nanoparticles are subjected to single-axial compressive stress, and the mechanical stress causes the rearrangement of the magnetic dipoles of the iron-based nanoparticles and places them parallel with the direction of the ceramic layer. Therefore, in human MRI, the degree of saturation magnetization along the magnetization direction depends on the hydrogen atoms, which are the main source of nuclei because the human body is mainly composed of water, and it is the hydrogen atoms in water that help in visualizing the image. As the magnetization vector of the atomic nucleus gradually increases and then stabilizes during the spinning process, the nucleus will resonate if disturbed by a fixed-frequency radio frequency (Figure 7). The resonance effect, which is limited by the ceramic material, brings higher saturation magnetization to the iron-based nanoparticles, thereby enhancing their ability for T2-weighted MRI diagnostic imaging.

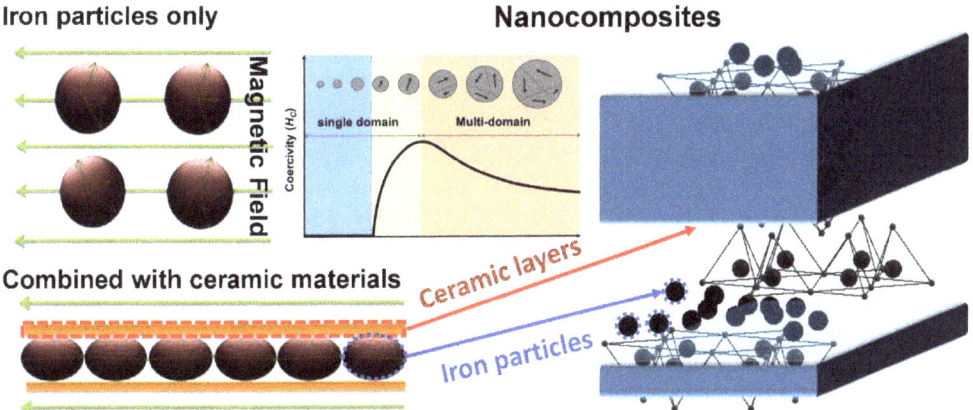

Figure 7. Schematic of possible mechanisms of layer-shaped ceramic materials limiting space of iron-based nanoparticles and with enhanced magnetic properties.

6. Magnetic Fluid Hyperthermia (MFH) with Ceramic Material Composite Iron Nanoparticles

Thermal treatments include laser treatment, focused ultrasound treatment, microwave treatment, and use of radiofrequency probes. These treatments aim to raise the temperature of the tumor to 43–46 °C to achieve the effect of thermal therapy [79–81].

However, the above-mentioned thermal therapy systems are macroscopic heating systems, which generally have the disadvantages of low thermal efficiency and being easily limited by the tumor volume, which result in uneven heat-field distribution [82]. In addition, some new methods have been developed, including pulsed laser, infrared, and magnetic-field-guided heat therapies [83]. Examples of heat sources include metal nanoshells, nanorods, and carbon nanotubes. In short, when these energy-absorbing materials reach the tumor, they can be irradiated from outside the body using strong energy sources (e.g., near-infrared laser). When the materials absorb this energy, it is converted into heat energy to increase the temperature of the tumor surface and destroy the tumor structure, thus achieving the effect of heat therapy [84]. However, this treatment method can only treat tumors close to the body surface and is inadequate for deeper tumors.

In recent years, several independent research groups have been developing a method termed magnetic fluid hyperthermia (MFH), which involves use of a magnetic fluid together with an alternating magnetic field to treat tumors [85]. This method improves upon the drawbacks mentioned above, killing cancer cells without affecting the adjacent normal tissues [86,87].

6.1. Principles of MFH

Magnetic nanoparticles exposed to alternating current (AC) magnetic fields generate heat by hysteresis loss [88,89]. However, not all magnetic nanoparticles generate heat in this way. For magnetic nanoparticles with multiple magnetic domains (e.g., 2- and 3-valent iron), the heat in an AC-field environment is generated through hysteresis loss, and for magnetic nanoparticles with single magnetic domains (e.g., single-domain ferric tetroxide nanoparticles), the heat is generated through Néel relaxation and Brownian relaxation. The reason heat is not generated by hysteresis loss for magnetic particles is that because of their superparamagnetic properties, they have a single magnetic domain and fixed magnetic moment direction [90].

Therefore, the heating principle can be divided into hysteresis loss, Néel relaxation, and Brownian relaxation [91]:

(A) Hysteresis loss: When a material has multiple magnetic domains, the direction of the magnetic moment becomes singular and the same as the magnetic field when an AC magnetic field is applied. When the magnetic-field strength changes, the resulting hysteresis curves do not overlap, which results in heat release;

(B) Néel relaxation: When a material is a single-domain superparamagnetic material, the inner nucleus rotates and overcomes the energy barrier $E = KV$ when an AC magnetic field is applied, where K is the anisotropy constant, and V is the volume of the particle. The thermal energy is released when it returns to the original magnetic moment direction;

(C) Brownian relaxation occurs in materials with multiple or single magnetic domains when an applied magnetic field is applied, which causes the particles to rotate and rub against the external medium and release thermal energy. Therefore, the characteristics of Brownian relaxation are related to the solution viscosity, as shown in Figure 8a.

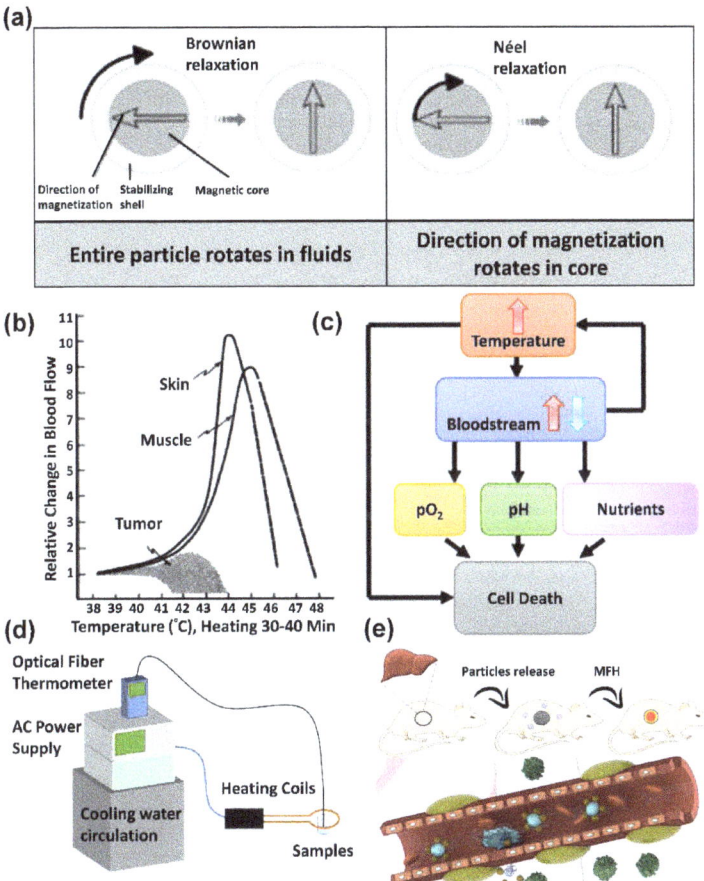

Figure 8. Thermal principles of magnetic fluid hyperthermia and physiological environmental heat therapy: (**a**) Brownian relaxation and Néel relaxation diagrams; (**b**) effect of temperature increase on tumor; (**c**) thermal cell-killing pathway; (**d**) high-frequency magnetic heating induction device; (**e**) iron-based nanoparticle accumulation in tumor tissue based on magnetic guidance, with a higher temperature produced than for normal tissue through the mechanism of enhanced permeability and retention.

The following equation is the heat loss (P) for a single-magnetic-domain material, as shown in Equation (2).

$$P = \frac{V(M_s H \omega \tau)^2}{2\tau k_b T(1+\omega^2 \tau^2)} \quad (2)$$

where V is the particle volume; M_S is the saturation magnetization value; H is the AC-electromagnetic-field strength; ω is the angular frequency of AC; τ is the relaxation time; and k_b is the Boltzmann constant. When $\omega\tau = 1$, we obtain the maximum heat loss value. When the saturation magnetization is more substantial, the heat loss is more extensive:

$$\frac{1}{\tau} = \frac{1}{\tau_B} + \frac{1}{\tau_N}; \quad \tau = \frac{3\eta V H}{kT}; \quad \tau_N = \tau_0 \exp\left(\frac{KV}{K_b T}\right) \quad (3)$$

where η is the medium viscosity; VH is the particle hydration volume; k_b is the Boltzmann constant; V is the particle volume; K is the anisotropy constant; T is the absolute temperature; and τ_0 is the time constant. We use the specific adsorption rate (SAR) to obtain the thermal energy generated by the predicted material. The efficiency of conversion from energy to thermal energy of the magnetic nanoparticles in an AC-magnetic-field environment is related to the AC-magnetic-field frequency, particle size and surface modification [91].

6.2. Treatment with MFH

When the local tumor temperature is increased to 41–46 °C by the magnetofluid in an AC-magnetic-field environment, the reason for using heat to treat tumor cells can be easily understood, as shown in Figure 8b,c below. One of the differences between tumor cells and normal tissues is that tumor cells receive more nutrients through continuous neovascularization [92]. However, most of these new blood vessels are disorganized and functionally abnormal; therefore, when heat is applied, tumor cancer cells, similarly to normal cells, increase their blood flow by vasodilatation to carry away the heat; however, this process is inefficient, and heat is retained in the tumor tissue. Therefore, as the temperature increases, neovascularization in the tumor tissue is continuously disrupted, which results in reduced blood flow and heat retention. Finally, the tumor cannot obtain nutrients to achieve the therapeutic effect. As shown in Figure 8e, after heat treatment in rats, the blood flow in the tumor cells is reduced, while the blood flow in normal cells is increased by 8–10 times. Therefore, poor heat dissipation ability may cause heat to become trapped inside the tumor, increasing the temperature, which further affects the pH, pO_2, and nutrient supply and leads to cell death [93].

7. Drug Delivery with Ceramic Material Composite Iron Nanoparticles

To reach the desired treatment site in clinical chemotherapy, high doses of drugs are usually required, increasing the risk of nonspecific toxic reactions and other physiological side effects that cause additional pain to patients. Therefore, how to efficiently deliver low-dose medications to the desired treatment site has long been a research direction for pharmaceutical companies and laboratories. The magnetic-drug-targeting technique, which uses magnetic nanoparticles in conjunction with an external magnetic field, has recently gained attention (Table 1). Magnetic nanoparticles are mainly used as drug carriers in this application. In general, magnetic nanoparticles containing drugs or antibodies are intravenously injected into the body, transported through the circulatory system, and finally concentrated at the site of the applied magnetic field, as shown in Figure 8d. In this way, more drugs can be directly focused on the lesion and then released through the drug-release mechanism. Lubbe published a study in 1996 in which they performed the first human clinical trial using magnetic drug targeting [94]. They used an intravenous infusion of magnetic particles (100 nm particle size; starch) immobilized with epirubicin (a tumor treatment drug) in solution and placed a permanent magnet with a magnetic flux density of 0.8 T close to the treatment site. According to the results, they could successfully guide the magnetic particles to the target area in more than half of the subjects. FeRx Inc. has attempted to commercialize this technology for cancer treatment, and it is currently undergoing clinical trials [95]. Biological applications of ceramic material composite iron nanoparticles depend on the carrier's biological toxicity and the composition of the ceramic structure, both of which necessitate the use of biocompatible materials. The main categories of application are biosensors, oxidative stress cytoprotection, bacterial disinfection, and cancer treatment.

Table 1. MFH bioapplications of ceramic composite iron-based nanomaterials.

Iron-Based Material	Ceramic	Cell Type	Biological Effect	Material Effect	Year	Ref.
Calcium zinc iron silicon oxide composite	Glass	Bone cancer	Promotes osteoblast proliferation	Supports nascent cell proliferation	2011	[96]
Fe/mesoporous bioactive glass	Glass	Human bone marrow mesenchymal stem cells	Improves local delivery of drug therapy and killing of infected tissue cells	Intensifies magnetization	2011	[97]
(Fe^{2+}/Fe^{3+})-doped hydroxyapatite	Hydroxyapatite	Osteoblast	Lower level of cytotoxicity achieved	Intensifies magnetization	2012	[98]
Fe_3O_4	Magnetic calcium phosphate cement	Breast cancer	Reduces tumor volume	Controlled timing of drug release	2016	[99]
Fe^{3+}	Hardystonite	Bone cancer	Enhances drug delivery and killing of tumor cells	Intensifies magnetization	2017	[100]
Ferrimagnetic	Glass	Fibroblast/bone cancer	Does not substantially affect cell morphology	Supports nascent cell proliferation	2017	[101]
Fe_3O_4	Hydroxypropyl methylcellulose	Breast cancer	Reduces tumor volume	Controlled timing of drug release	2017	[102]
Fe_3O_4	Akermanite	Osteosarcoma	Lower level of cytotoxicity achieved	Controlled timing of drug release	2019	[103]
Magnetic nanoparticles	Calcium phosphate	Mesenchymal stem cell	Increases metabolic activity and proliferation	Intensifies magnetization	2020	[104]
FePt	Kaolinite	Hepatocellular carcinoma	Enhances magnetic signal and killing of tumor cells	Intensifies magnetization	2020	[105]
Hematite nanocrystal	Glass	Fibroblast	Lower level of cytotoxicity achieved	Intensifies magnetization	2021	[106]
Single-atomic iron catalysts	Glass	Bone marrow mesenchymal stem cell	Efficacious osteosarcoma ablation	Supports nascent cell proliferation	2021	[107]
FePt	Montmorillonite	Hepatocellular carcinoma	Enhances magnetic signal and killing of tumor cells	Intensifies magnetization	2021	[108]
Superparamagnetic iron oxide nanoparticles	Glass	Mesenchymal stem cells	Does not affect cell proliferation	Intensifies magnetization	2022	[109]

7.1. Cancer Therapy

7.1.1. Bone Cancer

Currently, bone cancer is primarily treated by shaving the affected area. This approach is likely to cause disease recurrence because the cancer cells are not entirely eradicated. Therefore, the treatment process is usually combined with chemotherapy. However, most anticancer drugs have low solubility and severe drug side effects. These disadvantages have motivated the design of a controlled drug delivery system, as shown in Figure 9a [110]. The purpose in the research of Farzin et al. was to enhance the treatment impact. In their study, the researchers used iron oxide nanoparticles as a mechanism for controlled drug release, which can be combined with BGs to exploit the magnetic field to control the distribution of the anticancer drug in the bone tissue and prevent its release in other undesired locations [111]. To elaborate the use of BGs as a drug platform, various modified methods may be helpful in multiple medical applications, such as implantation in medical bone restoration, tracking postoperative surgery, and treating bone cancer [112]. To increase the accumulation of iron-based materials at the tumor site, researchers have developed modifications of the specific targeting molecules in ceramic materials. In native bone cancer, the folate receptor is not overexpressing; however, most bone tumors are metastatic. Therefore, the material with grafted folate molecules can still be used to treat bone cancer transferred from other cancers [113]. The MG63 (human osteosarcoma) cell line is supposedly a suitable in vitro test model for bone cancer. However, MG63 lacks the folate receptor; no noticeable difference in the endocytosis process was observed when folate molecules were grafted onto our material. This distinction between normal and cancer cells has made FA an attractive ligand for specific targeted bone cancer drug delivery [114].

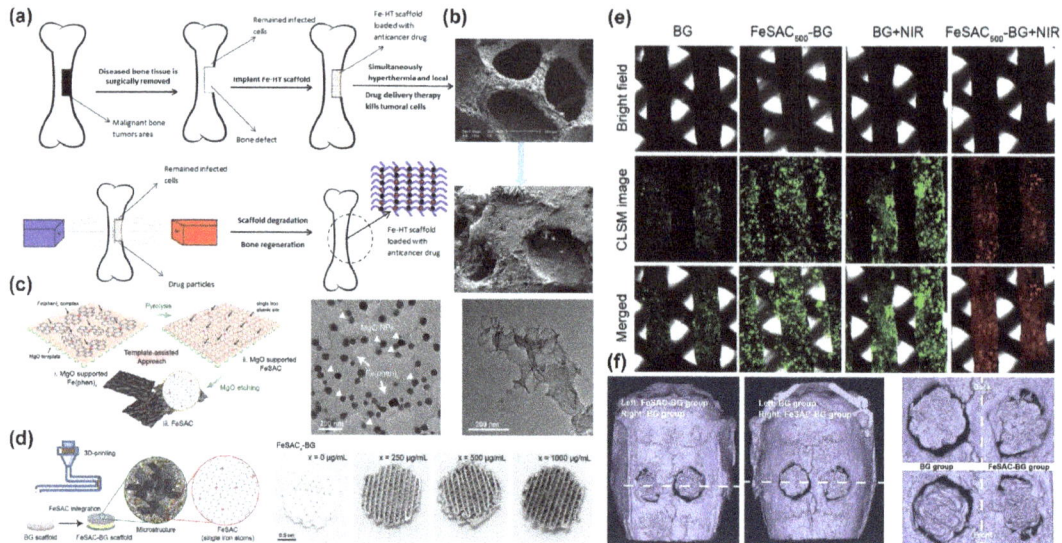

Figure 9. Bone marrow mesenchymal stem cell treatment and cell proliferation during bone cancer treatment: (**a**) schematic diagram of ceramic material containing iron-based nanoparticles bound as biological scaffolds (BGs) after bone cancer surgery; (**b**) BGs immersed in biomimetic body fluid to produce hydroxyapatite; (**c**) 3D mesh ceramic fibers with monocrystalline iron attached to the laminar surface; (**d**) BGs loaded with iron nanoparticles by 3D printing of muffin-like nanocomposite; (**e**) mesenchymal stem cell growth observed under confocal microscope analysis; (**f**) 3D muffin-like BGs embedded in bone to assist bone repair after surgical excision for bone cancer. Adapted with permission from [100,107]. Copyright 2017 Elsevier and 2021 John Wiley and Sons.

7.1.2. Liver Cancer

Hepatocellular carcinoma (HCC) is a primary malignant tumor of the liver cells. According to the National Cancer Institute SEER database, the average five-year survival rate for patients with HCC is 19.6%, and the survival rate for advanced metastases is as low as 2.5%. Following early diagnosis, treatment can be provided through local-area therapy, including surgical resection, radiofrequency ablation, transvenous chemoembolization, and liver transplantation. HCC is usually diagnosed at an advanced stage, when the tumor cannot be removed, which renders these treatments ineffective. Liver cancer is the fifth most common cancer and the fourth leading cause of cancer-related deaths worldwide [115]. There are two major types of primary liver cancer, HCC and intrahepatic cholangiocarcinoma (ICC), and less common cancers such as angiosarcoma, hemangiosarcoma, and hepatoblastoma. HCC accounts for more than 80% of primary liver cancer cases worldwide, and secondary liver cancer occurs when tumors from other parts of the body metastasize to the liver. Although breast, esophageal, stomach, pancreatic, lung, kidney, and several other cancers can metastasize to the liver, most secondary liver cancers originate from colorectal cancer. Approximately 70% of patients with colorectal cancer will develop secondary liver cancer [116].

HCC is the most common type of chronic liver cancer in adults and the most common cause of death in patients with cirrhosis. Unlike other organs or tissues in the human body, the nerves of the liver are distributed on the surface, with few inside the liver. Therefore, when a small tumor grows in the liver, it is almost painless and does not show any symptoms. Without regular checkups, it is easy to overlook the potential threat of the tumor tissue [117,118]. Among the various screening and diagnostic methods, MRI can provide high-resolution liver images without ionizing radiation. HCC exhibits a high-intensity pattern in T2-weighted images. Owing to the selective role of the hepatobiliary system, the application of iron-based nanoparticles leads to an increased accumulation of iron in the liver, thereby increasing the sensitivity of MRI for liver imaging. Chan et al. have developed a ceramic material compounded with FePt nanoparticles, which is a superparamagnetic iron-based nanomaterial contrast agent that is suitable for HCC diagnosis. With superparamagnetic, low-toxicity, biocompatible, and adaptable characteristics, iron-based nanocarriers are widely used in biomedical applications, such as imaging, differentiation, fluorescent labeling, clinical diagnosis, and drug delivery [105]. To enhance and optimize the application of FePt nanoparticles in MRI, a magnetic kaolinite and montmorillonite composite material is used to adsorb a large amount of FePt nanoparticles in realizing optimal MRI conditions (Figure 10a,c). The fine particles of kaolinite and montmorillonite have stable chemical structures, uniformly distributed pore structures, and high adsorption capacities. They can adsorb different substances in their layered structures, such as FePt nanoparticles or chemotherapeutic drugs. The novel ceramic-combined FePt nanocomposites exhibit enhanced magnetic flux, as seen in Figure 10b (according to the vibrating sample magnetometer, the magnetic field of the nanocomposites is approximately 78% higher than that of the FePt particles). FePt nanoparticles have excellent magnetocaloric effects. Their heating capacity can be substantially increased when combined with kaolinite and montmorillonite. The temperature can be increased to nearly 50 °C, and thus, HCC cancer cells can be killed by MFH [108]. In addition to MFH, HCC can also be diagnosed in mice using high-precision MRI after enhancement of the magnetic flux through composite materials (Figure 10d).

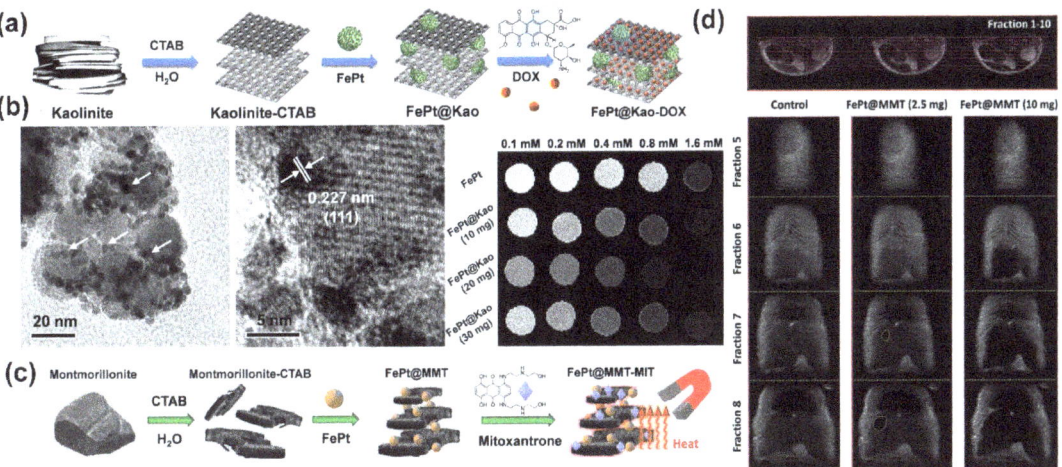

Figure 10. HCC treatment with FePt nanoparticle composite ceramic materials: (**a**) laminated kaolinite structure composite materials; (**b**) sandwich-structured nanoparticles under TEM; (**c**) laminated montmorillonite composite material; (**d**) T2-weighted MRI image of mouse liver tissue. Adapted with permission from Refs. [105,108]. Copyright 2020 ACS Publications and 2021 Springer Nature.

7.1.3. Breast Cancer

Medical research has led to the development of powerful treatments against breast cancer. Thanks to advances in science, we can pinpoint the specific weapons that are most effective for individual patients, which is a process that is referred to as precision medicine. Precision medicine is a growing trend in modern medicine, and it involves the creation of treatment plans that are best suited to each individual's disease, environment, and lifestyle. Selecting treatments for individual patients and developing care plans that are tailored to individual needs is not a new concept. The most dramatic changes have come from our knowledge of genetics and cancer biology, including that of breast cancer. Precision medicine is already being used in breast cancer treatment. For example, iron-based nanoparticles can detect whether a breast cancer tumor cell is making excessive amounts of HER2 protein. If it is, then the tumor is classified as HER2-positive, which can be effective if a drug-targeting HER2 is used.

Another example is genetic testing for women with a strong family history of breast cancer. Specific genetic mutations, such as *BRCA1* or *BRCA2*, can substantially increase the risk of developing breast cancer. Women with these genes can reduce the cancer risk by initiating preventive measures more often and earlier, such as through mammography and MRI using iron-based contrast for the observation of T2-weighted MRI images. In addition, we can use these modern genetic tests for breast cancer to determine the breast-cancer-recurrence rate and whether post-surgical chemotherapy would be beneficial. Increasingly, such tests are guiding physicians in making treatment decisions. As more biomarkers are identified and more treatments are developed, the precision of breast cancer care will become more accurate. When these biomarkers are used to guide iron-based materials into breast cancer cells, the iron nanoparticles can be used to thermally kill the tumor tissue by MFH to obtain targeted therapeutic results [119]. Wang et al. developed a heat-shrinkable, injectable biodegradable material composed of hydroxypropyl methylcellulose (HPMC), polyvinyl alcohol (PVA), and Fe_3O_4. The authors chose MB-231 for the in vitro experiments to show that the ablation of tumors is positively correlated with the weight of the HPMC/Fe_3O_4, iron content, and heating time. This novel, safe, and biodegradable material will facilitate the technological transformation of MFH, and it is also expected to introduce new concepts to the field of biomaterial research. Moreover, Tseng et al. used hydroxyapatite (HAP) as a drug carrier for breast cancer treatment via MFH and chemotherapy. The authors developed bifunctional nanoparticles (Pt–Fe–HAP) made of HAP containing iron and platinum ions for combination therapy [120].

7.2. Promotion of Osteoblast, Fibroblast, and Bone Marrow Mesenchymal Stem Cell Proliferation

Biocompatible synthetic bone grafting based on BGs is widely used in orthopedics and dentistry. Clinically, similar results to those shown in Figure 9b,f, can be achieved using BGs alone or in combination with other bone grafts for filling bone defects in periodontal surgery with transformation into HA via the body fluid immersion method [121]. A common ceramic material that contains calcium phosphate, HA is biocompatible and bone resorptive; hence, it is the bone substitute that is most widely used in bone tissue engineering, functioning as a platform facilitating bone regeneration [122–124].

The technological development of multifunctional materials has been the focus of the research in recent years. For example, silica materials embedded in a light-induced fever agent can be exploited in both photothermal therapy and near-infrared fluorescence imaging [125]. As another example, Fe_3O_4 nanoparticles are of use in thermal drug release and MRI when combined with a temperature-sensitive polymer and when folic acid (FA) molecules are grafted onto their surface [126]. HA nanoparticles are suitable for T1-weighted MRI when processed to contain europium (Eu^{3+}) and gadolinium (Gd^{3+}) ions, and they can also be modified with FA molecules to target cancer cells [127]. Moreover, researchers have also reported the use of multifunctional HA nanorods in actual practice [128]. The potential for great demand is beyond doubt, given the scarcity of ceramic substrates combined with iron-based nanoparticles. Wang et al. generated BGs using 3D printing after loading iron-based nanoparticles onto the surface, and they observed bone tissue repair and regeneration through MRI (Figure 9c). Through microscopy, they maintained the proliferation and growth state of the bone marrow mesenchymal stem cells by creating muffin-like 3D block structures and loading them with iron nanomaterials (Figure 9d,e). They confirmed that the ceramic material could be used to repaired the bone defect by generating HA under biomimetic body fluid.

7.3. Other Biological Applications Related to Drug Release

Owing to the sensitivity and detection limits, we cannot use conventional biochemical assays to distinguish slight differences. Zuo et al. produced monoatomic iron test strips by the dropwise addition of an aqueous hydrogen peroxide solution to detect the catalytic effect of butyrylcholinesterase in combination with image capture using a cellphone [129]. The combination of the cell phone-photo function to obtain fluorescent images is expected to promote further development in the field of portable detectors. Ma et al. synthesized four nitrogen–ligand monoatomic iron–carbon materials to mimic hydrogen peroxidase and superoxide dismutase to break down intracellular reactive oxygen species and prevent apoptosis [91]. Xu et al. used an organometallic framework containing monatomic iron to suppress the inflammatory response and accelerate tissue growth in a wound-healing experiment [130].

8. Conclusions

Of the substantial applications of magnetic nanoparticles combined with ceramic materials in the biomedical field that were introduced in this review, most are still in the phase of clinical testing or at the laboratory stage, except for contrast agents, which are currently available in commercial form and have been used in clinical diagnosis, indicating that there are still numerous bottlenecks to be overcome before magnetic nanoparticles can be practically applied in the biomedical field—examples of these challenges range from the selection of ceramic materials and the synthesis of magnetic nanoparticles to the functionalization of nanoparticle surfaces. In addition to the applications that we describe in this paper, new applications of magnetic nanoparticle composite ceramic materials include in vivo cell-specific material calibration, sensing and tracking, and tissue engineering for regulating and accelerating tissue or cell growth. In addition, the integration of magnetic guidance technology, magnetic thermal therapy technology, and MRI monitoring technology is bound to be among the future trends in development.

Author Contributions: Conceptualization, M.-H.C., C.-H.L. and M.H.; resources, M.-H.C.; data curation, M.-H.C., C.-H.L. and Y.-C.C.; writing—original draft preparation, M.-H.C. and C.-H.L.; writing—review and editing, M.-H.C., C.-H.L., Y.-C.C. and M.H.; supervision, M.H.; project administration, M.H. All authors have read and agreed to the published version of the manuscript.

Funding: This research was funded by Genomics Research Center, Academia Sinica, for Michael Hsiao.

Acknowledgments: The authors would like to express their gratitude to the Genomics Research Center, Academia Sinica, for supporting Michael Hsiao. Ming-Hsien Chan is grateful for the support of the Academia Sinica Postdoctoral Fellowship.

Conflicts of Interest: The authors declare no conflict of interest.

References

1. Nistico, R.; Cesano, F.; Garello, F. Magnetic Materials and Systems: Domain Structure Visualization and Other Characterization Techniques for the Application in the Materials Science and Biomedicine. *Inorganics* **2020**, *8*, 6. [CrossRef]
2. Bao, Y.P.; Wen, T.L.; Samia, A.C.S.; Khandhar, A.; Krishnan, K.M. Magnetic nanoparticles: Material engineering and emerging applications in lithography and biomedicine. *J. Mater. Sci.* **2016**, *51*, 513–553. [CrossRef]
3. Karimi, Z.; Karimi, L.; Shokrollahi, H. Nano-magnetic particles used in biomedicine: Core and coating materials. *Mat. Sci. Eng. C-Mater.* **2013**, *33*, 2465–2475. [CrossRef]
4. Cohen-Erner, M.; Khandadash, R.; Hof, R.; Shalev, O.; Antebi, A.; Cyjon, A.; Kanakov, D.; Nyska, A.; Goss, G.; Hilton, J.; et al. Fe_3O_4 Nanoparticles and Paraffin Wax as Phase Change Materials Embedded in Polymer Matrixes for Temperature-Controlled Magnetic Hyperthermia. *ACS Appl. Nano Mater.* **2021**, *4*, 11187–11198. [CrossRef]
5. Ghutepatil, P.R.; Salunkhe, A.B.; Khot, V.M.; Pawar, S.H. APTES (3-aminopropyltriethoxy silane) functionalized $MnFe_2O_4$ nanoparticles: A potential material for magnetic fluid hyperthermia. *Chem. Pap.* **2019**, *73*, 2189–2197. [CrossRef]
6. Deka, S.; Saxena, V.; Hasan, A.; Chandra, P.; Pandey, L.M. Synthesis, characterization and in vitro analysis of alpha-Fe_2O_3-$GdFeO_3$ biphasic materials as therapeutic agent for magnetic hyperthermia applications. *Mat. Sci. Eng. C-Mater.* **2018**, *92*, 932–941. [CrossRef]
7. Choi, H.; An, M.; Eom, W.; Lim, S.W.; Shim, I.B.; Kim, C.S.; Kim, S.J. Crystallographic and Magnetic Properties of the Hyperthermia Material $CoFe_2O_4$@$AlFe_2O_4$. *J. Korean Phys. Soc.* **2017**, *70*, 173–176. [CrossRef]
8. Wildeboer, R.R.; Southern, P.; Pankhurst, Q.A. On the reliable measurement of specific absorption rates and intrinsic loss parameters in magnetic hyperthermia materials. *J. Phys. D Appl. Phys.* **2014**, *47*, 495003. [CrossRef]

9. Bear, J.C.; Yu, B.; Blanco-Andujar, C.; McNaughter, P.D.; Southern, P.; Mafina, M.K.; Pankhurst, Q.A.; Parkin, I.P. A low cost synthesis method for functionalised iron oxide nanoparticles for magnetic hyperthermia from readily available materials. *Faraday Discuss.* **2014**, *175*, 83–95. [CrossRef]
10. Aslibeiki, B.; Kameli, P.; Salamati, H.; Concas, G.; Fernandez, M.S.; Talone, A.; Muscas, G.; Peddis, D. Co-doped $MnFe_2O_4$ nanoparticles: Magnetic anisotropy and interparticle interactions. *Beilstein J. Nanotech.* **2019**, *10*, 856–865. [CrossRef]
11. Jalili, H.; Aslibeiki, B.; Varzaneh, A.G.; Chernenko, V.A. The effect of magneto-crystalline anisotropy on the properties of hard and soft magnetic ferrite nanoparticles. *Beilstein J. Nanotech.* **2019**, *10*, 1348–1359. [CrossRef]
12. Zhu, Y.; Kekalo, K.; NDong, C.; Huang, Y.Y.; Shubitidze, F.; Griswold, K.E.; Baker, I.; Zhang, J.X.J. Magnetic-Nanoparticle-Based Immunoassays-on-Chip: Materials Synthesis, Surface Functionalization, and Cancer Cell Screening. *Adv. Funct. Mater.* **2016**, *26*, 3953–3972. [CrossRef]
13. Hergt, R.; Dutz, S.; Muller, R.; Zeisberger, M. Magnetic particle hyperthermia: Nanoparticle magnetism and materials development for cancer therapy. *J. Phys. Condens. Mat.* **2006**, *18*, S2919–S2934. [CrossRef]
14. Vurro, F.; Gerosa, M.; Busato, A.; Muccilli, M.; Milan, E.; Gaudet, J.; Goodwill, P.; Mansfield, J.; Negri, A.; Gherlinzoni, F.; et al. Doped Ferrite Nanoparticles Exhibiting Self-Regulating Temperature as Magnetic Fluid Hyperthermia Antitumoral Agents, with Diagnostic Capability in Magnetic Resonance Imaging and Magnetic Particle Imaging. *Cancers* **2022**, *14*, 5150. [CrossRef]
15. Lloyd, S.M.; Lave, L.B.; Matthews, H.S. Life cycle benefits of using nanotechnology to stabilize platinum-group metal particles in automotive catalysts. *Environ. Sci. Technol.* **2005**, *39*, 1384–1392. [CrossRef]
16. Weng, C.J. Nanotechnology copper interconnect processes integrations for high aspect ratio without middle etching stop layer. *Mat. Sci. Semicon. Proc.* **2010**, *13*, 56–63. [CrossRef]
17. Senior, L.; Ratcliffe, S.; Knight, M.; Perriman, A.; Mann, S.; Curnow, P. Silicon Transporters: From Membrane Proteins to Nanotechnology. *Protein Sci.* **2014**, *23*, 133.
18. Lee, J.S.; Cha, J.M.; Yoon, H.Y.; Lee, J.K.; Kim, Y.K. Magnetic multi-granule nanoclusters: A model system that exhibits universal size effect of magnetic coercivity. *Sci. Rep.* **2015**, *5*, 12135.
19. Shiroka, T. Introduction to solid state physics. *Contemp. Phys.* **2020**, *61*, 221–222. [CrossRef]
20. Aslibeiki, B.; Kameli, P.; Manouchehri, I.; Salamati, H. Strongly interacting superspins in Fe_3O_4 nanoparticles. *Curr. Appl. Phys.* **2012**, *12*, 812–816. [CrossRef]
21. Brollo, M.E.F.; Pinheiro, I.F.; Bassani, G.S.; Varet, G.; Guersoni, V.C.B.; Knobel, M.; Bannwart, A.C.; Muraca, D.; van der Geest, C. Iron Oxide Nanoparticles in a Dynamic Flux: Implications for Magnetic Hyperthermia-Controlled Fluid Viscosity. *ACS Appl. Nano Mater.* **2021**, *4*, 13633–13642. [CrossRef]
22. Sudame, A.; Kandasamy, G.; Maity, D. Single and Dual Surfactants Coated Hydrophilic Superparamagnetic Iron Oxide Nanoparticles for Magnetic Fluid Hyperthermia Applications. *J. Nanosci. Nanotechnol.* **2019**, *19*, 3991–3999. [CrossRef] [PubMed]
23. Kandasamy, G.; Sudame, A.; Luthra, T.; Saini, K.; Maity, D. Functionalized Hydrophilic Superparamagnetic Iron Oxide Nanoparticles for Magnetic Fluid Hyperthermia Application in Liver Cancer Treatment. *ACS Omega* **2018**, *3*, 3991–4005. [CrossRef] [PubMed]
24. Aslibeiki, B.; Kameli, P.; Salamati, H. The role of Ag on dynamics of superspins in $MnFe_{2-x}Ag_xO_4$ nanoparticles. *J. Nanopart. Res.* **2013**, *15*, 1430. [CrossRef]
25. Ito, A.; Tanaka, K.; Honda, H.; Abe, S.; Yamaguchi, H.; Kobayashi, T. Complete regression of mouse mammary carcinoma with a size greater than 15 mm by frequent repeated hyperthermia using magnetite nanoparticles. *J. Biosci. Bioeng.* **2003**, *96*, 364–369. [CrossRef]
26. Sun, S.H.; Murray, C.B.; Weller, D.; Folks, L.; Moser, A. Monodisperse FePt nanoparticles and ferromagnetic FePt nanocrystal superlattices. *Science* **2000**, *287*, 1989–1992. [CrossRef]
27. Kim, J.; Lee, Y.; Sun, S.H. Structurally Ordered FePt Nanoparticles and Their Enhanced Catalysis for Oxygen Reduction Reaction. *J. Am. Chem. Soc.* **2010**, *132*, 4996–4997. [CrossRef]
28. Bae, S.Y.; Shin, K.H.; Jeong, J.Y.; Kim, J.G. Feasibility of FePt longitudinal recording media for ultrahigh density recording. *J. Appl. Phys.* **2000**, *87*, 6953–6955. [CrossRef]
29. Rellinghaus, B.; Mohn, E.; Schultz, L.; Gemming, T.; Acet, M.; Kowalik, A.; Kock, B.F. On the L1(0) ordering kinetics in Fe-Pt nanoparticles. *IEEE Trans. Magn.* **2006**, *42*, 3048–3050. [CrossRef]
30. Varanda, L.C.; Jafelicci, M. Self-assembled FePt nanocrystals with large coercivity: Reduction of the fcc-to-L1(0) ordering temperature. *J. Am. Chem. Soc.* **2006**, *128*, 11062–11066. [CrossRef]
31. Lu, L.Y.; Wang, D.; Xu, X.G.; Zhan, Y.; Jiang, Y. Enhancement of Magnetic Properties for FePt Nanoparticles by Rapid Annealing in a Vacuum. *J. Phys. Chem. C* **2009**, *113*, 19867–19870. [CrossRef]
32. Nakaya, M.; Kanehara, M.; Teranishi, T. One-pot synthesis of large FePt nanoparticles from metal salts and their thermal stability. *Langmuir* **2006**, *22*, 3485–3487. [CrossRef] [PubMed]
33. Yu, C.H.; Caiulo, N.; Lo, C.C.H.; Tam, K.; Tsang, S.C. Synthesis and fabrication of a thin film containing silica-encapsulated face-centered tetragonal FePt nanoparticles. *Adv. Mater.* **2006**, *18*, 2312–2314. [CrossRef]
34. Burkert, T.; Eriksson, O.; Simak, S.I.; Ruban, A.V.; Sanyal, B.; Nordstrom, L.; Wills, J.M. Magnetic anisotropy of L1(0) FePt and $Fe_{1-x}Mn_xPt$. *Phys. Rev. B* **2005**, *71*, 13. [CrossRef]
35. Okamoto, S.; Kikuchi, N.; Kitakami, O.; Miyazaki, T.; Shimada, Y.; Fukamichi, K. Chemical-order-dependent magnetic anisotropy and exchange stiffness constant of FePt (001) epitaxial films. *Phys. Rev. B* **2002**, *66*, 024413. [CrossRef]

36. Aslibeiki, B.; Ehsani, M.H.; Nasirzadeh, F.; Mohammadi, M.A. The effect of interparticle interactions on spin glass and hyperthermia properties of Fe_3O_4 nanoparticles. *Mater. Res. Express* **2017**, *4*, 075051. [CrossRef]
37. Staunton, J.B.; Ostanin, S.; Razee, S.S.A.; Gyorffy, B.L.; Szunyogh, L.; Ginatempo, B.; Bruno, E. Temperature dependent magnetic anisotropy in metallic magnets from an ab initio electronic structure theory: L1(0)-ordered FePt. *Phys. Rev. Lett.* **2004**, *93*, 257204. [CrossRef]
38. Aslibeiki, B.; Eskandarzadeh, N.; Jalili, H.; Varzaneh, A.G.; Kameli, P.; Orue, I.; Chernenko, V.; Hajalilou, A.; Ferreira, L.P.; Cruz, M.M. Magnetic hyperthermia properties of $CoFe_2O_4$ nanoparticles: Effect of polymer coating and interparticle interactions. *Ceram. Int.* **2022**, *48*, 27995–28005. [CrossRef]
39. Rezanezhad, A.; Hajalilou, A.; Eslami, F.; Parvini, E.; Abouzari-Lotf, E.; Aslibeiki, B. Superparamagnetic magnetite nanoparticles for cancer cells treatment via magnetic hyperthermia: Effect of natural capping agent, particle size and concentration. *J. Mater. Sci. Mater. Electron.* **2021**, *32*, 24026–24040. [CrossRef]
40. Limthin, D.; Leepheng, P.; Klamchuen, A.; Phromyothin, D. Enhancement of Electrochemical Detection of Gluten with Surface Modification Based on Molecularly Imprinted Polymers Combined with Superparamagnetic Iron Oxide Nanoparticles. *Polymers* **2022**, *14*, 91. [CrossRef]
41. Lotfi, S.; Aslibeiki, B.; Zarei, M. Efficient Pb (II) removal from wastewater by TEG coated Fe_3O_4 ferrofluid. *J. Water Environ. Nanotechnol.* **2021**, *6*, 109–120.
42. Stolyar, S.V.; Krasitskaya, V.V.; Frank, L.A.; Yaroslavtsev, R.N.; Chekanova, L.A.; Gerasimova, Y.V.; Volochaev, M.N.; Bairmani, M.S.; Velikanov, D.A. Polysaccharide-coated iron oxide nanoparticles: Synthesis, properties, surface modification. *Mater. Lett.* **2021**, *284*, 128920. [CrossRef]
43. Aslibeiki, B.; Kameli, P.; Ehsani, M.H.; Salamati, H.; Muscas, G.; Agostinelli, E.; Foglietti, V.; Casciardi, S.; Peddis, D. Solvothermal synthesis of $MnFe_2O_4$ nanoparticles: The role of polymer coating on morphology and magnetic properties. *J. Magn. Magn. Mater.* **2016**, *399*, 236–244. [CrossRef]
44. Ebadi, M.; Bullo, S.; Buskaran, K.; Hussein, M.Z.; Fakurazi, S.; Pastorin, G. Dual-Functional Iron Oxide Nanoparticles Coated with Polyvinyl Alcohol/5-Fluorouracil/Zinc-Aluminium-Layered Double Hydroxide for a Simultaneous Drug and Target Delivery System. *Polymers* **2021**, *13*, 855. [CrossRef]
45. Lazzarini, A.; Colaiezzi, R.; Passacantando, M.; D'Orazio, F.; Arrizza, L.; Ferella, F.; Crucianelli, M. Investigation of physicochemical and catalytic properties of the coating layer of silica-coated iron oxide magnetic nanoparticles. *J. Phys. Chem. Solids* **2021**, *153*, 110003. [CrossRef]
46. Anila, I.; Lahiri, B.B.; Mathew, J.; Philip, J. Synthesis and magneto-structural properties of chitosan coated ultrafine cobalt ferrite nanoparticles for magnetic fluid hyperthermia in viscous medium. *Ceram. Int.* **2022**, *48*, 22767–22781. [CrossRef]
47. Nalluri, L.P.; Popuri, S.R.; Lee, C.H.; Terbish, N. Synthesis of biopolymer coated functionalized superparamagnetic iron oxide nanoparticles for the pH-sensitive delivery of anti-cancer drugs epirubicin and temozolomide. *Int. J. Polym. Mater. Polym. Biomater.* **2021**, *70*, 1039–1052. [CrossRef]
48. Khani, T.; Alamzadeh, Z.; Sarikhani, A.; Mousavi, M.; Mirrahimi, M.; Tabei, M.; Irajirad, R.; Abed, Z.; Beik, J. Fe_3O_4@Au core-shell hybrid nanocomposite for MRI-guided magnetic targeted photo-chemotherapy. *Laser Med. Sci.* **2022**, *37*, 2387–2395. [CrossRef]
49. Abdollahi, B.B.; Ghorbani, M.; Hamishehkar, H.; Malekzadeh, R.; Farajollahi, A.R. Synthesis and characterization of actively HER-2 Targeted Fe_3O_4@Au nanoparticles for molecular radiosensitization of breast cancer. *Bioimpacts* **2022**, *12*, 23682. [CrossRef]
50. Le, T.T.; Nguyen, T.N.L.; Nguyen, H.D.; Phan, T.H.T.; Pham, H.N.; Le, D.G.; Hoang, T.P.; Nguyen, T.Q.H.; Le, T.L.; Tran, L.D. Multimodal Imaging Contrast Property of Nano Hybrid Fe_3O_4@Ag Fabricated by Seed-Growth for Medicinal Diagnosis. *Chemistryselect* **2022**, *7*, e202201374. [CrossRef]
51. Singh, D.; Singh, S.; Sahu, J.; Srivastava, S.; Singh, M.R. Ceramic nanoparticles: Recompense, cellular uptake and toxicity concerns. *Artif. Cell Nanomed. B* **2016**, *44*, 401–409. [CrossRef] [PubMed]
52. Perez, R.A.; El-Fiqi, A.; Park, J.H.; Kim, T.H.; Kim, J.H.; Kim, H.W. Therapeutic bioactive microcarriers: Co-delivery of growth factors and stem cells for bone tissue engineering. *Acta Biomater.* **2014**, *10*, 520–530. [CrossRef] [PubMed]
53. Wu, C.T.; Chang, J. Mesoporous bioactive glasses: Structure characteristics, drug/growth factor delivery and bone regeneration application. *Interface Focus* **2012**, *2*, 292–306. [CrossRef] [PubMed]
54. Yan, X.X.; Yu, C.Z.; Zhou, X.F.; Tang, J.W.; Zhao, D.Y. Highly ordered mesoporous bioactive glasses with superior in vitro bone-forming bioactivities. *Angew. Chem. Int. Ed.* **2004**, *43*, 5980–5984. [CrossRef]
55. Avnir, D.; Coradin, T.; Lev, O.; Livage, J. Recent bio-applications of sol-gel materials. *J. Mater. Chem.* **2006**, *16*, 1013–1030. [CrossRef]
56. Habraken, W.J.E.M.; Wolke, J.G.C.; Jansen, J.A. Ceramic composites as matrices and scaffolds for drug delivery in tissue engineering. *Adv. Drug Deliver. Rev.* **2007**, *59*, 234–248. [CrossRef]
57. Liu, X.; Rahaman, M.N.; Hilmas, G.E.; Bal, B.S. Mechanical properties of bioactive glass (13-93) scaffolds fabricated by robotic deposition for structural bone repair. *Acta Biomater.* **2013**, *9*, 7025–7034. [CrossRef]
58. Bi, L.X.; Rahaman, M.N.; Day, D.E.; Brown, Z.; Samujh, C.; Liu, X.; Mohammadkhah, A.; Dusevich, V.; Eick, J.D.; Bonewald, L.F. Effect of bioactive borate glass microstructure on bone regeneration, angiogenesis, and hydroxyapatite conversion in a rat calvarial defect model. *Acta Biomater.* **2013**, *9*, 8015–8026. [CrossRef]
59. Vallet-Regi, M.; Balas, F.; Colilla, M.; Manzano, M. Bone-regenerative bioceramic implants with drug and protein controlled delivery capability. *Prog. Solid State Chem.* **2008**, *36*, 163–191. [CrossRef]

60. Arcos, D.; Greenspan, D.C.; Vallet-Regi, M. A new quantitative method to evaluate the in vitro bioactivity of melt and sol-gel-derived silicate glasses. *J. Biomed. Mater. Res. A* **2003**, *65A*, 344–351. [CrossRef]
61. Hench, L.L. The story of Bioglass (R). *J. Mater. Sci.-Mater. Med.* **2006**, *17*, 967–978. [CrossRef] [PubMed]
62. Yan, X.X.; Deng, H.X.; Huang, X.H.; Lu, G.Q.; Qiao, S.Z.; Zhao, D.Y.; Yu, C.Z. Mesoporous bioactive glasses. I. Synthesis and structural characterization. *J. Non-Cryst. Solids* **2005**, *351*, 3209–3217. [CrossRef]
63. Yu, C.Z.; Yan, X.X.; Huang, X.H.; Deng, H.X.; Wang, Y.; Zhang, Z.D.; Qiao, S.Z.; Lu, G.Q.; Zhao, D.Y. The in-vitro bioactivity of mesoporous bioactive glasses. *Biomaterials* **2006**, *27*, 3396–3403.
64. Xia, W.; Chang, J. Well-ordered mesoporous bioactive glasses (MBG): A promising bioactive drug delivery system. *J. Control. Release* **2006**, *110*, 522–530. [CrossRef] [PubMed]
65. Zhu, Y.F.; Shang, F.J.; Li, B.; Dong, Y.; Liu, Y.F.; Lohe, M.R.; Hanagata, N.; Kaskel, S. Magnetic mesoporous bioactive glass scaffolds: Preparation, physicochemistry and biological properties. *J. Mater. Chem. B* **2013**, *1*, 1279–1288. [CrossRef] [PubMed]
66. Zhou, P.Y.; Xia, Y.; Wang, J.; Liang, C.; Yu, L.; Tang, W.; Gu, S.; Xu, S.G. Antibacterial properties and bioactivity of HACC- and HACC-Zein-modified mesoporous bioactive glass scaffolds. *J. Mater. Chem. B* **2013**, *1*, 685–692. [CrossRef]
67. Wu, C.T.; Chang, J.; Fan, W. Bioactive mesoporous calcium-silicate nanoparticles with excellent mineralization ability, osteostimulation, drug-delivery and antibacterial properties for filling apex roots of teeth. *J. Mater. Chem.* **2012**, *22*, 16801–16809. [CrossRef]
68. Zhu, M.; Shi, J.L.; He, Q.J.; Zhang, L.X.; Chen, F.; Chen, Y. An emulsification-solvent evaporation route to mesoporous bioactive glass microspheres for bisphosphonate drug delivery. *J. Mater. Sci.* **2012**, *47*, 2256–2263. [CrossRef]
69. Vallet-Regi, M.; Izquierdo-Barba, I.; Colilla, M. Structure and functionalization of mesoporous bioceramics for bone tissue regeneration and local drug delivery. *Philos. Trans. R. Soc. A Math. Phys. Eng. Sci.* **2012**, *370*, 1400–1421. [CrossRef] [PubMed]
70. Baino, F.; Fiorilli, S.; Mortera, R.; Onida, B.; Saino, E.; Visai, L.; Verne, E.; Vitale-Brovarone, C. Mesoporous bioactive glass as a multifunctional system for bone regeneration and controlled drug release. *J. Appl. Biomater. Funct.* **2012**, *10*, 12–21.
71. Zhang, J.H.; Zhao, S.C.; Zhu, M.; Zhu, Y.F.; Zhang, Y.D.; Liu, Z.T.; Zhang, C.Q. 3D-printed magnetic Fe_3O_4/MBG/PCL composite scaffolds with multifunctionality of bone regeneration, local anticancer drug delivery and hyperthermia. *J. Mater. Chem. B* **2014**, *2*, 7583–7595. [CrossRef] [PubMed]
72. Willey, J.D.; Avery, G.B.; Manock, J.J.; Skrabal, S.A.; Stehman, C.F. Chemical analysis of soils—An environmental chemistry laboratory for undergraduate science majors. *J. Chem. Educ.* **1999**, *76*, 1693–1694.
73. Robinson, C.; Adewunmi, W.; Lindbo, D.; Moebius-Clune, B. Environmental Science, Soil Conservation, and Land Use Management. *Know Soil Know Life* **2012**, 109–138. [CrossRef]
74. Bastida, F.; Moreno, J.L.; Nicolas, C.; Hernandez, T.; Garcia, C. Soil metaproteomics: A review of an emerging environmental science. Significance, methodology and perspectives. *Eur. J. Soil Sci.* **2009**, *60*, 845–859. [CrossRef]
75. Celik, Y.; Suvaci, E.; Weibel, A.; Peigney, A.; Flahaut, E. Texture development in Fe-doped alumina ceramics via templated grain growth and their application to carbon nanotube growth. *J. Eur. Ceram. Soc.* **2013**, *33*, 1093–1100. [CrossRef]
76. Barcelos, K.A.; Tebaldi, M.L.; do Egito, E.S.T.; Leao, N.M.; Soares, D.C.F. PEG-Iron Oxide Core-Shell Nanoparticles: In situ Synthesis and In Vitro Biocompatibility Evaluation for Potential T-2-MRI Applications. *Bionanoscience* **2020**, *10*, 1107–1120. [CrossRef]
77. Meloni, A.; Pistoia, L.; Restaino, G.; Missere, M.; Positano, V.; Spasiano, A.; Casini, T.; Cossu, A.; Cuccia, L.; Massa, A.; et al. Quantitative T2*MRI for bone marrow iron overload: Normal reference values and assessment in thalassemia major patients. *Radiol. Med.* **2022**, *127*, 1199–1208. [CrossRef] [PubMed]
78. McKiernan, E.P.; Moloney, C.; Chaudhuri, T.R.; Clerkin, S.; Behan, K.; Straubinger, R.M.; Crean, J.; Brougham, D.F. Formation of hydrated PEG layers on magnetic iron oxide nanoflowers shows internal magnetisation dynamics and generates high in-vivo efficacy for MRI and magnetic hyperthermia. *Acta Biomater.* **2022**, *152*, 393–405. [CrossRef]
79. Hildebrandt, B.; Wust, P.; Ahlers, O.; Dieing, A.; Sreenivasa, G.; Kerner, T.; Felix, R.; Riess, H. The cellular and molecular basis of hyperthermia. *Crit. Rev. Oncol. Hematol.* **2002**, *43*, 33–56. [CrossRef]
80. Wu, W.; Jiang, C.Z.; Roy, V.A.L. Designed synthesis and surface engineering strategies of magnetic iron oxide nanoparticles for biomedical applications. *Nanoscale* **2016**, *8*, 19421–19474. [CrossRef] [PubMed]
81. Gupta, A.K.; Gupta, M. Synthesis and surface engineering of iron oxide nanoparticles for biomedical applications. *Biomaterials* **2005**, *26*, 3995–4021. [CrossRef] [PubMed]
82. DeNardo, S.J.; DeNardo, G.L.; Natarajan, A.; Miers, L.A.; Foreman, A.R.; Gruettner, C.; Adamson, G.N.; Ivkov, R. Thermal dosimetry predictive of efficacy of In-111-ChL6 nanoparticle AMF-induced thermoablative therapy for human breast cancer in mice. *J. Nucl. Med.* **2007**, *48*, 437–444. [PubMed]
83. Aslibeiki, B.; Kameli, P.; Salamati, H. The effect of grinding on magnetic properties of agglomereted $MnFe_2O_4$ nanoparticles. *J. Magn. Magn. Mater.* **2012**, *324*, 154–160. [CrossRef]
84. Aslibeiki, B.; Kameli, P. Magnetic properties of $MnFe_2O_4$ nano-aggregates dispersed in paraffin wax. *J. Magn. Magn. Mater.* **2015**, *385*, 308–312. [CrossRef]
85. Aslibeiki, B.; Kameli, P.; Salamati, H. The effect of dipole-dipole interactions on coercivity, anisotropy constant, and blocking temperature of $MnFe_2O_4$ nanoparticles. *J. Appl. Phys.* **2016**, *119*, 063901. [CrossRef]
86. Polevikov, V.; Tobiska, L. On the solution of the steady-state diffusion problem for ferromagnetic particles in a magnetic fluid. *Math. Model. Anal.* **2008**, *13*, 233–240. [CrossRef]

87. Ring, H.L.; Bischof, J.C.; Garwood, M. Use and Safety of Iron Oxide Nanoparticles in MRI and MFH. *eMagRes* **2019**, *8*, 265–277.
88. Ito, A.; Matsuoka, F.; Honda, H.; Kobayashi, T. Heat shock protein 70 gene therapy combined with hyperthermia using magnetic nanoparticles. *Cancer Gene Ther.* **2003**, *10*, 918–925. [CrossRef]
89. Ito, A.; Shinkai, M.; Honda, H.; Kobayashi, T. Heat-inducible TNF-alpha gene therapy combined with hyperthermia using magnetic nanoparticles as a novel tumor-targeted therapy. *Cancer Gene Ther.* **2001**, *8*, 649–654. [CrossRef] [PubMed]
90. Jabir, M.S.; Nayef, U.M.; Abdulkadhim, W.K.; Sulaiman, G.M. Supermagnetic Fe_3O_4-PEG nanoparticles combined with NIR laser and alternating magnetic field as potent anti-cancer agent against human ovarian cancer cells. *Mater. Res. Express* **2019**, *6*, 115412. [CrossRef]
91. Ma, M.; Wu, Y.; Zhou, H.; Sun, Y.K.; Zhang, Y.; Gu, N. Size dependence of specific power absorption of Fe_3O_4 particles in AC magnetic field. *J. Magn. Magn. Mater.* **2004**, *268*, 33–39. [CrossRef]
92. Ebrahimisadr, S.; Aslibeiki, B.; Asadi, R. Magnetic hyperthermia properties of iron oxide nanoparticles: The effect of concentration. *Phys. C* **2018**, *549*, 119–121. [CrossRef]
93. Hilger, I.; Fruhauf, K.; Andra, W.; Hiergeist, R.; Hergt, R.; Kaiser, W.A. Heating potential of iron oxides for therapeutic purposes in interventional radiology. *Acad. Radiol.* **2002**, *9*, 198–202. [CrossRef]
94. Lubbe, A.S.; Alexiou, C.; Bergemann, C. Clinical applications of magnetic drug targeting. *J. Surg. Res.* **2001**, *95*, 200–206. [CrossRef] [PubMed]
95. Williams, P.S.; Carpino, F.; Zborowski, M. Magnetic Nanoparticle Drug Carriers and Their Study by Quadrupole Magnetic Field-Flow Fractionation. *Mol. Pharm.* **2009**, *6*, 1290–1306. [CrossRef] [PubMed]
96. Jiang, Y.M.; Ou, J.; Zhang, Z.H.; Qin, Q.H. Preparation of magnetic and bioactive calcium zinc iron silicon oxide composite for hyperthermia treatment of bone cancer and repair of bone defects. *J. Mater. Sci. Mater. Med.* **2011**, *22*, 721–729. [CrossRef] [PubMed]
97. Wu, C.T.; Fan, W.; Zhu, Y.F.; Gelinsky, M.; Chang, J.; Cuniberti, G.; Albrecht, V.; Friis, T.; Xiao, Y. Multifunctional magnetic mesoporous bioactive glass scaffolds with a hierarchical pore structure. *Acta Biomater.* **2011**, *7*, 3563–3572. [CrossRef]
98. Tampieri, A.; D'Alessandro, T.; Sandri, M.; Sprio, S.; Landi, E.; Bertinetti, L.; Panseri, S.; Pepponi, G.; Goettlicher, J.; Banobre-Lopez, M.; et al. Intrinsic magnetism and hyperthermia in bioactive Fe-doped hydroxyapatite. *Acta Biomater.* **2012**, *8*, 843–851. [CrossRef]
99. Gao, W.; Zheng, Y.Y.; Wang, R.H.; Chen, H.R.; Cai, X.J.; Lu, G.M.; Chu, L.; Xu, C.Y.; Zhang, N.; Wang, Z.G.; et al. A smart, phase transitional and injectable DOX/PLGA-Fe implant for magnetic-hyperthermia-induced synergistic tumor eradication. *Acta Biomater.* **2016**, *29*, 298–306. [CrossRef]
100. Farzin, A.; Fathi, M.; Emadi, R. Multifunctional magnetic nanostructured hardystonite scaffold for hyperthermia, drug delivery and tissue engineering applications. *Mater. Sci. Eng. C* **2017**, *70*, 21–31. [CrossRef]
101. Bretcanu, O.; Miola, M.; Bianchi, C.L.; Marangi, I.; Carbone, R.; Corazzari, I.; Cannas, M.; Verne, E. In Vitro biocompatibility of a ferrimagnetic glass-ceramic for hyperthermia application. *Mat. Sci. Eng. C* **2017**, *73*, 778–787. [CrossRef] [PubMed]
102. Wang, F.J.; Yang, Y.; Ling, Y.; Liu, J.X.; Cai, X.J.; Zhou, X.H.; Tang, X.Z.; Liang, B.; Chen, Y.N.; Chen, H.R.; et al. Injectable and thermally contractible hydroxypropyl methyl cellulose/Fe_3O_4 for magnetic hyperthermia ablation of tumors. *Biomaterials* **2017**, *128*, 84–93. [CrossRef] [PubMed]
103. Saber-Samandari, S.; Mohammadi-Aghdam, M.; Saber-Samandari, S. A novel magnetic bifunctional nanocomposite scaffold for photothermal therapy and tissue engineering. *Int. J. Biol. Macromol.* **2019**, *138*, 810–818. [CrossRef]
104. Rodrigues, A.F.M.; Torres, P.M.C.; Barros, M.J.S.; Presa, R.; Ribeiro, N.; Abrantes, J.C.C.; Belo, J.H.; Amaral, J.S.; Amaral, V.S.; Banobre-Lopez, M.; et al. Effective production of multifunctional magnetic-sensitive biomaterial by an extrusion-based additive manufacturing technique. *Biomed. Mater.* **2021**, *16*, 015011. [CrossRef] [PubMed]
105. Chan, M.H.; Hsieh, M.R.; Liu, R.S.; Wei, D.H.; Hsiao, M. Magnetically Guided Theranostics: Optimizing Magnetic Resonance Imaging with Sandwich-Like Kaolinite-Based Iron/Platinum Nanoparticles for Magnetic Fluid Hyperthermia and Chemotherapy. *Chem. Mater.* **2020**, *32*, 697–708. [CrossRef]
106. Borges, R.; Mendonca-Ferreira, L.; Rettori, C.; Pereira, I.S.O.; Baino, F.; Marchi, J. New sol-gel-derived magnetic bioactive glass-ceramics containing superparamagnetic hematite nanocrystals for hyperthermia application. *Mater. Sci. Eng. C* **2021**, *120*, 111692. [CrossRef]
107. Wang, L.Y.; Yang, Q.H.; Huo, M.F.; Lu, D.; Gao, Y.S.; Chen, Y.; Xu, H.X. Engineering Single-Atomic Iron-Catalyst-Integrated 3D-Printed Bioscaffolds for Osteosarcoma Destruction with Antibacterial and Bone Defect Regeneration Bioactivity. *Adv. Mater.* **2021**, *33*, 2100150. [CrossRef] [PubMed]
108. Chan, M.H.; Lu, C.N.; Chung, Y.L.; Chang, Y.C.; Li, C.H.; Chen, C.L.; Wei, D.H.; Hsiao, M. Magnetically guided theranostics: Montmorillonite-based iron/platinum nanoparticles for enhancing in situ MRI contrast and hepatocellular carcinoma treatment. *J. Nanobiotechnol.* **2021**, *19*, 308. [CrossRef]
109. Borges, R.; Ferreira, L.M.; Rettori, C.; Lourenco, I.M.; Seabra, A.B.; Muller, F.A.; Ferraz, E.P.; Marques, M.M.; Miola, M.; Baino, F.; et al. Superparamagnetic and highly bioactive SPIONS/bioactive glass nanocomposite and its potential application in magnetic hyperthermia. *Biomater. Adv.* **2022**, *135*, 112655. [CrossRef]
110. Lee, J.; Kim, H.; Kim, S.; Lee, H.; Kim, J.; Kim, N.; Park, H.J.; Choi, E.K.; Lee, J.S.; Kim, C. A multifunctional mesoporous nanocontainer with an iron oxide core and a cyclodextrin gatekeeper for an efficient theranostic platform. *J. Mater. Chem.* **2012**, *22*, 14061–14067. [CrossRef]

111. Guardado-Alvarez, T.M.; Devi, L.S.; Vabre, J.M.; Pecorelli, T.A.; Schwartz, B.J.; Durand, J.O.; Mongin, O.; Blanchard-Desce, M.; Zink, J.I. Photo-redox activated drug delivery systems operating under two photon excitation in the near-IR. *Nanoscale* **2014**, *6*, 4652–4658. [CrossRef] [PubMed]
112. Lin, H.M.; Lin, H.Y.; Chan, M.H. Preparation, characterization, and in vitro evaluation of folate-modified mesoporous bioactive glass for targeted anticancer drug carriers. *J. Mater. Chem. B* **2013**, *1*, 6147–6156. [CrossRef] [PubMed]
113. Virk, M.S.; Lieberman, J.R. Tumor metastasis to bone. *Arthritis Res. Ther.* **2007**, *9*, S5. [CrossRef]
114. Zhou, Z.X.; Shen, Y.Q.; Tang, J.B.; Fan, M.H.; Van Kirk, E.A.; Murdoch, W.J.; Radosz, M. Charge-Reversal Drug Conjugate for Targeted Cancer Cell Nuclear Drug Delivery. *Adv. Funct. Mater.* **2009**, *19*, 3580–3589. [CrossRef]
115. Chen, B.W.; Chiu, G.W.; He, Y.C.; Huang, C.Y.; Huang, H.T.; Sung, S.Y.; Hsieh, C.L.; Chang, W.C.; Hsu, M.S.; Wei, Z.H.; et al. Extracellular and intracellular intermittent magnetic-fluid hyperthermia treatment of SK-Hep1 hepatocellular carcinoma cells based on magnetic nanoparticles coated with polystyrene sulfonic acid. *PLoS ONE* **2021**, *16*, e0245286. [CrossRef]
116. Chidambaranathan-Reghupaty, S.; Fisher, P.B.; Sarkar, D. Hepatocellular carcinoma (HCC): Epidemiology, etiology and molecular classification. *Adv. Cancer Res.* **2021**, *149*, 1–61.
117. Mazumder, A.; Dwivedi, A.; Assawapanumat, W.; Saeeng, R.; Sungkarat, W.; Nasongkla, N. In vitro galactose-targeted study of RSPP050-loaded micelles against liver hepatocellular carcinoma. *Pharm. Dev. Technol.* **2022**, *27*, 379–388. [CrossRef]
118. Choi, H.J.; Choi, B.S.; Yu, B.; Li, W.G.; Matsumoto, M.M.; Harris, K.R.; Lewandowski, R.J.; Larson, A.C.; Mouli, S.K.; Kim, D.H. On-demand degradable embolic microspheres for immediate restoration of blood flow during image-guided embolization procedures. *Biomaterials* **2021**, *265*, 120408. [CrossRef]
119. Suleman, M.; Riaz, S. 3D in silico study of magnetic fluid hyperthermia of breast tumor using Fe_3O_4 magnetic nanoparticles. *J. Therm. Biol.* **2020**, *91*, 102635. [CrossRef]
120. Tseng, C.L.; Chang, K.C.; Yeh, M.C.; Yang, K.C.; Tang, T.P.; Lin, F.H. Development of a dual-functional Pt-Fe-HAP magnetic nanoparticles application for chemo-hyperthermia treatment of cancer. *Ceram. Int.* **2014**, *40*, 5117–5127. [CrossRef]
121. Hayashi, A.; Yokoo, N.; Nakamura, T.; Watanabe, T.; Nagasawa, H.; Kogure, T. Crystallographic characterization of the crossed lamellar structure in the bivalve Meretrix lamarckii using electron beam techniques. *J. Struct. Biol.* **2011**, *176*, 91–96. [CrossRef]
122. Bose, S.; Tarafder, S. Calcium phosphate ceramic systems in growth factor and drug delivery for bone tissue engineering: A review. *Acta Biomater.* **2012**, *8*, 1401–1421. [CrossRef]
123. Lewandrowski, K.U.; Gresser, J.D.; Wise, D.L.; Trantolo, D.J. Bioresorbable bone graft substitutes of different osteoconductivities: A histologic evaluation of osteointegration of poly(propylene glycol-co-fumaric acid)-based cement implants in rats. *Biomaterials* **2000**, *21*, 757–764. [CrossRef]
124. Saikia, K.C.; Bhattacharya, T.D.; Bhuyan, S.K.; Talukdar, D.J.; Saikia, S.P.; Jitesh, P. Calcium phosphate ceramics as bone graft substitutes in filling bone tumor defects. *Indian J. Orthop.* **2008**, *42*, 169–172. [CrossRef]
125. Singh, A.K.; Hahn, M.A.; Gutwein, L.G.; Rule, M.C.; Knapik, J.A.; Moudgil, B.M.; Grobmyer, S.R.; Brown, S.C. Multi-dye theranostic nanoparticle platform for bioimaging and cancer therapy. *Int. J. Nanomed.* **2012**, *7*, 2739–2750.
126. Rastogi, R.; Gulati, N.; Kotnala, R.K.; Sharma, U.; Jayasundar, R.; Koul, V. Evaluation of folate conjugated pegylated thermosensitive magnetic nanocomposites for tumor imaging and therapy. *Colloids. Surf. B Biointerfaces* **2011**, *82*, 160–167. [CrossRef]
127. Ashokan, A.; Menon, D.; Nair, S.; Koyakutty, M. A molecular receptor targeted, hydroxyapatite nanocrystal based multi-modal contrast agent. *Biomaterials* **2010**, *31*, 2606–2616. [CrossRef] [PubMed]
128. Chen, F.; Zhu, Y.J.; Zhang, K.H.; Wu, J.; Wang, K.W.; Tang, Q.L.; Mo, X.M. Europium-doped amorphous calcium phosphate porous nanospheres: Preparation and application as luminescent drug carriers. *Nanoscale Res. Lett.* **2011**, *6*, 67. [CrossRef]
129. Zuo, Z.Y.; Song, X.M.; Guo, D.Y.; Guo, Z.R.; Niu, Q.F. A dual responsive colorimetric/fluorescent turn-on sensor for highly selective, sensitive and fast detection of Fe^{3+} ions and its applications. *J. Photochem. Photobiol. A Chem.* **2019**, *382*, 111876. [CrossRef]
130. Xu, C.J.; Sun, S.H. Monodisperse magnetic nanoparticles for biomedical applications. *Polym. Int.* **2007**, *56*, 821–826. [CrossRef]

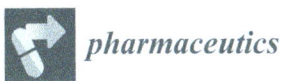

Systematic Review

Nanomedicine and Hyperthermia for the Treatment of Gastrointestinal Cancer: A Systematic Review

Lidia Gago [1,2,3], Francisco Quiñonero [1,3], Gloria Perazzoli [1,2,3], Consolación Melguizo [1,2,3], Jose Prados [1,2,3,*], Raul Ortiz [1,2,3,†] and Laura Cabeza [1,2,3,†]

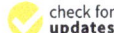

Citation: Gago, L.; Quiñonero, F.; Perazzoli, G.; Melguizo, C.; Prados, J.; Ortiz, R.; Cabeza, L. Nanomedicine and Hyperthermia for the Treatment of Gastrointestinal Cancer: A Systematic Review. *Pharmaceutics* **2023**, *15*, 1958. https://doi.org/10.3390/pharmaceutics15071958

Academic Editor: Constantin Mihai Lucaciu

Received: 9 June 2023
Revised: 8 July 2023
Accepted: 14 July 2023
Published: 15 July 2023

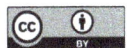

Copyright: © 2023 by the authors. Licensee MDPI, Basel, Switzerland. This article is an open access article distributed under the terms and conditions of the Creative Commons Attribution (CC BY) license (https://creativecommons.org/licenses/by/4.0/).

[1] Institute of Biopathology and Regenerative Medicine (IBIMER), Center of Biomedical Research (CIBM), University of Granada, 18100 Granada, Spain; lgago@ugr.es (L.G.); fjquinonero@ugr.es (F.Q.); gperazzoli@ugr.es (G.P.); melguizo@ugr.es (C.M.); roquesa@ugr.es (R.O.); lautea@ugr.es (L.C.)
[2] Department of Anatomy and Embryology, Faculty of Medicine, University of Granada, 18071 Granada, Spain
[3] Biosanitary Institute of Granada (ibs.GRANADA), SAS-University of Granada, 18014 Granada, Spain
* Correspondence: jcprados@ugr.es
† These authors contributed equally to this work.

Abstract: The incidence of gastrointestinal cancers has increased in recent years. Current treatments present numerous challenges, including drug resistance, non-specificity, and severe side effects, needing the exploration of new therapeutic strategies. One promising avenue is the use of magnetic nanoparticles, which have gained considerable interest due to their ability to generate heat in tumor regions upon the application of an external alternating magnetic field, a process known as hyperthermia. This review conducted a systematic search of in vitro and in vivo studies published in the last decade that employ hyperthermia therapy mediated by magnetic nanoparticles for treating gastrointestinal cancers. After applying various inclusion and exclusion criteria (studies in the last 10 years where hyperthermia using alternative magnetic field is applied), a total of 40 articles were analyzed. The results revealed that iron oxide is the preferred material for magnetism generation in the nanoparticles, and colorectal cancer is the most studied gastrointestinal cancer. Interestingly, novel therapies employing nanoparticles loaded with chemotherapeutic drugs in combination with magnetic hyperthermia demonstrated an excellent antitumor effect. In conclusion, hyperthermia treatments mediated by magnetic nanoparticles appear to be an effective approach for the treatment of gastrointestinal cancers, offering advantages over traditional therapies.

Keywords: gastrointestinal cancer; magnetic nanoparticles; hyperthermia; cytotoxic drugs

1. Introduction

The treatment of gastrointestinal cancer poses a significant challenge due to its increasing incidence in the population [1]. For example, colorectal cancer (CRC) ranks third in incidence and second in mortality, while stomach cancer (GC) and esophageal cancer (EC) rank fourth and sixth in mortality, respectively [2].

Current treatments encompass resection surgery along with chemotherapy, radiation therapy, and/or targeted therapies [3,4]. A broad range of drugs are utilized in various types of gastrointestinal cancer. These include 5-fluorouracil (5-FU), oxaliplatin (OXA), and irinotecan (IRI) in CRC; 5-fluorouracil combined with leucovorin, docetaxel, and oxaliplatin (FLOT) in GC [5]; and carboplatin and paclitaxel in EC, among others [6]. However, most drugs and their combinations generate side effects that can lead to treatment failure. For example, neurotoxicity is induced by OXA [7], cardiotoxicity by 5-fluorouracil [8], and severe neutropenia and hypersensitivity reactions follow paclitaxel treatment [9]. Additionally, drug resistance mechanisms induced by cytotoxins lead to poor response to chemotherapy and patient relapse [10]. Therefore, there is an essential need for new strategies to improve the prognosis of these diseases.

In this context, nanomedicine has emerged as a promising approach to cancer treatment and diagnosis. Numerous nanoformulations are available, with sizes ranging from 1 to 100 nm. Their inherent characteristics provide a drug delivery system with several advantages, such as reduced side effects of antitumor agents, improved targeting of the affected region, and increased drug levels in the tumor region, among others [10]. Both organic and inorganic nanoparticles (NPs) [11] have been employed to enhance cancer therapy. In fact, lipid-based nanoparticles have been the first clinically approved therapeutic nanoplatform against cancer by the FDA [12]. A classic example of their application is Doxil, a PEGylated liposome loaded with the drug Doxorubicin (DOXO) [13]. More recently, Onivyde, a liposome encapsulated with irinotecan, was approved by the FDA for the treatment of metastatic pancreatic cancer [14].

In this regard, magnetic NPs, a group of inorganic nanoformulations, have been proposed as an innovative strategy due to their physicochemical properties. They consist of a magnetic core and a polymeric coating, with iron oxide NPs being the most widely utilized. Magnetic NPs have superparamagnetic properties, which means that they are magnetized in the presence of an alternating external magnetic field (AMF), but lose magnetization without it, thereby reducing the potential for aggregation in the body and, consequently, the probability of embolization [15,16]. Among the advantages of these NPs is their ability to diffuse to the tumor region due to the application of a magnetic field near the target tissue [17]. Additionally, magnetic cores are used as contrast agents in various imaging techniques, such as magnetic resonance imaging (MRI), or newer techniques such as magnetic particle imaging. This allows for the tracking of these nanoformulations as they circulate within the organism, which is an interesting approach in terms of establishing targeted therapy [18].

Another major advantage derived from the use of magnetic NPs is their ability to generate high temperatures when an AMF is applied, which is known as hyperthermia. This property is considered one of the most intriguing and promising applications in the field of cancer nanomedicine, since it offers the possibility of applying a combined treatment, integrating the antitumor capacity of the drug loaded in the NPs and the hyperthermia generated [19]. Promising results have been obtained in various types of cancer after applying hyperthermia treatment alone or in combination with chemotherapy [20,21]. Recently, Narayanaswamy et al. (2022) utilized NPs with a $MnFe_2O_4$ core and an Fe_3O_4 shell against human colon and breast cancer cell lines (MDA-MB-231 and HT-29, respectively), increasing cell death by up to 70% [22]. Furthermore, Piehler et al. (2020) and Rego et al. (2020) demonstrated the applicability of hyperthermia in vivo using DOX-functionalized magnetic NPs and aminosilane-coated iron oxide NPs, respectively [23,24]. Dabaghi et al. (2021) developed 5-FU functionalized chitosan-coated magnetic NPs to deliver hyperthermia specifically against CRC-induced mice, showing a significant reduction in tumor volume and tumor vascularization [25]. In sum, many results support the benefits of hyperthermia therapy in cancer treatment.

In the present systematic review, we analyzed the most recently published studies on the application of hyperthermia based on magnetic NPs in gastrointestinal cancers. The review highlights crucial aspects of the emerging advancements in magnetic nanomaterials and provides a brief overview of the challenges and limitations of this therapeutic strategy.

2. Materials and Methods
2.1. Study Eligibility

The purpose of the present systematic review was to analyze the most recent and representative information on studies evaluating the therapeutic efficacy of NP-mediated hyperthermia in the treatment of various gastrointestinal cancers. This review was conducted following the criteria set out in the PRISMA guidelines [26]. To this end, only studies from the last 10 years were considered, deeming older ones obsolete. According to the Burton–Kebler index for obsolescence [27], more than half of the publications on this subject were included.

2.2. Inclusion Criteria

This systematic review included scientific publications between January 2013 and January 2023, with full text available and written in English. We also included works where hyperthermia treatment was applied through the use of an AMF on the NPs of interest as a therapy against any of the known gastrointestinal cancers.

2.3. Exclusion Criteria

Studies were excluded if hyperthermia, defined as an increase in temperature, was applied by any method other than the use of a magnetic field, such as water baths, lasers, ultrasound, etc. Furthermore, reviews, meta-analyses, systematic reviews, book chapters, or editorials were not considered for the review.

2.4. Data Sources

For the bibliographic search, the electronic databases Pubmed, SCOPUS, and Web of Science were used. The first established medical subject heading (MeSH) terms included: "Colorectal Neoplasms", "Gastrointestinal Neoplasms", "Esophageal Neoplasms", "Intestinal Neoplasms", "Stomach Neoplasms", "Cecal Neoplasms", "Duodenal Neoplasms", "Ileal Neoplasms", "Jejunal Neoplasms", "Nanoparticles", "Liposomes", and "Hyperthermia". The final search equation was ((("Colorectal Neoplasms" [MeSH Terms] OR "Gastrointestinal Neoplasms" [MeSH Terms] OR "Esophageal Neoplasms" [MeSH Terms] OR "Intestinal Neoplasms" [MeSH Terms] OR "Stomach Neoplasms" [MeSH Terms] OR "Cecal Neoplasms" [MeSH Terms] OR "Duodenal Neoplasms" [MeSH Terms] OR "Ileal Neoplasms" [MeSH Terms] OR "Jejunal Neoplasms" [MeSH Terms]) OR ((("colon" [Title/Abstract] OR "colorectal" [Title/Abstract] OR "colonic" [Title/Abstract] OR "Gastric*" [Title/Abstract] OR "Gastrointestinal" [Title/Abstract] OR "Esophageal*" [Title/Abstract] OR "Intestinal*" [Title/Abstract] OR "Stomach*" [Title/Abstract] OR "Cecal*" [Title/Abstract] OR "Duodenal*" [Title/Abstract] OR "Ileal*" [Title/Abstract] OR "Jejunal*" [Title/Abstract]) AND ("cancer*" [Title/Abstract] OR "tumor*" [Title/Abstract] OR "tumour*" [Title/Abstract] OR "neoplasm*" [Title/Abstract] OR "carcinoma*" [Title/Abstract]))) AND ("nanoparticles" [MeSH Terms] OR "nanoparticle*" [Title/Abstract] OR "nanoconjugate*" [Title/Abstract] OR "liposomes" [MeSH Terms] OR "liposome*" [Title/Abstract]) AND ("hyperthermia" [MeSH Terms] OR "hyperthermia*" [Title/Abstract]). Some minor modifications were made to adjust the search in the rest of the databases.

2.5. Study Selection

Two of the authors (L.G. and F.Q.) conducted the literature search. Initially, all articles were analyzed by title and abstract, with those meeting the inclusion criteria being selected. Both authors then reviewed all the selected articles through full-text analysis, considering the established inclusion and exclusion criteria.

2.6. Data Extraction

Following the study selection process, the same two authors separately analyzed the selected articles to extract data. The Cohen's kappa statistical test result exceeded 0.8 (Cohen, 1968), indicating good agreement between the two authors [28]. All discrepancies were resolved by consensus between authors F.Q. and L.G. and, when necessary, two other authors intervened. A specific questionnaire, divided into two evaluation phases, was used to establish the quality of the selected articles; those papers scoring less than 6 points were excluded from the systematic review. Table 1, which presents the data obtained after exhaustive analysis of each article, includes information on the types of nanoformulations used, the antitumor agents transported, the applied magnetic fields, and notable in vitro and in vivo results, in addition to the article references.

Table 1. Summary of the most relevant characteristics of the selected articles.

Nanoformulation	Antitumor Agent	AMF	In Vitro Assay	In Vivo Assay	Tumor Type	Main Results	Reference
$MnFe_2O_4$-Fe_3O_4 core–shell NPs	-	384.5 kHz, 27.85 kA/m	Cytotoxicity assay (HT29)	-	CRC	High cytotoxicity effect	[22]
Cs MNPs	5-FU	435 kHz, 15.4 kA/m	-	HT29 tumor-bearing mice	CRC	Decrease in tumor size	[25]
Exosome-FA-MNPs	DOXO	310 kHz	Cytotoxicity assay (HT29)	HT29 tumor-bearing mice	CRC	High cytotoxicity effect and decrease in tumor size	[29]
MNPs loaded Cs nanofibers	-	750–1150 kHz	Cytotoxicity assay (CT26)	-	CRC	High cytotoxicity effect	[30]
SPIONs loaded microrobots	5-FU	430 kHz, 45 kA/m	Cytotoxicity assay (HCT116)	-	CRC	High cytotoxicity effect	[31]
Fluorescent MNP labeled iPS	-	63 kHz, 7 kA/m	-	MGC803 tumor-bearing mice	GC	Decrease in tumor size and good MRI results	[32]
SPIO-APTES anti-CD133 MNPs	IRI	1.3–1.8 kHz	Cytotoxicity (Caco-2, HCT116, DLD1)	HCT116 tumor-bearing mice	CRC	High cytotoxicity assay, decrease in tumor size and good MRI results	[33]
anti-HER2 carboxydextran and amphiphilic polimer SPIONs	-	280 kHz, 31 kA/m	Cytotoxicity assay (NUGC-4)	-	GC	High cytotoxicity effect	[34]
Anti-131I-labeled CC49 SPIONs	-	252 kHz, 15.9 kA/m	-	LS174T tumor-bearing mice	CRC	Decrease in tumor size	[35]
MPVA-AP1 nanovehicles	DOXO	50–100 kHz	Liberation assay	-	CRC	High drug liberation and drug release	[36]
TAT/CSF1R inhibitor functionalized magnetic liposomes	-	288 kHz, 35 kA/m	-	CT26 tumor-bearing mice	CRC	Decrease in tumor size and increased magnetic targeting	[37]
PEG-PBA-PEG coated SPIONs	5-FU	13,560 kHz	Cytotoxicity assay (HT29, HCT116)	-	CRC	High cytotoxicity effect	[38]
Alginate coated MPNPs and QDs	DOXO	4–6.3 kA/m	-	CT26 tumor-bearing mice	CRC	Good MRI results	[39]
Agar encapsulated MNPs	DOXO	400 kHz, 0.45 kA/m	Cytotoxicity assay (HT29)	-	CRC	High cytotoxicity effect	[40]
APTES coated MNPs	-	300 kHz	-	VX2 tumor-bearing rabbits	EC	Decrease in tumor size	[41]
(maghemite/PLGA)/Cs NPs	-	250 kHz, 4 kA/m	Cytotoxicity assay (T84)	Healthy mice	CRC	High cytotoxicity effect and good MRI results	[42]

Table 1. Cont.

Nanoformulation	Antitumor Agent	AMF	In Vitro Assay	In Vivo Assay	Tumor Type	Main Results	Reference
PLGA SPIONs	DOXO	205 kHz, 2 kA/m	Cytotoxicity assay (CT26)	CT26 tumor-bearing mice	CRC	High cytotoxicity assay, drug release, decrease in tumor size and good MRI results	[43]
Bacteria derived MNPs	-	187 kHz, 23 kA/m	-	HT29 tumor-bearing mice	CRC	In vivo apoptotic and necrotic areas and good MRI results	[44]
Solid-lipid MNPs	-	250 kHz, 4 kA/m	Cytotoxicity assay (HT29)	-	CRC	High cytotoxicity effect	[45]
Bacteria-derived MNPs	5-FU	250 kHz, 4 kA/m	Liberation assay	-	CRC	High drug release	[46]
Bacteria-derived MNPs	OXA	197 kHz, 18 kA/m	Liberation assay	-	CRC	High drug release	[47]
Cobalt ferrite NPs	-	261 kHz, 8–19.8 kA/m	Cytotoxicity assay (CT26)	CT26 tumor-bearing mice	CRC	High cytotoxicity effect and decrease in tumor size	[48]
MNPs	CDDP	237 kHz, 20 kA/m	Cytotoxicity assay (Caco-2)	-	CRC	High cytotoxicity effect	[49]
PEG-PCL-PEG/FA MNPs	5-FU	13,560 kHz, 0.4 kA/m	Cytotoxicity assay (HT29)	-	CRC	High cytotoxicity effect	[50]
MNPs	-	100 kHz, 4 kA/m	MRI assay	-	CRC	Good MRI results	[51]
Iron oxide nanocubes	DOXO	182 kHz	Patient-derived CSCs	Patient-derived CSCs tumor-bearing mice	CRC	High cytotoxicity assay, decrease in tumor size	[52]
Iron oxide NPs/Au NPs core/shell nanohybrid	-	13,560 kHz	Cytotoxicity assay (CT26)	CT26 tumor-bearing mice	CRC	High cytotoxicity effect, decrease in tumor size, increased magnetic targeting and good MRI results	[53]
$ZnCoFe_2O_4$ and $ZnMnFe_2O_4$ NPs	-	1.35 kA/m	Cytotoxicity assay (CT26)	CT26 tumor-bearing mice	CRC	High cytotoxicity effect, decrease in tumor size and better targeting	[54]
Polymers functionalized MNPs	Niclosamide	405 kHz	Cytotoxicity assay (HCT116)	-	CRC	High Cytotoxicity effect	[55]
Magnetic solid lipid NPs coated with FA and Dextran	DOXO	Not specified	Cytotoxicity assay (CT26)	CT26 tumor-bearing mice	CRC	High cytotoxicity effect, decrease in tumor size and metastases	[56]

Table 1. Cont.

Nanoformulation	Antitumor Agent	AMF	In Vitro Assay	In Vivo Assay	Tumor Type	Main Results	Reference
Acid citric and EDC/NHC functionalized MNPs	-	87 kHz-340 kHz, 79.57 kA/m	Cytotoxicity assay (not specified)	-	CRC	High cytotoxicity effect	[57]
PMAO-PEG MNPs	-	650 kHz, 16.71 kA/m	Cytotoxicity assay (HCT116)	-	CRC	High cytotoxicity effect	[58]
APTS/PRO functionalized SPIONs loaded with TNF-alfa	-	110 kHz, 8.75 kA/m	Cytotoxicity assay (SW480, HepG2)	-	CRC	High cytotoxicity effect	[59]
Carboxydextran coated MNPs	-	390 kHz, 28 kA/m	Cytotoxicity assay (HCT116)	Peritoneal-dissemination mice	CRC	High cytotoxicity effect and metastases decrease	[60]
Carboxydextran coated MNPs	Bortezomib	233 kHz, 29.39 kA/m	Cytotoxicity assay (Caco-2)	-	CRC	High cytotoxicity effect	[61]
Liposome encapsulated citric acid-coated MNPs	DOXO	300 kHz, 59.3 kA/m	Cytotoxicity assay (CT26)	-	CRC	High cytotoxicity effect and drug release	[62]
Monosaccharides coated MNPs	-	292 kHz, 51.0 kA/m	Cytotoxicity assay (CT26)	-	CRC	High cytotoxicity effect	[63]
PLGA SPIONs	-	930 kHz, 13 kA/m	-	CT26 tumor-bearing mice	CRC	Increased magnetic targeting	[64]
PMAO MNPs	-	606 kHz, 14 kA/m	-	CC-531 tumor-bearing rats	CRC	Heterogeneous cytotoxicity results	[65]
Cs MNPs	5-FU	435 kHz, 15.4 kA/m	-	HT29 tumor-bearing mice	CRC	Sensitizes cells for further therapies and DNA damage	[66]

AP1 (atherosclerotic plaque-specific peptide-1); APTES (3-aminopropyltriethoxysilane); CRC (colorectal cancer); Cs (chitosan); CSCs (Cancer stem cells); CSF1R (Colony stimulating factor 1 receptor); DOXO (doxorubicin); EC (esophageal cancer); EDC (1-ethyl-3-(3-dimethylaminopropyl) carbodiimide); FA (folic acid); 5-FU (5-fluorouracil); GC (gastric cancer); iPS (Induced pluripotent stem cells); IRI (irinotecan); MNPs (magnetic nanoparticles); MPVA (magnetic poly(vinyl alcohol)-based nanovehicles); MRI (magnetic resonance imaging); NHC (N-hydroxysuccinimide); NPs (nanoparticles); OXA (Oxaliplatin); PEG (polyethylene glycol); PLGA (poly(lactic-co-glycolic acid)); PMAO (poly(maleic anhydride-alt-1-octadecene)); SPIONs (Superparamagnetic iron oxide nanoparticles); TAT (Transactivator of transcription peptide).

3. Results and Discussion

3.1. Study Description

After conducting the bibliographic search in the PubMed, SCOPUS, and Web of Science databases, a total of 672 articles were obtained. Subsequently, 193 duplicate articles were excluded and, once analyzed by title and abstract, another 429 articles were excluded, leaving 50 selected. Likewise, nine of the fifty articles did not meet the inclusion criteria and one of them had low quality values. Therefore, a total of 40 articles were finally included in the present systematic review. All the data concerning the search are represented in the flow diagram in Figure 1.

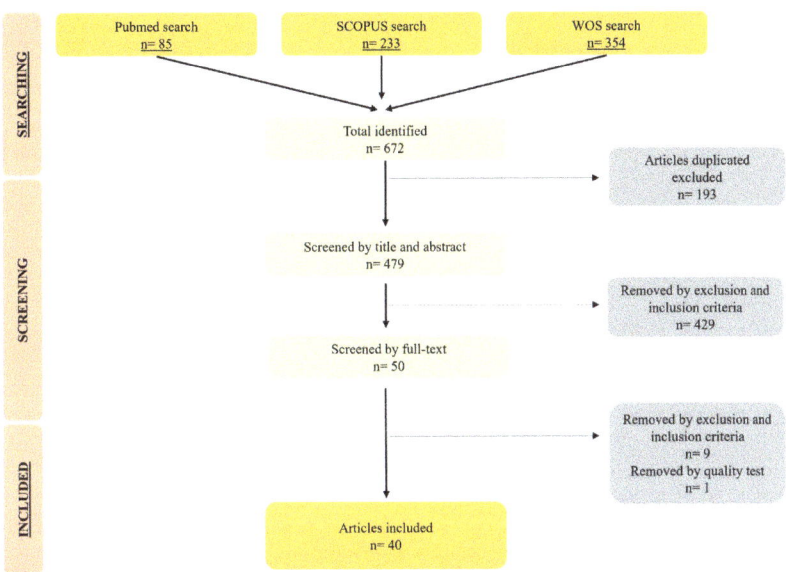

Figure 1. Flow diagram that represents the articles included in the systematic review.

3.2. Characteristics of Magnetic Nanoformulations

Table 1 shows the different nanoformulations used in each article and some of their main characteristics. Of the 40 articles analyzed, 100% of the nanoformulations were based on the magnetic properties of iron oxide nuclei or derivatives (magnetite or maghemite), indicating that iron was the preferred material for creating magnetic NPs. Furthermore, 36 out of 40 articles utilized an NP-based nanocarrier, while the remaining four articles employed more complex systems, including an exosome-based system [29], chitosan nanofibers [30], microrobots [31], and induced pluripotent stem cells [32]. Interestingly, three manuscripts featured antibody-functionalized NPs, including anti-CD133 [33], anti-HER2 [34], and radioactively labeled anti-CC49 [35]. Two articles used AP-1 [36] and TAT [37] peptides for functionalization. Regardless, the objective was to enhance the capabilities of the different nanoformulations (Figure 2). Approximately 47% of manuscripts combined hyperthermia therapy with drug usage. The most widely used chemotherapeutic agents were Doxorubicin (DOXO) and 5-Fluorouracil (5-FU), featured in eight and six articles, respectively. Other drugs included Oxaliplatin (OXA), Irinotecan (Iri), Cisplatin (CDDP), Bortezomib, and Niclosamide. Most of the selected articles analyzed the magnetic characteristics of the nanoformulations. Specifically, 25 articles highlighted the specific absorption rate (SAR) or magnetic saturation point (Ms), both of which are closely related to heat generation capacity after the application of an AMF. The value of the applied magnetic field and the duration of its application vary depending on the hyperthermia system. In fact, 30 of the 40 articles employed a field frequency within the range of 100 to 650 kHz. Conversely, two articles applied frequencies below 100 kHz, five used high frequencies such as Jahangiri et al. (2021) (13.56 MHz) [38], and three did not specify the frequency used. Ha et al. (2020) and Wang et al. (2021) demonstrated that functionalizations such as quantum dots [39] or the inclusion of NPs in gels [40] could impede temperature rise, suggesting that the choice of NPs is very relevant.

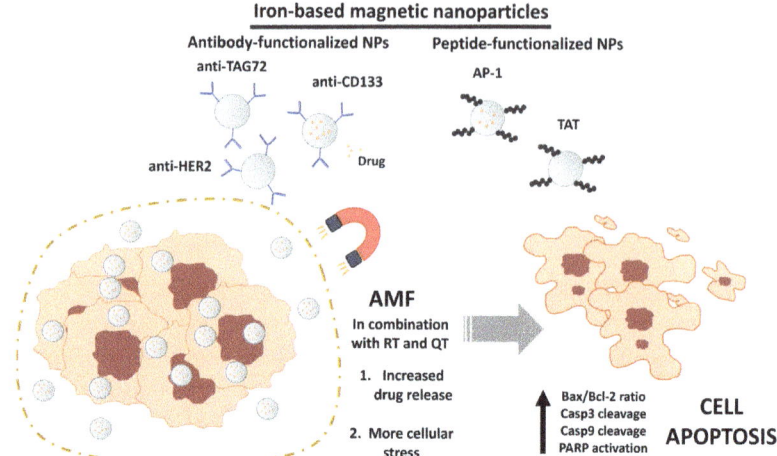

Figure 2. Use of magnetic nanoparticles in in vitro AMF hyperthermia application experiments. Magnetic nanoparticles, typically composed of iron, can be functionalized with antibodies (against HER2, TAG72, or CD133) or specific peptides to actively target a tumor population. AMF facilitates, in formulations that encapsulate drugs, a greater drug release into the cell and the induction of heightened cellular stress. These factors ultimately result in the death of tumor cells, triggering the activation of PARP and the cleavage of several caspases to activate the apoptotic pathway.

Moreover, and regarding the time of the treatment followed, the application of a 30 min treatment predominated, both in vitro and in vivo (13 of the 40 articles). The rest of the studies applied times ranging from 5 to 60 min. Likewise, in the case of in vivo tests, some authors applied a 30 min treatment continued over time, exposing the experimental animals to cycles of 30 min during the days established in each case [32,35,36]. Transfer to the clinic would involve the application of hyperthermia cycles alone or in combination with other treatments, depending on the approach. Due to the malignancy of the tumors and recurrences, it may be necessary to apply treatment cycles every certain time previously established. This is the case of the clinical trial conducted by Johannsen et al. (2005) for prostate cancer, in which patients were exposed to six weekly 60 min hyperthermia treatments [67]. Finally, concerning cell lines on which the NPs were tested, in vitro or in vivo, 38 articles were conducted on colon lines, notably the CT26 murine colorectal carcinoma line (11 articles) and HT29 human colorectal adenocarcinoma (9 articles). Only three of the forty articles used gastric [32,34] and esophageal [41] cancer lines. Therefore, the scarcity of investigations in some gastrointestinal cancers necessitates new research.

3.3. Biocompatibility of Hyperthermia Assays

Hyperthermia treatment safety is a major limitation in its clinical application. Interestingly, iron oxide was employed in the generation of NPs in all analyzed articles (40 articles) due to its biocompatibility [68], thereby avoiding damage to healthy cells. Fernández-Álvarez et al. (2021) used a non-tumor fibroblastic line and human blood samples to ensure no effect on normal tissue, erythrocytes, coagulation, and the complement system [42].

In addition, clinically accepted values of magnetic fields have been established, indicating that the product of the frequency and amplitude values must not exceed 5×10^9, as higher values can potentially harm DNA [69]. In fact, only 12 out of the 40 articles used magnetic fields within the clinically accepted range [32,35,40,43–51]. Conversely, 12 articles did not provide the necessary information to calculate this value [29,30,33,36,38,39,41,52–56]. Some authors have sought alternatives to generate magnetic NPs through a combustion system and varying concentrations of citric acid. These NPs induced high temperatures following an 87 kHz magnetic field, suggesting that a high Fe^{2+}/Fe^{3+} ratio can enhance the hyperthermic capacity of nanoformulations without the need to increase the field frequency [57]. Ninety-five percent of the selected articles with in vivo tests demonstrated that hyperthermia treatment with NP did not induce damage to healthy tissues. In fact, Shen et al. (2019) generated magnetic solid lipid NPs coated with folic acid (FA) and Dextran and performed biocompatibility assays in CT26 colorectal tumor-bearing mice. Following hyperthermia treatment, they analyzed blood values and potential histological damage, obtaining normal ratios in all cases, thus supporting the apparent safety of these treatments in vivo [56]. Furthermore, Fang et al. (2021) demonstrated that magnetic liposomes functionalized with TAT/CSF1R inhibitor did not cause changes in body weight or histopathological damage following hyperthermia treatment in CT26 tumor-bearing mice [37]. However, new nanoformulation approaches are required that allow for an increase in temperature without increasing the frequency and intensity of the applied AMF. In this regard, it has been described that shortening the distance between NPs can enhance temperature rise [70]. Yang et al. (2020) generated magnetic nanoparticles and assembled and packaged them into a magnetic complex, obtaining higher temperature rises at very low frequencies (1.3–1.8 kHz) compared to single NPs [33]. These results have also been supported by other authors, such as Hu et al. (2023), who developed a controlled intracellular aggregation of NPs in acidic environments, obtaining better overall heating results [71].

3.4. In Vitro Assays

Of the 40 articles analyzed, 26 conducted cell viability tests applying hyperthermia treatment with or without chemotherapy (Table 1). All studies displayed better results with AMF than without it. However, significant differences were observed in induced cell death relative to the nanoformulations and the applied hyperthermia protocol.

Castellanos-Rubio et al. (2020) underscored the importance of selecting an optimal iron concentration for generating hyperthermia. They noted that at a concentration of 0.25 mg/mL, no significant cell death was observed in the colorectal cancer cell line HCT116. Conversely, at 0.5 mg/mL, cell survival decreased drastically [58]. Similarly, some NP functionalizations not only enhance heating capabilities but also cytotoxic effects in vitro. For example, Teo et al. (2017) generated SPIONs functionalized with 3-aminopropyltriethoxysilane (APTS) and/or protamine sulfate (PRO) loaded with TNF-α. They demonstrated that PRO increases NP toxicity in tumor cell lines, such as HepG2 and SW480, after AMF application compared to an APTS coating [59].

In certain cases, the molecular characteristics of the tumor cell line enable the selection of the appropriate NP functionalization, as demonstrated by Kagawa et al. (2021), who used anti-HER2 antibodies for treating the NUGC-4 cell line from gastric cancer, not showing any toxicity in healthy human fibroblasts due to their selectivity for internalization in cells with high HER2 expression, characteristic of gastrointestinal tumors such as gastric and esophageal tumors [34,72]. Among our selected articles, four reported complete cell death derived from the treatment [34,52,60,61]. Interestingly, three of these articles applied NP functionalized with carboxydextran. Both Fernandes et al. (2021) and Álvarez-Berríos et al. (2014) employed hyperthermia therapies in combination with chemotherapy, demonstrating the synergy that can result from applying both therapeutic approaches. Specifically, Fernandes et al. (2021) used polymer-coated iron oxide nanocubes loaded with DOXO, applying hyperthermia treatment from 10 to 90 min (3 cycles of 30 min) (182 kHz AMF) on patient-derived tumor stem cells (CSCs) [52]. After 24 h of exposure to treatment, more than 50% cell death was observed, reaching 100% at 7 days with a significant increase in the percentage of apoptosis and necrosis. These authors demonstrated that the heat generated by AMFs enhanced drug release and stimulated internalization in cells, thereby sensitizing them to chemotherapy. Similarly, five additional articles demonstrated significant drug sensitization, corroborating the enhanced release of some chemotherapeutics, such as 5-FU, OXA, and DOXO, following the use of AMF [36,43,46,47,62].

It has been proposed that the improvement following combined hyperthermia-chemotherapy treatment is due solely to the increase in temperature. However, interestingly, three of the selected articles demonstrated that less cell death was induced when water baths were applied (at the same temperature as those induced by AMF) [43,61]. Specifically, Álvarez-Berríos et al. (2013) used cisplatin-loaded iron oxide NPs and increased the temperature using a water bath or 237 kHz AMF. Hyperthermia generated 50% cell death in the Caco-2 CRC cell line compared to the 40% induced by the water bath. They hypothesized that AMF generates additional cellular stress that enhances membrane fluidity and ultimately results in cell death [49]. Therefore, hyperthermia generated by magnetic NPs appears to be a superior option for improving anticancer therapies compared to other systems.

Finally, hyperthermia associated with chemotherapy was not the only therapeutic approach against gastrointestinal cancer. Mirzaghavami et al. (2021) employed a combined treatment of chemotherapy, hyperthermia, and radiotherapy, inducing a greater decrease in the percentage of cell viability (45%) in the colorectal cancer cell line HT29 compared to individual treatments [50]. Additionally, a significant increase in apoptosis and necrosis was observed in the treated cell lines, increasing the Bax/Bcl2 ratio. Hyperthermia therapies induce more pronounced apoptosis than necrosis (Figure 2). Apoptosis was analyzed in nine of the forty selected articles. In fact, Jahangiri et al. (2021) provided an extensive description of this process, noting the overexpression of proapoptotic factor Bax, cleaved caspase-3, cleaved caspase-9, and PARP after treatment on HT29 and HCT116 colorectal cancer cell lines [38]. A similar increase in cleaved caspase-3 was shown in HCT116 by Ahmad et al. (2020) [55]. Moreover, Wydra et al. (2015) observed an increase in the generation of ROS after the application of AMF [63].

3.5. In Vivo Assays

A total of 50% (20) of the selected manuscripts carried out in vivo experiments, as shown in Table 1. The most commonly used animals were mice (90%), with CT26 tumor-bearing mice being the cancer model most frequently chosen by the authors. The utilization of magnetic NPs yielded beneficial results in all instances. In fact, Beyk and Tavakoli (2019) utilized nanohybrids of iron oxide and gold NPs, applying a magnet to the tumor region in CT26-tumor bearing mice for 3 h prior to hyperthermia treatment [53]. The results exhibited a higher temperature increase (49 °C) in the tumor area compared to treatment without a magnet (46 °C). This temperature increase led to significant inhibition of tumor size (92%). With regard to the generated temperature, most of the experiments achieved temperatures ranging from 41 to 50 °C [32,60]. However, after removal of the organs and application of MHT, it was observed that in mice with tumors induced from gastric lines, a large increase in temperature (up to 60 °C) was produced by applying ex vivo magnetic hyperthermia for 5 min, while in mice without tumors this high increase occurred in the liver, the organ in which the accumulation of these NPs took place [32]. Garanina et al. (2020) examined the impact of different temperatures on treatment. They noticed effective reduction in tumor growth in CT26 tumor-bearing mice at 42–43 °C. However, in 4T1 breast cancer tumor-bearing mice, which have a more resistant cell line, the tumor cells recurred after 20 days. In this case, effective treatment occurred at 46–48 °C. Furthermore, temperatures of 58–60 °C were tested, but these caused weight and motility losses, although recovery was observed over time [48]. These findings underscore the importance of personalizing treatments based on the tumors to be treated, whenever feasible, and avoiding excessively high temperatures that might lead to adverse effects.

Alternatively, magnetic steering was also reported by Wang et al. (2020) following magnet application (1 h) with positive outcomes [64]. Similarly, Beyk and Tavakoli observed MRI targeting due to these NPs' ability to act as contrast agents, as was shown in seven other articles (Figure 3) [53]. These results hence signify the possibility of externally enhancing in vivo targeting to the tumor thanks to the magnetic capabilities of NPs. Additionally, Kwon et al. introduced the potential of improving targeting by functionalizing NPs. They applied an FA polymer to the shell of their nanoformulations, achieving improved tumor targeting in HT29 colorectal cancer tumor-bearing mice [29]. However, FA receptors are also found in the small intestine. That is why Shen et al. coated their nanoformulations with dextran, circumventing this compound's recognition, thus directing more NPs to the colon region where the dextran was degraded by the dextranase produced there [56].

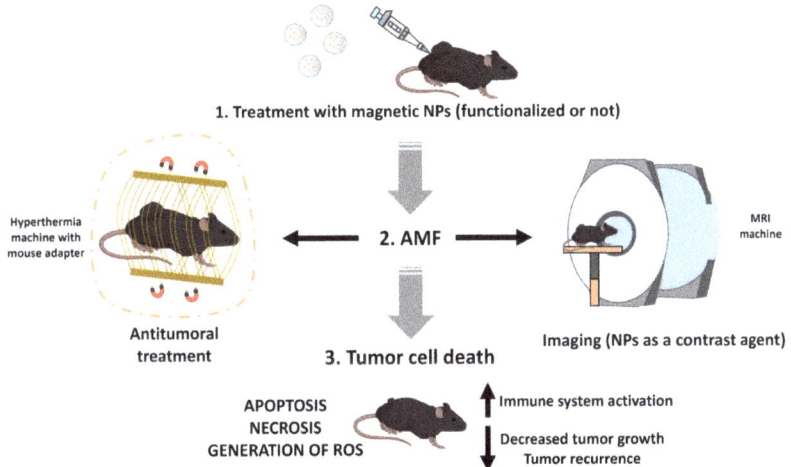

Figure 3. Use of magnetic hypothermia in in vivo experiments. Typically, the assays involve an intravenous administration of the NPs into the mouse such that once they reach the tumor, they are capable of: (1) generating hyperthermia when exposed to an AMF, serving as an antitumor therapy alone or in combination with chemotherapeutic drugs; or (2) acting as contrast agents, creating negative contrast and potentially being used for tumor diagnosis and monitoring. Following the generation of hyperthermia, tumor cell death can occur through several pathways, with apoptosis, necrosis, or extensive oxidative stress being the most notable.

Although most in vivo studies were performed in mice or rats, Liu et al. (2013) conducted an in vivo model of esophageal cancer by injecting VX2 cells into the esophageal mucosa. The authors employed two hyperthermia models: one using a magnetic stem introduced into the esophagus of mice and the other by introducing magnetic NPs into the tumor mass. The results showed that, after the application of a 300 kHz field, both treatments showed a proven anti-tumor efficacy, although it was necessary to control both the temperature and the time of exposure to hyperthermia to avoid causing damage to healthy tissue [41].

All analyzed articles demonstrated positive outcomes in terms of tumor volume reduction when applying hyperthermia and NPs together compared to the application of the AMF or the nanoformulation alone. Nonetheless, it is worth noting that Arriortua et al. (2016) displayed highly varied results, as some tumors in the animal models used (CC-531 colon adenocarcinoma tumor-bearing rats) were almost obliterated while in other cases cell death was minor [65]. Moreover, eight of the twenty-one articles including in vivo analysis examined the apoptotic and necrotic effect induced by hyperthermia at the histological or genetic level. In fact, Beyk and Tavakoli (2019) and Kwon et al. (2021) revealed increases in the expression of some genes indicating apoptosis (cleaved PARP, Bax or cleaved Caspase-3) (Figure 3) [29,53]. These results were confirmed at the histological level in three more articles [35,43,65]. Conversely, Dabaghi et al. (2020) did not demonstrate any modulation in apoptosis gene expression, suggesting a cell death mediated by an increase in ROS [66]. Therefore, the mechanism through which tumor cell death is accomplished could be related to the type of NP and the hyperthermia treatment system. Additionally, three articles assessed the decrease in tumor metastases following treatment. Stankovic' et al. (2020)

did not exhibit dissemination of tumor cells after treatment in histological sections, while Matsumi et al. (2021) and Shen et al. (2019) observed a significant decrease in the number of metastatic nodules and ascites in murine models [35,56,60]. Finally, Fang et al. (2021) transplanted tumor cells from a mouse to other regions post hyperthermia treatment, but no tumor recurrence was noticed, implying activation of immune memory [37]. These results were validated by Jiang et al. (2022) using a CRC model surrounded by bacteria. In this case, immune system activation occurred after hyperthermia, resulting in an increase in cytokines, re-polarization of macrophages, and an increase in antigen presentation [54]. Therefore, hyperthermia treatments also have the ability to activate the immune response, which is typically suppressed in cancer (Figure 3). Likewise, the combination of hyperthermia and immunotherapy is another combined treatment option that may have very promising results. One of the selected articles used a magnetic liposomal system possessing the penetrating TAT peptide by which they administered the CSF1R inhibitor, so that it was possible to repolarize M2 macrophages, thus reducing immunosuppression in the tumor region [37]. It has previously been described that hyperthermia and immunotherapy have synergistic effects, giving rise to the possibility of triggering immunogenic cell death or reversing the immunosuppressive environment of tumors [73]. Thus, after tumor ablation by hyperthermia treatment, antigenic remnants would be released into the environment so they could be used as autologous vaccines against cancer. An example of this is presented in the work carried out by Pan et al. (2020), in which they applied magnetic NPs in combination with the programmed death ligand α-PD-L1 against a breast cancer model. Briefly, the generation of cytotoxic T cells against tumor antigens is achieved and α-PD-L1 prevents tumor immunosuppression, ultimately increasing the number of T cells and the immune response [74]. These results have been confirmed in other articles, demonstrating the potential of this therapeutic approach [75,76].

The benefits observed in in vitro and in vivo trials encourage the transfer of these treatments to the clinic. Currently, the application of magnetic hyperthermia as a possible treatment has been tested in clinical trials against prostate cancer (NCT02033447) and glioblastoma (DRKS00005476). In the first case, patients treated with magnetic nanoparticles received six cycles of therapy for 1 h during phase I of the study and showed tolerance and efficacy as antitumor therapy. Nevertheless, this therapy is still in phase II clinical trials. Regarding the hyperthermia treatment itself, its major limitations lie in the control of the local temperature reached in the tissue, which can negatively affect healthy cells, in addition to the heterogeneous distribution of the temperature in the tumor mass [77]. Additionally, one of the major problems in bringing this therapy to the clinic is the biosafety of the nanoformulations, which must have an exhaustive control of the size and components, making their production totally controlled [69]. Furthermore, another problem is the frequent parenteral administration of nanoparticles, as opposed to the simpler traditional oral administration. This fact generates a more expensive treatment, so that the commercial production of these treatments must be justified by greater efficacy or safety (including side effects) compared to the therapy traditionally used. Finally, many of the results obtained in preclinical studies (in vitro and in vivo models) are not subsequently retained in clinical trials, since certain characteristics, such as specific functionalization against a target, do not act in the same way in these models as in the human body [78].

For all the above reasons, the future of this line of research implies the need to expand the current research in order to solve the drawbacks encountered and finally allow the existence of a novel treatment that improves the quality of life of the affected patients.

4. Conclusions

Magnetic NP-driven hyperthermia treatment offers an innovative and promising therapeutic strategy for gastrointestinal cancers. Numerous magnetic NPs, capable of inducing heat and exhibiting varying biological properties, have been developed in recent years. These have been applied to some gastrointestinal cancers, although most assays have been conducted in vitro on CRC. As for the magnetic characteristics of NPs, iron oxide has predominantly been used as the magnetic core, with magnetic fields ranging between 100 and 600 kHz. Nearly half of the tests were conducted using combination therapies with drugs (chemotherapy), with DOXO being notably prominent. The outcomes have been very promising both in vitro and in vivo, reducing metastasis and tumor recurrence in certain cases. However, it has become evident that there is a need to broaden studies to encompass other cancers within the gastrointestinal tract. Further investigation will be necessary to affirm the benefits of hyperthermia application using magnetic NPs in the treatment of gastrointestinal cancer and to overcome barriers to clinical application.

Author Contributions: Conceptualization, J.P., R.O. and L.C.; methodology, L.G. and F.Q.; software, G.P.; validation, C.M. and G.P.; formal analysis, L.G. and F.Q.; investigation, L.G., F.Q. and G.P.; data curation, C.M.; writing—original draft preparation, C G., F.Q. and G.P.; writing—review and editing, C.M. and J.P.; visualization, C.M.; supervision, L.C. and R.O.; funding acquisition, C.M and J.P. All authors have read and agreed to the published version of the manuscript.

Funding: This work was supported by the PI19/01478 and PMPTA22/00136 (Instituto de Salud Carlos III) (FEDER). In addition, it was partially supported by Project P20_00540, A-CTS-666-UGR20, B-CTS-122-UGR20 and PYC20 RE 035 (Proyectos I + D + i Junta de Andalucía 2020) (FEDER). LG acknowledges FP-PRE grant (2021) from the Junta de Andalucia (Spain).

Institutional Review Board Statement: Not applicable.

Informed Consent Statement: Not applicable.

Data Availability Statement: Not applicable.

Acknowledgments: We thank Instrumentation Scientific Center (CIC) from University of Granada for technical assistance.

Conflicts of Interest: The authors declare no conflict of interest.

References

1. Arnold, M.; Abnet, C.C.; Neale, R.E.; Vignat, J.; Giovannucci, E.L.; McGlynn, K.A.; Bray, F. Global Burden of 5 Major Types of Gastrointestinal Cancer. *Gastroenterology* **2020**, *159*, 335–349.e15. [CrossRef]
2. Sung, H.; Ferlay, J.; Siegel, R.L.; Laversanne, M.; Soerjomataram, I.; Jemal, A.; Bray, F. Global Cancer Statistics 2020: GLOBOCAN Estimates of Incidence and Mortality Worldwide for 36 Cancers in 185 Countries. *CA Cancer J. Clin.* **2021**, *71*, 209–249. [CrossRef] [PubMed]
3. Huang, F.L.; Yu, S.J. Esophageal Cancer: Risk Factors, Genetic Association, and Treatment. *Asian J. Surg.* **2018**, *41*, 210–215. [CrossRef] [PubMed]
4. Machlowska, J.; Baj, J.; Sitarz, M.; Maciejewski, R.; Sitarz, R. Gastric Cancer: Epidemiology, Risk Factors, Classification, Genomic Characteristics and Treatment Strategies. *Int. J. Mol. Sci.* **2020**, *21*, 4012. [CrossRef]
5. Sexton, R.E.; Al Hallak, M.N.; Diab, M.; Azmi, A.S. Gastric Cancer: A Comprehensive Review of Current and Future Treatment Strategies. *Cancer Metastasis Rev.* **2020**, *39*, 1179–1203. [CrossRef]
6. Watanabe, M.; Otake, R.; Kozuki, R.; Toihata, T.; Takahashi, K.; Okamura, A.; Imamura, Y. Recent Progress in Multidisciplinary Treatment for Patients with Esophageal Cancer. *Surg. Today* **2020**, *50*, 12–20. [CrossRef]
7. Knowlton, C.A.; Mackay, M.K.; Speer, T.W.; Vera, R.B.; Arthur, D.W.; Wazer, D.E.; Lanciano, R.; Brashears, J.H.; Knowlton, C.A.; Mackay, M.K.; et al. Cancer Colon. In *Encyclopedia of Radiation Oncology*; Springer: Berlin/Heidelberg, Germany, 2013; p. 77.
8. Shiga, T.; Hiraide, M. Cardiotoxicities of 5-Fluorouracil and Other Fluoropyrimidines. *Curr. Treat. Options Oncol.* **2020**, *21*, 27. [CrossRef] [PubMed]
9. Al-Mahayri, Z.N.; AlAhmad, M.M.; Ali, B.R. Current Opinion on the Pharmacogenomics of Paclitaxel-Induced Toxicity. *Expert. Opin. Drug Metab. Toxicol.* **2021**, *17*, 785–801. [CrossRef]
10. Garbayo, E.; Pascual-Gil, S.; Rodríguez-Nogales, C.; Saludas, L.; Estella-Hermoso de Mendoza, A.; Blanco-Prieto, M.J. Nanomedicine and Drug Delivery Systems in Cancer and Regenerative Medicine. *Wiley Interdiscip. Rev. Nanomed. Nanobiotechnol.* **2020**, *12*, e1637. [CrossRef]
11. Aghebati-Maleki, A.; Dolati, S.; Ahmadi, M.; Baghbanzadeh, A.; Asadi, M.; Fotouhi, A.; Yousefi, M.; Aghebati-Maleki, L. Nanoparticles and Cancer Therapy: Perspectives for Application of Nanoparticles in the Treatment of Cancers. *J. Cell Physiol.* **2020**, *235*, 1962–1972. [CrossRef]
12. Chaudhuri, A.; Kumar, D.N.; Shaik, R.A.; Eid, B.G.; Abdel-Naim, A.B.; Md, S.; Ahmad, A.; Agrawal, A.K. Lipid-Based Nanoparticles as a Pivotal Delivery Approach in Triple Negative Breast Cancer (TNBC) Therapy. *Int. J. Mol. Sci.* **2022**, *23*, 10068. [CrossRef] [PubMed]

13. Gonzalez-Valdivieso, J.; Girotti, A.; Schneider, J.; Arias, F.J. Advanced Nanomedicine and Cancer: Challenges and Opportunities in Clinical Translation. *Int. J. Pharm.* **2021**, *599*, 120438. [CrossRef] [PubMed]
14. Milano, G.; Innocenti, F.; Minami, H. Liposomal Irinotecan (Onivyde): Exemplifying the Benefits of Nanotherapeutic Drugs. *Cancer Sci.* **2022**, *113*, 2224–2231. [CrossRef] [PubMed]
15. Vurro, F.; Jabalera, Y.; Mannucci, S.; Glorani, G.; Sola-Leyva, A.; Gerosa, M.; Romeo, A.; Romanelli, M.G.; Malatesta, M.; Calderan, L.; et al. Improving the Cellular Uptake of Biomimetic Magnetic Nanoparticles. *Nanomaterials* **2021**, *11*, 766. [CrossRef]
16. Wu, K.; Su, D.; Liu, J.; Saha, R.; Wang, J.-P. Magnetic Nanoparticles in Nanomedicine: A Review of Recent Advances. *Nanotechnology* **2019**, *30*, 502003. [CrossRef]
17. Farzin, A.; Etesami, S.A.; Quint, J.; Memic, A.; Tamayol, A. Magnetic Nanoparticles in Cancer Therapy and Diagnosis. *Adv. Heal. Healthc. Mater.* **2020**, *9*, 1901058. [CrossRef] [PubMed]
18. Li, Y.; Xin, J.; Sun, Y.; Han, T.; Zhang, H.; An, F. Magnetic Resonance Imaging-Guided and Targeted Theranostics of Colorectal Cancer. *Cancer Biol. Med.* **2020**, *17*, 307–327. [CrossRef]
19. Jose, J.; Kumar, R.; Harilal, S.; Mathew, G.E.; Parambi, D.G.T.; Prabhu, A.; Uddin, M.S.; Aleya, L.; Kim, H.; Mathew, B. Magnetic Nanoparticles for Hyperthermia in Cancer Treatment: An Emerging Tool. *Environ. Sci. Pollut. Res.* **2020**, *27*, 19214–19225. [CrossRef]
20. Acar, M.; Solak, K.; Yildiz, S.; Unver, Y.; Mavi, A. Comparative Heating Efficiency and Cytotoxicity of Magnetic Silica Nanoparticles for Magnetic Hyperthermia Treatment on Human Breast Cancer Cells. *3 Biotech* **2022**, *12*, 313. [CrossRef]
21. Minaei, S.E.; Khoei, S.; Khoee, S.; Mahdavi, S.R. Sensitization of Glioblastoma Cancer Cells to Radiotherapy and Magnetic Hyperthermia by Targeted Temozolomide-Loaded Magnetite Tri-Block Copolymer Nanoparticles as a Nanotheranostic Agent. *Life Sci.* **2022**, *306*, 120729. [CrossRef]
22. Narayanaswamy, V.; Jagal, J.; Khurshid, H.; Al-Omari, I.A.; Haider, M.; Kamzin, A.S.; Obaidat, I.M.; Issa, B. Hyperthermia of Magnetically Soft-Soft Core-Shell Ferrite Nanoparticles. *Int. J. Mol. Sci.* **2022**, *23*, 14825. [CrossRef]
23. Piehler, S.; Dähring, H.; Grandke, J.; Göring, J.; Couleaud, P.; Aires, A.; Cortajarena, A.L.; Courty, J.; Latorre, A.; Somoza, Á.; et al. Iron Oxide Nanoparticles as Carriers for DOX and Magnetic Hyperthermia after Intratumoral Application into Breast Cancer in Mice: Impact and Future Perspectives. *Nanomaterials* **2020**, *10*, 1016. [CrossRef]
24. Rego, G.; Nucci, M.; Mamani, J.; Oliveira, F.; Marti, L.; Filgueiras, I.; Ferreira, J.; Real, C.; Faria, D.; Espinha, P.; et al. Therapeutic Efficiency of Multiple Applications of Magnetic Hyperthermia Technique in Glioblastoma Using Aminosilane Coated Iron Oxide Nanoparticles: In Vitro and In Vivo Study. *Int. J. Mol. Sci.* **2020**, *21*, 958. [CrossRef]
25. Dabaghi, M.; Rasa, S.M.M.; Cirri, E.; Ori, A.; Neri, F.; Quaas, R.; Hilger, I. Iron Oxide Nanoparticles Carrying 5-Fluorouracil in Combination with Magnetic Hyperthermia Induce Thrombogenic Collagen Fibers, Cellular Stress, and Immune Responses in Heterotopic Human Colon Cancer in Mice. *Pharmaceutics* **2021**, *13*, 1625. [CrossRef] [PubMed]
26. Muka, T.; Glisic, M.; Milic, J.; Verhoog, S.; Bohlius, J.; Bramer, W.; Chowdhury, R.; Franco, O.H. A 24-Step Guide on How to Design, Conduct, and Successfully Publish a Systematic Review and Meta-Analysis in Medical Research. *Eur. J. Epidemiol.* **2020**, *35*, 49–60. [CrossRef]
27. Száva-Kováts, E. Unfounded Attribution of the "Half-Life" Index-Number of Literature Obsolescence to Burton and Kebler: A Literature Science Study. *J. Am. Soc. Inf. Sci. Technol.* **2002**, *53*, 1098–1105. [CrossRef]
28. Wanden-Berghe, C.; Sanz-Valero, J. Systematic Reviews in Nutrition: Standardized Methodology. *Br. J. Nutr.* **2012**, *107*, S3–S7. [CrossRef] [PubMed]
29. Kwon, S.-H.; Faruque, H.A.; Kee, H.; Kim, E.; Park, S. Exosome-Based Hybrid Nanostructures for Enhanced Tumor Targeting and Hyperthermia Therapy. *Colloids Surf. B Biointerfaces* **2021**, *205*, 111915. [CrossRef] [PubMed]
30. Lin, T.-C.; Lin, F.-H.; Lin, J.-C. In Vitro Characterization of Magnetic Electrospun IDA-Grafted Chitosan Nanofiber Composite for Hyperthermic Tumor Cell Treatment. *J. Biomater. Sci. Polym. Ed.* **2013**, *24*, 1152–1163. [CrossRef]
31. Park, J.; Jin, C.; Lee, S.; Kim, J.; Choi, H. Magnetically Actuated Degradable Microrobots for Actively Controlled Drug Release and Hyperthermia Therapy. *Adv. Healthc. Mater.* **2019**, *8*, 1900213. [CrossRef]
32. Li, C.; Ruan, J.; Yang, M.; Pan, F.; Gao, G.; Qu, S.; Shen, Y.L.; Dang, Y.J.; Wang, K.; Jin, W.L.; et al. Human Induced Pluripotent Stem Cells Labeled with Fluorescent Magnetic Nanoparticles for Targeted Imaging and Hyperthermia Therapy for Gastric Cancer. *Cancer Biol. Med.* **2015**, *12*, 163. [CrossRef]
33. Yang, S.-J.; Tseng, S.-Y.; Wang, C.-H.; Young, T.-H.; Chen, K.-C.; Shieh, M.-J. Magnetic Nanomedicine for CD133-Expressing Cancer Therapy Using Locoregional Hyperthermia Combined with Chemotherapy. *Nanomedicine* **2020**, *15*, 2543–2561. [CrossRef]
34. Kagawa, T.; Matsumi, Y.; Aono, H.; Ohara, T.; Tazawa, H.; Shigeyasu, K.; Yano, S.; Takeda, S.; Komatsu, Y.; Hoffman, R.M.; et al. Immuno-Hyperthermia Effected by Antibody-Conjugated Nanoparticles Selectively Targets and Eradicates Individual Cancer Cells. *Cell Cycle* **2021**, *20*, 1221–1230. [CrossRef]
35. Stanković, A.; Mihailović, J.; Mirković, M.; Radović, M.; Milanović, Z.; Ognjanović, M.; Janković, D.; Antić, B.; Mijović, M.; Vranješ-Đurić, S.; et al. Aminosilanized Flower-Structured Superparamagnetic Iron Oxide Nanoparticles Coupled to 131I-Labeled CC49 Antibody for Combined Radionuclide and Hyperthermia Therapy of Cancer. *Int. J. Pharm.* **2020**, *587*, 119628. [CrossRef] [PubMed]
36. Kuo, C.Y.; Liu, T.Y.; Chan, T.Y.; Tsai, S.C.; Hardiansyah, A.; Huang, L.Y.; Yang, M.C.; Lu, R.H.; Jiang, J.K.; Yang, C.Y.; et al. Magnetically Triggered Nanovehicles for Controlled Drug Release as a Colorectal Cancer Therapy. *Colloids Surf. B Biointerfaces* **2016**, *140*, 567–573. [CrossRef]

37. Fang, Y.; He, Y.; Wu, C.; Zhang, M.; Gu, Z.; Zhang, J.; Liu, E.; Xu, Q.; Asrorov, A.M.; Huang, Y. Magnetism-Mediated Targeting Hyperthermia-Immunotherapy in "Cold" Tumor with CSF1R Inhibitor. *Theranostics* **2021**, *11*, 6860–6872. [CrossRef]
38. Jahangiri, S.; Khoei, S.; Khoee, S.; Safa, M.; Shirvalilou, S.; Pirhajati Mahabadi, V. Potential Anti-Tumor Activity of 13.56 MHz Alternating Magnetic Hyperthermia and Chemotherapy on the Induction of Apoptosis in Human Colon Cancer Cell Lines HT29 and HCT116 by up-Regulation of Bax, Cleaved Caspase 3&9, and Cleaved PARP Proteins. *Cancer Nanotechnol.* **2021**, *12*, 34. [CrossRef]
39. Ha, P.T.; Le, T.T.H.; Ung, T.D.T.; Do, H.D.; Doan, B.T.; Mai, T.T.T.; Pham, H.N.; Hoang, T.M.N.; Phan, K.S.; Bui, T.Q. Properties and Bioeffects of Magneto–near Infrared Nanoparticles on Cancer Diagnosis and Treatment. *New J. Chem.* **2020**, *44*, 17277–17288. [CrossRef]
40. Wang, Y.-J.; Lin, P.-Y.; Hsieh, S.-L.; Kirankumar, R.; Lin, H.-Y.; Li, J.-H.; Chen, Y.-T.; Wu, H.-M.; Hsieh, S. Utilizing Edible Agar as a Carrier for Dual Functional Doxorubicin-Fe3O4 Nanotherapy Drugs. *Materials* **2021**, *14*, 1824. [CrossRef]
41. Liu, J.; Li, N.; Li, L.; Li, D.; Liu, K.; Zhao, L.; Tang, J.; Li, L. Local Hyperthermia for Esophageal Cancer in a Rabbit Tumor Model: Magnetic Stent Hyperthermia versus Magnetic Fluid Hyperthermia. *Oncol. Lett.* **2013**, *6*, 1550–1558. [CrossRef]
42. Fernández-Álvarez, F.; Caro, C.; García-García, G.; García-Martín, M.L.; Arias, J.L. Engineering of Stealth (Maghemite/PLGA)/Chitosan (Core/Shell)/Shell Nanocomposites with Potential Applications for Combined MRI and Hyperthermia against Cancer. *J. Mater. Chem. B* **2021**, *9*, 4963–4980. [CrossRef] [PubMed]
43. Thirunavukkarasu, G.K.; Cherukula, K.; Lee, H.; Jeong, Y.Y.; Park, I.-K.; Lee, J.Y. Magnetic Field-Inducible Drug-Eluting Nanoparticles for Image-Guided Thermo-Chemotherapy. *Biomaterials* **2018**, *180*, 240–252. [CrossRef] [PubMed]
44. Mannucci, S.; Ghin, L.; Conti, G.; Tambalo, S.; Lascialfari, A.; Orlando, T.; Benati, D.; Bernardi, P.; Betterle, N.; Bassi, R.; et al. Magnetic Nanoparticles from Magnetospirillum Gryphiswaldense Increase the Efficacy of Thermotherapy in a Model of Colon Carcinoma. *PLoS ONE* **2014**, *9*, e108959. [CrossRef] [PubMed]
45. Muñoz de Escalona, M.; Sáez-Fernández, E.; Prados, J.C.; Melguizo, C.; Arias, J.L. Magnetic Solid Lipid Nanoparticles in Hyperthermia against Colon Cancer. *Int. J. Pharm.* **2016**, *504*, 11–19. [CrossRef]
46. Clares, B.; Biedma-Ortiz, R.A.; Sáez-Fernández, E.; Prados, J.C.; Melguizo, C.; Cabeza, L.; Ortiz, R.; Arias, J.L. Nano-Engineering of 5-Fluorouracil-Loaded Magnetoliposomes for Combined Hyperthermia and Chemotherapy against Colon Cancer. *Eur. J. Pharm. Biopharm.* **2013**, *85*, 329–338. [CrossRef]
47. Jabalera, Y.; Garcia-Pinel, B.; Ortiz, R.; Iglesias, G.; Cabeza, L.; Prados, J.; Jimenez-Lopez, C.; Melguizo, C. Oxaliplatin–Biomimetic Magnetic Nanoparticle Assemblies for Colon Cancer-Targeted Chemotherapy: An In Vitro Study. *Pharmaceutics* **2019**, *11*, 395. [CrossRef]
48. Garanina, A.S.; Naumenko, V.A.; Nikitin, A.A.; Myrovali, E.; Petukhova, A.Y.; Klimyuk, S.V.; Nalench, Y.A.; Ilyasov, A.R.; Vodopyanov, S.S.; Erofeev, A.S.; et al. Temperature-Controlled Magnetic Nanoparticles Hyperthermia Inhibits Primary Tumor Growth and Metastases Dissemination. *Nanomedicine* **2020**, *25*, 102171. [CrossRef]
49. Torres-Lugo, M.; Castillo, A.; Mendez, J.; Rinaldi, C.; Soto, O.; Alvarez-Berrios, M.P. Hyperthermic Potentiation of Cisplatin by Magnetic Nanoparticle Heaters Is Correlated with an Increase in Cell Membrane Fluidity. *Int. J. Nanomed.* **2013**, *8*, 1003–1013. [CrossRef]
50. Mirzaghavami, P.S.; Khoei, S.; Khoee, S.; Shirvalilou, S.; Mahdavi, S.R.; Pirhajati Mahabadi, V. Radio-Sensitivity Enhancement in HT29 Cells through Magnetic Hyperthermia in Combination with Targeted Nano-Carrier of 5-Flourouracil. *Mater. Sci. Eng. C* **2021**, *124*, 112043. [CrossRef]
51. Pawlik, P.; Blasiak, B.; Depciuch, J.; Pruba, M.; Kitala, D.; Vorobyova, S.; Stec, M.; Bushinsky, M.; Konakov, A.; Baran, J.; et al. Application of Iron-Based Magnetic Nanoparticles Stabilized with Triethanolammonium Oleate for Theranostics. *J. Mater. Sci.* **2022**, *57*, 4716–4737. [CrossRef]
52. Fernandes, S.; Fernandez, T.; Metze, S.; Balakrishnan, P.B.; Mai, B.T.; Conteh, J.; De Mei, C.; Turdo, A.; Di Franco, S.; Stassi, G.; et al. Magnetic Nanoparticle-Based Hyperthermia Mediates Drug Delivery and Impairs the Tumorigenic Capacity of Quiescent Colorectal Cancer Stem Cells. *ACS Appl. Mater. Interfaces* **2021**, *13*, 15959–15972. [CrossRef]
53. Beyk, J.; Tavakoli, H. Selective Radiofrequency Ablation of Tumor by Magnetically Targeting of Multifunctional Iron Oxide–Gold Nanohybrid. *J. Cancer Res. Clin. Oncol.* **2019**, *145*, 2199–2209. [CrossRef] [PubMed]
54. Jiang, H.; Guo, Y.; Yu, Z.; Hu, P.; Shi, J. Nanocatalytic Bacteria Disintegration Reverses Immunosuppression of Colorectal Cancer. *Natl. Sci. Rev.* **2022**, *9*, nwac169. [CrossRef]
55. Ahmad, A.; Gupta, A.; Ansari, M.M.; Vyawahare, A.; Jayamurugan, G.; Khan, R. Hyperbranched Polymer-Functionalized Magnetic Nanoparticle-Mediated Hyperthermia and Niclosamide Bimodal Therapy of Colorectal Cancer Cells. *ACS Biomater. Sci. Eng.* **2020**, *6*, 1102–1111. [CrossRef]
56. Shen, M.Y.; Liu, T.I.; Yu, T.W.; Kv, R.; Chiang, W.H.; Tsai, Y.C.; Chen, H.H.; Lin, S.C.; Chiu, H.C. Hierarchically Targetable Polysaccharide-Coated Solid Lipid Nanoparticles as an Oral Chemo/Thermotherapy Delivery System for Local Treatment of Colon Cancer. *Biomaterials* **2019**, *197*, 86–100. [CrossRef] [PubMed]
57. Ramirez, D.; Oliva, J.; Cordova-Fraga, T.; Basurto-Islas, G.; Benal-Alvarado, J.J.; Mtz-Enriquez, A.I.; Quintana, M.; Gomez-Solis, C. High Heating Efficiency of Magnetite Nanoparticles Synthesized with Citric Acid: Application for Hyperthermia Treatment. *J. Electron. Mater.* **2022**, *51*, 4425–4436. [CrossRef]
58. Castellanos-Rubio, I.; Rodrigo, I.; Olazagoitia-Garmendia, A.; Arriortua, O.; Gil de Muro, I.; Garitaonandia, J.S.; Bilbao, J.R.; Fdez-Gubieda, M.L.; Plazaola, F.; Orue, I.; et al. Highly Reproducible Hyperthermia Response in Water, Agar, and Cellular

Environment by Discretely PEGylated Magnetite Nanoparticles. *ACS Appl. Mater. Interfaces* **2020**, *12*, 27917–27929. [CrossRef] [PubMed]
59. Teo, P.; Wang, X.; Chen, B.; Zhang, H.; Yang, X.; Huang, Y.; Tang, J. Complex of TNF-α and Modified Fe_3O_4 Nanoparticles Suppresses Tumor Growth by Magnetic Induction Hyperthermia. *Cancer Biother. Radiopharm.* **2017**, *32*, 379–386. [CrossRef]
60. Matsumi, Y.; Kagawa, T.; Yano, S.; Tazawa, H.; Shigeyasu, K.; Takeda, S.; Ohara, T.; Aono, H.; Hoffman, R.M.; Fujiwara, T.; et al. Hyperthermia Generated by Magnetic Nanoparticles for Effective Treatment of Disseminated Peritoneal Cancer in an Orthotopic Nude-Mouse Model. *Cell Cycle* **2021**, *20*, 1122–1133. [CrossRef]
61. Alvarez-Berríos, M.P.; Castillo, A.; Rinaldi, C.; Torres-Lugo, M. Magnetic Fluid Hyperthermia Enhances Cytotoxicity of Bortezomib in Sensitive and Resistant Cancer Cell Lines. *Int. J. Nanomed.* **2014**, *9*, 145–153. [CrossRef]
62. Hardiansyah, A.; Huang, L.Y.; Yang, M.C.; Liu, T.Y.; Tsai, S.C.; Yang, C.Y.; Kuo, C.Y.; Chan, T.Y.; Zou, H.M.; Lian, W.N.; et al. Magnetic Liposomes for Colorectal Cancer Cells Therapy by High-Frequency Magnetic Field Treatment. *Nanoscale Res. Lett.* **2014**, *9*, 497. [CrossRef] [PubMed]
63. Wydra, R.J.; Rychahou, P.G.; Evers, B.M.; Anderson, K.W.; Dziubla, T.D.; Hilt, J.Z. The Role of ROS Generation from Magnetic Nanoparticles in an Alternating Magnetic Field on Cytotoxicity. *Acta Biomater.* **2015**, *25*, 284–290. [CrossRef]
64. Wang, J.T.-W.; Martino, U.; Khan, R.; Bazzar, M.; Southern, P.; Tuncel, D.; Al-Jamal, K.T. Engineering Red-Emitting Multi-Functional Nanocapsules for Magnetic Tumour Targeting and Imaging. *Biomater. Sci.* **2020**, *8*, 2590–2599. [CrossRef]
65. Arriortua, O.K.; Garaio, E.; Herrero de la Parte, B.; Insausti, M.; Lezama, L.; Plazaola, F.; García, J.A.; Aizpurua, J.M.; Sagartzazu, M.; Irazola, M.; et al. Antitumor Magnetic Hyperthermia Induced by RGD-Functionalized Fe_3O_4 Nanoparticles, in an Experimental Model of Colorectal Liver Metastases. *Beilstein J. Nanotechnol.* **2016**, *7*, 1532–1542. [CrossRef] [PubMed]
66. Dabaghi, M.; Quaas, R.; Hilger, I. The Treatment of Heterotopic Human Colon Xenograft Tumors in Mice with 5-Fluorouracil Attached to Magnetic Nanoparticles in Combination with Magnetic Hyperthermia Is More Efficient than Either Therapy Alone. *Cancers* **2020**, *12*, 2562. [CrossRef] [PubMed]
67. Johannsen, M.; Gneveckow, U.; Eckelt, L.; Feussner, A.; Waldöfner, N.; Scholz, R.; Deger, S.; Wust, P.; Loening, S.A.; Jordan, A. Clinical Hyperthermia of Prostate Cancer Using Magnetic Nanoparticles: Presentation of a New Interstitial Technique. *Int. J. Hyperth.* **2005**, *21*, 637–647. [CrossRef]
68. Sharifi, I.; Shokrollahi, H.; Amiri, S. Ferrite-Based Magnetic Nanofluids Used in Hyperthermia Applications. *J. Magn. Magn. Mater.* **2012**, *324*, 903–915. [CrossRef]
69. Liu, X.; Zhang, Y.; Wang, Y.; Zhu, W.; Li, G.; Ma, X.; Zhang, Y.; Chen, S.; Tiwari, S.; Shi, K.; et al. Comprehensive Understanding of Magnetic Hyperthermia for Improving Antitumor Therapeutic Efficacy. *Theranostics* **2020**, *10*, 3793–3815. [CrossRef]
70. Giustini, A.J.; Ivkov, R.; Hoopes, P.J. Magnetic Nanoparticle Biodistribution Following Intratumoral Administration. *Nanotechnology* **2011**, *22*, 345101. [CrossRef]
71. Hu, A.; Pu, Y.; Xu, N.; Cai, Z.; Sun, R.; Fu, S.; Jin, R.; Guo, Y.; Ai, H.; Nie, Y.; et al. Controlled Intracellular Aggregation of Magnetic Particles Improves Permeation and Retention for Magnetic Hyperthermia Promotion and Immune Activation. *Theranostics* **2023**, *13*, 1454–1469. [CrossRef]
72. Abrahao-Machado, L.F.; Scapulatempo-Neto, C. HER2 Testing in Gastric Cancer: An Update. *World J. Gastroenterol.* **2016**, *22*, 4619. [CrossRef]
73. Stephen, Z.R.; Zhang, M. Recent Progress in the Synergistic Combination of Nanoparticle-Mediated Hyperthermia and Immunotherapy for Treatment of Cancer. *Adv. Healthc. Mater.* **2021**, *10*, 2001415. [CrossRef] [PubMed]
74. Pan, J.; Hu, P.; Guo, Y.; Hao, J.; Ni, D.; Xu, Y.; Bao, Q.; Yao, H.; Wei, C.; Wu, Q.; et al. Combined Magnetic Hyperthermia and Immune Therapy for Primary and Metastatic Tumor Treatments. *ACS Nano* **2020**, *14*, 1033–1044. [CrossRef] [PubMed]
75. Chao, Y.; Chen, G.; Liang, C.; Xu, J.; Dong, Z.; Han, X.; Wang, C.; Liu, Z. Iron Nanoparticles for Low-Power Local Magnetic Hyperthermia in Combination with Immune Checkpoint Blockade for Systemic Antitumor Therapy. *Nano Lett.* **2019**, *19*, 4287–4296. [CrossRef]
76. Liu, X.; Zheng, J.; Sun, W.; Zhao, X.; Li, Y.; Gong, N.; Wang, Y.; Ma, X.; Zhang, T.; Zhao, L.-Y.; et al. Ferrimagnetic Vortex Nanoring-Mediated Mild Magnetic Hyperthermia Imparts Potent Immunological Effect for Treating Cancer Metastasis. *ACS Nano* **2019**, *13*, 8811–8825. [CrossRef] [PubMed]
77. Hedayatnasab, Z.; Abnisa, F.; Daud, W.M.A.W. Review on Magnetic Nanoparticles for Magnetic Nanofluid Hyperthermia Application. *Mater. Des.* **2017**, *123*, 174–196. [CrossRef]
78. Metselaar, J.M.; Lammers, T. Challenges in Nanomedicine Clinical Translation. *Drug Deliv. Transl. Res.* **2020**, *10*, 721–725. [CrossRef]

Disclaimer/Publisher's Note: The statements, opinions and data contained in all publications are solely those of the individual author(s) and contributor(s) and not of MDPI and/or the editor(s). MDPI and/or the editor(s) disclaim responsibility for any injury to people or property resulting from any ideas, methods, instructions or products referred to in the content.

MDPI
St. Alban-Anlage 66
4052 Basel
Switzerland
www.mdpi.com

Pharmaceutics Editorial Office
E-mail: pharmaceutics@mdpi.com
www.mdpi.com/journal/pharmaceutics

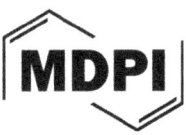

Disclaimer/Publisher's Note: The statements, opinions and data contained in all publications are solely those of the individual author(s) and contributor(s) and not of MDPI and/or the editor(s). MDPI and/or the editor(s) disclaim responsibility for any injury to people or property resulting from any ideas, methods, instructions or products referred to in the content.

www.ingramcontent.com/pod-product-compliance
Lightning Source LLC
LaVergne TN
LVHW070453100526
838202LV00014B/1714